Critical Care Nursing

Carolyn M. Hudak, R.N., Ph.D.

Adult Nurse Practitioner
Formerly Associate Professor of Nursing and
Assistant Professor of Medicine
University of Colorado Health Sciences Center
Denver, Colorado

Thelma "Skip" Lohr, R.N., M.S.

Nursing Consultant, Educator
Assistant Director, Psychodrama, Sociometry, Sociatry
Staff Nurse, Adult Services
National Jewish Hospital
Denver, Colorado

Barbara M. Gallo, R.N., M.S.

Assistant Director
Visiting Nurse and Home Care Services of Greater Hartford, Inc.
Hartford, Connecticut

J. B. Lippincott Company Philadelphia Toronto

Third
Edition

Critical Care Nursing

For information address J. B. Lippincott Company, East
Washington Square, Philadelphia, Pennsylvania 19105.

6 5 4

Library of Congress Cataloging in Publication Data
Main entry under title:

Critical care nursing.

    Includes bibliographies and index.
    1. Intensive care nursing.   I. Hudak, Carolyn M.
II. Lohr, Thelma.   III. Gallo, Barbara M.
RT120.I5C74 1982   610.73′61   81-12375
ISBN 0-397-54353-0   AACR2

The authors and publisher have exerted every effort to
ensure that drug selection and dosage set forth in this text
are in accord with current recommendations and practice
at the time of publication. However, in view of ongoing
research, changes in government regulations, and the
constant flow of information relating to drug therapy and
drug reactions, the reader is urged to check the package
insert for each drug for any change in indications and
dosage and for added warnings and precautions. This is
particularly important when the recommended agent is a
new or infrequently employed drug.

Printed in the United States of America

To my husband, John, with love,
Carolyn

To my family and family of friends,
Skip

To Mom,
Bobbie

Contents

Unit Four
Specific Crisis Situations

Unit Five
Professional Practice in the Critical Care Unit

Contributors

Patricia D. Barry, R.N., B.S.N.E., M.S.N.
Psychiatric Liaison/Clinical Nurse Specialist, St. Francis Hospital; and Adjunct Faculty, University of Hartford, Hartford, Connecticut

Ann T. Bobal, R.N., B.S.
Nursing Supervisor, Medical Service, Veterans Administration Medical Center, Denver, Colorado

H. L. Brammell, M.D.
Associate Professor of Physical Medicine and Rehabilitation, University of Colorado Health Sciences Center, Denver, Colorado

Patricia K. Brannin, R.N., M.S.N., A.A.R.T.
Pulmonary Nurse Clinician/Adult Nurse Practitioner, Director Adult and OPD Nursing Services, National Jewish Hospital, Denver, Colorado

Eileen Brent, R.N., M.S.
Coordinator, Respiratory Department, National Jewish Hospital and National Asthma Center, Denver, Colorado

Barbara Fuller, R.N., M.S., Ph.D.
Professor of Nursing, University of Colorado School of Nursing, Denver, Colorado

Joseph O. Broughton, M.D.
Clinical Instructor in Medicine, University of Colorado Health Sciences Center; and Medical Director, Inhalation Therapy Department, Mercy Hospital, Denver, Colorado

Helen Busby, R.N.
Critical Care Practitioner, Supervisor, Critical Care Areas, West Nebraska General Hospital, Scottsbluff, Nebraska

Karen D. Busch, R.N., M.S.
Ph.D. Candidate, University of Texas, Austin, Texas

Donald E. Butkus, M.D.
Colonel, MC, Chief, Department of Nephrology, Director, Division of Medicine, Department of the Army, Walter Reed Army Institute of Research, Walter Reed Army Medical Center, Washington, DC

Corinne A. Cloughen, R.N.
Neuro Trauma ICU/CCU, Swedish Medical Center, Englewood, Colorado

Lane D. Craddock, M.D.
Associate Clinical Professor of Medicine, University of Colorado School of Medicine; and Director, Cardiopulmonary Department, General Rose Memorial Hospital, Denver, Colorado

Maureen Cushing, J.D., R.N.
Attorney at Law, Boston, Massachusetts

Cynthia Johnson Dahlberg, M.A., C.C.C.-Sp.
Director, Department of Speech and Language Pathology, Craig Hospital, Englewood, Colorado

Frank Davidoff, M.D.
Chief, Division of General Medicine, Department of Medicine, University of Connecticut School of Medicine, Farmington, Connecticut

Patricia Diehl, R.N., B.S.N., M.A. Educ.-Nursing
Associate Professor, School of Nursing, Medical Center, West Virginia University, Morgantown, West Virginia

Robert W. Hendee, Jr., M.D.
Assistant Clinical Professor of Neurosurgery, University of Colorado School of Medicine; and Chairman, Department of Surgical Specialties, Children's Hospital, Denver, Colorado

Shirley J. Hoffman, R.N., B.S.N.
Cardiovascular Clinical Specialist, Presbyterian Denver Hospital, a Division of Presbyterian/St. Luke's Medical Center, Denver, Colorado

Judith Ives, R.N., B.S.N., M.S.N.
Critical Care Instructor in Staff Development, University of Colorado Health Sciences Center, Denver, Colorado

Carole Kravec, M.A.T., C.C.C.-Sp.
Speech Pathologist, Craig Hospital, Englewood, Colorado

Barbara Lockwood, R.N., M.S.N.
Flight Nurse and Critical Care Practitioner; and Director of Nursing, St. Anthony's Hospital, Denver, Colorado

Cary Lou Martinson, R.N., B.S.N.
Assistant Head Nurse, Orthopedic Unit, Swedish Medical Center, Denver, Colorado

Mary Ellen McManus, R.N.
Staff Nurse, Poison Control Lab, Denver General Hospital, Denver, Colorado

Naomi Domer Medearis, R.N., M.A., M.B.A.
Educational Consultant and Vice President, Associates for Continuing Education, Inc., Denver, Colorado

Joan Mersch, R.N., M.S.
Clinical Nursing Coordinator, CCU, Stanford Medical Center, Palo Alto, California

Marilynn Mitchell, R.N., M.S.N.
Head Nurse, Neurology—Neurosurgical ICU and Neuro Step-Down Unit, Denver General Hospital, Denver, Colorado

Deborah Moisan, R.N.
Staff Nurse, Poison Control Lab, Denver General Hospital, Denver, Colorado

Ann Marie Powers, R.N., B.S., M.S.
Clinical Nurse Specialist/Transplant Coordinator, Yale–New Haven Hospital, New Haven, Connecticut

Karen Robbins, R.N., B.S.N., M.S.
Nurse Clinician in Transplantation, Hartford Transplant Service in Affiliation with Hartford Hospital, Hartford, Connecticut

William A. Seiffert, M.D.
Internal Medicine, Medical Director, Critical Care Areas, West Nebraska General Hospital, Scottsbluff, Nebraska

Julie A. Shinn, R.N., M.A., C.C.R.N.
Educational Coordinator, Critical Care Units, Stanford University Hospital, Stanford, California

Janice S. Smith, R.N., M.S.
Instructor, Medical–Surgical Nursing, Community College of Denver, North Denver, Colorado

Rae Nadine Smith, R.N., M.S.
Clinical Nursing Specialist, Sorenson Research Company, Salt Lake City, Utah

Marilynn J. Washburn, R.N., B.S.N.
Supervisor, Patient Transport, Samaritan Health Services, Phoenix, Arizona

Phillip S. Wolf, M.D.
Associate Clinical Professor of Medicine, University of Colorado; and Director, Coronary Care Unit, General Rose Memorial Hospital, Denver, Colorado

Preface

What started out to be a routine revision of *Critical Care Nursing* turned out to be a major rewriting. We blew the budget, but we ended up with a comprehensive, sophisticated text on current critical care nursing practice. In essence, the book has become a resource unto itself. Repetition of material may occur where we think it is advantageous to learning, or the reader may be referred to an in-depth discussion elsewhere in the book.

This edition continues our original emphasis on a holistic approach with the specific purpose of impacting nursing care by providing a broader scope to practice. This broadened scope includes the patient, family, technology, and the nurse.

The unit on core body systems underwent a major workover. So many changes have occurred in even our basic knowledge of anatomy and physiology that these sections were completely rewritten. Responding to reader suggestions, we added significant chunks of new material on ventilatory support and ventilators, cardioversion, intra-aortic balloon pumping, direct cardiac output measurement, and assessment of the comatose patient.

The material on artificial cardiac pacing, cardiac drugs, arrhythmias, serum enzymes and electrolytes, respiratory diseases and management including adult respiratory distress syndrome, peritoneal dialysis, renal transplantation, and care of the brain-injured and the spinal cord-injured patient has been heavily revised. Invasive Neurological Assessment Techniques has been updated and includes a section on induced barbiturate coma.

The unit on specific crisis situations also underwent major rewriting. Completely rewritten are the chapters on burns and disseminated intravascular coagulation. Heavily revised are the chapters on hepatic failure (which now contains information on a number of liver diseases), acute gastrointestinal bleeding, and hyperalimentation. New to this section are a comprehensive chapter on diabetic emergencies and a chapter on drug and poison overdose.

Discussion of the problem of burnout and its particular affinity for the critical care nurse is new to this edition. When our personal, social, work, and life goals are out of balance, our effectiveness and sense of wholeness are affected. Work and life stresses culminate in the critical care unit. The chapter on adverse effects of the critical care unit on the nurse speaks to these issues.

Also new is the perspective of the patient as a person with a social history that influences his behavior in the CCU. This concept is dealt with in a chapter on sociometric impact on the patient.

Because of the ongoing concern with legal issues related to nursing practice, we included a completely new chapter on the legal responsibilities of the critical care nurse.

The final chapter on the training and development of the critical care nursing staff is a monograph on the subject. It will walk you through the steps involved in providing innovative and economically feasible strategies for developing personnel in the unit or for your own personal growth.

As in the first and second editions of *Critical Care Nursing,* we are grateful to our contributing authors who have persevered with us through deadlines, revisions, and delays. Some of our contributors have been with us through all three editions and remain special friends. Contributors new to this edition came to our attention in a variety of ways and to them we give a special welcome and thanks for their excellent work.

We are indebted to Charlene A. Lark, R.N., M.S., Assistant Director of Nursing at Denver General Hospital, Denver, Colorado, for keeping us apprised of reactions to the book and for suggesting areas of content for inclusion in this and past editions of the book.

Photographs for the material on artificial cardiac pacing and direct cardiac output measurement were provided courtesy of Presbyterian Denver Hospital, a division of Presbyterian/St. Luke's Medical Center, Denver, Colorado. We are grateful for their support and cooperation.

Carolyn M. Hudak, R.N., Ph.D.
Thelma "Skip" Lohr, R.N., M.S.
Barbara M. Gallo, R.N., M.S.

Thelma "Skip" Lohr

Introduction: Crisis Care Versus Critical Care

Two words, *intensive* and *critical,* are commonly used to describe care offered to seriously ill patients. As units and services have become more sophisticated, different yet descriptive terms have been selected to distinguish one type of care from the other. Some terms originate from the environment and the process involved (intensive, dialysis); others originate from the patient's status (crisis, critical); and still others originate from the body system involved (coronary, renal). We have even combined words to differentiate the units from the general services (neuro-intensive care). No matter how hard we try to find terms which accurately portray what we mean, words have limitations. They are static and cannot convey the process that makes up the care.

Critical and *crisis* are two static terms which have had a close association. They are so frequently interchanged in nursing discussions that many practitioners are cognizant only of the similarities, not the differences. Webster defines each of these terms as follows:

crisis—an emotionally significant event or radical change of status in a person's life . . . an unstable state of affairs in which a decisive change is impending.

critical—exercising or involving careful judgment or judicious evaluation; discriminating, careful, exact . . . indispensable for the weathering, the solution, or the overcoming of a crisis . . . of doubtful issue: attended by risk or uncertainty.

Although both of these terms broaden the activities of nursing to include more of the nurse's intellect and decision-making processes, the essence of the difference begins with the purpose and the way it is achieved — that is, through the steps of the nursing process. The chart below delineates the differences between crisis care and critical care as related to purpose, orientation, focus, and the essential steps of the nursing process.

Crisis Care vs Critical Care within a Nursing Process Framework

	CRISIS CARE	**CRITICAL CARE**
Purpose	Lifesaving	Life-maintaining
Orientation	Treat the presenting crisis symptoms and stabilize	Treat the first presenting symptoms and prevent a crisis
Focus	On body systems in failure — to reverse the failure or maintain the system	On all body systems — to support those in trouble and to maintain those in health
Assessment	Discriminating for presenting signs and symptoms	Discriminating, exact, careful for subtle signs and symptoms before they become grossly presenting
Planning	Established protocol and procedures	Established protocol and procedures are constantly adjusted and adapted to patient's individuality and frequently changing status (days/weeks)
Interventions	Continuous until life is stabilized for transportation to a unit, or until death occurs (hours)	Continuous with a wider range, until adaptation to a higher level of wellness is attained, or until death occurs
Evaluation	Immediate for effectiveness of treatment	Immediate and long-term for effectiveness of each therapy procedure, planned and frequent assessment of each body system with a variety of tools, continuous adjustment of short-term and long-range goals as the patient's status changes

---

At first, when specialty units were first developed, they were added to the corresponding department of medicine, and each had a physician for director and supervisor. The physicians were responsible for the care given, which also made them responsible for training the nurses and supervising the unit's activities.

As nurses became qualified and certified in critical care, which spans all clinical areas, they reestablished their roles as supervisors of patient care and staff educators. Along with this, nurses gradually accepted the responsibility for the quality of care given in the unit. What started with *audit* and *peer review* continues today with *quality assurance councils* whose members are staff nurses from each of the units. Now, many hospitals have combined their specialty units under one major heading — critical care areas — with a physician director who acts also as an adviser and resource person. We have elected not to include crisis (emergency) and surgical nursing, for each is an entity of its own with a definite bank of knowledge and skills based on the same physiology and pathophysiology of the body.

The following chapters are mostly "words" about critical care knowledge, skills, and processes, and we wish our readers the energy to translate their learning into their own nursing process for quality care.

Unit One

Critical Care Nursing Process

The Fantasy
1

THE REALITY OF FANTASY

The Fantasy described below was first presented in 1973 as Margaret Berry visualized what the future *could* be like. Today this fantasy continues to ring true — it is timeless; it is still pertinent! Over the past decade, the theme of "people caught in their technical world" has become ever so common, as the tools of our everyday life become part of our everyday medical world — tools which include helicopter emergency rooms, analyzer computers, and sophisticated medical equipment. Thus, The Fantasy continues to have a place in current discussions.

Margaret Ann Berry

FANTASY?

The sun shone on the gleaming white edifice called *The Hospital*. The telerecorder rang sharply in the receiving heliport and the teletype began its nervous chatter. The receiving room nurse walked over to read the message: "Caucasian, male; fifty-five years of age; shortness of breath; crushing chest pain; collapsed over desk; history of two previous similar attacks." She punched out the message on the electronic call board, indicating the estimated time of arrival.

When the sound of the helicopter blades increased to a deafening level, the nurse moved out to the landing pad. As the copter touched down, the doors in the fuselage opened and the life-support capsule was lowered into the waiting cradle car on the track. As soon as the nurse removed the sky hooks from the ends of the capsule, the helicopter lifted off with a pulsing roar. The nurse activated the electronic conveyor track and the capsule moved into the receiving room.

Once inside, the nurse quickly opened the capsule and took from the pocket the field-punched computer cards. As she passed the call board, she activated the call switches from The Learned Ones who would be concerned with #125–A–70–90056, the newly arrived case. While she awaited their arrival, she fed the cards into a computer and the information was instantaneously displayed on the video screen in all four corners of the receiving room and at the diagnosis console. Suddenly the doors marked "Biological, Psychological, and Sociological" burst open and The Learned Ones and their assistants quickly entered the room. Glancing furtively at the video printouts, each addressed his attention to the problems of #125–A–70–90056 which were in the area of his specialty. One by one they took their respective problem area in its minicapsule and left by way of the doors "Bio-

logical, Psychological, and Sociological." When all had left and only the capsule and clothing of #125–A–70–90056 remained at the diagnostic console, the nurse signaled for the sanitation specialist to prepare the room for the next arrival.

In white coveralls and armed with a collection of aerosols filled with various sanitizers, the specialist began to clean the life-support capsule, assisted by the receiving room attendant. The two chatted cheerfully as they did their work. After they had folded the clothing left inside the capsule they noticed an ethereal cloud inside the capsule. Selecting a stronger sanitizer, the specialist sprayed the cloud more thoroughly. Much to his dismay the cloud did not disappear. A second glance showed that the clothing was no longer neatly folded.

The specialist summoned the nurse from the receiving room office. She too tried without success to disperse the cloud and fold the clothes. Then she notified the offices of the director of nurses and the supervisors of biological, psychological, and sociological nursing problems. They arrived from the various areas, but they too were unsuccessful. The Learned Ones were recalled, but again all efforts met with failure. As the crowd of professionals stood pondering over the puzzling conditions inside the capsule, a small voice was heard:

"But what about me? I am MORE than the sum total of my parts!"

Carolyn M. Hudak,
Thelma L. Lohr,
and Barbara M. Gallo

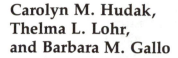

Critical Care Nursing: What Makes It Special?
2

It is our contention that the essence of critical care nursing lies not in special environments or amid special equipment but rather in the decision-making process of the nurse and a willingness to act upon the decisions made.

Critical care nurses have been pioneers in what is now called the "expanded role." From the days of the 24-hour recovery room which substituted for an intensive care unit, nurses in these areas have had to look beyond just "taking vital signs." Before the term *critical care nursing* evolved, the critical care nurse was the one who could see beyond the patient's blood pressure, pulse, and respiration. She felt a pulse and noted its quality, made a mental note of the temperature of the skin and its state of hydration, compared the pulse rate with the temperature and blood pressure, and asked "Why?" if the anticipated correlation was not there. In short, she functioned according to her intellect. She anticipated events based on what she knew about normal physiology and her patient's condition, and if findings other than those she anticipated materialized, she asked herself "Why?" and proceeded to gather additional clinical data to answer that question. If she failed to answer the question, her response was based merely on intuition, "That patient just doesn't look good to me!" We believe that predictability based on intuition actually involved a response to clinical cues which nurses had not attempted to identify concretely. For example, the patient doesn't "look good" because

- His respirations are more shallow.
- His color is duskier than previously.

- His eyes have an anxious stare.
- He is more restless now.
- He is perspiring.

The critical care nurse of today seeks the *rational base* for all her interpretations and actions.

THE NURSING PROCESS IN CRITICAL CARE

What are the processes a nurse follows to arrive at a decision which serves as a guide for intervention?

1. Appropriate information is collected.
2. An assessment is made based on the data collected.
3. A plan of action is decided upon.
4. The results of these actions are evaluated.

For example, a postoperative patient has a blood pressure of 88/60, pulse 100, respirations 28, and diaphoresis. Perhaps these symptoms are the result of pain . . . or hemorrhage. Further information is needed to support either premise.

- Does he complain of pain?
- Does he "splint" the area when he moves?
- Is his dressing wet?
- Is urine output diminished?
- Is there any evidence of bleeding into the incisional area?
- What is the pulse quality?
- Does the CVP lend any clues?

After analyzing these findings, the nurse makes an assessment. If the assessment indicates that pain control is necessary, the plan will be to medicate the patient for pain. Next, the outcome of the intervention is evaluated. For example, after medicating the postoperative patient, the nurse will anticipate a given outcome. If the vital sign parameters noted above are due to pain, the nurse will anticipate that the patient's vital signs will return to "normal" if pain is relieved. If this anticipated outcome does not occur, the nurse then asks "Why?" and proceeds to gather additional data to answer that question. This leads to reassessment, further planning, and reevaluation. The process is continuous until the problem is resolved.

We believe that the essence of critical care nursing is to be found in the decision-making process that is based on a sound understanding of physiological and psychological entities. It requires the ability to deal with critical situations with a rapidity and precision not usually necessary in other health-care settings. It requires

adeptness at integrating information and establishing priorities, for when illness strikes one body system, other systems become involved in the effort to cope with the disequilibrium. The person admitted to a critical care unit usually receives excellent care for the affected body system, but problems in other systems are not recognized early, if at all. Critical illnesses will always endanger and involve the respiratory, cardiovascular, renal, and central nervous systems as well as the self-esteem of each person.

We believe that the nurse needs to actively engage a mental image of the person and his body processes to gather all the data possible for the decision-making process. Therefore, the framework outlined in Figure 2-1 is proposed as a basis for the study of persons with critical illnesses and of critical care nursing.

HUMAN NEEDS AND CRITICAL CARE NURSING

Individuals seek to preserve their lives by directing all their energies toward the most basic unmet needs. For example, all the compensatory mechanisms of a person with inadequate cardiac output will work to maintain the circulation of oxygen, thus meeting the most basic requirement for life. In this situation, energy is directed away from subsystems such as the gastrointestinal, skin, and kidney functions, creating a degree of *physiological amputation*.

The need for a sense of security to allay anxiety is always present, but it is not the most basic need at this time. Later, when needs for air, cellular nutrition, and elimination are met, the efforts of the individual are directed toward seeking security, a sense of belonging, and self-esteem.

Although each of us has physiological and psychological mechanisms which compensate for disequilibrium, there are situations in which we cannot adapt without outside intervention. It is in these situations that the critical care nurse becomes the patient's advocate and fosters adaptation.

Adaptive Nursing and Patient Advocacy

The individual's attempts to cope with the environment include avoidance, in which one flees from the situation; counteraction, in which body defenses try to destroy the stressor, often at the expense of other systems; and adaptation, in which one seeks to establish a compatible response to the stress and still retain a steady state.

Although all mechanisms foster self-preservation, nursing intervention is aimed at adaptation. By fostering responses that encourage useful functioning both physiologically and emotionally, nurses enhance adaptation and aid the patient in conserving energy. On the other hand, when nursing intervention or lack of it does not foster adaptation, the patient's energy is wasted and a state of *entropy* exists; that is, the patient will have a diminished capacity to deal with a changing situation. Thus, entropy is increased when a patient's energy is devoted to maladaptive functioning which perpetuates the disequilibrium, and entropy is minimized when the patient expends energy which fosters adaptation to the disequilibrium.

An example of maladaptation versus adaptation is seen in the patient with restrictive lung disease who develops a lung infection resulting in $\uparrow CO_2$ and $\downarrow O_2$. This patient cannot compensate because of his restrictive lung disease; thus, his established pattern of breathing is maladaptive, perpetuating the problem of gas exchange. On the other hand, adaptive nursing intervention involves helping the patient to breathe more deeply and fostering the drainage of secretion either by having him do breathing exercises or by use of mechanical aids. Although the energy is still expended, it is expended usefully. This concept of minimizing entropy is consistent with the ultimate goal of health care: to restore the person to a steady state with minimal stress to the rest of the body.

Because of the degree of patient contact, critical care nurses have more influence than other health-care personnel in either fostering adaptation or encouraging entropy. That influence may be a burden as well as a challenge. It does not, however, negate the responsibility of other health-care personnel to act on behalf of patient adaptation.

Fostering adaptive functioning means that the nurse negotiates for the patient. She becomes his advocate. Because the critically ill patient often cannot effectively cope with both the physiological problem and the rest of his environment, it becomes necessary for the nurse to do for the patient what he is unable to do for himself so that his energy is conserved. As negotiator, the nurse must refrain from adding burdens which increase the patient's need to interact when such interaction will not foster adaptation. For example, patient energy spent in fearful suspense about the equipment nearby is not as help-

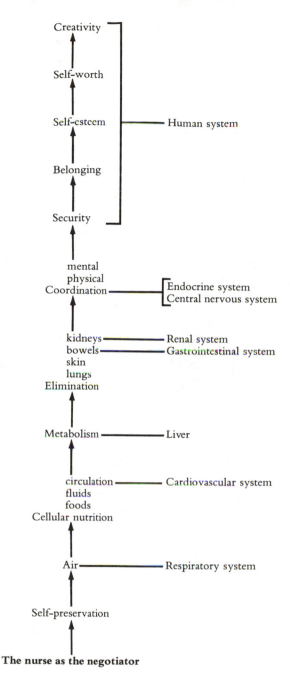

The nurse as the negotiator

FIGURE 2-1.
Hierarchy of human needs for critical care nursing.

ful as energy spent in asking about it and then listening to a reply. Or, energy spent in persistently requesting a loved one to be present may not be as helpful as energy spent interacting with that person.

Fostering safety for the critically ill patient involves decreasing his vulnerability both physiologically and emotionally. The feeling of security is lost or at least significantly decreased whenever there is a decrease in one's control of body functions. Loss of control may vary from fatigue and weakness to paralysis. It may result from pathology, from the environment (*e.g.,* restraint by IV tubing or machinery), or both; from fatigue and sleeplessness caused by physical discomfort; or from physiological fatigue (*e.g.,* dyspnea and sensory overload). Regardless of the decrease or loss of control, the nurse intervenes in order to increase the patient's feeling of safety. This may be accomplished by using technical skill, tools, medication, interaction; by providing assisted breathing with a respirator; by encouraging breathing exercises; or by staying with the patient during a time of anxiety or loneliness. Recognizing a patient's safety needs is an important element in the holistic approach to patient care. In addition, it is this very consideration of the "whole" patient which allows us to establish priorities as patient negotiators.

Negotiating for the patient is not without its hazards. This kind of caring and giving requires our energies in place of those which the patient is temporarily lacking. Therefore, to maintain our own emotional reserves, we also need to support one another as colleagues in the critical care unit and to enhance one another's feelings of belonging and self-esteem. Other hazards involve speaking on behalf of the patient often as a minority voice and in the face of administrative, physician, or peer pressure. It means experiencing the joy of patients who recover or the sadness and anger of those who do not.

It is apparent to us that this philosophy of nursing need not and should not be confined to critical care areas. It is every patient's right to expect this type of intelligent care; it is the nurse's responsibility and challenge to provide it.

The increasing use of *primary nursing* in which one nurse coordinates the care of specific patients over the 24-hour day also reiterates the nurse's role as patient negotiator. This method of patient assignment further expresses the responsibility and accountability of nursing and its need to provide continuity of care.

In the first edition of *Critical Care Nursing* we predicted that the responsibilities then defined as the expanded role would soon be the standard level of practice for the professional nurse. This has indeed happened. Meanwhile, we continue to develop the *thinking* part of nursing while also blending it with the *doing* part of patient care.

Unit
Two
Holistic Approach
to Critical Care Nursing

Thelma "Skip" Lohr

Sociometric Impact on the Patient 3

Over the past 3 decades, researchers from many health fields have been investigating the role of psychosocial factors in the pathogenesis and prognosis of physical illness. Now, it is a commonly accepted fact that these factors do indeed play an important role. A search of the literature* leads one to discover that not only are these factors elusive and unpredictable, but traditional research techniques and tools do not reveal their contribution to illness and health.

Researchers, realizing the experimental uniqueness of life events data, are undertaking to design new tools and techniques. In 1976, Tennant and Andrew designed a stress measurement scale for life events.[1] One premise of this scale is that some of life's events are inherently more stressful and thus will have a greater impact. In a recent study of patients suffering from myocardial infarctions, Byrne and Whyte found that it is not just the event, but how the person perceives it, and thus, his emotional response to it that determine the impact.[2]

Just organizing this wealth of diverse information apparently is a struggle.[3-7] In writing about the stress response theories, Burchfield states, ". . . despite advances in our understanding of the physiological correlates of the stress response, the field is still lacking an integrative framework which can explain the majority of research results in a logical, theoretical manner."[8]

*A vast majority of the reported studies and research conducted during the past 10 years can be found in the *Journal of the American Psychosomatic Society, Psychosomatic Medicine,* and the *Journal of Psychosomatic Research.*

I have found a framework in the works of Moreno.[9,10] What follows is as old as man and as contemporary as this moment. What the reader will discover is an exciting, viable theory that allows him to "see" the invisible structures of our everyday lives which foster health and creativity. It will also be discovered that critical care nurses are in pivotal positions to aid both patients and families in maintaining or building these invisible structures of life and health. A few examples from current research that lend themselves to the discussion are noted through the reference numbers.

Early in the 1900s, Jacob Moreno moved from the traditional sociometry of *macro*scopic study of social structures to become the creator of a new system of sociometry. He began to study the *micro*scopic dynamics of people within groups. As a result, he sculpted a new framework of sociometry based on two positive aspects of people and groups—spontaneity and creativity. Hollander concludes, ". . . sociometry is based on the concept that individuals must have a specific number of people with whom they can meaningfully relate or feel close to in order to experience their creativity and power: i.e., self-confidence."[11]

With Moreno's new framework, a new language emerged, a language with energy words such as *social atom, tele,* and *social equilibrium.*

THE SOCIAL ATOM

The word *atom* suggests an awesome source of powerful energy—a suggestion which holds true for the social atom. The social atom is a powerful energy source of each individual's life. It is also a fact of life that we *live.* Moreno defined it as "the smallest functional unit within our social group."[12] This social unit, which exists at birth and continues and expands into adulthood, is formed by numerous relationships that Moreno called "tele" structures. Originating from a Greek concept, *tele* is a term he used to describe the far-reaching transmission of a feeling, positive or negative, from one person to another—the instinctive ability that allows one to know another intuitively. Tele is always mutual, while one-way tele is *empathy.* People have given it mystical and magical qualities, and teenagers who recognize their ability to "feel another" call it "picking-up vibes."

Through their work with Moreno's concepts, the Hollanders have further clarified the social atom concept.[13-15]

The Psychological Social Atom

This atom is the smallest number of people each person requires to maintain social equilibrium and, thus, a healthy and creative life. The number each person requires usually varies from two to five. Generally, these people are family members and/or friends who are vital to the person's life. (There are some individuals who have replaced people with plants, animals, or objects.) Although these relationships seem to "just happen," they are the result of mutual tele selection by both individuals. They allow for the expression of human feelings (*e.g.,* warmth, love, anger, joy, sorrow, sexuality) and endure over long periods of time.

When the psychological social atom drops below the required number resulting from events of separation, social disequilibrium results, and the person experiences shock and grief. This is evidenced in inappropriate behaviors (*i.e.,* forgetfulness, thoughtlessness, disorganization) or symptoms of ill health (*i.e.,* colds, headaches, angina, cancer). The person *must* regain social equilibrium and will search to fill the void. The void, however, cannot truly be filled until grieving is complete.

If the person's atom is comprised of only one, all energy will be directed toward maintaining this member. Living examples of this were Richard and Ann, two elderly people living in a nursing home. They had become very good friends and were inseparable. Ann broke her hip in a fall, and following surgery, she remained in a coma for several weeks. When Ann was taken to the hospital, Richard wanted to follow, but nursing home personnel thought it would be inappropriate and so detained him. He faked sleep and waited until 2 A.M. to leave "out the back way." He came to the hospital to "be with her!" He was so unobtrusive that several shifts passed before people began to mention the old man in the room. Then the staff became aware of and concerned for Richard's health and hygiene. He had neither eaten (Ann was on IVs and receiving no trays) nor bathed. He absolutely refused to return to the nursing home for anything. The unit's staff quietly and spontaneously began caring for Richard, too. He joined them in the dining room (he had very little vision) and shared their trays, which always seemed to have "too much food." Although he beamed from the attention, he remained quietly content just to be in Ann's room. When physicians and nurses were finished with their cares, he could be found gently stroking her arm or forehead and softly reminiscing about their life and his love for her — very private and intimate moments that caused the staffs' eyes to tear as they appreciated this gift of caring. Staff, well-aware that it was against unit visiting policies, found nonverbal consensus through others' behaviors.

This continued for 3 to 4 weeks, and as the social worker prepared to assist Richard's reentry into the nursing home upon Ann's death, Ann came out of coma. She got progressively stronger and walked with a walker, and together they returned to the home.

This old gentleman's behaviors were most understandable and appropriate, for Ann was the last significant person in his life. His social atom was about to hit zero, with his own survival at stake. In a psychological social atom of two, it is not uncommon that when one dies, the other follows within a short period of time.[16]

The Collective Social Atom

This collective is one's cultural atom. It is the smallest number of groups or affiliations in which a person must have membership. Collectives are the tele structures in which people assume roles and counterroles of their culture for the expression of their creativity and productivity. They provide one's identity (*i.e.,* mother-child, husband-wife, teacher-student, nurse-patient). Collectives that are common for most people are family, work, social, recreational, educational, and religious.[17]

The relationships within a collective begin the sociometric network that links the collective to other social groups and the community. One example is the critical care nurse who designs and presents cardiopulmonary resuscitation (CPR) learning experiences for her husband's realtor group and then is asked by other realtor groups to do the same for them. Another network pattern is the collective of hospital nurses who have membership in the district nurse's association, which is part of the state's association, which is part of the national organization.

Although a person may have numerous collectives, only one or two will be vital for homeostasis. If membership is terminated in one of these, the person will again experience shock and grief and will begin a search to replace the collective.

The Individual Social Atom

This atom is the smallest number of people within a collective that one needs to feel a sense of belonging. These are the people who respond positively, negatively, or indifferently to our many needs — from sharing our creativity to supporting our efforts or comforting our hurts. These people are a source for our motivation and energy, and although many are important, only a few are vital to our survival within a collective.

As in the previous two atoms, should the number drop below what is required, a sociometric crisis develops for the person. He will "look" in crisis and may not be able to function. Soon his energies will be directed toward searching for replacements. If people are not available, death within the collective occurs, and the person will then terminate his position and search for a new collective, as well. All critical care units have staff members who stand-out — "stars." Should one of these people resign, it is but a short period of time until statements such as, "It just isn't the same," "I feel burned-out," and "I'd like to try something different," are heard. Either someone moves in to fill the void, or the statement makers resign also. The new staff members, given time and opportunity, will change the undercurrent of turmoil to one of belonging by building their own telic structure of relationships.

Three distinct atoms within one, yet they are not separate and isolated entities in one's life. What happens in one atom affects the total. For example: Tony lost his job. He was very upset and irritable — with his children, his wife, and his friends — until he found employment and replaced his work collective with another.

SUMMARY

A diagram of Richard's sociometric network may best portray the social atom concept. Prior to moving to the nursing home, Richard's social atom had been decreasing gradually, and his physical and emotional energy waned with each loss. Figure 3–1 starkly illustrates that Richard's collective of friends, which included Ann, was his only remaining network for living. He was literally dying from without — social atom death.

Together, Richard and Ann chose to move into the nursing home, for Ann had grown to be a close companion who lovingly cared for him. Figure 3–2 indicates that the nursing home folk replaced his collective of friends. There, Richard had many individual relationships, while Ann grew stronger as his psychological and individual atom.

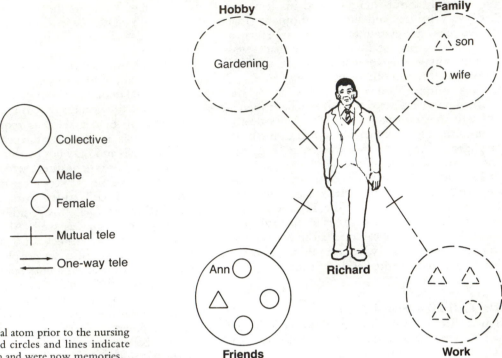

FIGURE 3-1.
Richard's social atom prior to the nursing home. Dotted circles and lines indicate what *had* been and were now memories.

SOCIOMETRIC IMPACT ON CRITICAL CARE

According to Hollander, the sociometry of one's social atom answers "three of the most important questions each person asks throughout life:

1. Who am I?
2. Where do I fit?, and
3. How well am I functioning?"[18]

These three questions become paramount when a person is removed from the uniqueness of his social atom for hospitalization. The effect is momentary termination of one's usual life processes and sensory deprivation of familiar sounds, sights, and experiences —*plus* the addition of a new collective with its unique individuals and environment. Figure 3-3 illustrates such a move. The staff members who care for the patient upon admission do in fact become his individual atom within his new collective. The primary nurse becomes one of the required few necessary to maintain homeostasis within the collective.

Individuals from within his atom, also at loose ends, follow him to the hospital, seeking to keep their connections. One or two of these individuals, usually family members or close friends, become extensions of the patient and have a vital role in establishing and maintaining the patient's relationships (and theirs) within the unit. The most common behaviors that accomplish this are for the family members to ask the questions the patient cannot, to seek the explanations the patient cannot, and to contribute information when the patient does not.

The nurse, however, has a hospital collective that she maintains with the required number of people for belonging and homeostasis.[19] She also has (as does everyone) an expansiveness for accommodating others, including the critical care patients. The patient-others are usually short-term and frequently leave without notice —by transfer or death. For the nurse to invest in each new patient means constantly coping with pain and loss of relationships. Continually investing in new patients without completing terminations with the previous patients is exhausting. The nurse's social atom overexpands, resulting in disequilibrium. When this occurs, the nurse will seek ways to return to homeostasis. A frequent way is to give token investment to the patient, while more completely focusing on her own work relationships and activities.

Khan beautifully describes this very real dilemma in this statement: "We were so intent on saving Mark's arm, it was all we saw. When we got him up in a chair, I think we could have

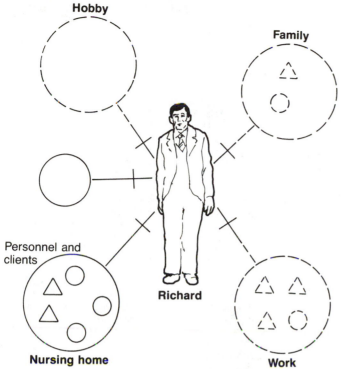

FIGURE 3-2.
Richard's social atom in the nursing home.

accidently left Mark in bed and carried his arm across the room without ever noticing the difference."[20]

It has long been accepted that critical care environments can precipitate a wide variety of feelings and mental states, including isolation, confinement, boredom, relief, fear, confusion, hallucinations, and paranoia. For the patient, the cause is paradoxical — sensory overload from the new environment's persistent lights, sounds,

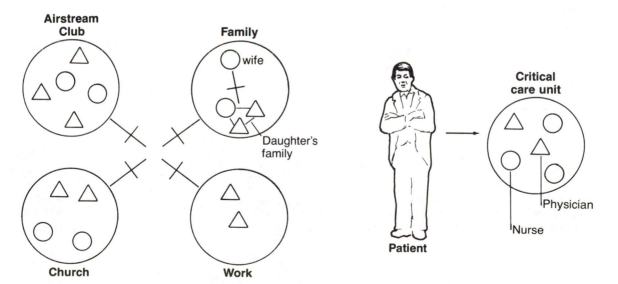

FIGURE 3-3.
A diagram of a social atom upon hospitalization.

and noises and sensory deprivation from loss of familiar sensory stimuli and periods of time that keep the person oriented.[21,22] People stimuli in the form of family, friends, and nurses are discovered most times to be the solution, for people need to feel connected to prevent feeling "crazy."

Many critical care nurses also experience isolation, confinement, boredom, and fear. The unit is not part of mainstream traffic; the patient's room is small and compact; patient assignments absorb hours of time; unresponsive, unchallenging patients provoke nursing by habit. The intensity and duration of these feelings are of a lesser degree for the nurse than for the patient. The nurses seek relief through the people in their collective atom with comments such as, "Relieve me for a moment, will you? I've got to get out of there before I go crazy." or "I'm so bored—do you (nurse) need any help?" These solutions are most important, for when the nurse has minimized the environment's effects on her own self, she is then available to do the same for the patient.

Transfer from critical care is another paradox for the patient. The stress and fears of going into a new collective can be overwhelming; at the same time, the knowledge of getting better is reassuring.[23] Linkage to this new collective is through the nurse and physician. A vital connection is the nurse who accompanies the patient to the next unit and introduces him to the new individuals. To start with, the new collective of individuals will at least know his name and that he now belongs to them. Yet in that same moment, he experiences a great loss, and again the need and importance of family members increase.

Many nurses are indeed searching for ways to minimize their unit's impact and are finding solutions. I believe the answers are in both what the patient and the nurse experience. When staff must constantly rotate shifts and units, their individual and collective atoms will be in constant crisis. Their emotional energies will go toward making and renewing relationships, and they will have very little energy available for the patient. However, in a unit in which the staff is stable and its members have had time to develop high cohesion, the nurse is free to be emotionally available to her patients. In this unit, the patient will be able to find a powerful energy source in his primary nurse and nurse advocate.

REFERENCES

1. Tennant C, Andrew G: A scale to measure the stress of life events. Aust NZ J Psychiatry 10:27–33, 1976
2. Byrne DG, Whyte HM: Life events and myocardial infarctions revisited: The role of measures of individual impact. J Human Stress 42, No. 1:1–9, 1980
3. Rogertine GN Jr et al: Psychological factors in the prognosis of malignant melanoma: A prospective study. Psychosom Med 41, No. 8:647–656, 1979
4. Theorell T: Life events and disease: Psychosocial precipitators of episodes of clinical coronary heart disease. J Psychosom Res 23:403–404, 1979
5. Matus I, Bush D: Asthma attack frequency in a pediatric population. Psychosom Med 41, No. 8:629–635, 1979
6. Monteiro L: Cardiac Patient Rehabilitation: Social Aspects of Recovery. New York, Springer Publishing, 1979
7. Lloyd C et al: Life events as predictors of academic performance. J Human Stress 6, No. 3, 15–25, 1980
8. Burchfield S: The stress response: A new perspective. Psychosom Med 41, No. 8:661, 1979
9. Moreno JL: Who Shall Survive, 3rd ed. Beacon, Beacon House, 1978
10. Moreno JL: Sociometry and the Science of Man. Beacon, Beacon House, 1956
11. Hollander CE: Psychodrama, role playing, and sociometry: Living and learning processes. In Kurpous D (ed): Learning: Making Learning Environments More Effective, p 220. Muncie, Accelerated Development, 1978
12. Moreno JL: Who Shall Survive, p 69
13. Hollander CE: Psychodrama, pp 170–241
14. Hollander CE, Hollander SL: Action Relationships in Learning. Denver, Snow Lion Press, 1978
15. Hollander SL: Social Atom: An Alternative to Imprisonment. Denver, Snow Lion Press, 1974
16. Cottingham E et al: Environmental events preceding sudden death in women. Psychosom Med 42, No. 6:569–573, 1980
17. Orth-Gomer K: Ischemic heart disease and psychological stress in Stockholm and New York. J Psychosom Res 23:403–404, 1979
18. Hollander CE: Psychodrama, p 219
19. Northouse PG: Interpersonal trust and empathy in nurse-nurse relationships. Nurs Outlook, November–December 1979, pp 365–368
20. Khan B et al: Trauma care: Don't forget the patient. AJN, August 1979, p 51
21. Lindemuth JE et al: Sensory overload. AJN, January 1981, pp 1456–1458
22. Kroner K: Dealing with the confused patient. AJN, November 1979, pp 71–78
23. Minckly B et al: Myocardial infarct stress-of-transfer inventory: Development of a research tool. Nurs Res, January–February 1979, pp 3–10

Karen D. Busch,
and Barbara M. Gallo

Emotional Response to Illness 4

When an individual's dynamic stability is threatened or impinged upon and his usual coping mechanisms begin to fail him, he enters a state of illness. Much of this book is focused on supporting and implementing the patient's response to the threat of illness through physiological maintenance and adjustments. It is the purpose of this chapter to consider the intimate relationship between one's emotional response to illness and its effect upon one's adaptation to temporary or permanent limitations. Concepts of anxiety, grief, and adaptation to illness will be presented for the purpose of developing related nursing interventions based on principles of sound theory.

STRESS AND ILLNESS

Illness, or the threat of it, acts as a stressor that leads to an ambient state of tension. The existence of tension produces a response toward adaptation, and this tension state is known as *entropy*. For example, if a person is dehydrated, he drinks when he becomes aware of his thirst. The tension state of thirst activates his response of drinking. If he drinks salt water, neither the stressor nor the tension state of thirst will be relieved, and his state of entropy will increase. If he drinks fresh water, his dehydration will be relieved and therefore his thirst, and he will place himself in a state of negative entropy, thus freeing his energies to cope with other stressors of life (Fig. 4-1).

Just as thirst is the motivating tension state to relieve dehydration, the phenomenon of anxiety

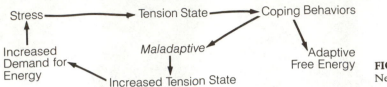

FIGURE 4-1.
Negative entropy.

is the tension state which activates one's response to the threat of illness. When energy is channeled toward reducing the stressor, it minimizes entropy. But energy is often directed toward merely relieving the tension state and may only perpetuate entropy, as with the thirsty, dehydrated person who drinks salt water.

ANXIETY

The relationship among stress, anxiety, and coping is a complex one, which manifests itself continuously in any critical care setting. Stress has been defined as any stimulus condition that results in a disequilibrium of psychological functioning. In turn, this disequilibrium initiates attempts to restore the original state of dynamic equilibrium.

Anxiety, in this sense, can be viewed as a state of disequilibrium or tension that prompts attempts at coping. Coping can then be viewed as a transaction between the person and his environment. Successful transactions have the quality of reducing tension and promoting a sense of well-being.

Any stress that threatens one's sense of wholeness, containment, security, and control will bring anxiety into play. Illness is one such stress. The physiological responses of rapid pulse rate, increased blood pressure, increased respirations, dilated pupils, dry mouth, and peripheral vasoconstriction may go undetected in the seemingly cool, calm, self-controlled patient. These autonomic responses to anxiety are frequently the most reliable index of the degree of anxiety when behavioral responses do not conform to the nurse's expectations. Behavioral responses indicative of anxiety are often familial and culturally learned. They vary from quiet composure in the face of disaster to panic in the presence of a mouse.

Nevertheless, such extremes of control or panic use valuable energy, and when this energy is not directed toward eliminating the stressor, it serves only to perpetuate the state of entropy. The goal of nursing care is always to promote physiological and emotional equilibrium, thereby minimizing entropy and freeing the patient's energy resources for healing and recuperation.

Whenever possible the threatening stress is reduced or eliminated. When this is done the problem is quickly resolved and the patient is returned to a state of equilibrium. Usually, however, the stress is not so easily eliminated; instead, many other stresses are introduced to remedy the original problem. For most people, hospitalization is that kind of secondary stress. To find oneself as a patient in a critical care unit is tangible proof that one's life is in jeopardy. For most, fears that one's life is being threatened are justified, as is the feeling of being wholly at the mercy of strangers. A sense of inadequacy or inferiority results as the individual is unable to understand what is happening to his body or how the personnel and machinery that surround him will return him to his previous state of health.

It is not often possible for the nurse to simply remove the noxious stimulus condition which evokes anxiety. In these circumstances, the nurse must assess the effectiveness of the patient's coping behaviors and either support them, help the patient to modify them, or teach new coping behaviors. Frequently, levels of anxiety are so high that the anxious state becomes the stimulus condition that demands additional coping responses.

Coping behaviors may be directed toward eliminating either the stress of illness or the stress of the anxiety state itself. The nurse must evaluate each behavior in the light of whether or not it functions to restore a steady state. Those behaviors that are consistent with movement toward a steady state can then be supported and encouraged. More likely, the nurse may need to help the patient modify or find substitutes for those coping devices which are disruptive or threatening to homeostasis. At times, it may be necessary to teach or introduce new coping behaviors to enhance movement toward the overall goal of homeostatic equilibrium.

For example, in a critical period a patient may be more capable of experiencing concern and worry over the variety of equipment that surrounds him rather than of focusing on the threat to his life. This activity may allow him some necessary denial of the reality of the crisis, but the worry itself may drain him of needed energy. Information and explanation of the machinery may serve to reduce his secondary anxiety, while expert nursing care may serve to reassure him nonverbally of his security without stripping him of his defense of denial.

Anxiety is commonly experienced when there is a threat of helplessness or lack of control. Thus, nursing measures that reinforce a sense of control help to increase the patient's sense of autonomy and reduce the overpowering sense of loss of control. Providing order and predictability allows the patient to anticipate and prepare for what is to follow. Perhaps it creates only a mirage of control, but anticipatory guidance keeps the patient from being caught off guard and allows him to muster those coping mechanisms which he can bring to bear.

Allowing small choices when the patient is willing and ready decreases the patient's feeling that he is totally at the mercy of others. Is he ready for pain medication? Would he prefer to lie on his right or left side? In which arm would he like his IV? How high does he want the head of his bed? Does he want to cough now or in 20 minutes following pain medication? All serve to let the patient participate in ways that allow him to exert a certain amount of control and predictability. It may also help him accept his lack of control of procedures for which he has little choice. Minute decisions like these allow him to exercise some controls in a way designed to help reduce the anxiety-provoking sense of helplessness.

A second overriding cause of anxiety is a sense of isolation. Rarely is one more lonely than in the midst of a socializing crowd of strangers. In such a situation individuals either attempt to include themselves, remove themselves, or distance themselves with feigned interest in a magazine, scenery, or anything else that offers them relief from the sense of not belonging. The sick person surrounded by active and busy persons is in a similar situation but with fewer available resources to reduce his sense of isolation. Serious illness and the fear of dying separate the patient from his family. The reassuring cliché "You'll be all right" serves to reinforce the sense of distance the patient is experiencing. It shuts off his expression of fears and his questions of what is to come next. The efficiency and activity engulfing him increase his sense of separateness as he lies isolated in his bed.

A third category of anxiety-provoking stimuli includes those that threaten the individual's security. Needless to say, entrance into the critical care unit serves as dramatic confirmation to the family and patient that their security on all levels is being severely threatened. Most individuals associate the critical care unit with a life-and-death crisis; many associate it with the deaths of relatives and friends.

But to the nurse, the unit may represent a closer and safer vigilance of life, with attention directed more to the preservation of life than to the fears of and preparations for dying that may be occupying the minds of the patient and his family. Upon the patient's admission to the unit, insecurity is undoubtedly about life itself. Later, questions of length of hospitalization, return to work, well-being of the family, permanent limitations, and the like arise, so that the state of insecurity is ever present.

Techniques That Deal With Anxiety

Techniques that have evolved from cognitive theories of learning may offer help to anxious patients and their families. These techniques are promising because they can be initiated by the patient and are not dependent on complex insight or understanding of one's own psychological makeup. They can also be employed to reduce anxiety in a way that avoids probing into the individual's personal life. Furthermore, the patient's friends and family members can be taught these techniques to help them and the patient reduce tension.

POSITIVE THINKING

Most likely, the highly anxious person is giving himself messages which serve to increase or perpetuate his anxiety. These messages are conveyed in one's continuously running "self-talk" or *internal dialogue*.[1] The individual in the critical care unit may be saying to himself things such as, "I can't stand it in here. I've got to get out." or, "I can't handle this pain." By asking the patient to share aloud what is going on in his internal dialogue, the nurse can bring to the patient's attention those messages which are distracting him from rest and relaxation. Substitute messages should be suggested to the patient. It is important to ask the patient to substitute rather than delete messages because the internal dialogue is continually operating and will not turn off, even if the individual wills it so. Therefore, asking the patient to substitute constructive, assuring comments is more likely to help him significantly reduce his level of tension. Comments like, "I'll handle this pain just one day at a time." or, "I've been in tough spots before, and I am capable of making it through this one!" will automatically reduce anxiety as well as help the patient shape his coping behavior accordingly. Any message that enhances the patient's confidence in himself and puts him in an active role rather than in the passive role of a victim will increase his sense of coping and well-being.

A similar method can be applied to the patient's *external conversation* with others. By simply requiring the individual to speak accurately about himself to others, the same goals can be accomplished. For example, the patient who exclaims that he can't do anything for himself should be asked to identify the things that he is able to do, such as lift his weight, turn on his side, make a nurse feel good with a rewarding smile, or help his wife to understand what is happening. Even the smallest movement in the weakest of patients should be acknowledged and claimed by the patient. This technique is useful in helping individuals correct their own misconceptions of themselves and the way others see them. In this way, a patient's sense of helplessness, and therefore anxiety, is reduced.

MENTAL IMAGERY AND RELAXATION

Teaching the patient to use *mental imagery* and *relaxation* are two other useful techniques to help the patient reduce his own tension state. The nurse can encourage the patient to imagine himself being in a very pleasant place he has been before or taking part in a very pleasant experience he has had or would like to have. The patient should be instructed to focus and linger on the sensations that he experiences. Questions such as, "What colors do you see? What sounds are present? How does the air smell? How does your skin feel? Is there a breeze in the air?" all help to increase the intensity of the fantasy and thereby promote relaxation through escape.

Guided mental imagery can also be used to help reduce unpleasant feelings of depression, anxiety, and hostility. Patients who must relearn life-sustaining tasks like walking or feeding themselves can use imagery to mentally prepare themselves to successfully take on the challenge. In these instances, patients should be taught to visualize themselves moving through the task and successfully completing it. If this method seems trivial or silly to the patient, he can be reminded that this is a method commonly used by athletes to improve their performance and to prepare themselves mentally before an important event.

Techniques which induce *deep muscle relaxation* can also be used by the nurse to help the patient decrease anxiety and avoid the use of tranquilizing drugs when they are contraindicated. The patient is first directed to find as comfortable a position as possible and then to take several deep breaths and let them out slowly. Next, the patient is asked to clench a fist or curl his toes as tightly as possible, to hold the position for a few seconds, then to let go, while focusing on the sensations of the releasing muscles. The patient should practice this technique beginning with the toes and moving upward through the body—through the feet, calves, thighs, abdomen, chest, and so on. This procedure is done slowly, with the patient giving nonverbal signals, like lifting a finger, to indicate when each new muscle mass has reached a state of relaxation. Special attention can be given to the back, shoulders, neck, scalp, and forehead because these are the areas in which many people experience physical tension.

Once the patient has achieved a state of relaxation, the nurse can suggest to him that he fantasize or sleep as deeply as he chooses for a few moments. A moderately dark room and a soft voice will facilitate the mood of relaxation. Asking the patient to relax is frequently nonproductive compared with directing him to release a muscle mass, to let go of his tension, or to imagine his tension draining through his body and sinking deeply into the mattress.

Despite the employment of the above methods of reducing anxiety, many patients in critical care units are confronted with especially intense problems relating to loss of health, body parts, or physiological functions. The nurse's acute awareness of the patient's vacillating adaptation to his new condition, through the process of grief, will help both the nurse and the patient deal with the challenge ahead of them.

RESPONSE TO LOSS

The threat of illness precipitates the coping behaviors associated with loss. For some patients it is an adaptation to dying; for others it is the loss of health or loss of a limb, a blow to one's self-concept, or the necessity to change one's lifestyle. All of these require a change in one's self-image—a loss of the familiar self-image and its replacement with an altered self-image. Nevertheless, the dynamics of grief present themselves in one form or another.

The response to loss can be described in four phases: shock and disbelief, development of awareness, restitution, and resolution. Each phase has characteristic and predictable behaviors which fluctuate among the various phases in an unpredictable way. Through the recognition and assessment of the various behaviors and an understanding of their underlying dynamics, the nurse can plan nursing interventions to support the healing process.

Shock and Disbelief

In this stage of responding to loss, the patient demonstrates the behaviors characteristic of denial. He fails to comprehend and experience the emotional impact and rational meaning of his diagnosis. Because the diagnosis has no emotional meaning, the patient often fails to cooperate with precautionary measures. For example, the patient may attempt to get out of bed against the doctor's orders, may deviate from his diet, may fail to inform the nurse of minor pain, and may assert that he is there for a *rest!* Denial may go so far as to allow the patient to project his difficulties onto what he perceives as ill-functioning equipment, mistaken lab reports, and — more likely — onto the sheer incompetence of physicians and nurses.

When such blatant denial occurs, it is apparent that the problem is so anxiety-provoking to the patient that it cannot be handled by the more sophisticated defense mechanism of rational problem solving. Thus, the stressor is obliterated. This phase of denial may also serve as the period when the patient's resources, temporarily blocked by the shock, can now be regrouped for the battle ahead. The principle of intervention consists not in stripping away the defense of denial but in supporting the patient and acknowledging his situation through nursing care.

The nurse accepts and recognizes the patient's illness by watching the monitor or changing the dressings. She communicates acceptance of the patient through tone of voice, facial expression, and the use of touch. She can reflect back to the patient his statements of denial in a way that allows him to hear them — and eventually to examine their incongruity and apply reality — as by saying, "In some ways you believe that having a heart attack will be helpful to you?" She can also acknowledge the patient's difficulty in accepting his restrictions by such comments as, "It seems hard for you to stay in bed." By verbalizing what the patient is expressing the nurse gently confronts his behavior but does not cause anxiety and anger by reprimanding and judging him. Thus, in this phase the nurse supports denial by allowing for it but does not perpetuate it. Rather she uses herself to acknowledge, accept, and reflect the patient's new circumstance.

It is interesting to note that although denying illness can prevent adaptation at a new level, denial also has its advantages. High deniers with myocardial infarctions have been shown to have a higher survival rate than moderate or low deniers.[2] They also often return to work sooner and reach higher levels of rehabilitation. This points out the effectiveness of denial as a coping mechanism as well as the hazards of stripping it away before the patient is ready.

Development of Awareness

In this stage of grief, the patient's behavior is characteristically associated with anger and guilt. The anger may be expressed overtly and may be directed at the staff for oversights, tardiness, and minor insensitivities. At this time the ugliness of reality has made its impact. Displacement of the anger on others helps to soften the impact. The expression of anger itself helps give the patient a sense of power in a seemingly helpless state. A demanding manner and a whining tone often characterize this stage and are attempts at regaining the control that appears to be lost. However, such behavior often serves to alienate the nurse and other personnel. The patient who does not demand or whine has probably withdrawn into depression. He will demonstrate verbal and motor retardation, will have difficulty sleeping, and may prefer to be left alone. The depression is characteristic of other depressions, such as anger turned inward.

During this phase the nurse is likely to hear irrational expressions of guilt. The patient seeks to answer, "Why me?" He will attempt to isolate his human imperfections and attribute the cause of his malady to them. He and his family may participate in looking for a person or object to blame.

Guilt feelings around one's own illness are difficult to understand unless one examines the basic dynamic of guilt. Guilt arises when there is a decrease in the feeling of self-worth or when the self-concept has been violated. In this light, the nurse can understand that what is behind an expression of guilt is a negatively altered self-concept. Blame thus becomes nothing more than projection of the unbearable feeling of guilt.

Nursing intervention in this phase must be directed toward supporting the patient's basic sense of self-worth and allowing and encouraging the expression of direct anger. Nursing measures that support a patient's sense of self-worth are numerous: calling the patient by name, introducing him to strangers (particularly when they are to examine him), talking *to* rather than *about* him, and most of all providing and respecting his need for privacy and modesty. The nurse needs to guard against verbal and nonverbal expressions of pity. It is better to empathize with the patient's specific feelings of anger, sadness, and guilt rather than with his condition.

The nurse can create outlets for anger by listening and by refraining from defending either herself, the doctor, or the hospital. A nondefensive, accepting attitude will decrease the patient's sense of guilt, and the expression of anger will avert some of the depression. Later, when the patient is apologetic for his irrational outburst, the nurse can interpret the necessity of this kind of verbalization as a step toward rehabilitation.

Restitution

In this stage the griever puts aside his anger and resistance and begins to cope constructively with his loss. He tries new behaviors consistent with his limitations. His emotional level is one of sadness, and much of his time may be spent crying. As he adapts himself to his new image, he spends considerable time going over and over significant memories relevant to his loss. Behaviors in this stage include the verbalization of fears regarding his future. Often these go undetected because they are unbearable for the family to hear. After severe trauma, which may have resulted in scarring or removal of a body part or loss of sensation, the patient may question his sexual adequacy and the future response of his mate to his changed body. He probably also questions his new role in his family and job and has a variety of concerns that are specific to his own life-style.

Thus, in the mourning process such manifestations as reminiscing, crying, questioning, expressing fears, and trying out new behaviors serve to help the patient modify his old self-concept and begin working with and experiencing his revised concept.

Nursing intervention in this stage should again be supportive to allow this adaptation to occur. Listening to the patient for lengthy periods of time will be necessary. If the patient is able to verbalize his fears and questions about the future, he will be better able to define his anxiety and to solve his problems. Furthermore, hearing himself talk about his fears will help him put them into a more rational perspective. He may require privacy, acceptance, and encouragement

to cry so that he can find respite from his sadness.

During this stage the nurse might have the patient consider meeting someone who has successfully adapted to similar trauma. This measure would provide the patient with a role model as he begins to take on a new identity, which often occurs after the crisis period.

Additionally, the patient, with appropriate support from the nurse, will begin to identify and acknowledge changes that are arising out of his adaptation to illness. Relationships can and do change. Because friends respond to an invalid differently than they do to a healthy person, the patient will not feel or believe that he is being treated like his old self.

During this time the family has also been going through a similar process. They too have experienced shock, disbelief, anger, and sadness. When they are ready to try to solve their problems, their energies will be directed toward wondering how the changes in the patient will affect their mutual relationship and their life-style. They too will experience the pain of turmoil and uncertainty. Nurses must help the family also. By providing ventilation and acceptance of their feelings of repulsion and fear, the nurse can help the family to be more useful to and accepting of the patient. Through intensive listening the nurse provides a sounding board and then redirects the members of the family back to each other so that they can give and receive support.

Resolution

Resolution is the stage of identity change. At first the patient can be observed to be overidentifying himself as an invalid. He may discriminate against himself and make derogatory remarks about his body. Another method is to detach the traumatized part such as a stoma, prosthesis, scar, or paralyzed limb by naming it and referring to it in a simultaneously alienated and affectionate way. The patient is alert to the ways in which health-care workers respond to his body and to his comments about himself and may be testing out their acceptance before he ventures into the outside world. Chiding him or telling him that many others share his problem will be less helpful than acknowledging his feelings and indicating acceptance by continuing to care for and talk with him.

As time passes and the patient adapts, the sting of the endured hurt abates, and the patient moves toward identifying himself as an individual who has certain limitations due to his illness, rather than as a "cripple" or "invalid." He no longer uses his defect as the basis of his identity. As the resolution is reached, the patient is able to depend on others when necessary, and he should not need to push himself beyond his endurance or to overcompensate for his inadequacy. Often the individual will look back upon the crisis as a growing period. Hopefully, he will have achieved a sense of pride at accomplishing the difficult adaptation. He is able to reflect back realistically upon his successes and disappointments without discomfort. At this time he may find it useful and gratifying to help others by sharing himself as a role model for those who, in the stage of restitution, are experiencing their own identity crises.

Unfortunately, the hospital nurse is rarely in a position to observe the successful outcome. It is useful for her to know the process in order that she may work with and communicate an attitude of hope, especially when her patient is most self-disparaging.

The goal of nursing care in this stage is to help the patient attach a sense of self-esteem to his rectified identity. Nursing intervention revolves around helping the patient find the degree of dependence that he needs and can accept. She must accept and recognize with the patient his vacillation between independence and dependence, and she must encourage a positive emotional response to his new state of modified dependence. Certainly she can support and reinforce his growing sense of pride in his rehabilitation. For those nurses who have had the experience of working through the process with one individual, the problem will be to stand back and allow the patient to move away from them.

ADAPTATION TO ILLNESS
Another method of assisting and evaluating a patient's response to his illness is described by Martin and Prange.[3] By comparing emotional adaptation with physical state of illness or well-being, it is easy to identify problem areas.

Martin and Prange theorize that there is an emotional lag by which a person becomes physically ill before he adapts emotionally; it follows then that in the process of recuperation the person becomes well before he adapts emotionally. Thus, in the shaded area of Figure 4-2, the patient is likely to be denying his illness. Again, he is likely to be uncooperative in his treatments and resist restrictions placed upon him. As he adjusts to his sick role, things should go fairly smoothly. Then, as the patient improves physically, the nurse and others begin to raise their expectations for his activity and independence. However, because his emotional adaptation has not caught up with his physical state, the patient will move forward only with trepidation. He will demonstrate greater concern over his physical state and will increase his demands for help. Preparation for his return to health, acknowledgment of his concerns about increased activity, and the reassurance of watchful eyes will help alleviate his anxiety as he progresses.

One principle that greatly affects understanding of the patient's response is the fact that during stress the patient will regress in an attempt to conserve his energies. Thus, during times of acute exacerbation or the raising of expectations, or during any significant change, the initial response will be to regress to an earlier emotional position of safety. Weaning from a respirator, removal of monitor leads, or increased activity and reduction in medication often trigger anxiety and regression. This regression may even include a retreat into increased dependency, depression, and anger. At that time comfort may be found in regressing into a state the patient has already discovered he can live through or master. The regression is usually temporary and brief and serves to pinpoint the cause of anxiety. At this time health personnel may become disappointed, anxious, or angry with the patient's backsliding and may wish to retreat from him. It is more helpful, however, to acknowledge that

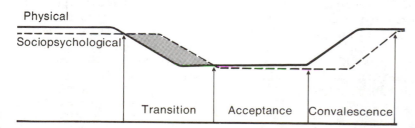

FIGURE 4-2.
The solid line represents a normal level of physical well-being, the broken line a corresponding degree of sociopsychological integration.

regression is inevitable and to support the patient with intervention appropriate in earlier stages.

Each person's electrocardiogram has common characteristics as well as individual differences. Similarly, each person's response to illness, if put into a graph, would have both common and unique points. There will be variations in time and in the congruence between physical and sociopsychological responses, but the stages will occur predictably. Like the electrical events of the heart, responses to illness, both adaptive and maladaptive, can be anticipated and hopefully minimized.

The prevalence of anxiety and depression as part of the response to illness is documented in a study by Cassem and Hackett.[4] During this research project, any patient whose outlook or behavior endangered his physical or emotional well-being was referred for psychiatric consultation. Of 441 patients who were admitted to the coronary care unit because of myocardial infarction, 145 (32.7%) were referred because of anxiety, depression, or behavior problems. Referrals because of anxiety were highest on the patients' first and second days in the unit, with referrals for depression peaking on days three and four. Behavior problems were the third most common reason for consultation. The greatest number were referred on day two, with fewer on day four. The behaviors included denying illness by threatening to leave the hospital, euphoria, sexually suggestive comments, and conflicts about hospital or treatment restrictions. This supports the premise that anxiety accompanies transition into illness and that depression emerges as people recognize the impact of the illness.

Although these responses occurred in patients who had had myocardial infarctions, they may be generalized to include other persons who have a sudden onset of illness and who need intensive care. In addition, the authors noted that the interventions that helped patients deal with their situation did not have to be carried out by psychiatrists alone.

Both doctors and nurses were invited to make referrals. Not only did nurses make more referrals than doctors, but all those referred by doctors had already been referred earlier by nurses. This fact points out that nurses made early and astute observations about coping mechanisms. Because of their expertise and proximity to the patient, nurses should continue both to intervene and to make referrals.

TEACHING AND LEARNING

Recognizing the patient's response to illness helps predict the time at which information will be best absorbed and most helpful to him. Learning is most likely to occur during quiet stages when the patient's emotional outlook corresponds to his physical condition. This can be seen in Figure 4-2 (the stage of acceptance) in which the lines representing sociopsychological and physical functioning are in close proximity. This means that the patient feels just about as sick (or well) as he is. Providing information in this phase of illness will help him move on to the next phase of recovery. When there is less congruence between the patient's emotional outlook and his physical condition, the lines representing sociopsychological and physical functioning are farther apart. Providing information at this time may increase the patient's vulnerability and either reinforce his defenses, causing resistance, or diminish them enough to cause regression. Both responses result from anxiety and will further increase the gap between sociopsychological and physical functioning.

As the patient adjusts to the sick role, he will be receptive to learning about his illness. Because progress heightens anxiety, teaching is usually more effective during the period of acceptance than during the times in which the patient is moving either into or out of the sick role. Whenever there is movement forward or backward on the health-illness continuum, there is likely to be an emotional response of anxiety, worry, or depression which will interfere with concentration and learning. Therefore, admission, transfer, or readmission to the critical care unit, as well as hospital discharge, are poor times for learning to occur. During periods of anxiety, it is useful to ascertain the patient's perceptions of what is happening so that misunderstandings that may cause unnecessary worry can be corrected.

Informal teaching and the provision of information which serves to enhance equilibrium while promoting a minimum of entropy are best woven into the other nursing procedures occurring throughout the patient's stay in the critical care unit. For effective learning to take place, the high levels of anxiety commonly found in critical care units must be decreased to no more than mild anxiety states in which the patient demonstrates alertness without fear, motivation to learn, and interest. The more facts there are to absorb and the more behavior change is implied by the information, the more likely the patient is to respond with increased levels of anxiety, and therefore, the greater the need to teach during periods of only mild anxiety.

Anxiety levels, physiological function, and the patient's own priorities must be assessed when the readiness of the patient-learner is evaluated. Anxiety, worry, pain, and some medications will interfere with the patient's ability to learn.

Informal teaching and rehabilitation programs that may involve structure and extended periods of time should occur after the crisis, when the patient has reached a fairly stable period of adjustment. In order to provide this type of essential health teaching, hospital-based personnel can conduct programs for patients to return to after hospital discharge. In addition, community-based classes can be conducted, and teaching can be done in the home. Follow-up learning sessions are necessary regardless of where they take place.

With the trend of early hospital discharge, individualized teaching in the home is often necessary to carry out that which was begun in the hospital. At home, in their own surroundings and with their own routines, the patient's and family's knowledge and their ability to apply it can be evaluated by community health nurses.

Most of the learning required of patients who are recovering from critical illness involves a change in behavior that will alter their life-style. Dietary changes that restrict calories, sodium, cholesterol, or carbohydrate are common. A change in activity level may be imposed, exercise may be prescribed, and a decrease in smoking may be imperative. None of these changes are easy to make. Providing information is rarely enough to alter behavior.

Group teaching is a well-suited technique for learning which involves life-style changes. Group process can provide support, offer encouragement and motivation, and reinforce information and accomplishments.

An effective approach to learning includes a combination of informal teaching, group instruction, and individualized learning and evaluation at home. Teaching can be started during the hospital stay, but it can rarely be completed.

The hierarchy of needs described in Figure 2-1 is another guide to keep in mind when predicting receptivity to teaching. During the stage of severe physiological limitations, when the patient's energies are directed at maintaining basic physiological functions, teaching which involves upper levels of functioning will probably be unsuccessful. Learning occurs more easily when security, a sense of belonging, and self-esteem are high. Often learning about illness means that the patient and family must not only learn facts and techniques but must also synthesize, apply, and adapt what is said to their own lives. This will be difficult when there are high degrees of anxiety, depression, or acute physical dysfunction. It will be impossible for patients to respond creatively while they are struggling to maintain basic physiological needs.

When the teachable moment appears, the following reminders will help keep communication open:

- Find out about the patient's concerns before teaching.
- Ask for his ideas and perceptions of what is happening.
- Avoid judgmental statements.
- Then, ask yourself: "Is what he wants to learn what I want to teach him?"

The nursing process will help you answer that question. This process can be used to determine the teaching plan just as it is used to determine any other nursing action. It involves collecting information, making an assessment, determining a teaching plan, and evaluating the outcome.

TRANSFERENCE

There are some types of irrational behavior directed toward nurses which cannot be explained by adaptation or grieving. It appears that in times of stress, as well as at other times, some patients attribute to the nurses feelings, desires, characteristics, attitudes, and fears that they have encountered in the past. This phenomenon is called *transference*. Exhibitionism, extreme dependency, and irrational demands are some behaviors that can often be accounted for by transference.

It may be that in times of crisis and regression, reality testing is impaired, and the patient is more likely to act and react to the irrational fears and feelings that originated when he was a helpless child. In such instances, the patient must be treated and addressed as an adult and helped to test reality in the current environment. For example, if the patient fears that the nurses do not care about him, he can be encouraged to ask specific nurses how they feel or he can be helped to identify what it is about the nurses that suggests to him that they do not care for him. At that time, specific explanations can be given about nurses' behavior. This type of intervention satisfies the patient's need to be cared about far better than global reassurance and generalizations that the nurses do care about him.

Just as patients may transfer feelings which originated from their earlier experiences, so too do nurses. This process is called *countertransference* and should be considered whenever a nurse's behavior toward a particular patient differs from her usual pattern. Inappropriate or intense feelings, including anger, the desire to argue, and extreme protectiveness, should signal the possibility that countertransference is occurring.

TRANSFER FROM THE CRITICAL CARE UNIT

Regression is often elicited when the patient is told that he is ready to be transferred to the general unit. The stage of illness greatly influences the patient's response to transfer. If the patient is transferred while he is denying his illness, the move will be done with ease because it further fortifies his feeling that he isn't very sick. On the other hand, if the patient is transferred when he is improving physically more than he acknowledges emotionally, then anxiety will be heightened. The patient is saying, "I'm sick, and being transferred means you think I'm getting better when I'm not." In trying to cope with the anxiety generated by the move, he will regress and become more dependent. Transferring a patient when he first acknowledges the severity of his illness may create discomfort for nurses because the patient is likely to be frightened, angry, uncooperative, and demanding.

Preparing the Transfer

Regardless of the timing, in preparing for transfer both the nurse and the patient need to accept the fact that their relationship with each other will be ending. This may be done by reminiscing over an initial meeting or a special moment and by talking about the move.

If the patient is feeling dependent, then more time may be needed to talk about how it will be to leave. Often, because of discomfort at saying goodbye, nurses withdraw under the guise that it is easier for the patient when the nurse ignores the termination process. This unexplained withdrawal may be interpreted by the patient as a lack of interest or as anger over earlier unre-

solved outbursts when he had been experiencing a change in body image and lowered esteem because of his illness.

The news of transfer often comes without warning or preparation. Even though the patient may be pleased with his progress, he is at the same time concerned about losing the reassurance of special equipment, close surveillance, and the presence of familiar faces. It has long been advocated that continuity of care be provided by thoughtful preparation. Introduction to the new nurses who will take over care of the patient, as well as follow-up visits by the critical care nurses, will increase familiarity, enhance security, and let the patient know that he is important. Removing equipment before the time of transfer will lessen the strain of having to give up his room, equipment, and nurse all at the same time.

Family members can provide valuable support during the transfer process when they know what will happen and when they have had their questions answered and their concerns addressed. Family members who either accompany patients during the transfer or meet them at the new room and then stay with them during the remainder of the day can lessen the stress associated with the change. This was validated in a study reported by Schwartz and Brenner which examined the use of nursing interventions to reduce patient stress.[5]

In this experiment, 30 patients hospitalized in coronary care units owing to acute myocardial infarction were randomly put into three groups: two experimental and one control. In one experimental group, nurses provided families information about transfer and encouraged them to maintain contact with the patient similar to that described above. In the second experimental group, the patient met and developed a relationship with the nurse to whom he would be transferred. The usual transfer procedure was used for the control group. The hypothesis was that either of the two experimental nursing approaches would reduce the stress associated with transfer, decrease cardiovascular complications, and result in fewer reports of stress by the subjects. Overall, experimental patients in both groups scored lower than the control group on patient stress as reported by patient, family, and nurse and on cardiovascular complications for 72 hours after transfer. No difference was found in the physical complaints reported the evening of transfer. In addition, the authors noted that patients in both experimental groups were more likely to comply with physician orders, had fewer readmissions to the coronary care unit, and spent fewer days hospitalized on the nursing unit.[6]

In another study reported by Klein et al, urine catecholamine studies on patients transferred to a general unit from a coronary care unit indicated that increased stress with transfer occurred in five of seven patients.[7] All five of these patients had a cardiovascular complication such as arrhythmia. In a follow-up study, however, seven patients were prepared for transfer from the beginning of their stay. They had follow-up visits by the nurse and care by the same physician. No cardiovascular complications occurred, and only two had a rise in urine catechols at the time of transfer. Even with preparation for transfer, regression and anxiety may occur; however, by acknowledging his concerns and receiving support from the nurse, the patient will again mobilize his energy.

Because these processes have proved predictable, they give the nurse a basis for her care and provide rationale for appropriate intervention. In spite of the predictability of these responses in human behavior, they still have an impact upon the individual and are unique to him. By the time they are modified by his personality and by sociocultural and economic variables, they have become a significant part of his life and are indeed made unique as they become a historical and living part of his identity.

REFERENCES

1. Meichenbaum D: Cognitive-Behavior Modification. New York, Plenum Press, 1977
2. Hackett T, Cassem NH, Wishnie H: The coronary care unit: An appraisal of its psychological hazards. N Engl J Med 279, No. 25:1365–1370, 1968
3. Martin HW, Prange AJ: Adaptation to illness. Nurs Outlook 10:168–171, 1962
4. Cassem NH, Hackett TP: Psychiatric consultation in a coronary care unit. Ann Intern Med 75, No. 1:9–11, 1971
5. Schwartz LP, Brenner ZR: Critical care unit transfers: Reducing patient stress through nursing interventions. Heart Lung 8:540–546, 1979
6. *Ibid.*
7. Klein F et al: Transfer from a coronary care unit: Some adverse responses. Arch Intern Med 122:104–108, 1968

Karen Busch

Families in Crisis
5

A holistic approach to critical care nursing must include the patient's family. For the purposes of this chapter, *family* means any persons who share intimate and routine day-to-day living with the critical care patient—in other words, those persons whose social homeostasis is altered by the patient's entrance into the arena of critical illness or injury, and who are a significant part of the patient's normal life-style and therefore must be a part of holistic care.

STRESS AND FAMILY ADAPTATION

The patient's entrance into a life-death sick role threatens and alters the family's homeostasis for many reasons. The patient's responsibilities will now have to be added to the responsibilities of others and therefore will demand an alteration in their schedules and activities. When these responses are left undone, the members experience various degrees of discomfort and annoyance. Financial concerns are usually major; also, daily activities which previously were of little consequence to family members now become important and often difficult to manage. Such activities as packing school lunches for children, keeping the family car filled with gasoline, taking out the garbage, and balancing the checkbook can, when unfulfilled, all become critical incidents with the right timing.

In addition to the responsibilities the patient normally carries, the social role the patient plays in the family will also be missing. Disciplinarian, provider of affection, lover, humorist, time keeper, motivator, comforter, and so on are all important roles; when they are missing, considerable havoc and even grief in the family may ensue.

The family enters into a crisis situation under the following conditions:

- A stressful event occurs, which threatens lasting changes for the family.
- Usual problem-solving activities are inadequate and therefore do not lead rapidly to the previous state of balance.
- The present state of family disequilibrium cannot be maintained and will lead either to improved family health and adaptation or to decreased family adaptability and increased proneness to crisis events.

By using these conditions to identify and define families in crisis, the stress of normal maturational events of family life such as marriage, pregnancy, enrollment in school, and retirement can be appreciated in a different light. Holmes and Rahe have scored stressful life events which can be predictors of illness.[1] These life events all require readjustment and include such things as marital reconciliation, change in finances, and trouble with the in-laws or the boss. Thus, it is not only situations of disease and injury that propel families into crisis. A family who has been coping adequately with unemployment may not be able to deal with the added stress of a critically ill family member. What appears to be a family's overreaction to a small stress may be explained as having a "last straw" effect added onto a maturational crisis.

Some families experience many more crises than others. Often the challenges and demands that face these families are similar to the ones that present themselves to all families. There appears to be an additional factor of *cognitive appraisal* which must be considered. Some persons or families appear to assign catastrophic meaning to some events that others would not. If family members appraise a situation by giving it the proportions and labels of crisis events, then the emotions, stress, and anxiety associated with a crisis, as well as attempts to cope, will follow.[2] This phenomenon then implies that crises based on cognitive appraisal are individual and unique—that is, a crisis for one family is not necessarily a crisis for another. The wide range of family behaviors and reactions observed by critical care nurses can in large part be explained by this concept. Cultural and age variables can also be accounted for in this way.

Brose makes four important generalizations about crises which can form a basis for nursing care of families dealing with them:

1. Whether a person emerges stronger or weaker as a result of a crisis is not based so much on his previous character as on the kind of help he receives during the actual crisis.
2. People become more amenable to suggestions and open to help during actual crises.
3. With the onset of a crisis situation, old memories of past crises may be evoked. If maladaptive behavior was used to deal with previous situations, the same type of behavior may be repeated in the face of a new crisis.
4. The only way to survive a crisis is to be aware of it.[3]

Roberts states, "Families of patients in a critical care unit attempt to continue in a steady state. They accomplish this goal either by minimizing the significance of the patient's illness, or by being overprotective of him. The critically ill patient enters the hospital in biological crisis. Unlike the patient, the family enters the same hospital, or critical care unit, in psychological crisis."[4] Roberts also makes the point that as stress increases, the family system at first improves; as stress continues, disintegration of the family system may occur.[5]

Reactions to crisis situations are difficult to categorize because they depend upon individual responses to stress, and within a family, several mechanisms to handle stress and anxiety will be employed. In general, the nurse may observe behaviors which indicate emotions signifying helplessness and urgency. An inability to make decisions and mobilize resources can be noted. A sense of fear and panic pervades. Irrational acts, demanding behavior, withdrawal, perseveration, and fainting all have been observed by critical care nurses. Just as the patient is experiencing shock and disbelief about his illness, so too is the family. A nurse must perceive the feeling that a crisis victim is experiencing, particularly when that person cannot identify the problem or feeling to himself or others.

NURSING INTERVENTION

Nursing intervention must be designed to help families do the following:

- Reach a higher level of adaptation by learning from the crisis experience

• Regain a state of equilibrium
• Experience the feelings involved in the crisis to avoid delayed depressions and allow for future emotional growth

Assessment

The critical care nurse can expect to deal with large numbers of persons who can be defined as being in a crisis. Almost all patients and families who populate the waiting room will fit the crisis conditions described above. The problem will be to assess the immediate events causing the disruption and then to help the families assign priorities to their needs so that they can act accordingly.

The nurse will need to identify current methods of coping and to evaluate them in terms of adaptation (see Chapter 4). The nurse will need to determine, and sometimes point out to the clients, chronic problems resulting from the threatening crisis. When the situational crisis seems inconsequential or obscure, the nurse must attempt to discern and understand the meaning the clients have attributed to the event. Furthermore, it will help to evaluate current maturational problems with which the family may be attempting to cope. Understanding the parameters of the crisis may give the direction for action.

The Use of the Relationship

Establishing an emotionally meaningful relationship with people in crisis tends to be easier than at any other time. Persons in crisis are highly receptive to an interested and empathic helper. In the first meeting with the patient's family, the nurse must demonstrate an ability to help.

The family must be prepared for their experience in the critical care unit. The patient's condition, alertness, and appearance should be described in terms suitable to the family's level of understanding. Any equipment should be explained before the family views the patient. At the bedside further explanation can be made.

Other specific help can be given at this time to demonstrate the nurse's interest. Looking up telephone numbers can be extremely difficult for the highly anxious family member. Even deciding who is to be notified of the patient's status can be an overwhelming decision at these times.

With this kind of timely intervention, the family will begin to trust and depend on the nurse's judgment. This process then allows family members to believe the nurse when she conveys a feeling of hope and confidence in their ability to deal with whatever is ahead of them in the days to come. It is important to avoid giving false reassurance; rather, the reality of the situation can be expressed in statements like, "This is a complicated problem; together we can work on it."

Defining the Problem

As the relationship develops from one interaction to another, the nurse can formulate the dynamics of the problem. The formulations would include such items as the following:

• The meaning the family has attached to the event
• Other crises with which the family may be already coping
• The coping mechanisms previously used in times of stress, with an idea of why these behaviors are or are not working at this time
• The normal resources of the family, which may include friends, neighbors, relations, colleagues, and so forth. The nurse, having identified these areas, will best use them with the family to help them deal with their predicament.

A vital part of the problem-solving process is to help the family clearly state what their immediate problem is. Often people feel overwhelmed and immobilized by the free-floating anxiety or panic caused by acute stress. Stating the problem in words helps the client achieve a degree of *cognitive mastery*. Regardless of the difficulty or threat the problem implies, being able to state it as such reduces anxiety by helping the family to feel that they have achieved some sort of understanding of what is happening.

Defining and redefining the problem or problems must occur many times before resolution of the crisis occurs. Stating the problem clearly automatically helps the family to assign priorities and direct the needed actions. For example, finding a baby-sitter may become the number one priority, superseding notification of close relatives of a tragic accident. Goal-directed activity will further help to decrease anxiety and the irrational acts that sometimes go with it.

In high levels of stress, some people expect themselves to react differently. Rather than turning to the resources they use daily, they become reluctant to involve them. Simply asking people who it is that they usually turn to when they are upset and finding out what has gotten in the way of turning to these people now helps direct the client back to the normal mechanisms that he uses to maintain homeostasis. When the client is reluctant to call on a friend, the nurse can help with the indecision by asking, "Wouldn't you want to help her if she were in your place?" Most families are truly not without resources; they have only failed to recognize and call on them.

Defining and redefining the problem may also help to put the problem in a different light. It is possible in time to view a tragedy as a challenge and the unknown as an adventure.

The nurse can also help the family call on their own strengths. How have they handled stress before? Have they used humor, escape, exercise, or friendship? Do they telephone close friends and relatives who are far away? Even though the family may be threatened financially at this time, some expenditures of this sort may be well worth the money.

Problem Solving

A problem-solving technique which emphasizes choices and alternatives will help the family achieve a sense of control over part of their lives. It will also serve to remind them, as well as clarify to them, that they are ultimately responsible for dealing with the event, and that it is they who must live with the consequences of their decisions.

Helping the family focus on feelings is extremely important in order to avoid delayed grief reactions and protracted depressions later on. The nurse can give direction to the family to help each other cry and to share their fear and sadness. Reflection of feelings or active listening will be necessary throughout the crisis. If the nurse can start a statement by saying, "You feel . . .," she will be reflecting a feeling. If she says, "You feel *that* . . .," she will be reflecting a judgment instead of a feeling. Describing and recognizing one's feelings will decrease the need to look for someone to blame. Valuing the expression of feelings may help the clients avoid the use of tranquilizers, sedatives, and excessive sleep to escape painful feelings. In sad and depressing times the nurse can authentically promise the family that they will feel better with time. Depression is self-limiting.

During the difficult days that a person is critically ill, the family may become very dependent on the judgment of professionals. It may be difficult for them to identify the appropriate areas in which to accept others' judgments. The nurse can best handle inappropriate expectations like, "Tell me what I should do?" by acknowledging the feelings involved in an accepting manner and stating the reality of the situation; for example, "You wish I could make that difficult decision for you, but I can't, because you are the ones who will have to live with the consequences." This type of statement acknowledges the clients' feelings and recognizes the complexity of the problem, while emphasizing each individual's responsibility for his or her own feelings, actions, and decisions.

Once the problem has been defined and the family begins goal-directed activity, the nurse may help further by asking them to identify the steps they must take. This anticipatory guidance will help reduce anxiety and make things go more smoothly.

Crisis victims must always be left with a specific plan of action. This plan may be as simple as, "Call me tomorrow at 2:00 P.M."; regardless of its simplicity, it implies hope, responsibility, and a reason to get through the night.

The critical care nurse's time with families is often limited due to the nature of her work, so it is important to make every interaction as useful to the family as possible. She will have to take responsibility for directing the conversation and focusing on the here and now. She will need to avoid the temptation of giving useless advice in favor of emphasizing a problem-solving approach. However, she must use her judgment and recognize those moments when direction is vital to health and safety. It is often necessary to direct families to return home to rest. This can be explained by saying that by maintaining their own health they will be more helpful to the patient at a later time. To make each interaction meaningful, the nurse must focus on the crisis situation and avoid getting involved in long-term chronic problems and complaints. For example, she would help the family of the overdose patient deal with the events immediately preceding the suicide attempt rather than with long-standing family problems.

Referral

Regardless of the nurse's ability in this area, there will be some families who will profit most by referral to a mental health nurse clinician, a social worker, a psychologist, or a psychiatrist. A nurse can best help the client accept help from others by emphatically acknowledging the difficulty of the problem and providing a choice of names and phone numbers. At times it even may be appropriate for the nurse to set up the first meeting; however, the chances of follow-through are greater when the client makes his own arrangements.

WHEN THE PATIENT IS DYING

For the most part, the goals of the critical care nurse are to preserve life and facilitate healing. Too often nurses experience a sense of disappointment and failure —even anger with the patient —when the patient does not recover. When a patient dies, whether unexpectedly or as the inevitable end of a tragic and painful illness, the family of the patient becomes intimately involved in a crisis that will shape their memories, feelings, and attitudes about death for the rest of their lives.

The challenge for nurses working with the dying patient and the family is to turn an often painful and trumatic experience into one that is also constructive and positive. When there is time, the last days of life can be a time of resolution, reconciliation, and termination.

An attitude of mutual trust among the staff, the patient, and the patient's family is essential to meet this challenge. To promote trust, the nurse must develop the courage to answer the patient's and the family's questions honestly but with a sensitivity that allows the family members to maintain hope and integrity. Cassem identifies nine treatment recommendations for the care and management of the dying patient.[6] These areas of recommendation, described in the following pages, contribute to nursing strategies directed toward establishing an atmosphere in which trust and communication among the staff, the patient, and the family are most likely to occur.

Competence

Critical care nurses will be quick to recognize the amount of comfort and care which is conveyed through absolute technical competence. Even though extreme lifesaving measures may be withheld, ". . . being good at what one does brings emotional as well as scientific benefits to the patient."[7] Being lifted and handled by competent hands is reassuring to both patient and family. Likewise, sloppy and shortcut techniques will be interpreted by the family as a devaluing of life because it is ending.

Concern

Concern or compassion is conveyed to the family when the staff is actively involved with them. Often nurses attempt to defend themselves against the pain of involvement by trying to hide or cover their sensitivity. The problem with this defense is that it is interpreted as callousness by the patient and his family. For some nurses, lack of involvement is a way of protecting themselves from becoming overly involved. Overinvolvement occurs for most nurses from time to time and, in fact, can threaten their competence and judgment. However, it can be managed with understanding supervision, good listening, and personal insight.[8] Perhaps a greater problem for many nurses is that other nurses and colleagues may interpret the signs of compassion and healthy involvement as signs of overinvolvement. A nurse whose eyes become filled with tears at a sensitive moment conveys a sense of empathy to clients, not a loss of control. The major goal for many nurses is to learn to demonstrate comfortably the concern and compassion that are already an integral part of their emotional makeup.

Comfort

The aggressive pursuit of comfort is a primary nursing goal for the dying patient.

When a decision to limit or stop certain treatment measures has been made, overall treatment must be intensified, if anything, so that the patient and family are enabled to meet the patient's death as peacefully and comfortably as possible.[9]

Pain relief is an important part of providing comfort for many critical care patients. The nurse must communicate closely with the patient and the physician to create a regimen in which the patient's integrity and peace of mind are not reduced by pain or the need to beg for medication. When a patient is in continuous pain, it is more appropriate to give medication on a predetermined schedule (*e.g.,* q3h) rather than as needed (*e.g.,* prn).[10] Furthermore, Cassem, referring to the work of Marks and Sachar, states, "Fewer than 1% of hospitalized medical patients given narcotics for pain develop a serious problem of addiction."[11] In the terminal patient, concern for comfort supersedes concern for the problems of addiction. Knowing the patient's concern and desires about his pain experience is of utmost importance. For example, some patients will elect not to trade alertness for pain reduction. Many nurses will want to medicate these patients because working with people in excruciating pain is trying and frustrating. It also increases the nurse's feelings of helplessness, and therefore, anxiety.

In addition, nurses should be made aware that staff attitudes appear to have much to do with the ordering and giving of analgesic medication. In general, patients who are young and female tend to receive more powerful analgesics than others. In a research study, nurses tended not to use their own initiative in giving older patients the more powerful analgesics. However, they had little difficulty implementing the prn orders for the more powerful drugs for younger patients.[12] Thus, age, rather than physical condition, degree of pain, or other variables, appeared to be the determining factor relating to the nurses' implementation of prn medication orders for patients with pain. This points out that nurses must be careful to assess the individual's need and capacity for pain medication and separate this assessment from other factors that are not relevant to the individual.

Finally, *every possible comfort measure* which can be employed without greatly increasing discomfort should automatically be taken. Mouth care can be easily overlooked in a patient who is not eating. Dryness, drooling, odor, and poor nutrition may cause pain and discomfort. The family can be involved in applying lip balm to the patient's lips and washing saliva from the skin. Positioning, skin care, and massage are all useful measures in promoting comfort. Some family members will choose to participate in this type of care, while others may be uncomfortable or fear they will hurt the patient. Sometimes the family's participation means more work for the nurse; however, this participation in care can be a highly significant and useful experience for the grieving family.

Promoting comfort for the dying requires constant and judicious decision making. Should a febrile patient be covered when he is cold? Should someone with depressed respirations be sedated when he is restless and anxious? Comfort measures that break the usual protocol of the critical care unit may be required. Honest and direct communication with the patient and the family will help guide the actions of nurses and physicians on complicated matters.

Communication
Listening, and listening well, is the cornerstone of effective communication. Some patients do not wish to talk about dying. To do so will strip them of whatever hope they are holding. Others will deal with death in a symbolic way. They will speak of autumns and winters and other subjects which may symbolize endings. This is an effective way of terminating one's life, and no interpretation is necessary.

Family members may elect to use the time to go over special memories, reconcile past misunderstandings, and forgive each other for past transgressions. Hopefully they will have the time and atmosphere to say the things they need to say.

The nurse's role is to establish an atmosphere in which this type of communication can occur. What does the family need to be comfortable on the unit—a cup of coffee, a pillow, a place to sit, permission to leave? Does the family wish to be present at the time of death? How can they be reached? All of these questions take sensitive timing and a straightforward approach on the part of the nurse. When words escape the nurse, as they often may in difficult moments, or if words seem inadequate, much can be conveyed by touching a shoulder or an arm.

Children
Allowing children to visit a critical care unit may require special arrangements on the part of the staff. If the patient wishes to see his child or grandchild and if the child wishes to see the patient in a critical care unit, then the child should be offered short, simple explanations concerning the patient's condition. Answering the child's questions in terms the child will understand will help to reduce possible fears. The person taking care of the child should be made aware that invasive procedures and equipment such as nasogastric tubes will most likely upset small children. If a visit from the child is not possible, then arrangements for a telephone visit might be made.

Family Cohesion and Integration
The family in crisis is vulnerable to all types of other stresses. As has been stated previously, helping family members provide support for one another is of paramount importance. If they wish to have some member of the family stay with the patient, they can support one another by providing meal and rest breaks. Being together and being available to one another will be sufficient for many families. The nurse may choose to say to some family members that even though they are not doing anything for the patient, their presence seems to relax or comfort the patient or the patient's wife.

Cheerfulness

Not even dying people like a sad and grumpy nurse. Keeping one's sense of humor and expressing it appropriately offer relief in a difficult situation. Generous smiles and a sense of humor will also help the family to relax and share themselves in their usual ways. A good joke can also be appreciated by a dying patient.

Sensitivity to the patient's mood and a sense of timing are useful in assessing a patient's receptivity to light-heartedness. Talking to the patient in one's typical fashion will help the family relax and communicate more easily with one another and the patient. In turn, the patient should feel less isolated and alone in this final crisis.

Consistency and Perseverance

During times of crisis, complaints and criticisms are frequently directed toward the nurse. A non-defensive, tolerant attitude and a willingness to continue working with the patient and family are the most effective ways of conveying compassion and understanding. Continued interest in a patient and family demonstrates a sense of worth and respect to those involved.

As patients get closer to death, nurses are likely to spend less time with them.[13] This decreased contact may evoke feelings of abandonment, sadness, and hopelessness in both patients and family. Moreover, changes in staff shifts increase the patient's sense of isolation and use up his energy adjusting to new people. Providing consistent staff who do not withdraw helps the patient and family develop trust and a sense of belonging that can become a rewarding experience for everyone involved.

Equanimity

Cassem describes equanimity as the "capacity to be comfortable with the dying patient."[14] For many nurses, being comfortable about death is dependent upon the ability to modify goals that are aimed at preserving life with goals that are designed to preserve personal integrity and family stability when a patient is dying. Thus, rather than considering death as a symbol of failure, nurses can view it as a life-enriching and professionally gratifying experience.

The Critical Care Nurse

The nature of critical care nursing is such that the nurse is exposed to repeated losses. When the nurse has experienced this type of loss as a result of death in her personal life, then dealing with dying patients may at times reactivate feelings and memories associated with these personal losses. Therefore, it is essential that the nursing staff support one another, especially by listening in a tolerant way when a colleague is expressing what is generally considered to be unacceptable feelings. As Quint implies, a supportive relationship is necessary to acquire the ability to communicate with dying patients.[15]

Few nurses come to the critical care unit with these abilities. It will be necessary for most nurses to request specific educational experiences, as well as consultation and supervision from appropriate resources. The intensity of emotion and involvement demanded by a nursing role in critical care makes these nurses particularly vulnerable to the "burnout" syndrome (see Chapter 31).

Crisis intervention for families undergoing acute stress is an important preventive mental health function that nurses can provide. Their knowledge of and proximity to the problem allow them to be first-line resource professionals. As patient advocates, their role will be to realize and point out that dealing with a psychological crisis in the family greatly affects the recovery and well-being of the patient, as well as decreases the chances for further disequilibrium in the family unit.

REFERENCES

1. Holmes TH, Rahe RH: Social readjustment rating scale. J Psychosom Res 2:213–218, 1967
2. Lazarus RS: Cognitive and personality factors underlying threat and coping. In Levine S, Schotch NA (eds): Social Stress, pp 143–164. Chicago, Aldine, 1970
3. Brose C: Theories of family crisis. In Hymovich D, Barnard MU (eds): Family Health Care, pp 279–282. New York, McGraw-Hill, 1973
4. Roberts SL: Behavioral Concepts and the Critically Ill Patient, p 359. New Jersey, Prentice-Hall, 1976
5. *Ibid.*, p 355
6. Cassem N: The dying patient. In Hackett TP, Cassem N (eds): Handbook of General Hospital Psychiatry, pp 300–318. St. Louis, C.V. Mosby, 1978
7. *Ibid.*, p 305
8. Shubin S: Burnout: The professional hazard you face in nursing. Nursing 8, No. 7:22–27, 1978
9. Cassem N: Treatment decisions in irreversible illness. In Hackett TP, Cassem N (eds): Handbook of General Hospital Psychiatry, pp 562–575. St. Louis, C.V. Mosby, 1978
10. Cassem: The dying patient, p 306
11. *Ibid.*
12. Pilowsky I, Bond MR: Pain and its management in malignant disease: Elucidation of staff-patient transactions. In Weisenberg M (ed): Pain, pp 332–335. St. Louis, C.V. Mosby, 1975
13. Glaser B, Strauss A: Awareness of Dying, p 227. Chicago, Aldine, 1965
14. Cassem: The dying patient, p 310
15. Quint JC: The Nurse and the Dying Patient, p 199. New York, Macmillan, 1967

Janice S. Smith

Adverse Effects of Critical Care Units on Patients
6

The necessity of employing highly technical and precise measures to preserve life in a crisis situation commonly found in critical care units can create an environment totally alien and life-threatening to the patient. The complicated equipment necessary for maintaining life requires unquestionable expertise on the part of personnel involved in patient care. However, if life-preserving measures are to have any value for the patient, the nurse must be aware of aspects of care beyond the patient's physical needs and the mechanical workings of the ever increasing array of machines that medical technology is producing.

The psychosocial support needed by the patient in the critical care unit demands more than assistance in dealing with a critical illness. The sounds and activities of the unit are bombarding the patient 24 hours a day; in addition, the patient must cope with the effects of fear concerning illness. Normal defense mechanisms that allow us to cope with threatening situations are diminished in all patients and probably absent in the unresponsive patient. The ability to run from a frightening or painful stimulus is gone, as is the ability to analyze a situation objectively and take action to control it.

To appreciate how devastating confinement to a critical care unit can be, the nurse needs only to think of her own feelings about reversing roles with a patient. When asked if they would volunteer to spend 24 hours in the patient role in the crisis care unit, nurses respond readily with a definite "No!" In view of their awareness of the environmental threats of such units, nurses must function as the negotiator for the patient. To be an effective negotiator the nurse must acquire knowledge about the effects of sensory input on the human organism.

SENSORY INPUT

The broad concept of sensory input deals with stimulation of all of the five senses: visual, auditory, olfactory, tactile, and gustatory. Stimuli to all of the senses may be perceived in a qualitative manner as pleasant or unpleasant, acceptable or unacceptable, desirable or undesirable, soothing or painful. Individual perceptions of stimuli may vary drastically. Some individuals may consider the sounds and smells of a metropolitan business section to be pleasant, acceptable, desirable — or painful.

Everyday activities including the choice of food or drink are based on the individual's perception of what is liked or disliked. Thus, people tend to choose, whenever possible, the environment or stimuli from the environment most acceptable to them. Patients in the critical care unit, however, have no control over the choice of their environment or most of its stimuli.

In addition to the quality of a stimulus, the nurse must also consider the quantity. Too much of a desirable stimulus can become as unacceptable as too little stimulation. For example, gorging oneself with a favorite food to the point of revulsion is "too much of a good thing." In the critical care unit, too much undesirable stimuli such as excessive and constant noise, bright light, and hyperactivity can be as distorting and bothersome as too little stimuli such as gloom, silence, and inactivity.

In trying to control environmental stimuli in a critical care unit, the nurse must therefore be aware of both the type and the amount of sensory input. If sensory stimuli are diminished too drastically, the patient is exposed to *sensory deprivation,* which can cause severe disorganization of normal psychological defenses.[1] When sensory stimuli occur in excessive quantity, the phenomenon of *sensory overload* will create an equally undesirable response to the environment, including confusion and withdrawal.

Sensory Deprivation

Sensory deprivation is a general term used to identify a variety of symptoms which occur following a reduction in the quantity or the degree of structure or quality of sensory input.[2] Other terms used to denote sensory deprivation

or some form of it include *isolation, confinement, informational underload, perceptual deprivation,* and *sensory restriction.* A variety of symptoms or changes in behavior have been noted in normal adults following exposure to sensory deprivation for varying lengths of time. These include loss of sense of time; presence of delusions, illusions, and hallucinations; restlessness; and any of the types of behavior or symptoms present in psychoses.

Sensory deprivation need not be present for a period of days or weeks for psychopathologic reactions to occur. In one study conducted on a normal young male subject, an 8-hour period of sensory deprivation elicited an acute psychotic reaction followed by continuation of delusions for several days and severe depression and anxiety for a period of several weeks.[3]

The degree of sensory deprivation possible in a laboratory setting is greater than that likely in a critical care unit. We must remember, though, that laboratory subjects are aware of the time involved in the experiment and have the ability to stop anytime they wish. They also possess clinically normal defense mechanisms. Hospital patients do not have these advantages.

STRESS AND SENSORY DEPRIVATION

It is not presently known how the stress of illness will affect human subjects exposed to sensory deprivation. There is no reason to assume that such stress will make patients any less susceptible to adverse reactions to such deprivation. On the contrary, it would appear more logical that patients faced with coping with illness would have increased susceptibility to and more severe responses to sensory deprivation. The main types of patients most susceptible to the adverse effects of sensory deprivation would appear to be the unresponsive or unconscious patient, the very young patient, the very old patient, and the postoperative patient.

It has been known for more than 25 years that sensory deprivation can lead to psychotic behavior. In spite of this insight, little has been done to apply this knowledge to planning for patients in critical care units. Hospital personnel have long demonstrated at least a passing concern over the control of excessive noise causing sensory overload by the use of the familiar "Quiet, Please" signs in hospitals and other health-care facilities, but a survey of the literature and an examination of many critical care units fails to demonstrate a similar concern for creating an environment intended to diminish the effects of sensory deprivation.

SOUND—QUALITY AND QUANTITY

If unstructured sound or noise were all that was necessary to prevent the phenomenon of sensory deprivation, most crisis care units would never need to be concerned with the concept at all. It is not, however, *quantity* alone that must be considered. Even more important is the inclusion of planning the *quality* of stimuli in the external environment. A British investigator supports such a conclusion by stating, "Reality testing can only occur when there is a continual input of meaningful information from the outside world. When this is markedly reduced, as under experimental conditions of sensory deprivation, reality testing is impaired and internal mental events are taken to be events in the external world."[4] This could easily explain why some critical care patients appear to have hallucinations, and it points out the need to provide *meaningful* information to all patients in such a threatening setting.

REALITY TESTING

For reality testing to occur there must be familiar environmental stimuli. However, the sounds of the critical care unit cannot be said to be familiar to more than a few medical and nursing personnel who spend long periods of their working life in such an environment. Therefore, the nurse in the critical care unit should be certain that the environment offers the patient adequate stimuli to provide for reality testing.

As human beings we take our physical environment for granted, but if we suddenly awoke in a world without grass or sunlight or the sounds of traffic or human speech, we would not have the necessary stimuli to keep our minds in contact with reality. We would try to interpret the unknown stimuli on the basis of that with which we have always been familiar. In reality, however, our interpretations may be wrong. This is especially true of patients who suffer temporary loss of any of the senses, particularly vision or hearing, since we normally employ a combination of senses to interpret our environment.

This lack of reality testing may offer at least partial explanation for the high incidence of psychosis in patients commonly assigned to critical care units for long-term care due to an "unconscious state." The fact that no physical reason has ever been identified to explain posttraumatic psychosis offers additional support to such an assumption.[5,6]

Nursing is limited in its consideration of the unconscious patient who is often found in critical care units because authorities in the field have perpetuated the concept that such patients are insensitive to their environment and have perceptual disturbances that affect their responses to the environment. In view of the necessity of reality testing and the lack of meaningful information to allow such testing in the critical care unit, it is reasonable to explain some of the reactions of patients, including even the unconscious patient, as being caused by the lack of meaningful input which can be referred to as sensory deprivation. There is more empirical data to support this assumption than there is evidence for believing that posttraumatic psychosis is due to physical phenomena.

Patient Situation. One example of such a situation caused by sensory deprivation in the critical care unit occurred during an experiment I conducted with an unresponsive patient assumed to be unconscious by both the medical and nursing team members. Carol was a 20-year-old college student with severe basal skull trauma and multiple injuries who was unresponsive throughout the 8-day period she spent in a critical care unit.

When Carol began responding verbally, her first words to her mother were: "Am I free now? I was in the hands of the Soviet Union!" An immediate interpretation of such a statement could reasonably be that she was totally out of contact with reality due to the injury and had dreamed such an episode. It is just as reasonable to assume that she could have perceived that the actions in the unit and treatments she received due to her condition were related to torture, and she was the victim for some unknown reason.

Carol had no noticeable motor control of her facial muscles, so she was "blind." She had a tracheostomy that required frequent suctioning. She was almost immobile because of fractures and spasticity necessitating plaster casts or cloth restraints on all extremities. It is reasonable to assume that such a situation could cause her to believe she was being tortured, since she had no means of interpreting her experience realistically from meaningful cues in the environment.

Planning for Sensory Stimulation. Many other situations and case histories can be reported to stress the importance of planning for and providing meaningful sensory stimulation for the patients cared for in all hospital units, but especially the ones in critical care units.[7] Nurses can play a significant role in alleviating the unnecessary stress caused by sensory deprivation by recognizing the need for the structuring of sensory input.

The use of auditory stimuli such as the explanation of any treatment or procedure to be performed on a patient is a basic requirement and must not be overlooked as insignificant. But explanation alone is not adequate to prevent adverse effects of sensory deprivation. This type of communication can be considered a minimal requirement in a broader area of communication called *security information*.

Providing for Security Information. Security information helps prevent unnecessary anxiety and disorientation regarding date, time, and place. It also includes explanation of treatment and procedures. This is particularly important for patients with deviations in levels of consciousness due to trauma, drugs, or toxicity. Orientation to date and time can be encouraged not only by including the information in conversation but by providing large-faced clocks that are readily visible to the patient and large calendars that display the day, month and year in large figures. The simplicity of such information sometimes causes it to be overlooked, but it can affect the patient's comfort by providing information we take for granted. In addition, it is essential to provide this information because an assessment of the patient's state of orientation is often based on his answers to questions concerning time and place.

USING THE NURSING HISTORY

A nursing history included in the initial phase of planning can help make nursing intervention an effective part of the total care. Such a history requires that individualized questions be asked of both patient and family members. A brief outline of a normal 24-hour period of activity and sleep habits gives a good starting point in compiling a useful nursing history. A simple rule to use in collecting a nursing history is to determine what is significant or familiar to the patient and expose him to it, if possible.

Additional information which may be included in the nursing history could be anything from food likes and dislikes to favorite type of music or TV programs. It would be desirable to provide exposure to familiar stimuli such as playing a favorite record from home or finding the right radio station to listen to or requesting a taped message sent from a loved one who cannot visit. Such action will offer meaningful sensory stimulation to the patient in an otherwise unfamiliar environment. The family and friends should be involved in planning and providing

such sensory input, especially for unresponsive patients. The potential value of a familiar voice in giving information or encouragement to a patient was vividly demonstrated by a recent incident.

Critical Incident I

A young woman was admitted to a critical care unit shortly after Christmas. She had a diagnosis of viral encephalopathy and a guarded prognosis. She became unresponsive within a few hours and her husband was told she was not expected to live. In spite of this she held on to life for 2 months, during which the hopeless prognosis remained. Twice more the husband was told that death was imminent.

Finally with the last contact from the hospital that his wife was dying, the young husband told his 2½-year-old son that his mother was dying. The child repeatedly told his father not to worry because his mommy wouldn't die. The father took the boy to the critical care unit to see his mother for the last time.

While there the boy said, "I love you, Mommy." To the shock of all except the boy, his mother opened her eyes for the first time. The young woman later told everyone, "I had forgotten everything until I heard his voice say 'I love you, Mommy.' " She is well on the road to recovery now.

One of the most agonizing feelings must be that of uselessness on the part of a family member or friend at the bedside of an unresponsive loved one. During a survey conducted in critical care units preceding a research project on unresponsive patients, I was repeatedly impressed by the scene of a mother, father, husband, wife, or other close relative standing at the bedside and staring with a variety of emotions at the unresponsive patient. A simple direction, or granting of permission in some cases, to touch the patient's hand and talk to him brought a look of relief and gratitude to their faces. With further assistance on what to say to the patient, the visitor became very effective in diminishing sensory deprivation by discussing familiar people or subjects and topics of interest to the patient.

The value of simple conversation about everyday activities is underestimated in the care of the unresponsive patient in critical care units. This is pointed out vividly in the following incident.*

Critical Incident II

Interest in nursing implications inherent in care of the unconscious patient beyond the physical dimensions was initiated while caring for a patient in her late

*Smith JS: A Study of Sensory Response in the Unconscious Patient. Thesis submitted to the faculty of the Graduate School of the University of Colorado in partial fulfillment of the requirements for the degree of Master of Science, School of Nursing, 1970

fifties, comatose as a result of metastatic carcinoma of the brain. The investigator carried on a one-sided conversation about many things, including a daily introduction of self, explanations of care to be given, and discussion of the day and the weather. There was no perceptible response from the patient. Her condition appeared to be slowly deteriorating. Contact with the patient was lost after four days due to an assignment change.

About two months later while boarding a train, the investigator was approached by a woman on crutches who called the investigator's name and asked if she were a nurse. Following an affirmative response and recognition of the previous nurse-patient interaction the investigator and the patient conversed for several hours. The discussion revealed much about the initial relationship between them. The patient expressed how she had felt during the days she lay in the hospital bed totally defenseless and at the mercy of those on the nursing team and that the investigator had been the only person who had identified herself and talked to the patient.

Of particular interest to the patient was information as to the nurse's time of leaving and when she would return. When the investigator had informed her she would be leaving for another assignment she said she had felt like crying because she anticipated receiving no further information about the outside world. The patient recalled much more about the interaction than the investigator.

Such experiences indicate that even in today's modern nursing world the little things, such as consideration of the patient as an individual deserving common courtesies, are still important to patients. It cannot be taken for granted that such behavior is automatic; nurses are conditioned to be comfortable around the hectic environment of a critical care unit and quickly forget the sense of awe or fear that was present the first time they saw the unit.

It might be helpful for the nurses in the critical care unit to stop for a moment each day and project themselves mentally into the patient's role to determine what information or activity might be desirable. Such an act might be effective in salvaging whatever human dignity is left for a patient who has been subjected to the regressive procedures of being bathed, fed, and forced to meet toileting needs in bed, shielded from other patients only by a cloth curtain with wide openings at top and bottom.

Sensory Overload

The area of sensory overload has not received as much attention as that of sensory deprivation, but some of its effects on humans are known. One of the best-documented adverse effects is that of decreased hearing following long-term exposure to high noise levels such as those found in factories or machine shops. It is also recognized that tension and anxiety increase when an individual is exposed to noise for continuous periods of time without quiet periods of rest. Edgar Allan Poe capitalized on such knowledge in horror stories dealing with the effect of continuous rhythmic sounds such as the dripping of water or the whirring of machinery, as in "The Pit and the Pendulum." In more modern settings we have heard of the use of continuous noise as a means of torturing prisoners of war. We too must capitalize on this information. When patients become increasingly anxious or restless, environmental causes such as noise as well as physiological reasons such as hypercarbia must be considered in trying to determine the cause of such behavior.

Many years ago Florence Nightingale expressed her awareness of the effects of noise on patients: "Unnecessary noise is the most cruel absence of care which can be inflicted on either sick or well."[8]

Clues about the significance of both the quantity and quality of noise are offered by a study conducted in a recovery room. It was found that high levels of noise increased the need for pain medication. It is interesting to note, however, that the most pronounced reaction on the part of the recovery room patient was that of resentment of the sound of occasional laughter from the recovery room personnel.[9]

The normal egocentricity of persons facing an illness crisis must be recognized by the nurse. With this knowledge it is easy to understand that transient paranoia will cause the patient to interpret all action around him as pertaining to him. The laughter of the staff is laughter at him. The patient who overhears a discussion by staff members may interpret it as meaning, "I am dying, but they won't tell me." Hospital personnel should be certain that all talking and laughing in the patient care areas is intended to be heard by the patients. If patients do not have soundproof areas, the staff must modify their behavior and go to another area to socialize.

The presence of continuous noise in critical care units must be minimized at certain times in every 24-hour period.[10] The cardiac monitors should not be kept in areas where patients must hear their beeping continuously. The physical planning for units must provide facilities where patients on continuous respirators are not in the same open area as other patients. However, ways have not yet been devised for protecting patients who are on the respirator from the machine's incessant cycling noise. Nor is it presently known how or if the sound of the machine has any adverse psychological effect on the patient. In view of the recent and ongoing advancement in technical methods necessary for retention of life, problems such as this will continue. As technology becomes more advanced and heroic lifesaving measures succeed in significant numbers of patients, we will then be able to focus attention on their less apparent psychological needs in order to preserve quality of life.

Continuous Sound. The effect of continuous sound on the intricate physiological functions of the human organism is not fully known, but intelligent assumptions can be made that a variety of adverse responses can be expected. Even without such empirical data to support the need to control unnecessary noise, we can look at our own life-style to see how we react to continuous or loud noise. It is normal to attempt to plug our ears in the presence of a loud noise such as a firecracker, and it is just as normal to choose to sleep in a quiet room with the sounds of the outside world shut out by well-constructed walls or special soundproofing. It is perhaps not feasible to control noise in the environment of critical care units to the same extent to which the patient is accustomed, but it is both feasible and essential that nurses exert a conscious effort to avoid unnecessary noise in such an environment.

Preventing Exhaustion. Another facet of controlling unnecessary noise involves preventing exhaustion. There is adequate knowledge available in the areas of sleep research to prove that sleep is essential for both physical and mental well-being.[11] Therefore, nurses need to plan for and provide an environment which will not only allow but also encourage sleep for patients in critical care units. This sounds deceptively simple until one realizes what is necessary in meeting such a need. A darkened room makes it impossible to visually observe the critically ill patient, but few people can sleep in a lighted room even if the lighting level is low or soft. Normal practice is to sedate many patients in such a unit, but the nurse must realize the drug-induced or interrupted sleep is not adequate for any significant period of time. The human organism must have normal uninterrupted periods of sleep that are long enough to allow all stages of sleep to occur. This normally means a period of a minimum of 2 to 3 hours, but even that is probably not adequate for most people for a period of more than a day or two.

The Hospital Phenomenon

The hospital environment is one that should be conducive to rest and recuperation from illness, but it is no surprise to any nurse that such a myth has long been dispelled. A bitter joke frequently heard from patients is that a hotel room is cheaper, has better food and service, and provides a better chance to get a rest.

The fact is that the hospital environment is one that deprives the patient of normal sensory stimuli while it bombards him with continuous strange sensory stimuli not found in the average home environment. This situation is a combination of sensory deprivation and sensory overload which will be referred to as the *hospital phenomenon*.

Normal sounds at home include voices of loved ones and friends; barking of neighborhood dogs, automobile, bus and train traffic and horns, the television or radio on a familiar station, children at play; the washing machine or dishwasher; the daytime telephone calls; and many other sounds and sights which diminish when night comes. On the other hand, sounds in critical care units include voices of strangers in large numbers; movement of bed rails; beeping of cardiac monitors; paging systems calling strange names; suctioning of tracheostomies; telephones ringing at all hours; whispers, laughter, and muffled voices. These are accompanied by continuous lighting, strange views of equipment, fear, and pain.

The combination of the loss of familiar stimuli and continuous exposure to strange stimuli elicits varying types of defensive responses from the patient. Withdrawal is one defense mechanism used, and it may cause a patient to be erroneously labeled confused or disoriented. Additional research is needed in this area, but it is fairly safe to assume that some degree of withdrawal from the frightening reality of the situation is common. On the assumption that many patients cope by withdrawing, nurses should anticipate a delayed response when calling the patient's name and should provide extra environmental objects to orient the patient to time, date, and place.

PERIODICITY

Another area of knowledge necessary for the nurse in the critical care unit deals with the broad concept of periodicity. Other terms include *circadian rhythm, biological clock, internal clock,* and *physiological clock.* It has been recognized for a number of years that all living creatures have not only an identifiable life cycle but also short-term cycles which are rhythmical in nature; disruption of that rhythm can cause deviations from the normal or cessation of life.

Daily Cycle. The human organism possesses a 24-hour cycle that is resistant to change, and long-term disruption can be fatal. Each of the biochemical and biophysical processes of the human body possesses a rhythm with peaks of function or activity which occur in consistent patterns within the normal, customary 24-hour day.

Physiological Variations. Knowledge of when physiological functions are at their lowest level would allow for more intelligent assessment of the significance of vital-sign fluctuation. For example, normal variations in the quantity of urine output should be expected, since the kidneys possess their own unique rhythm as demanded by sleep and activity patterns. Drug dosage, sleep periods, and stressful procedures such as surgery may also someday be based on knowledge of individual circadian rhythms, thus avoiding further stress in the most vulnerable part of the cycle and capitalizing on the strongest parts of the cycle.

Sleep. Even though the critical care environment traditionally shows lack of regard for the 24-hour cycle of the human organism by ignoring the need for a period of undisturbed sleep, the fact remains that the human organism cannot adapt to any other cycle. There are both physiological and psychological necessities for sleep that affect humans' potential for maximal recovery from illness in minimal time. Probably the most significant sleep deprivation is in the area of rapid eye movement (REM) sleep because it occurs later in the sleep cycle. REM sleep is necessary for mental restoration and occurs mainly in the last cycles of an uninterrupted night of sleep. The normal person has four or five cycles of sleep lasting about 90 minutes each. Disrupting the continuity of sleep cycles in the critical care unit probably causes most deprivation in the REM stage. This further threatens the psychological well-being of the patient.[12]

Adverse side effects are numerous in individuals who are deprived of the stages of deep sleep and REM sleep for even a few days. The adverse effects include irritability and anxiety, physical exhaustion and fatigue, and even disruption of metabolic functions, including adrenal hormone production.

Such adverse effects indicate the necessity for providing an environment conducive to all stages of sleep including the REM stage. Because a cycle of sleep measured from REM stage to REM stage requires from 90 to 100 minutes, it is important to provide periods of a minimum of 2 hours of uninterrupted sleep during the night.[13] More frequent arousal can cause enough disruption to deprive the patient of essential cyclic rest and activity periods and create a situation incompatible with life.

When assessing the patient's condition, consider whether or not there have been adequate uninterrupted time periods for all stages of sleep to occur. The plan must provide such periods as early as possible following admission to the unit. The necessity of taking vital signs every 1 or 2 hours during the night must be weighed against the damage caused to the human organism when it is deprived of sleep. Physiological functions reach their lowest levels in the middle of the night, whereas in the early morning hours functions are beginning to reach a maximum level. Therefore, normal fluctuations in vital signs should be expected and patients should not be subjected to activity or stressful procedures in the early morning hours.

Conflicts With Hospital Policy. The practice of bathing critically ill patients between the hours of 2 A.M. and 5 A.M. because staff have time available is an example of uninformed and cruel care. The night hours must be treated in such a way as to provide the human organism its essential rest at the optimum time. Only absolutely essential life-preserving activities should be allowed to disturb the patient at night.

The equally harmful and unnecessarily rigid policy of allowing visitors 5 minutes with the patient every hour should be seriously reconsidered. For the patient to be disturbed every hour is certainly more harmful than using knowledge of sleep research and periodicity in planning visiting times and nursing care activities. Longer periods of time with the patient could be provided during the nonsleeping hours as one way of individualizing visiting policies.

Such visiting restrictions often produce hostility from family members as they struggle to maintain some time with the patient. Sharing knowledge of sleep research and periodicity with family members in a proper manner will probably elicit a willingness to work out an acceptable arrangement for sharing time with the patient. The nurse who believes routine nursing care measures should always take priority over time for relatives or significant others needs to seriously reevaluate her ability to give optimum care to the patient in critical care units.

Only the most critical condition could warrant ignoring the equally fatal outcome when exhaustion causes disequilibirum of physiological functions. Intelligent nursing care will provide rest periods for the patient with the same emphasis as providing assessment of cardiac status or other aggressive physical measures of care.

The usual critical care environment disregards the need to control the 24-hour sounds, light, and activity by having open units for six to ten patients who require care at variable times. Commitment to controlling the activity of the environment can diminish the constant level of noise, but additional measures may be necessary. If the patient is receptive to wearing darkened eyeshades and ear plugs to shut out light and sound, he may be able to tolerate the environment with less stress. This is the least we can offer a patient to minimize the adverse effects of the environment until units can be developed that consider rest and sleep for the critically ill patient. No patient needs such consideration more, but the irony of the situation is that the critically ill patient is placed in the least desirable environment for meeting such needs. Perhaps our intense efforts to improve care through the development of special critical care units is causing us to endanger the well-being of the patients.[14]

NUTRITION

Starvation

Critically ill patients are frequently unable to eat adequately. Recent and continuing advances in preventing actual starvation in these patients present many challenges to the critical care staff. The inadequate attempts at fluid and electrolyte replacement of the past have been superseded by the development of intravenous hyperalimentation (IVH).

Death due to the negative nitrogen balance produced by starvation has been well documented.[15] Until 1968, when IVH was developed, there was no alternative available when the patient was unable to ingest sufficient proteins and fats. The stress of trauma and illness places additional nutritional demands on the body. When food intake was not feasible or was significantly diminished, the patient faced starvation.

The complexities of total parenteral nutrition (TPN) itself pose threats to the lives of patients if not managed correctly. Possible life-threatening complications include septicemia, hyperosmolar coma, hypokalemia, hypophosphatemia, hypoglycemia, pneumothorax, and volume overloads.[16,17]

While TPN is an essential and vital part of the comprehensive care of patients in critical care units and while it will prevent starvation, it cannot prevent the problem of stomach ulceration in patients who are unable to eat.

Stress Ulcers

It is common knowledge that the human stomach requires food bulk or some substance to absorb its secretions of gastric juices. The amount of hydrochloric acid increases when stress occurs, as is the case in illness or trauma.[18] This means that most patients in critical care units are more susceptible to the formation of stomach ulceration.[19]

Most critical care patients are unable to eat normal quantities of food. Many are unable to eat any food at all, yet they all have increased quantities of secretions working on the gastric mucosa when food is not present.

In view of these facts, all critical care patients should be monitored for symptoms of bleeding ulcers. Reports of stomach pain should be recorded and further evaluated. A periodic hemetest on stools should be done.

In situations allowing administration of oral fluids, it is possible to give preventive doses of antacids. In other cases the use of anticholinergics (such as Pro-Banthine) or histamine antagonists (such as cimetidine) may be indicated.

PATIENTS WITH SPECIAL PROBLEMS

Patients assigned to critical care units are known to have special problems that cannot be safely cared for in the usual hospital setting. They need almost constant observation or special lifesaving equipment requiring specialized training and knowledge. Some patients have additional needs because they are especially susceptible to the environmental influences of the critical care unit.

As previously noted, the patients most likely to be adversely affected by the environment include (1) the unresponsive or defenseless patient,

(2) the very young, (3) the elderly, and (4) the postoperative patient.

With some variation in degree of significance, the areas of care discussed in this chapter are relevant to the child; however, further discussion is outside the scope of this book.

The information also applies to patients coming out of anesthesia in the recovery room. The main difference is that the time in the recovery room does not usually exceed a few hours, while patients in intensive care units stay for days and in some instances for weeks. Special emphasis will thus be given to the elderly patient and to the defenseless or unresponsive patient.

The Elderly Patient in Critical Care

Because of the large number of elderly people who need intensive care, critical care nurses need to be knowledgeable about the special problems of the elderly. Since the elderly often have some deterioration of their senses, nurses who are not aware of and sensitive to these problems can contribute to the stresses that these patients have already experienced.

In order to diminish the potentially adverse effects of the critical care environment for the elderly it is necessary for the nurse to

- assess the senses
- recognize the symptoms of acute brain syndrome
- use reality orientation therapeutically
- use touch in a therapeutic way
- understand the concept of territoriality as it relates to aging
- know the views on death and dying commonly held by elderly people

ASSESSMENT OF SENSES

It is essential to assess fully the senses of each elderly person, particularly for a history of visual and auditory deficits.[20] If the elderly patient is unable to filter out environmental sounds in order to hear soft-spoken words, talking louder or asking the patient to use a hearing aid may help. It will not help, however, to talk loudly (or yell) at the elderly person whose hearing is intact but whose motor responses are diminished or blocked by injury such as from a cerebral vascular accident.

If an elderly patient wears glasses, it is important to provide a clean pair even if he does not request them. Clean glasses will enable the patient to familiarize himself with the environment and see what is going on around him. And if the patient must rely upon lip reading to understand what is being said to him, glasses will enhance his ability to communicate.

Older people may also require more time to respond to verbal requests because motor responses tend to slow with age. This, along with the tendency to withdraw from the hyperactivity of the critical care unit, may further delay the response time. Because of these factors, it may be necessary when asking questions to allow a longer period of time for any motor or vocal response. It is reasonable to wait a full minute before repeating a request.

DISORIENTATION

Actions that appear to denote disorientation of a pathologic nature may be prematurely labeled *chronic brain syndrome* when they may actually be *acute brain syndrome*. In view of the grave consequences of hopelessness projected on the patient with chronic brain syndrome, it is imperative that adequate historic data be collected to differentiate between the two conditions. The primary difference between acute and chronic brain syndromes is that acute brain syndrome has a rapid onset but is considered reversible, while chronic brain syndrome is slow in onset and is irreversible. The significance of such differences has a great impact upon nursing care.

Symptoms of acute brain syndrome include

- fluctuation in the level of awareness
- visual hallucinations (auditory hallucinations are not present)
- misidentification of persons (usually in the form of thinking a nurse is some close relative such as a sister or daughter)
- severe restlessness[21]

A sudden change in the elderly person's life, such as removal from familiar surroundings or administration of certain sedative and tranquilizing drugs, can precipitate these symptoms. The following situation reported by Kiely illustrates these points.[22]

A 78-year-old retired schoolteacher was knocked down by a purse snatcher while on her way to a neighborhood grocery store. There was no physical injury evident but the event triggered an episode of paroxysmal tachyarrhythmia accompanied by vascular collapse with a blood pressure of 79/30 mm. Hg.

At the emergency room she was able to coherently recount her experience and seemed more upset by the loss of her eyeglasses than her purse. She seemed mildly disoriented about time and place. A comprehensive physical and laboratory exam revealed only a low blood pressure and atrial flutter. With treatment, both of these returned to normal.

The patient's mental status, however, continued to deteriorate. She became increasingly disoriented and demanded that nursing personnel explain their presence in her "apartment." She became restless, climbed over the bedrails and when soft restraints were applied, became even more restless. Then she heard voices and screamed that people were trying to kill her. Sodium Amytal, 500 mg IM, initially sedated her but later heightened her arousal.

The very close correlation of these symptoms with the symptoms of sensory deprivation discussed earlier creates a situation that makes it impossible to differentiate the cause initially. A concerted effort at reality orientation by the nursing staff must be started immediately as a primary treatment for either condition.

REALITY ORIENTATION

Reality orientation requires a rigid, repetitive regime of giving security information at predetermined times around the clock. The monotony of the procedure may make nurses want to give up the regime when there is no positive response after a few days. For the benefit of the patient, however, the regime must continue until the patient can repeat the information on request (or until death releases the nurse from the responsibility). After a few days, repetition is more comfortable if the information is prefaced by a statement to the patient that you know the information has been stated many times, but that it is important to repeat it until the patient is able to say it to you. Such repetition should continue until the patient recovers or dies.

The elderly patient must adapt to a major change in spatial perception and territory when placed in the critical care unit. The frequently existing problems related to diminished vision and hearing combined with disruption of territory create greater vulnerability to adverse effects from sensory deprivation and sensory overload.

USING TOUCH

Touch is a highly therapeutic tool that the nurse should use to alleviate the fear an elderly patient often has when faced with an illness crisis. Even the person who normally rejects touching may feel the need for such contact at this time.

Elderly patients who have verbal or sensory impairment may benefit greatly from supportive touch.[23] It is easy to determine the patient's receptivity by gently touching his or her hand or arm. If the arm is not withdrawn, it is a cue of acceptance. Take care to speak to patients with impaired sight before touching them to avoid startling them unnecessarily.

TERRITORIALITY

At a time in life when adapting to change becomes increasingly difficult and painful, the patient is confronted with an extreme limitation of territory. Even the patient coming from a long-term care facility has had more space to claim and greater freedom to organize it in the manner so desired. The historically diminishing size of the territory possessed and controlled by the elderly creates psychological pain and a decrease in self-esteem. The nurse in a critical care unit can be sensitive to this by avoiding unnecessary intrusion into the patient's now further diminished territory.

Limitation of the space available to the patient in the critical care unit is severe enough, but even further limits occur because extensions of territoriality are usually not available in this setting. Examples of extensions frequently used by the elderly patient include radio, television, and telephones. Both televisions and telephones are normally denied to the patients in these units. However, the availability of small television sets with earplugs for sound control and telephones with wall jacks makes it more feasible to use both items in a critical care unit. Nursing assessment can determine the patient's ability to benefit from their use without harmful effects.[24]

It is possible that a telephone contact from a special person will do more than any medication to help a patient relax. Certainly the judicious use of ear phones to enjoy a favorite radio program will help counteract the adverse effects of the strange sounds of the critical care unit. The nurse who recognizes the potentially great therapeutic effect of such territorial extensions will incorporate them into the humanistic plan of care for all patients, with special awareness of the unique needs of the elderly.

Further intrusions also occur in the form of impersonal equipment kept at the bedside (*e.g.,* suction machines, monitors, oxygen equipment, IV equipment) which the patient does not view as personal possessions. This creates a situation in which spatial orientation is limited to the confines of the bed and possibly a bedside stand. For this reason, the patient usually clusters all personal possessions in the bed or on the small stand. Nurses should tolerate such space-occupying items since their importance to the patient far exceeds the degree to which they interfere with nursing activities.

A visit to the home or room of an elderly person characteristically reveals the presence of multiple treasures on walls, tables, and shelves, including pictures, books, glass items, and so forth. No matter how poverty-stricken the person is, there will be some highly prized items. These objects develop increased value for the elderly as the years pass, and the nurse must protect such possessions brought to the unit and allow the patients to position them wherever they wish within the pathetically small territory allotted to them.

The informed and sensitive nurse will preface any intrusion into the personal territory of the patient with appropriate conversation, including an explanation of the reason for invading the space, and then await the cue that the patient is ready and receptive. Such cues can be vocal or projected through body language, including facial expressions and body posturing. A receptive cue could be in the statement, "Well, if it has to be done then go ahead," or a beginning movement to turn over to expose the area for the shot. Cues that you are rushing too much may include the question, "Why do I have to have that?" or a movement to pull the covers near the neck. Such cues demand more explanation and less haste.

DEALING WITH DEATH

The inevitability of death must be accepted at times in the critical care unit.[25] Being aware that many elderly people accept dying as the final stage and natural outcome of life may help the staff when it has been decided that the patient should be allowed to die without further intervention. While this question of when to withhold further intervention is certainly not unique to the elderly, there are certain aspects of the problem which are generally more common in older people. Certainly the healthy 80-year-old with a history of a CVA will have dealt more directly with his feelings of dying (and his family with their feelings of losing him to death) than will have the 18-year-old and his family. No implication is intended, however, that age alone is the criterion for determining the extent of the heroic effort to sustain life. Age is, however, a highly significant factor to be considered along with factors such as previous state of health and current cause of illness.

It is important that whenever possible the patient's feelings about dying be listened to, and the family must be included in discussions and decisions (see Chap. 5). Enforcement of restrictive visiting rules should be ignored in such a situation to prevent further adverse effects of isolation on the patient and to assist the family in dealing with the common feelings of guilt at such a time. The family also suffers from adverse effects caused by the critical care environment. Hospital policy must not be allowed to remove humanistic values from nursing care.

Roberts has expressed an opinion that perhaps we ignore the patient's wishes and prolong the process of dying rather than the process of living.[26] She also reminds us that many aged patients have control over their lives until they lose control when admitted to the critical care unit. The role of the nurse becomes vital, and she must resolve her own feelings about death as she works with the patient and family in an advocacy role. Perhaps the elderly see what we cannot when they plead with us to let them die. It is wrong to project our personal fear of death on the patient who repeatedly pleads with us to stop our heroic efforts to sustain a poor quality of life manifested many times by constant pain and exhaustion. The right to die while human dignity is still present must be considered seriously.

The Unresponsive Patient

The patient most likely to suffer greatest psychological trauma related to the adverse effects of the environment is the patient traditionally labeled "unconscious." The disease processes causing this pathologic state are widely diversified. The more common causes are usually related to trauma of extracranial or intracranial origin. Such primary disease processes are frequently accompanied by multiple traumas such as fractures, lacerations, and unknown soft-tissue damage. This patient requires care that considers both physical and psychological needs, given by a nurse who believes that human dignity is a basic right to be preserved.

Few patients place as many significant and continuous demands on the nurse as the unconscious patient. Too often the only emphasis of care is on the patient's physical needs. There is no intent to minimize the physical needs, since the patient depends totally on the nurse and other members of the health-care team for life preservation. In order to give optimal care, however, more concern must be focused on the psychosocial needs of unconscious patients in critical care units.

Use of the erroneous label *unconscious* creates a psychological set for care givers that fosters attitudes of hopelessness. Such attitudes may be modified to benefit the patient by use of the more valid descriptive term *unresponsive*. The first precept that must be developed is that this is the most descriptive diagnostic label for such a patient. It is the only condition that can be demonstrated by assessment methods currently used in the health-care fields. The term *unresponsive* means that motor and sensory coordinated responses cannot be elicited from a particular patient. The term *unconscious* denotes a lack of sensory awareness that cannot currently be measured in the absence of concurrent motor response.

Replacing the label *unconscious* with the term *unresponsive* removes the connotation of lack of awareness which is automatically associated with the term *unconscious*. Taber's *Cyclopedic Medical Dictionary* gives a literal translation of unconscious as "not aware." It further defines the word as, "A state of being insensible or without conscious experiences." A survey of other such reference books by current health-care authorities reveals similar definitions. This mental set is being perpetuated in spite of documented incidents that invalidate such a definition for many patients who are labeled unconscious. (See the Critical Incidents earlier in this chapter.)

The probability that some unresponsive patients are also unconscious is very likely. However, in view of the current lack of ability to make such an assessment, the only logical approach for nurses to take is that *no patient is unconscious*. From that assumption the care required is the same as that needed by the patient with an intact communication process.

PAIN

The assessment and control of pain is a major problem area in nursing. Pain is rarely acknowledged as existing in unresponsive patients who are totally defenseless due to the lack of meaningful motor activity. That such a patient is defenseless is clearly evidenced by the fact that he cannot demand something for pain or refuse any invasive procedure that is performed regardless of how severe the pain may be. The author has observed a physical debridement of tissue, through a window cut in the cast, from the site of an open fracture of the proximal end of the radial bone on an "unresponsive" patient. No anesthesia or pain medication was administered. This could never be tolerated by any person with the ability to manifest a motor response by vocally rejecting it (loudly!) or by fleeing from the procedure.

In view of the knowledge that pain can be severe enough to be fatal in instances in which the injury itself is not lethal, it appears that such procedures are contraindicated without appropriate pain control measures. Much more investigation of pain is needed for the development of a safe and humane plan of care for such a patient. The current assumption that the patient who does not scream with pain is not capable of feeling pain is inhumane. It must be replaced by the more likely assumption that pain is felt, but response to it is blocked. Then, survival rates of multiple trauma patients may improve.

APPROACH TO CARE

Due to the inability to prove the *absence* of sensory functioning in the unresponsive patient, it is imperative that nursing care be planned in the context that sensory function exists in some form. All senses should be considered rather than just hearing. The traditional belief that hearing may be the last sense lost may have prevented some unnecessary conversations in the presence of the patient. Historically it has done very little, however, to develop a theoretic framework of nursing care which acknowledges the existence of sensory functioning.

Use of the more logical term *unresponsive* for the patient who cannot respond to commands due to motor-sensory pathology should initiate a refreshingly new positive approach to care. It is certainly the word best suited for directing nursing care.

FUTURE HOPE

Effective planning can reverse the current traumatic situation present in most critical care units. Total control of the sounds and activities is not possible in the physical setting present in most units used in hospitals today, but the nurse can exert her influence in the knowledgeable planning of future units. It is not possible to give concrete solutions that will fit all situations, but it is important to know that sensory input can be hazardous if it is excessive, meaningless, or too continuous. This knowledge, combined with the awareness that the patient is probably not familiar with the lifesaving but noisy technical machinery, will make the nurse in the critical care unit a knowledgeable and effective practitioner and negotiator for the patient.

A great number of nursing measures are presently possible. Identifying and using them will result in a significant advance in the area of individualization of care. Nursing has used the phrase "individualization of care" for a long time but now needs to apply it to the critical care units more extensively than ever before. The area of individualization of physical care has been more tangible and has therefore been the initial area of care focused on. However, the psychological care of the patient should now receive more emphasis. Some of our actions have been traditional rather than logical with empirical data supporting them. Knowledge available today indicates that actions must be justified. We must weigh their potential adverse effects against their validity and necessity. In other words, it is necessary to determine whether or not the omission of the act is more threatening than its commission, as in arousing a patient to take a blood pressure at the expense of disrupting the REM stage of sleep. The robot action of following a routine without theoretic knowledge involved in decision making is no longer an acceptable role of the nurse. Instead, it is necessary to make decisions based on sound rationale, with knowledge of the consequences and evaluation of the effects.

The near future should see many important improvements in the care provided the patient in critical care units. Rapidly developing technology will undoubtedly reach levels that only a few of the most creative dreamers will foresee. Four areas needing major change and for which adequate knowledge and technology appear already available are

- Use by nurses of a method of measuring physiological activity in order to assess the unresponsive patient's awareness of the environment. This is no more impossible than the use of the ECG appeared to the nurse 2 decades ago. Such assessment will significantly enhance care of the patient who has loss of coordinated motor response necessary for communication in the current movement-bound manner.
- Use of the term *unresponsive* rather than *unconscious*. As assessment techniques advance, so too will the description of our findings. Meanwhile, unresponsive is the term which better describes a total lack of motor response.
- Provision for all critically ill patients of environmentally controlled units offering full control of sound, light, and temperature. With the sophistication of patient monitoring equipment rapidly advancing, it will be possible to assess and monitor life signs without the use of contact instrumentation such as blood pressure cuffs and thermometers. Such procedures now normally require disturbing the patient on a 24-hour basis or not collecting such data during the periods of sleep which are necessary for restoring energy.
- Application by nurses of new data resulting from patient research, with increased involvement in initiating research in the patient-care setting. Quality of care can be improved only through research by nurses directly involved in patient-care activities.

When soundproof units with life-function monitoring devices of a noninvasive nature are a reality, nurses can focus on providing therapeutic structuring of the environment, since they will be free from the routine, repetitive functions now consuming a significant amount of time in each 24-hour period. Patients will not have to suffer the adverse effects of the hospital phenomenon to the same degree, and can receive the benefits of care planned to fit within their personal 24-hour cycle of biologic rhythmicity. Advanced technology must release nurses from these repetitive actions if it is to be of value to the patient.

REFERENCES

1. Curtis GC et al: A psychopathological reaction precipitated by sensory deprivation. Am J Psychiatry 125:255–260, 1968
2. Adams HB et al: Sensory deprivation and personality change. J Nerv Ment Dis 113:256, 1966
3. Curtis GC et al: Psychopathological reaction
4. Leff JP: Perceptual phenomena and personality in sensory deprivation. Br J Psychiatry 114:1499–1508, 1968
5. Adams M et al: The confused patient: Psychological responses in critical care units. Am J Nurs 78, No. 9:1504–1512, 1978
6. Gowan NJ: The perceptual world of the intensive care unit: An overview of some environmental considerations in the helping relationship. Heart Lung 8, No. 2:340–344, 1979
7. Wisser SH: When the walls listened. Am J Nurs 78, No. 6:1016–1017, 1978
8. Hurst TW: Is noise important in hospitals? Int J Nurs Stud 3:125–131, 1966
9. Minckley B: A study of noise and its relationship to patient discomfort in the recovery room. Nurs Res 17, No. 3:247–250, 1968
10. Whitfield S: Noise on the wards at night. Nurs Times 71:408–412, 1975
11. Helton MC et al: The correlation between sleep deprivation and the intensive care unit syndrome. Heart Lung 9, No. 3:464–468, 1980
12. Hayter J: The rhythm of sleep. Am J Nurs 80, No. 3:457–461, 1980
13. Luce GG: Body Time: Psychological Rhythms and Social Stress, p 86. New York, Pantheon, 1971
14. Mukheibir SC: Man's inhumanity to man: Intensive care may threaten the human life. Curationis 1:9–11, 1978
15. Blackburn GL et al: Nutrition in the critically ill patient. Anesthesiology 47, No. 2:181–194, 1977
16. Lumb PD et al: Aggressive approach to IV feeding of the critically ill patient. Heart Lung 8, No. 1:71–80, 1979
17. Blackburn GL: Hyperalimentation in the critically ill patient. Heart Lung 8, No. 1:67–70, 1979
18. Elrod RE: The patient with gastrointestinal disease. In Meidel HC et al (eds): Nursing Care of the Patient with Medical-Surgical Disorders, 2nd ed, pp 726–777. New York, McGraw-Hill, 1976
19. Taber RE: Preventing ulcer bleeding in multiple systems failure. Arch Surg 3:93, 1976
20. Burnside IM: The special senses and sensory deprivation. In Burnside IM (ed): Psychosocial Nursing Care of the Aged, pp 387–394. New York, McGraw-Hill, 1976

21. Butler RN, Lewis ML: Aging and Mental Health, pp 71–72. St. Louis, C.V. Mosby, 1973
22. Kiely WF: Critical care psychiatric syndrome. Heart Lung 2, No. 1:54–55, 1973
23. Murray RB et al: The Helping Relationship with Nurse and Elderly Client, pp 51–81. Englewood Cliffs, Prentice-Hall, 1980
24. Roberts SL: Territoriality: Space and the aged patient in intensive care units. In Burnside IM (ed): Psychosocial Nursing Care of the Aged, pp 72–83. New York, McGraw-Hill, 1973
25. Robertson S: Them lot won't let me go. Nurs Times 74:34, 1978
26. Roberts SL: To die or not to die: Plight of the aged patient in ICU. In Burnside IM (ed): Psychosocial Nursing Care of the Aged, pp 96–106. New York, McGraw-Hill, 1973

BIBLIOGRAPHY

Adams HB et al: Sensory deprivation and personality change. J Nerv Ment Dis 143:256–265, 1966

Benoliel JQ et al: As the patient views the ICU and CCU. Heart Lung 4, No. 2:260–264, 1975

Bentley S et al: Perceived noise in surgical wards and an intensive care area: An objective analysis. Br Med J 2:1503–1506, 1977

Blake FG: Immobilized youth. Am J Nurs 69, No. 11:2364–2369, 1969

Brock-Utnes JG et al: Psychiatric problems in intensive care: Five patients with acute confusional states and depressions. Anaesthesia 31, No. 3:380–384, 1976

Catlin F: Noise and emotional stress. J Chron Dis 18:509–518, 1965

Cesarano FL et al: The spaghetti syndrome: A new clinical entity. Crit Care Med 7, No. 4:182–183, 1979

Comer NL, Madow L, Dixon JJ: Observations of sensory deprivation in a life-threatening situation. Am J Psychiatry 125:164–169, 1967

Curtis GC et al: A psychopathological reaction precipitated by sensory deprivation. Am J Psychiatry 125:255–260, 1968

Dosset SM: Stress: II. The patient in the intensive therapy unit. Nurs Times 74, No. 21:890–891, 1978

Greenburg AG et al: Neglected components of intensive care. J Surg Residency 26, No. 5:494–498, 1979

Hoover MJ: Intensive care for relatives. Hospitals 53, No. 14:219–220, 222, 1979

Johnson P: The long hard dying of Joe Rodriquez. Am J Nurs 77, No. 1:54–57, 1977

Mappes TA, Zembaty JS: Biomedical Ethics. New York, McGraw-Hill, 1981

Milholland K: Family participants in the care of patients in the intensive care unit. Heart Lung 7, No. 5:866, 1978

Schwartz LP et al: Critical care unit transfer: Reducing patient stress through nursing interventions. Heart Lung 8, No. 3:540–546, 1979

Shenkin A: Monitoring the nutritional status of critically ill patients. Intensive Care Med 4:171–181, 1979

Stephenson CA: The stress response: Stress in critically ill patients. Am J Nurs 77, No. 11:1806–1808, 1977

Tinnin L: The intensive care psychosis: Ego boundary diffusion treatment and prevention. Md State Med J 26, No. 11:68–70, 1977

Vanson SR et al: Stress effects on patients in critical care units from procedures performed on others. Heart Lung 9, No. 3:494–497, 1980

Woodward JA: An ICU is a place to live . . . not just survive. RN 41, No. 1:62, 1978

Core Body Systems

A. Cardiovascular System
B. Respiratory System
C. Renal System
D. Nervous System

Section A   Cardiovascular System

Barbara Fuller

Normal Structure and Function of the Cardiovascular System
7

During the 70 years in the life of the average individual, the heart will pump approximately 5 quarts of blood per minute, 75 gallons per hour, 57 barrels a day, and 1.5 million barrels in a lifetime. The work accomplished by this organ is completely out of proportion to its size, but the surprising thing is that for most people the heart presents no illness problem. It functions normally throughout their life spans. For the individual who does develop a cardiac problem, however, the result is much different. When a pathologic condition manifests itself in this vital organ, the effects may be extremely dramatic and the outcome often drastic. The information contained in this chapter and the one following is therefore concerned with the normal structure and function of the heart, with the pathogenic variables which lead to the development of coronary heart disease as well as those which progressively produce more dysfunction in the circulatory system.

This chapter will deal with cardiac microstructure, the anatomic and physiological basis for contraction, and the physiological basis for events of the cardiac cycle. Next, factors influencing cardiac output and system, including cardiac perfusion, are presented. Finally, atherosclerotic heart disease is discussed. The reader who wishes more anatomic detail is referred to the many excellent books on this subject.

MICROSTRUCTURE AND CONTRACTION

Microscopically, cardiac muscle contains visible striations similar to those found in skeletal muscle. The ultrastructural pattern also resembles that of striated muscle. The cells branch and anastomose freely, as can be seen in Figure 7-1, *B,* and they form a three-dimensional complex network. The elongated nuclei, like those of smooth muscle, are found deep in the interior of the cells and not adjacent to the sarcolemma.

Unlike skeletal muscle, which is a morphologic syncytium, cardiac muscle fibers are completely surrounded by a cell membrane. At the point where two fibers meet, the two membranes become elaborately folded into a structure known as an *intercalated disk.* These intercalated disks provide strong connections among all the fibers of the cardiac muscle.

Although cardiac muscle is not a morphologic syncytium, it functions as one. Because of the presence of the intercalated disks, whose electrical potentials are extremely low, the rapid spread of excitation from cell to cell is possible. With each contractile impulse generated at the pacemaker, the spread of excitation is so rapid that there is essentially simultaneous contraction of the entire muscle.

Yet another difference (perhaps the most important difference between cardiac muscle and skeletal muscle cells) is that of *automaticity,* whereby cardiac muscle cells are capable of initiating rhythmic action potentials, and thus waves of contraction, without any outside humoral or nervous intervention.

Within each cell lie the thousands of contractile elements: overlapping actin and myosin filaments. Figure 7-2 illustrates these elements and the changes seen during diastole and systole. Not shown in the illustration are the many cross bridges that extend like rows of oars from the surface of the thicker myosin filaments. During diastole these bridges are unattached to other filaments.

Before contraction, the action potential causes a release of *calcium ions* from their sites on the sarcoplasmic reticulum of the myocardial cell. These ions then travel to the sarcomere (the basic contractile unit) where they attach to binding sites that are located at regular intervals along the length of each actin filament. This action of calcium uncovers the myosin cross-bridge binding sites on the actin filaments. The myosin cross bridges (oars) then can attach to these binding sites or actin. With a release of energy stored in adenosine triphosphate (ATP), these cross bridges move unidirectionally in a folding manner (like an oar stroke). This movement slides the actin and myosin filaments past each other, thereby increasing their interdigitation. Rapid, successive uncoupling of cross bridges and their reattachment to new actin binding sites serve to increase the interdigitation of these filaments even more.

The moving of the actin and myosin filaments past each other causes the sarcomere to shorten (see Fig. 7-2). This shortening is the essence of myocardial contraction (systole). Contraction ceases when the calcium ions return to their storage sites on the sarcoplasmic reticulum, thereby causing the binding sites on the actin filaments to be covered again. The separated actin and myosin filaments then slip past each other in the reverse direction, decreasing their interdigitation and thereby again lengthening the sarcomere to its relaxed state.

As can be seen, contraction requires both calcium and energy. Calcium that is loose in the sarcoplasm (cytoplasm of muscle cells) can cause contraction. Hence, calcium in excess of sarcoplasmic reticular storage sites could cause "perpetual contraction" or calcium rigor of the heart. Insufficient intracellular calcium can potentially weaken contractions.

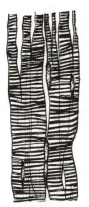
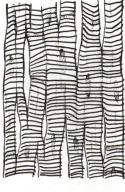
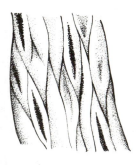

A. Striated Muscle   B. Cardiac Muscle   C. Smooth Muscle

FIGURE 7-1.
Histologic features of the three types of contractile tissue.

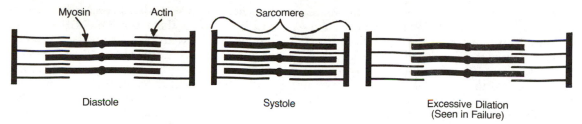

FIGURE 7-2.
Contractile elements lying inside a single sarcomere of a myocardial cell.

ELECTRICAL CHANGES AND CONTRACTION

Membranes of all the cells in the human body are charged—that is, they are polarized and therefore have electrical potentials. This means simply that there is a separation of charges at the membrane. In humans, all cell membranes regardless of type are positively charged, there being more positively charged particles at the outer surface of the cell membrane than at the inner surface.

Figure 7-3, *A* illustrates this "resting stage." This does not mean that there is a lack of negatively charged particles at the outer surface, nor that there is a lack of positively charged particles at the inner surface. It merely means that there is a net difference in the number and kind of charged particles at the outer surface as compared with the inner surface.

Cardiac muscle membranes are polarized, and the electrical potential can be measured, as it can in any of the cells in the human body. The potential results from the difference of intracellular and extracellular concentrations of electrolytes. The electrolyte mainly responsible for the charge at the membrane is potassium, with some contribution from sodium and chloride. When compounds of salts of the elements are dissolved in aqueous solutions, they dissociate into their charged particles called *ions*. It is through the selective control of the concentrations of these ions on either side of membranes that the electrical membrane potential is maintained.

Since the cell membrane is permeable to certain ions whose concentration gradient favors diffusion into the cell, energy must be expended to remove them from the cytoplasm and out through the cell membrane by means of a chemical carrier. The process is called *active transport*. For each molecule of an ion pumped from the cell, one molecule of ATP is required to provide the energy necessary to affect the chemical bond between the ion and the chemical carrier. The process of maintaining membrane potentials in living cells is an *endergonic* (energy-consuming) phenomenon.

When a stimulus is applied to the polarized cell membrane, the membrane which ordinarily is only slightly permeable to sodium permits sodium ions to diffuse rapidly into the cell. This occurs because of inactivation of the sodium active transport enzymes ("pumps"). The result is a reversal of net charges. The outer surface is now more negative than positive, and the membrane is said to be *depolarized* (Fig. 7-3, *B*). As soon as the impulse moves along the membrane, the separation of charges is restored by way of the sodium pump and potassium diffusion, restoring the original state or *repolarizing* the membrane. This is not unique to myocardial tissue but occurs in all nervous and muscular tissue.

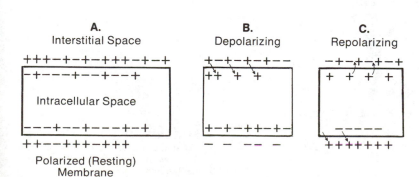

FIGURE 7-3.
The nature of cellular membranes in the human body.

As long as the electrical potential (difference) across the cell membrane remains below a critical point for that tissue, the depolarization remains localized and is called a *local depolarization.* Such a local event does not stimulate myocardial contraction. If the potential crosses this critical point or *threshold,* this depolarization will inactivate adjacent sodium pumps. This can cause depolarization in these areas. Thus, the original depolarization has become self-propagating and is termed an *action potential.* In a myocardial cell the occurrence of an action potential also triggers the release of intracellular calcium from its storage sites, thereby initiating systole, as previously described.

MACROSTRUCTURE AND CONDUCTION

The heart chambers and specialized tissues are diagrammed in Figure 7-4. In the wall of the right atrium is the sinoatrial *(SA) node.* This specialized tissue acts as normal cardiac pacemaker. In the lower right portion of the interatrial septum lies the *atrioventricular (AV) node.* This tissue acts to conduct, yet delay, the atrial action potential before it travels to the ventricles. Such a delay is necessary in order to allow separate atrial and ventricular contractions.

Although the myocardium is syncytial in nature, the atria are physically discontinuous from the ventricles. A specialized conduction system exists to conduct the action potential into and throughout the ventricles. From the AV node, the impulse travels down the *bundle of His* in the interventricular septum into either a right or left bundle branch and then through one of many *Purkinje fibers* to the ventricular myocardial tissue itself. An action potential can traverse this conducting tissue three to seven times more rapidly than it can travel through the ventricular myocardium. Hence the bundle, branches, and Purkinje fibers enable a near simultaneous contraction of all portions of the ventricle, thereby enabling a maximal unified pump action to occur.

Electrocardiograms

Let us now examine these events as they are depicted by an electrocardiogram (ECG) (see Fig. 7-5). ECG's will be extensively covered in a later chapter; hence, discussion here will be brief:

- The P wave represents the atrial depolarization that occurs with atrial systole.
- The P-Q interval represents the duration required for the impulse to reach the ventricular myocardium.
- The QRS complex denotes the electrical events concurrent with ventricular systole. This wave hides the electrical representation of atrial repolarization.

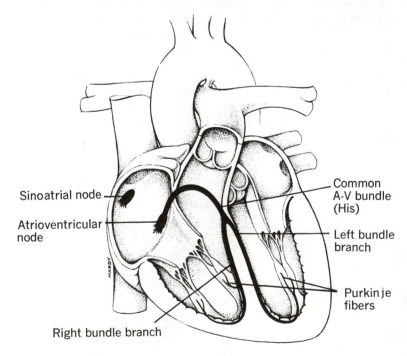

Sinoatrial node

Atrioventricular node

Right bundle branch

Common A-V bundle (His)

Left bundle branch

Purkinje fibers

FIGURE 7-4.
Distribution of the Purkinje system and the location of the sinoatrial node in the human heart.

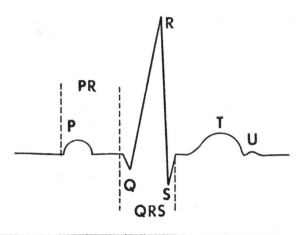

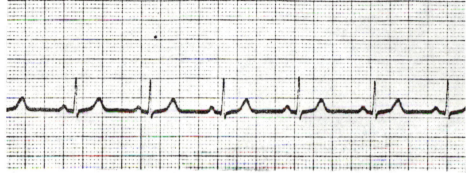

FIGURE 7-5.
Normal electrocardiogram tracing.

- The QT interval represents the length of time taken by ventricular depolarization and repolarization.
- The T wave represents repolarization and is caused in part by a reentry of potassium ions.
- The U wave depicts a supernormal phase that occurs during the beginning of ventricular recovery.

Rhythmicity and Pacing

An inherent property of myocardial cells is a spontaneous and rhythmic inactivation of their sodium pumps. Thus, any portion of atrial or ventricular cells can produce their own rhythmic series of action potentials and, hence, their own stimulus for contraction. However, if there were no coordination of these activities, the heart could not function as a pump.

Fortunately, rates of spontaneous discharge vary throughout the heart. The sinoatrial node, a specialized piece of cardiac tissue located between the openings of the inferior and superior vena cavae in the wall of the right atrium, discharges at a resting rate of 90 to 100 times per minute. Regular atrial myocardial cells have a discharge rate of about 60 to 70 per minute. The remainder of the conduction system and ventricles have progressively slower rates of discharge culminating in an idioventricular rhythm of about 40 per minute. Were the actions of the various parts of the heart independent and uncoordinated, effective pumping could never occur. This does not happen because the fastest area paces the remainder — provided intact conduction pathways exist between them. Normally, the SA node will act as the pacemaker. Without modification, however, this would result in an *unregulated* heart rate of 100 beats per minute because that is the rhythmic discharge rate of SA nodal time. However, in the healthy person, continued parasympathetic influences lower this spontaneous nodal rhythm to about 70 to 80 beats per minute. (This will be discussed further in the section on regulation of cardiac output.)

Should the normal conduction pathways be interrupted, the fastest pacemaker tissue on both sides of this interruption will govern their respective areas, and the ECG may evidence two independent such rhythms. Atrial systole is not needed in order for the ventricle to fill with blood. The important rhythm, clinically, is that of the ventricles. They are the chambers that supply the lungs and the rest of the body with blood. Their systolic rate helps to determine true perfusion. The slower the rate, the less able are the ventricles to meet the perfusion needs of the body during exercise or activities of daily living.

THE CARDIAC CYCLE

In the foregoing sections, the more subtle and less typically measurable features of cardiac function have been discussed. Pulse, blood pressure, and heart sounds are very important indicators of cardiac function and will now be discussed in light of the characteristics which have just been presented. Figure 7-6 summarizes the events during this cycle.

During diastole, blood enters the relaxed atria and flows passively into the relaxed ventricles. Diastole typically lasts 0.4 seconds (in a heart rate of 70 beats/min). Then the SA node discharges and atrial systole occurs, with a duration of 0.1 second. This atrial contraction is not responsible for most of ventricular filling. It squeezes just a small amount of remaining blood into the ventricles. Then the ventricles contract (the delay is due to the time needed for the action potential to traverse the AV node and conduction system). Ventricular systole elevates the pressure within the chambers, forcing both (1) the blood out into the pulmonary artery and aorta and (2) the tricuspid and bicuspid valves

shut. The slamming shut of these valves comprises the *"lub" heart sound.*

At the same time as the lub sound there is a surge of fluid pressure against the walls of the major arteries as a result of increased volume of blood pumped from the ventricles. This surge is felt in the peripheral circulation and is known as the *pulse.* The contractile phase or period is known as *systole,* and thus the blood pressure of this period of ventricular systole is called the *systolic pressure.*

Ventricular systole lasts about 0.3 seconds. After this, the ventricles relax, which causes the arterial pressure to exceed the intraventricular pressure, closing the semilunar valves. The closing of these valves (pulmonary and aortic) is heard as the *"dub" cardiac sound,* denoting the onset of ventricular diastole.

Since there is no pushing of blood into the arteries during ventricular diastole, blood pressure falls, and the diastolic blood pressure is lower than the systolic blood pressure.

CARDIAC OUTPUT

Cardiac output (CO) is a traditional measure of cardiac function. It equals the product of heart rate (HR) and stroke volume (SV):

$$CO = (HR) \times (SV)$$

Although it is approximately 4.8 liter per minute at rest, cardiac output can be altered to meet changing bodily demands for tissue perfusion. Since the latter is a function of body size, a newer more accurate measure of cardiac function is the

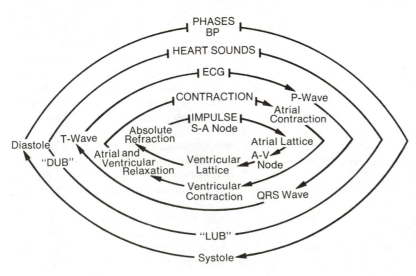

FIGURE 7-6.
The cardiac cycle.

cardiac index. This index is the cardiac output divided by the surface area of the body. It typically averages 3.0 ± 0.2 liter per minute.

$$\text{cardiac index} = \frac{\text{CO}}{\substack{\text{surface area} \\ (\text{M}^2)}}$$

Because of the relationship of stroke volume and heart rate on cardiac index, let us examine these further.

Regulation of Heart Rate

Although the heart possesses the ability to beat independently of any extrinsic influence, cardiac rate is under autonomic and adrenal catecholamine influence. Both parasympathetic and sympathetic fibers innervate the SA and AV nodes. In addition, there are sympathetic fibers that terminate in myocardial tissue. Figure 7-7 illustrates this innervation.

Parasympathetic stimulation releases acetylcholine near the nodal cells. This decreases their rate of depolarization, thereby slowing cardiac rate. Stimulation of sympathetic fibers causes them to release nonepinephrine (NE). This chemical increases the rate of nodal depolarization. It also has ionotropic effects upon myocardial fibers, which will be discussed later. Thus, sympathetic stimulation increases heart rate. The adrenal medulla also releases norepinephrine and epinephrine into the bloodstream. These catecholamines act upon the heart in the same way as sympathetic stimulation.

There are two reflexes that adjust heart rate to blood pressure: the aortic and Bainbridge reflexes. In the aortic reflex, a rise in arterial blood pressure stimulates aortic and carotid sinus baroreceptors to fire sensory impulses to the cardioregulatory center in the medulla. This causes an increase in parasympathetic or a decrease in sympathetic stimulation to the heart. Thus, a rise in arterial blood pressure reflexively causes a slowing of cardiac rate. That results in a decrease in cardiac output which, in turn, can decrease arterial blood pressure. Conversely, a fall in arterial blood pressure, such as in shock, will reflexively increase heart rate. This aortic reflex is an ongoing regulatory mechanism for homeostasis of arterial blood pressure.

The *Bainbridge reflex* utilizes receptors in the vena cavae. An increase in venous return stimulates these receptors, which then fire sensory impulses that travel to the cardioregulatory center. These reflexively cause a decrease in parasympathetic and an increase in sympathetic cardiac stimulation, thereby increasing cardiac rate. A fall in venous return causes a decrease in heart rate. Thus, the Bainbridge reflex adjusts cardiac rate to handle venous return.

Regulation of Stroke Volume

Three factors are involved in stroke volume: (1) preload, (2) afterload (or wall tension), and (3) inherent ionotropic myocardial contractility. Let us examine each in turn.

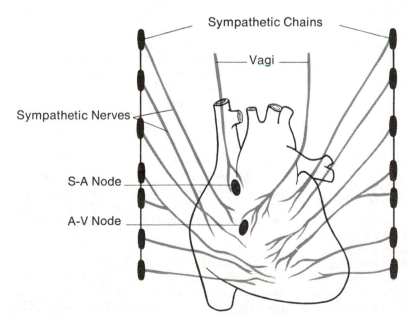

FIGURE 7-7.
Distribution of autonomic nerve fibers to the human heart.

Preload. This refers to *Starling's law of the heart.* The more a myocardial fiber is stretched immediately prior to contraction, the stronger it will contract. Stretch is determined by the volume of blood in a heart chamber at the end of diastole, referred to as *end diastolic volume (EDV).* Hence, increased venous return will increase the EDV, which will result in a more forceful systole (within normal limits). In this way, ventricular emptying (cardiac output) is automatically adjusted to venous return. Generally, the most clinically important EDV is that of the left ventricle, and by convention EDV is ventricular unless otherwise specified.

Anatomically, stretch decreases the overlap between actin and myosin filaments. This increases the number of "empty" or potential cross-bridge binding sites that can be involved per contraction (see Fig. 7-2). Overstretch caused by ventricular dilation in heart failure is thought to decrease contractile force by decreasing overlap too much. As a result, there are too few actual binding sites (so that only a few cross bridges can operate) to produce much of an initial contractile force. By the time the filaments interdigitate sufficiently, so that more myosin cross bridges can be induced, contraction is almost over. Thus, overstretch reduces the force of systole and can actually decrease ventricular emptying, thereby exacerbating the problem.

Afterload or Wall Tension. This is the second factor affecting stroke volume. It is the *force* required by the ventricles in order to open the aortic and pulmonary valves during systole (systolic ejection force). The higher the arterial pressure, the more force that is required (to push against this) by the ventricles. Also, the larger the ventricular diameter, the greater the required force. These relationships are described by the equation:

$$AL = VEF = AP \times VA$$

Where

    Al   represents *afterload*

    VEF   represents *ventricular ejection force* (wall tension)

    AP   represents *arterial pressure*

    VA   represents *ventricular cross-sectional area*

Some sources equate afterload with diastolic blood pressure. As can be seen from this equation, this is not strictly the case. Diastolic blood pressure can only roughly provide an index of afterload. Afterload increases the work that the heart must perform. In cases in which the heart cannot meet the necessary wall tension (force) requirements, afterload will then reduce stroke volume. This is most often seen in the failing heart.

Inherent (Ionotropic) Capabilities. This last factor involves intracellular processes that may act to increase or decrease contraction. These processes operate independently of Starling's law or extrinsic stimuli. Cellular stores of calcium and norepinephrine can be such factors. Also, sympathetic stimulation or β-adrenergic drugs may increase inherent contractility. Much remains to be learned about these capabilities.

CORONARY CIRCULATION

Blood supply to the myocardium is derived from the two main coronary arteries that originate from the aorta, immediately above the aortic valve. The left coronary artery supplies the major portion of the left ventricle, while the right coronary artery supplies the major portion of the right ventricle.

Shortly after its origin, the left coronary vessel branches into the anterior descending artery, which traverses the groove between the two ventricles on the anterior surface of the heart, and the circumflex artery, which passes to the left and posteriorly in the groove between the left atrium and the left ventricle. The circumflex branch may terminate before reaching the posterior side of the heart, or it may continue into the posterior groove between the left and right ventricles. The coronary circulation is referred to as *dominant left* if this branch of the left coronary artery supplies the posterior aspect of the heart, including the septum.

Eighty percent of human hearts are *dominant right.* When this situation prevails, the right coronary artery passes posteriorly and is responsible for the blood supply to the posterior side of the heart and the posterior portion of the interventricular septum.

Because of their anatomic deviation from the aorta (above the aortic valve) and the fact that they lie between myocardial fibers, blood flow through the coronary arteries occurs during ventricular diastole, not systole. Therefore, anything that decreases the diastolic time (*e.g.,* tachycardia) will decrease coronary perfusion.

PERIPHERAL CIRCULATION

The biologic significance of the cardiovascular system is tissue perfusion. Such perfusion supplies the cells with oxygen and nutrients while carrying away metabolic wastes, including carbon dioxide. Tissue perfusion is indirectly proportional to the rate of blood flow, which, in turn, is dependent upon several factors. One such factor is the difference between the mean arterial blood pressure and right atrial pressure (usually represented by the central venous pressure). The greater this difference, the faster the flow rate (all else being unchanged). Conversely, if the arterial pressure falls or the central venous pressure rises, flow rate, and hence tissue perfusion, will be decreased.

Another factor affecting flow rate is vessel resistance. This resistance is due in part to the friction of the fluid along the sides of the vessel. As such, it is inversely proportional to the fourth power of the radius of the vessel. The equation is

$$\text{vessel resistance} = \frac{1}{\text{vessel radius}^4}$$

Hence, the more constricted or narrower the vessel lumen, the greater the resistance. Vessel dilation decreases resistance and, as a result, increases the rate of blood flow. The relationship between vessel radius and blood flow has two general applications. One is to describe the flow rate through vessels of differing diameters (*e.g.*, arteries, capillaries). The other application concerns the ongoing regulation of blood flow by means of adjustments in arteriole diameters (*i.e.*, constriction and dilation). Arteriole constriction reduces the radius, thereby increasing resistance and thus decreasing the flow rate. Arteriole dilation, conversely, increases the flow rate.

The other two factors which can affect the flow rate are normally held constant. They are (1) the sum of all vessel lengths and (2) blood viscosity. Because they do not normally change significantly, they are usually omitted from flow rate considerations. Their relationships are obvious, though. The greater the length of a vessel, the more resistance, and thus the slower the flow rate. Also, the more viscous the blood, the slower the rate of its flow. The complete equation that describes all four factors is:

flow rate =

$$\frac{\text{mean arterial pressure} - \text{central venous pressure}}{\text{resistance} \times \text{viscosity} \times \text{vessel length}}$$

PATHOGENESIS OF CORONARY HEART DISEASE

Atherosclerosis

It is estimated that 95% of all cases of myocardial damage are due to intrinsic disease of the coronary vessels as a result of arteriosclerotic changes in the vessel walls. Arteriosclerotic changes in coronary vessels do not absolutely parallel systemic sclerotic changes and thus may be more severe than the observed peripheral alterations would indicate.

The most common characteristic of the diseased vessel is the presence of patchy atheromatosis scattered in the lining of the vessels and projecting into the lumen. Because of this propensity for atherosclerotic vessel changes, it is imperative that a brief discussion of the etiology of these vascular changes be included, as well as the correlation of vascular dysfunction and its effect upon functional anatomy of the myocardium.

Precursors to the atherosclerotic lesions are thought to be "fatty streaks" within the tunica intima endothelium of various arteries. They seem to occur as a normal feature early in life. Autopsies have shown them in the aortas of infants and in the cerebral and coronary arteries of adolescents dying of other causes. Next, the fatty streak evolves into a fibrous plaque, which spreads into the tunica media as well. Plaque formation involves hyperplasia of the smooth muscle cells of the tunica media layer and deposition of cholesterol-rich lipoproteins. These changes seem to occur during the first 2 decades of adult life. Later, these plaques become more complex *atheromas*, which are characterized by calcification, increased lipid and collagen deposition, and vascularization. These atheromas may also show degenerative changes such as cell debris, bleeding, and coagulation products.

Disturbance in circulation may result from various final causes. First, the plaque may progressively occlude the lumen of the vessel. Secondly, the rough plaque surfaces can attract platelets, which then initiate thrombus formation. Thirdly, pieces may break off from the thrombus or plaque itself and embolitically obstruct smaller vessels. Lastly, the plaque or factors involved with it may trigger an arterial spasm that can obstruct the vessel totally. All or some of these factors may be involved in a particular patient.

The current major theory of atherosclerosis states that the fatty streak is converted into a fibrous plaque because of damage to the endothelial lining (tunica intima), which allows plasma lipoprotein to invade the smooth muscle layer (tunica media) and to perhaps stimulate hyperplasia of this layer. Both cholesterol-containing lipoprotein and hypoxia such as can result from tobacco smoking (carbon monoxide rather than oxygen is bound to hemoglobin molecules) may stimulate local hyperplasia of the smooth muscle layer. It has also been demonstrated that the vessel wall can secrete cholesterol in response to breaks in the tunica intima.

Endothelial damage can result from a variety of factors including the physical trauma of "wear and tear," immunologic injury, hyperlipidemia, and hypoxia.

Atherosclerotic lesions typically occur in the epicardial regions of the main arteries and occur more often in the left coronary artery system. Plaques develop more often at points of increased wear and tear—areas of curvature and branching.

Coronary atherosclerosis results in a dminished ability of the coronary circulation to supply oxygen and nutrients to heart tissue. So long as this supply meets cardiac demands, there is no problem. Clinical impairment and signs are evident only when cardiac demand exceeds coronary supply (on a unit/time basis). Mild impairment may only be noticed when the cardiac demand is artificially and severely increased by a cardiac exercise stress test. More severe impairment may be evident as *angina* when the subject's ordinary daily exertions cause cardiac demand to exceed coronary supply. More severe impairment may trigger an *infarct*.

The ontogeny of atherosclerotic plaques is a long, silent process often lasting 2 to 4 decades. Its presence is not noted clinically until a critical (usually greater than 70%) obstruction produces signs and symptoms of ischemic heart disease, disrhythmias, or exercise stress-test abnormalities. Atherosclerosis was once considered an unavoidable result of normal aging. This is no longer regarded as true.

NONMODIFIABLE RISK FACTORS

Several risk factors have now been identified—some modifiable and some not. There are four nonmodifiable ones: sex, race, family history, and age. Atherosclerosis occurs most often in black males having a positive family history of coronary heart disease before the age of 50. The presence of estrogens seems to reduce the risk in premenopausal women. After menopause both males and females are at equal risk. The genetic nature of the family involvement is not currently known, but it may be polygenic. The family history also may well reflect environmental influences or familial life-styles that potentiate modifiable risk factors (*e.g.*, smoking, diet, tension). Although atherosclerotic heart disease is atypical in persons under 40 years of age, the risk increases with age beyond this point. Such risk

may simply reflect the time needed for full plaque development or an increased length of exposure to other potentiating factors (*e.g.*, tobacco).

MODIFIABLE RISK FACTORS

Modifiable risk factors which have been currently elucidated are sixfold. They are (1) hypertension, (2) hyperlipidemia, (3) tobacco smoking, (4) impaired glucose tolerance test or diabetes, (5) psychosocial stress, and (6) a dietary intake that is high in saturated fats, cholesterol, or calories.

Hypertension. Persons with blood pressure that chronically exceeds 140/90 torr are at risk, with the degree of risk proportional to the degree of hypertension, especially in the elderly.

Hyperlipidemia. The parameter of hyperlipidemia that seems to be a risk factor is the low density lipoprotein (LDL) fraction of the plasma lipoproteins. The LDL fraction is the one that contains most of the plasma cholesterol (bound to plasma proteins).

Risk seems to be associated with elevated plasma triglyceride levels and with plasma cholesterol levels in excess of 250 mg/dl. Persons with more than 250 mg/dl cholesterol levels are three to four times as likely to have atherosclerotic heart disease than those whose plasma cholesterol levels are less than 220 mg/dl.

Many factors may contribute to hyperlipidemia in general and hypercholesterolemia in particular. Major possibilities are (1) levels of endogenous cholesterol synthesis by normal body cells; (2) genetic factors that may increase the above mentioned cholesterol synthesis or prevent the degradation and elimination of cholesterol from the plasma; (3) dietary intake of saturated fats, calories, or alcohol; and (4) a sedentary life-style. Regular vigorous exercise may (indirectly) enhance hepatic degradation of cholesterol. Hyperlipidemia seems to be a major risk factor for the middle-aged person. In the elderly, it plays less of an etiologic role than does hypertension.

Smoking. The role of tobacco smoke is not clearly delineated, but its place as a risk factor is well established. One possible mode of action lies in the carbon monoxide contained in the smoke. This chemical competes with oxygen for transport sites on hemoglobin molecules. Hence, tobacco smoke can produce hypoxemia. Another hypothesis states that tobacco smoke may stimulate catecholamine secretions.

Other mechanisms probably exist. Which, if any, of these hypotheses are valid and the extent to which they or other factors affect atherogenesis await further study. A recent report states that tobacco smokers have a 70% greater chance of developing atherosclerotic heart disease than do nonsmokers. The degree of risk is directly related to the number of cigarettes smoked per day. The risk does not seem to be cumulative. Ex-smokers (after several months) have the same low risk as nonsmokers.

Impaired Glucose Tolerance or Diabetes.
Females seem to be more at risk from impaired glucose tolerance or diabetes than are males. Although the exact mechanism is unknown, hyperglycemia itself seems to impair vascular integrity and may thus facilitate atheroma formation. Indeed, a myocardial infarct in a 30-year-old may be the first noted sign of diabetes.

Psychosocial Stress.   Psychosocial stress, or more specifically, a *type A personality,* has been recently promulgated as a risk factor for atherosclerotic heart disease. This personality, characterized by an intense competitiveness, a need to be better than others, and a sense of time urgency, may exacerbate or provoke environmental stressors. However, the link between stress or this personality and atherogenesis *per se* has yet to be established. These factors may predispose to excessive cardiac demands (for oxygen and nutrients) rather than to a decreased coronary supply.

BIBLIOGRAPHY

Guyton AC: Textbook of Medical Physiology, 5th ed. Philadelphia, WB Saunders, 1976

Jensen D: The Principles of Physiology. New York, Appleton-Century-Crofts, 1976

Levine HJ (ed): Clinical Cardiovascular Physiology. New York, Grune & Stratton, 1976

Price SA and Wilson LM: Pathophysiology: Clinical Concepts of Disease Processes. New York, McGraw-Hill, 1978

Ross WS: You Can Quit Smoking in 14 Days. California, Berkeley, 1976

Stephens G: Pathophysiology for Health Practitioners. New York, Macmillan, 1980

H. L. Brammell

Pathophysiology of Heart Failure
8

The heart, a complex structure composed of fibrous tissue, cardiac muscle, and electrical conducting tissue, has a single function: to pump blood. In order to do its job well, a good heart pump requires good functioning muscle, a good valve system, and an efficient pumping rhythm. An abnormality of sufficient severity of any component of the pump can affect its pumping efficiency and may cause the pump to fail.

RESERVE MECHANISMS OF THE HEART: RESPONSES OF THE HEART TO STRESS

When the heart is stressed, several reserve mechanisms can be called upon to maintain good pumping function, that is, to provide a cardiac output sufficient to meet the demands of the body. These mechanisms are increased heart rate, dilatation, hypertrophy, and increased stroke volume.

Increased Heart Rate

The first response is an increase in *heart rate* . This adjustment is rapid and has been experienced by everyone during periods of exercise or anxiety. Increasing the heart rate is an excellent way to quickly increase the cardiac output and meet the demands of the body for blood. Its utility and effectiveness, however, are functions of age, the

Supported by a Research and Training Center Grant (16–P-56815) from the Rehabilitation Services Administration, Department of Health, Education and Welfare, Washington, D.C.

functional state of the myocardium, and the amount of obstructive coronary artery disease, if any.

The maximum heart rate which can be achieved is related to age.[1] For example, a 20-year-old will plateau at approximately 200 beats per minute at maximum effort, whereas at age 65, maximum heart rate is about 153 beats per minute. After age 25, maximum heart rate capability drops approximately 6 beats for each 5 years. There is, of course, considerable spread around these mean maximum heart rates for each age — some persons will exceed and some fail to achieve the average value. As heart rate increases, the time for diastolic ventricular filling decreases, and at high heart rates the time available for ventricular filling may be so small that filling is inadequate and cardiac output starts to fall.

In addition to advancing age, the functional state of the heart muscle (how capable it is of maintaining repeated rapid contractions) and the state of the coronary circulation are important determinants of the effectiveness of heart rate as a response to stress. In persons with coronary artery disease and significant obstruction to one or more coronary arteries, a substantial increase in heart rate can be a potentially dangerous event. Coronary artery blood flow to the left ventricle takes place primarily in diastole. With increasing heart rates, decreased diastolic filling time, and increased demands of the heart for oxygen (heart rate being one of the major determinants of myocardial oxygen demand), coronary blood flow may become critical, and angina pectoris, congestive failure, or occasionally myocardial infarction may be produced. Furthermore, if the heart muscle contracts poorly and cannot sustain strong contractions at moderate or rapid rates, then heart failure may follow.

Heart rate, then, is an immediate response to stress that is effective in maintaining or increasing cardiac output but whose value depends on the patient's age, functional state of the myocardium, and amount of obstructive disease in the coronary arteries.

Dilatation

The second reserve mechanism of the heart is *dilatation*. With dilatation the muscle cell stretches. The relationship between the cardiac output (the amount of blood the heart pumps in each unit of time) and the length of the heart muscle cell at the end of diastole is expressed in the well-known *Starling relationship,* which states that as the end-diastolic fiber length increases, so does the cardiac output.

Like heart rate, however, the usefulness of dilatation is self-limiting. There is a point beyond which the stretching of the muscle cell leads not to an increase in cardiac output but to a decrease. This is partly explained by the *Laplace relationship,* which states that the tension in the wall of a chamber such as the left ventricle is directly related to the pressure in that chamber and its radius. Put another way, as the radius of the chamber increases (dilatation), so does the wall tension, as long as the pressure in the chamber rises or does not fall.

Since wall tension is directly related to the demand of the myocardium for oxygen, it is not difficult to see that eventually the radius will dilate to such a degree that the demand of the heart for oxygen cannot be met. In this instance, dilatation has advanced to the point where it is no longer providing an increase in cardiac output, and the pump has started to fail.

Hypertrophy

Third, individual cardiac muscle cells may *hypertrophy*. The process of hypertrophy requires time and is not an acute adjustment to stress. However, if the stress is applied long enough, such as with systemic or pulmonary hypertension or significant stenosis of the aortic or pulmonic valve (pressure loads), the muscle of the chamber pumping against the resistance may hypertrophy to such a degree that it effectively outgrows its blood supply and becomes ischemic. When this happens, hypertrophy ceases to be a useful compensatory mechanism, and the heart's pumping ability decreases. A similar situation may occur with the imposition of a volume load on the pumping ventricle, for example, as occurs with mitral or aortic regurgitation.

Stroke Volume

A fourth reserve mechanism of the heart is to increase its *stroke volume,* the amount of blood that it ejects into the circulation with each systole. It can do this either by increasing the percentage of the end-diastolic volume ejected with each beat (increase the ejection fraction through an increase in contractility) or by increasing the amount of blood presented to the heart (increased venous return). This is commonly accomplished by the reflexive increase of sympathetic nervous system activity which increases venous tone. Venous pressure is then raised, and thus venous return to the heart is increased.

Venous return is also increased by elevated body temperature, which shortens the time required for blood to completely circulate through the body; by recumbency, in which case the volume of blood that is held in the legs as a result of gravity is largely returned to the central circulation and presented to the heart; or by taking a deep breath, which increases intrathoracic negativity, thereby "sucking" more blood into the chest. Also, any increase in intravascular volume will increase venous return. By either an increase in ejection fraction (contractility) or venous return (volume), stroke volume and cardiac output will increase. As with other mechanisms of response to stress, increased venous return ("preload" to the physiologist) and increased contractility may not function to increase cardiac output. For example, the myocardium may be so fatigued (depressed contractility) that it cannot respond to further attempts to improve its force of contraction. Similarly, an increase in venous return may cause increased dilatation and decrease, rather than improve, cardiac output.

This simplistic review of cardiovascular responses to stress is designed to promote a basic understanding of the topic and to indicate how the responses can be overwhelmed. In addition, it will assist in generating an appreciation for approaching clinical situations, both diagnostic and therapeutic, from a physiological cause-and-effect point of view.

HEART FAILURE

When the normal cardiac reserves for responding to stress are inadequate to meet the metabolic demands of the body, the heart fails to do its job as a pump, and heart failure results. Also, as stated earlier, dysfunction of any of the components of the pump may ultimately result in failure. Heart failure was very simply and appropriately defined many years ago by Lewis as "a condition in which the heart fails to discharge its contents adequately."[2] This definition is as good today as it was in the 1930s.

Causes of Failure

HEART MUSCLE ABNORMALITIES

Abnormalities of the *muscle* causing ventricular failure include myocardial infarction, ventricular aneurysm, extensive myocardial fibrosis (usually from atherosclerotic coronary heart disease or prolonged hypertension), endocardial fibrosis, primary myocardial disease (cardiomyopathy), or excessive hypertrophy due to pulmonary hypertension, aortic stenosis, or systemic hypertension.

Myocardial Rupture. In acute myocardial infarction, *myocardial rupture* presents as a dramatic and often catastrophic onset of pump failure and is associated with a high mortality. Rupture usually occurs during the first 8 days following infarction, during the period of greatest softening of the damaged myocardium. Fortunately, myocardial rupture is a relatively rare complication of infarction. *Rupture of a papillary muscle,* of the interventricular septum, or of the free wall of the left ventricle may occur.

There are two papillary muscles in the left ventricle which are thumblike projections of muscle to which the restraining "guidewires" of the mitral valve, the chordae tendineae, are attached. The papillary muscle may be involved in the infarction process and very occasionally may rupture. When it does, there is a sudden loss of restraint of one of the leaflets of the mitral valve, and free mitral regurgitation occurs with each contraction of the left ventricle. This sudden profound pressure and volume load on the left atrium is reflected back through the pulmonary veins to the pulmonary vascular bed, and the acute onset of symptoms of pulmonary vascular congestion is noted. This is usually manifested as severe dyspnea and frank pulmonary edema. At the bedside, a loud murmur lasting throughout systole is present. Very often nothing can be done to save the patient, although occasionally emergency mitral valve replacement can be successfully accomplished.

Sudden heart failure is seen occasionally in acute myocardial infarction as a result of *rupture of the interventricular septum.* Like rupture of the papillary muscle, septal rupture is uncommon, but when it does appear is also usually noted in the first week after damage. Septal rupture is clinically characterized by chest pain, dyspnea, shock, and a rapid onset of evidence of pump failure. There is a loud murmur that lasts throughout systole at the lower left sternal border and is often accompanied by a thrill which can be felt by placing the hand over the precordium at the left sternal border. As with all myocardial ruptures, the prognosis of septal rupture is poor. However, it is possible to occasionally repair these ventricular septal defects by emergency surgery using cardiopulmonary bypass.

Ruptures of a papillary muscle and the interventricular septum are virtually indistinguishable at the bedside, with both presenting as sudden onset of left ventricular failure, a new murmur, and occasionally a palpable thrill. The location of the infarction is not helpful, and the clinical course in each is rapidly downhill. Emergency cardiac catheterization is the only way to clearly differentiate the two.[3]

Mechanical failure of the heart seen in acute myocardial infarction is another relatively rare event and is due to *rupture of the free wall of the left ventricle* and the spilling of blood into the pericardial cavity. This results in acute compression of the heart or tamponade and the inability of both chambers to fill adequately. There is then very sudden pumping failure with associated shock and death.

Rupture of the free wall may be preceded by or associated with a return of chest pain as the blood dissects through the necrotic myocardial wall. Sudden vascular collapse as occurs with ventricular fibrillation, but with an unchanged rhythm on the electrocardiogram (electromechanical dissociation), suggests rupture of the ventricular free wall. As with rupture of the papillary muscle and interventricular septum, rupture of the free wall of the left ventricle carries with it an extremely poor prognosis.

VALVE MALFUNCTION

Valve malfunction can lead to pump failure by causing either obstruction to outflow of the pumping chamber, such as valvular aortic stenosis or pulmonary stenosis (pressure load), or the valve may be regurgitant as with mitral or aortic insufficiency which present an increased volume of blood to the left ventricle (volume load).

Valve abnormalities that impose either a pressure or a volume load on one or more chambers usually are slowly progressive conditions that cause the heart to use its long-term defense mechanisms of dilatation and hypertrophy. Both these mechanisms can be overcome, with resultant pump failure.

Less commonly, an acute volume load is imposed on the heart, causing a rapid onset of pump failure. Bacterial endocarditis of the aortic or mitral valves, rupture of a portion of the mitral valve apparatus (papillary muscle or chordae tendineae), or rupture of the interventricular septum is the usual cause. In these cases, initial therapy is designed to support the heart during the period of acute insult so that the long-term compensatory mechanisms can be used. However, if this is not successful, emergency replacement of the abnormal valve or closure of the sepal defect is indicated.

ARRHYTHMIAS

Disorders of the cardiac *rhythm* can produce or contribute to failure in several ways. *Bradycardia* allows for increased diastolic filling and myocardial fiber stretch with an associated increase in stroke volume (Starling relationship). Cardiac output is therefore preserved. This is well tolerated in healthy persons; resting bradycardia is, in fact, a result of high levels of aerobic physical conditioning. However, in the diseased heart contractility is decreased, the useful limits of the Starling relationship are exceeded, and cardiac output may be diminished.

On the other hand, with *tachycardia,* diastolic filling time is decreased, myocardial oxygen demand is increased, and the diseased myocardium or the heart with significant coronary artery disease may tolerate the burden poorly and fail or develop ischemia, injury, or infarction. Furthermore, frequent premature contractions may decrease the cardiac output, a circumstance that may be poorly tolerated in a patient with marginal pump function.

Responses to Failure

When the heart's normal reserves are overwhelmed and failure occurs, certain physiological responses to the decrease in cardiac output are important. All of these responses represent the body's attempt to maintain a normal perfusion of vital organs.

The primary acute adjustment to heart failure is an increase in sympathetic nervous system influence on the arteries, veins, and heart. This results in an increase in heart rate, an increase in venous return to the heart, and increased force of contraction; in addition, sympathetic tone helps to maintain a normal blood pressure. The price extracted for this adjustment is an increase in myocardial oxygen demand and oxygen consumption, a request that may inadequately be met in the patient with significant coronary artery obstructive disease or poor pump contractility.

As a result of the autonomic nervous changes and other factors, the blood flow to the essential organs, specifically the brain and heart, is maintained at the expense of less essential organs such as the skin, gut, and kidneys. With severe congestive heart failure, there is sufficient decrease in blood flow to the skeletal muscles to cause a *metabolic acidosis* that must be considered when a treatment program is planned.

When the kidneys sense a decreased volume of blood presented for filtration, they respond by retaining sodium and water and thereby try to do their part in increasing the central blood volume and venous return. With an increase in circulating blood volume and venous return to the heart, there is an increase in end–diastolic fiber length (dilatation) and, within limits, an increase in stroke volume and cardiac output. However, with a failing heart, an increased circulatory volume may be too great a burden for the ventricle, and failure may be worsened.

In some patients with prolonged failure, remaining heart cells will hypertrophy, increasing pumping efficiency, and the clinical findings of heart failure may improve or disappear.

Assessment of Failure

LEFT VENTRICULAR FAILURE

It is useful to think of the clinical features of heart failure as coming from failure of either the left ventricle, the right ventricle, or both. When the *left ventricle* fails, its inability to discharge its contents adequately results in dilatation, increased end–diastolic volume, and increased intraventricular pressure at the end of diastole. This results in the inability of the left atrium to adequately empty its contents into the left ventricle, and pressure in the left atrium rises. This pressure rise is reflected back into the pulmonary veins which bring blood from the lungs to the left atrium. The increased pressure in the pulmonary vessels results in pulmonary vascular congestion, which is the cause of the most specific symptoms of left ventricular failure.

Pulmonary Vascular Congestion. The symptoms of pulmonary vascular congestion are dyspnea, orthopnea, paroxysmal nocturnal dyspnea, cough, and acute pulmonary edema.

Dyspnea, characterized by rapid, shallow breathing and a sensation of difficulty in obtaining adequate air, is distressing to the patient. Occasionally a patient may complain of insomnia, restlessness, or weakness, which is caused by the dyspnea.

Orthopnea, the inability to lie flat because of dyspnea, is another common complaint of left ventricular failure related to pulmonary vascular congestion. It is important to determine if the orthopnea is truly related to heart disease or whether elevating the head to sleep is merely the patient's custom. For example, if the patient states that he sleeps on three pillows, one might hasten to believe that he is suffering from orthopnea. If, however, when asked why he sleeps on three pillows, he replies that he does this because he likes to sleep at this elevation and

has done so since before he had symptomatic heart disease, the condition does not qualify as orthopnea.

Paroxysmal nocturnal dyspnea (PND) is a well-known complaint characterized by the patient's awakening in the middle of the night because of intense shortness of breath. Nocturnal dyspnea is thought to be caused by a shift of fluid from the tissues into the intravascular compartment as a result of recumbency. During the day the pressure in the veins is high, especially in the dependent portions of the body, due to gravity, increased fluid volume, and increased sympathetic tone. With this increase in hydrostatic pressure, some fluid escapes into the tissue space. With recumbency, the pressure in the dependent capillaries is decreased, and fluid is resorbed into the circulation. This increased volume represents an additional amount of blood which is presented to the heart to pump each minute (increased preload) and places an additional burden on an already congested pulmonary vascular bed, with acute onset of dyspnea the resultant symptom.

An *irritating cough* is one symptom of pulmonary vascular congestion that is often overlooked, but which may be a dominant symptom. It may be productive but is usually dry and hacking in character. This symptom is related to congestion of bronchial mucosa and an associated increase in mucus production.

Acute pulmonary edema is the most florid clinical picture associated with pulmonary vascular congestion. It occurs when the pulmonary capillary pressure exceeds the pressure which tends to keep fluid within the vascular channels (around 30 torr). At these pressures, there is transduction of fluid into the alveoli, which in turn diminishes the area available for the normal transport of oxygen into and carbon dioxide out of the blood within the pulmonary capillary bed. Acute pulmonary edema is characterized by intense dyspnea, cough, orthopnea, profound anxiety, cyanosis, sweating, noisy respirations, and very often chest pain and a pink, frothy sputum from the mouth. It constitutes a genuine medical emergency and must be managed vigorously and promptly.

Decreased Cardiac Output. In addition to the symptoms that result from pulmonary vascular congestion, left ventricular failure is also associated with nonspecific symptoms that are related to decreased cardiac output. The patient may complain of weakness, fatigability, apathy, lethargy, difficulty in concentrating, memory deficit, or diminished exercise tolerance. These symptoms may be present in chronic low output states and may dominate the patient's complaints. Unfortunately, these symptoms are nonspecific and are often ascribed to depression, neurosis, or functional complaints. Therefore, these potentially important indicators of deteriorating pump function are often not recognized for their true value, and the patient is either inappropriately reassured or placed on a tranquilizer or mood elevating preparation. Remember, the presence of the nonspecific symptoms of low cardiac output demands a careful evaluation of the heart as well as the psyche — an examination that will yield the information that will dictate proper management.

Heart Sounds and Rales. Physical signs associated with left ventricular failure that are easily recognized at the bedside include third and fourth heart sounds and rales in the lungs.

The fourth heart sound, or *atrial gallop,* is associated with and follows atrial contraction and is best heard with the bell of the stethoscope very lightly applied at the cardiac apex. The left lateral position may be required to elicit the sound. It is heard just before the first heart sound and is not always a definitive sign of congestive failure but may represent decreased compliance (increased stiffness) of the myocardium. It therefore may be an early, premonitory indication of impending failure. A fourth heart sound is common in patients with acute myocardial infarction, and likely does not have prognostic significance, but it may represent incipient failure.

On the other hand, a third sound, or *ventricular gallop,* is an important sign of left ventricular failure and in adults is almost never present in the absence of significant heart disease. Most physicians would agree that treatment of congestive failure is indicated upon the appearance of this sign.

The third sound is heard in early diastole following the second heart sound and is associated with the period of rapid passive ventricular filling. It is also best heard with the bell of the stethoscope applied lightly at the apex, with the patient in the left lateral position, and at the end of expiration.

The fine *moist rales* most commonly heard at the bases of the lungs posteriorly are often recognized as evidence of left ventricular failure, as indeed they may be. Before these rales are ascribed to pump failure, the patient must be instructed to cough deeply in order to open any basilar alveoli that may be compressed as a result of recumbency, inactivity, and compression from the diaphragm beneath. Rales that fail to clear after cough (posttussic) need to be evaluated; those that clear following cough are probably clinically unimportant. It is, however, important to note that the patient may have good evidence of left ventricular failure on the basis of a history of symptoms suggesting pulmonary vascular congestion or the finding of a third heart sound at the apex and yet have quite clear lung fields. It is not appropriate to wait for the appearance of rales in the lungs before instituting therapy for left ventricular failure.

Arrhythmias. Since an increase in heart rate is the heart's initial response to stress, sinus tachycardia might be expected and is often found in the examination of a patient with pump failure. Other rhythms associated with pump failure include atrial premature contractions, paroxysmal atrial tachycardia, and ventricular premature beats. Whenever a rhythm abnormality is detected, one must attempt to define the underlying pathophysiological mechanism; therapy can then be properly planned and instituted.

Other Signs. Other signs of left ventricular failure that may be noted in addition to a third heart sound, rales in the lungs, and supraventricular rhythms include: wheezing breath sounds, pulsus alternans (an alternating greater and lesser volume of the arterial pulse), a square-wave response to a standard Valsalva maneuver (see below), weight gain, and Cheyne-Stokes respirations. Indeed, patients may awaken at night during respiratory height of a Cheyne-Stokes cycle, a situation that may falsely be interpreted as PND but which may have the same pathophysiological significance. Weight gain resulting from retention of salt and water by the kidneys is a useful sign that the patient may follow at home. Daily weight should be recorded, the observation made in the morning after voiding and before breakfast.

Radiographic Findings. Radiographic examination of the chest is often helpful in making a diagnosis of heart failure. Careful evaluation of the chest roentgenogram may demonstrate changes in the blood vessels of the lungs that result from an increase in pulmonary venous pressure. Radiographic findings may be present in the absence of rales, and careful examination of the chest film is necessary if left ventricular failure is suspected.

RIGHT VENTRICULAR FAILURE

Failure of the *right ventricle* alone is often the result of severe underlying lung disease and such conditions as severe pulmonary hypertension (primary or secondary), stenosis of the pulmonary valve, or a massive pulmonary embolus. The right ventricle tolerates a volume load well, and pure right ventricular failure is usually due to resistance to outflow (pressure load). More commonly, however, right ventricular failure is the result of failure of the left ventricle. In this situation, symptoms and signs of both left and right ventricular failure are present, and the symptoms of left ventricular failure may improve as the right ventricle fails, through relief of left ventricular preload and decrease in pulmonary vascular congestion.

Low Cardiac Output. In contrast to left ventricular failure, in which specific symptoms can usually be related to a single underlying mechanism—pulmonary vascular congestion—the symptoms of right heart failure are not so specific, and many are related to a low cardiac output. Fatigability, weakness, lethargy, or difficulty in concentrating may be prominent. Heaviness of the limbs, especially the legs, an increase in abdominal girth, inability to wear previously comfortable shoes, and weight gain reflect the ascites and edema associated with right ventricular failure.

In addition, symptoms of the underlying pulmonary disease usually dominate complaints if failure is due to a primary pulmonary problem, usually chronic bronchitis or emphysema. Occasionally bronchiectasis or restrictive lung disease may be the primary pulmonary problem, but chronic bronchitis and emphysema are by far the most common pulmonary causes of right ventricular failure.

Engorgement of Jugular Veins. When the right ventricle decompensates, there is dilatation of the chamber, an increase in right ventricular end–diastolic volume and pressure, resistance to filling of the ventricle, and a subsequent rise in right atrial pressure. This increasing pressure is in turn reflected upstream in the venae cavae and can be recognized by an increase in the jugular venous pressure. This is best evaluated by looking at the veins in the neck and noting the height of the column of blood. With the patient lying in bed and the head of the bed elevated between 30° and 60°, the column of blood in the external jugular veins will be, in normal individuals, only a few millimeters above the upper border of the clavicle, if it is seen at all.

When an observation of venous pressure is recorded, the height of the column of blood above the sternal angle and the elevation of the head of the bed should be included. This will then provide a useful basis for comparison of future observations.

Edema. Edema is often considered a reliable sign of heart failure, and, indeed, it is often present when the right ventricle has failed. However, it is the least reliable sign of right ventricular dysfunction. Many people, particularly the elderly, spend much of their time sitting in a chair with the legs dependent. As a result of this body position, the decreased turgor of subcutaneous tissue associated with old age, and perhaps primary venous disease such as varicosities, ankle edema may be produced that reflects these factors rather than right ventricular failure.

When edema does appear related to failure of the right ventricle, it is dependent in location. If the patient is up and about, it will be noted primarily in the ankles and will ascend the legs as failure worsens. When the patient is put to bed, the dependent portion of the body becomes the sacral area, and edema should be looked for there. In addition, other signs of right ventricular failure should be present before the diagnosis is made. Dependent edema alone is inadequate documentation of the status of the right ventricle. With congestion of the liver, this organ may enlarge and become tender, ascites may be present, and jaundice may be noted.

Other Signs. As with left ventricular failure, sinus tachycardia and the other rhythms associated with pump failure may be present. In addition, right ventricular third and fourth heart sounds are not uncommon. They are best heard at the lower left sternal border, with the bell of the stethoscope applied lightly to the chest, and can be recognized by an increase in intensity with inspiration. Finally, signs of any underlying cause of right ventricular failure may be present, such as hyperresonance with percussion, low immobile diaphragms, decreased breath sounds, increased anteroposterior chest diameter, and use of the accessory muscles of respiration in patients with severe pulmonary emphysema.

VALSALVA MANEUVER IN DIAGNOSIS

The Valsalva maneuver has been used in the diagnosis of heart failure and has a long and interesting history.[4] It is discussed here more for its general clinical interest rather than as an important diagnostic maneuver in suspected heart failure.

The Valsalva maneuver has also been implicated as causing an occasional fatality either through the production of a cardiac arrhythmia or through the dislodging of venous thrombi, producing massive pulmonary embolization.

A standard Valsalva maneuver is produced by blowing into a mercury manometer to a pressure of 40 torr and sustaining this effort for 10 seconds. Naturally, a patient does not do this on his own during the day but may closely simulate the maneuver during a prolonged effort of straining at stool. Intermittent positive pressure breathing may produce short periods of a similar type of strain, as may a cough or sneeze.

In the normal response to the Valsalva maneuver there are four phases.

Phase I occurs with the onset of strain at which time there is an increase in intrathoracic pressure, which is transmitted to the great vessels (aorta and pulmonary artery) and leads to a rise in arterial blood pressure.

During *phase II,* as a later result of the increased intrathoracic pressure and limitation of venous return to the heart, there is a decrease in right atrial filling and a decrease in left ventricular stroke volume, producing a fall in arterial blood pressure and pulse pressure (the difference between the systolic and diastolic pressures). This fall in pressure stimulates the receptors in the carotid sinus, aortic arch, and common carotid artery, which are sensitive to pressure and which in turn cause an increase in sympathetic activity, resulting in an increase in heart rate and peripheral vasoconstriction. At the bedside, phase II is characterized by an increase in heart rate and a fall in blood pressure.

With *phase III,* or release of the strain, there is an increased venous return to the right heart and an increase in blood volume in the pulmonary vascular bed. This is ultimately transmitted to the left side of the heart, with an associated increase in the left ventricular stroke volume as the left ventricle once again fills. Because it takes a few seconds for the pulmonary vascular bed to fill with blood before it reaches the left heart, there may be a continuous fall in cardiac output and blood pressure for 2 to 3 seconds immediately upon the release of the strain.

Phase IV is called the *overshoot* and is characterized by bradycardia and a rise in blood pressure over the resting observed values. This occurs because the increased left ventricular stroke volume is ejected into a constricted peripheral vascular bed. This constricted bed causes an increase in peripheral resistance, and the pressure therefore rises. The pressure-sensitive receptors in the carotid body sense the higher pressure, and parasympathetic activity through the vagus nerve is stimulated, causing a reflex slowing of the heart. The overshoot period is then characterized by blood pressure that is greater than the initial resting values and by bradycardia.

In *heart failure,* the response to the Valsalva maneuver is quite different. As the strain begins, there is a rise in intrathoracic pressure. This rise in pressure is transmitted and is noted as an increase in the peripheral arterial pressure. However, as the strain continues, there is no decrease in pressure and no increase in the heart rate. Upon release of the maneuver, the blood pressure returns to the baseline values, and there is no overshoot.

This kind of response, in which there is only a rise in arterial pressure without any heart-rate changes and no overshoot response, has been called *the square-wave response* and is due to the fact that the failing myocardium, with its already maximized preload, will not change total stroke volume enough to decrease cardiac output further and stimulate the pressor receptors. The same kind of response is seen in patients with a significant atrial septal defect, since the preload to the right ventricle remains high because of the shunt from the left to the right atrium.

A pilot study designed to serially evaluate the Valsalva maneuver in 51 postinfarction patients showed it to be an insensitive indicator of an impending acute event.*

Management of Heart Failure

Heart failure may be present in varying degrees of severity. In acute myocardial infarction, heart failure has been simply and usefully classified by Killip into four classes: I, no failure; II, mild to moderate failure; III, acute pulmonary edema; and IV, cardiogenic shock.[5]

Early, moderate (Killip class II) and chronic failure are often characterized by a third heart sound, increased heart rate (usually sinus rhythm), and possibly fine posttussic crackling rales at the lung bases. In addition, evidence of pulmonary vascular congestion (often without

*HL Brammell: unpublished observations

pulmonary edema) is often present on the chest roentgenogram, and arrhythmias may be present: atrial premature contractions, atrial fibrillation, atrial flutter, paroxysmal atrial tachycardia, and junctional rhythms. The patient may be reasonably comfortable at rest or may have symptoms of low cardiac output or pulmonary vascular congestion. Symptoms are increased with activity.

Acute pulmonary edema (Killip class III) is a life-threatening situation characterized by transudation of fluid from the pulmonary capillary bed into the alveolar spaces, with associated extreme dyspnea and anxiety. Immediate care is required if the patient's life is to be saved.

Cardiogenic shock (Killip class IV) is the most ominous pump failure syndrome and has the highest mortality, even with aggressive care. Cardiogenic shock is recognized clinically by

- A systolic blood pressure less than 80 torr (often it cannot be measured)
- A feeble pulse that is often rapid
- Pale, cool, and sweaty skin that is frequently cyanotic
- Restlessness, confusion, and apathy
- Possible coma, although not usual
- Decreased or absent urine output

These manifestations of shock are a reflection of the profound inadequacy of the heart as a pump and usually reflect a large amount of muscle damage (40% or more of the left ventricular mass).

Some patients with significant, long-standing arterial hypertension will have manifestations of cardiogenic shock at relatively normal pressures. These people require a higher pressure to perfuse vital organs and maintain viability. Knowledge of the preceding blood pressure history is of great importance in recognizing these people. Not all clinical circumstances of cardiogenic shock are associated with an inadequate cardiac output, however. Depending on modifying circumstances, such as fever, the cardiac output may occasionally be normal or even increased.

The failure to decrease coronary care unit mortality below 10% to 15% is largely due to only modest improvement in the management and mortality of severe pump failure syndromes, especially cardiogenic shock.

PLAN

The physiological responses to heart failure form a rational basis for treatment. The goals of the management of congestive heart failure are to reduce the work of the heart, to increase car-diac output and myocardial contractility, and to decrease retention of salt and water.

Bed Rest. Since the heart cannot be put to complete rest to heal in the same fashion as a broken bone, the best that can be done is to put the entire patient to rest; thereby, through inactivity the overall pumping demand on the heart is decreased. *Bed rest* is therefore an important part of the treatment of congestive heart failure, especially in acute and refractory stages.

In addition to decreasing the overall work demands made on the heart, bed rest assists in lowering the work load by decreasing the intravascular volume through a recumbency-induced diuresis.[6] Studies of prolonged bed rest have demonstrated that within 48 to 72 hours of inactivity there is a decrease of plasma volume of 300 ml or more. While this is not a great volume in terms of the overall intravascular fluid compartment, it does assist in decreasing the volume load that is presented to the failing heart. It therefore assists in decreasing dilatation of the heart chambers and establishing a compensated state. This effect results from stimulation of atrial stretch receptors that sense the increased volume of blood returning to the right side of the heart, which would be sequestered in the lower extremities if the patient were upright. These receptors then "turn off" the production of antidiuretic hormone, and a diuresis follows. By decreasing intravascular volume and therefore the amount of blood presented to the heart to pump (preload), compensation of the heart may be enhanced.

Diuretics. In addition to bed rest, *salt and water restriction* and *diuretics,* either oral or parenteral, will also decrease preload and the work of the heart.

All diuretics, regardless of the route of administration, may cause significant changes in the serum electrolytes, especially potassium and chloride. Therefore, regular determination of serum electrolytes is important in patient follow-up. This is particularly true when the patient is also receiving digitalis, because low potassium produced by diuretics predisposes to digitalis toxicity, a life-threatening but avoidable complication. Because of this possibility, potassium supplements are customarily ordered when potassium-depleting diuretics are given, especially when digitalis is given as well.

The choice of route of administration of the diuretic is largely a function of the gravity of the clinical situation: mild to moderate left ventricular failure (manifested by sinus tachycardia, posttussic rales, and a third heart sound) can usually be managed with oral preparations. On the other hand, acute pulmonary edema, a life-threatening situation, demands more drastic approaches, and the parenteral route should be chosen.

Other modifiers of preload and afterload are valuable approaches to the management of acute and chronic failure states. Both pharmacologic and mechanical methods are useful.

Morphine. *Morphine* is the single most useful drug in the treatment of pulmonary edema. It achieves its primary physiological usefulness through a peripheral vasodilating effect, forming a peripheral pool of blood (bloodless phlebotomy) that decreases venous return and decreases the work of the heart. In addition, morphine allays the great anxiety associated with severe dyspnea and quiets the patient, thereby decreasing the respiratory pump mechanism for increasing venous return. Morphine also decreases arterial blood pressure and resistance, lessening the work of the heart (decreased afterload).

Reduce Circulating Blood Volume. An even more dramatic method for decreasing preload and the work of the heart is *phlebotomy,* a procedure that is often useful in the patient with acute pulmonary edema because it immediately removes a volume of blood from the central circulation, decreases venous return and filling pressure, and provides rather prompt reversal of some basic hemodynamic problems.

Phlebotomy may be bloodless *(rotating tourniquets),* or whole blood may be directly removed from the circulation. Tourniquets are less effective than direct removal of blood.

While often helpful in managing acute pulmonary edema, phlebotomy may be dangerous in the patient who does not have an increased intravascular volume. This situation most commonly occurs in patients with acute myocardial infarction in whom there is extensive muscle damage and rapid onset of pulmonary edema before the kidneys can compensate for a diminished cardiac output by sodium and water retention.

Patients with normal blood volume and pulmonary edema usually have a normal-sized heart on chest roentgenogram. Removing a unit of blood from the circulation either by use of tourniquets or by venesection may cause a significant drop in blood pressure in these patients. On the other hand, the person with more chronic congestive heart failure with an increased intravascular volume and dilatation of the heart in association with pulmonary edema is often an excellent candidate for rotating tourniquets or venesection.

Nitrates. The use of *nitrates,* both acutely and chronically, has been advocated in the management of heart failure.[7] By causing peripheral vasodilatation, the heart is "unloaded" (decreased afterload), with a subsequent increase in cardiac output, decrease in pulmonary artery wedge pressure (a measurement which reflects the degree of pulmonary vascular congestion and the severity of left ventricular failure), and decrease in myocardial oxygen consumption. This form of therapy has been found useful in mild to moderate failure and acute pulmonary edema failure associated with myocardial infarction, chronic refractory left ventricular failure, and failure associated with severe mitral regurgitation. At the present time, the use of parenteral vasodilator therapy (sodium nitroprusside) requires accurate hemodynamic monitoring of arterial and pulmonary wedge pressure (arterial cannula and Swan-Ganz catheter) and use of an infusion pump to carefully titrate the dose delivered.

Nitroprusside must be used with care. Long-acting nitrate therapy is usually given with isosorbide dinitrate (sublingual or oral, the former being preferred) or nitroglycerin ointment. Some patients who have received maximum benefit from other forms of therapy for left ventricular failure have been substantially improved by vasodilator treatment.

Digitalis. While modification of the work of the heart through decreasing preload and afterload is indicated in heart failure and at times permits avoidance of drugs that increase the force of myocardial contraction, inotropic agents remain important therapeutic tools.

Digitalis is the primary drug for increasing contractility. This inotropic drug has a multiplicity of uses in cardiology and is also potentially one of the most dangerous, a fact recognized in 1785 by William Withering, discoverer of the pharmacologic value and toxicity of digitalis (foxglove): "Foxglove when given in very large and quickly repeated doses occasions sickness, vomiting, purging, confused vision, objects appearing green or yellow, increased secretion of urine with frequent motions to part with it and sometimes inability to retain it; slow pulse even as low as 35 in a minute, cold sweats, convulsions, syncope and death."[8] In the failing heart, digitalis slows the ventricular rate and increases the force of contraction, increasing cardiac efficiency. As cardiac output increases, a greater volume of fluid is presented to the kidneys for filtration and excretion, and intravascular volume decreases.

In early failure with acute myocardial infarction, digitalis may increase the potential amount of damaged myocardium by causing increased contractility and therefore increased myocardial oxygen demand. Treatment of failure in this circumstance is probably best if preload or afterload is decreased through the use of diuretics or nitrates. Of course, if either agent causes a significant drop in central aortic pressure, coronary artery perfusion may fall and the area of damage increase. The key lessons here are that any medication has potentially ominous side-effects, that a management regimen must be selected with care and with a full understanding of potential adverse effects, and that close patient monitoring is mandatory.

Other Measures. Cardiogenic shock unfortunately is not a completely understood situation at this time. Accordingly, the management of cardiogenic shock is generally unsatisfactory. At the very least, treatment requires administration of bicarbonate to correct the metabolic acidosis, oxygen, and agents to elevate the blood pressure. The most commonly used pressor agents at this time are dopamine, norepinephrine, and glucagon. Depending upon the pulmonary artery wedge pressure (left ventricular filling pressure), the administration of small amounts of fluid may be indicated. Mechanical life-support devices such as intra-aortic balloon counterpulsation, direct ventricular assistors, or left heart bypass are occasionally used. The intra-aortic balloon assist device has been the most

successful to date and has established a place in cardiac care.

The general outlook for patients with cardiogenic shock is poor for both the short and the long term. Heart failure, with its accompanying symptoms of low cardiac output and/or pulmonary vascular congestion, is one of the major sources of disability in cardiovascular disease. Its recognition and pathophysiologically based management are of paramount importance if a patient's functional capacity and vocational and community viability are to be optimized and maintained.

REFERENCES

1. Fox SM, Gazes PC, Blackburn HW et al: Exercise and stress testing workshop report. J SC Med Assoc 65:74, 1969
2. Lewis T: Diseases of the Heart. New York, Macmillan, 1933
3. Longo EA, Cohen LS: Rupture of interventricular septum in acute myocardial infarction. Am Heart J 92:81, 1976
4. Judson WE, Hatcher, JD, Wilkins RW: Blood pressure responses to the Valsalva maneuver in cardiac patients with and without congestive failure. Circulation 11:889, 1955
5. Killip T, Kimball JT: Treatment of myocardial infarction in a coronary care unit: A two-year experience with 250 patients. Am J Cardiol 20:457, 1967
6. Miller PB, Johnson RL, Lamb LE: Effects of four weeks of absolute bed rest on circulatory function in man. Aerospace Med 35:1194, 1964
7. DaLuz PL, Forrester JS: Influence of vasodilators upon function and metabolism of ischemic myocardium. Am J Cardiol 37:581, 1976
8. Withering W: An Account of the Foxglove and its Medical Uses, with Practical Remarks on Dropsy and Other Diseases. London, C.G.J. and J. Robinson, 1785

SUGGESTED READING

Mason DT (ed): Congestive Heart Failure: Mechanisms, Evaluation and Treatment. New York, Yorke Medical Books, 1976

Management Modalities: Cardiovascular System

9

Shirley J. Hoffman
Alva R. Degner

CARDIAC MONITORING

Monitoring the patient with cardiac disturbances is now accepted as routine practice. Since the first hard wire bedside monitor, modern electronics has made constant sophisticated advances in monitoring equipment. Remote display systems currently incorporate features such as *nonfade scopes,* which keep the electrocardiogram (ECG) pattern visible across the screen; *freeze* modes, which allow the ECG pattern to be held for more detailed examination; *storage capability,* either by tape loops or an electronic memory, which permits retrieval of arrhythmias from 8 to 60 seconds after their occurrence; *automatic chart documentation,* in which the ECG recorder is activated by alarms or at preset intervals; *heart rate monitors,* which display the rate either by meter or by digital display (the alarm system is incorporated into the heart-rate monitor with adjustments for both the high and low settings); *multiparameter displays,* which offer display of pressures, temperature, electroencephalogram (EEG), respirations, and so forth; and *computer systems,* which store and analyze ECG data. The information can then be retrieved at any time to aid in diagnosis and to note trends in the patient's status.

Two types of patient monitoring equipment presently in use are hard wire devices and telemetry. Hard wire monitors require an electrical cable between the patient and the ECG display device. Telemetry simply requires the patient to carry a small battery-operated transmitter. No wire connection is needed between the patient and the ECG display device. In addition to the *transmitter,* which has a frequency similar to radio stations, telemetry systems require *receivers,* which pick up and display the signal on a scope, and *antennas,* which are built into the receiver and which may be mounted in the vicinity of the receiver to widen the range of signal pick-up. Batteries are the power source for the transmitter, thus making it possible to avoid electrical hazards by isolating the monitoring system from potential current leakage and accidental shock.

Manufacturers of hard wire and telemetry monitoring systems provide operating instructions, which should be followed to insure proper and safe functioning of the equipment.

ELECTRODE APPLICATION

A high quality trace will exhibit a narrow, stable baseline, absence of distortion or "noise," and sufficient amplitude of the QRS complex to properly activate the rate meters and alarm systems and to allow for identification of P waves.

Figures 9-1 and 9-2 show suggested electrode placements for hard wire monitoring. Since telemetry requires no ground electrode, two electrodes are placed in the positive and negative positions for the limb leads or for MCL_1.

Types of Electrodes

Needle electrodes are placed under the skin and thus eliminate variations caused by skin resistance. However, they are traumatic and provide a source of infection because of the break in skin integrity, and therefore they are not appropriate for long-term use. Metal disk electrodes are cumbersome and restricting to the patient. Considerable artifact occurs because of the inability to seal the disk adequately to the skin.

Disposable silver- or nickle-plated electrodes centered in a circle of adhesive paper or foam rubber are currently used for cardiac monitoring. Most electrodes are pre-gelled by the manufacturer. They may have disposable wires attached to the electrodes or nondisposable wires that snap onto the electrodes. They are comfortable for the patient, but if not properly applied, undue artifact and false alarms may result.

Portable monitor-defibrillators are now available in which the defibrillator paddles can be used as electrodes for rapid institution of monitoring in emergencies. The two paddles are placed on the chest and act as positive and negative electrodes. This provides a tracing on the oscilloscope and allows for immediate treatment of arrhythmias.

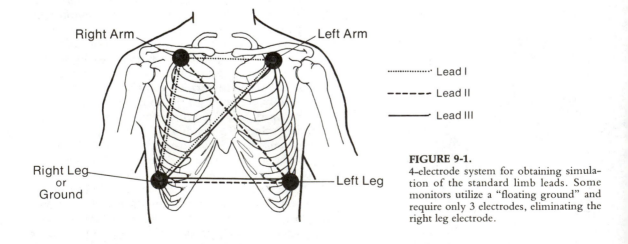

FIGURE 9-1.
4-electrode system for obtaining simulation of the standard limb leads. Some monitors utilize a "floating ground" and require only 3 electrodes, eliminating the right leg electrode.

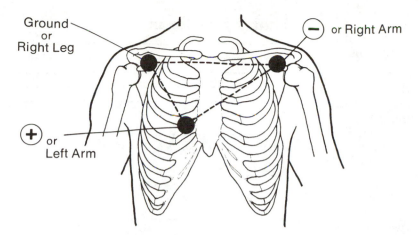

Ground
or
Right Leg

⊖ or Right Arm

⊕ or
Left Arm

FIGURE 9-2.
Marriott's MCL$_1$. (Use Lead I selection.)

ECG MONITOR PROBLEM SOLVING

Baseline But No ECG Trace
- Is the size (gain or sensitivity) control properly adjusted?
- Is appropriate lead selector being used on monitor?
- Is the patient cable fully inserted into ECG receptacle?
- Are electrode wires fully inserted into patient cable?
- Are electrode wires firmly attached to electrodes?
- Are electrode wires damaged?
- Is the patient cable damaged?
- Call for service if trace is still absent.

Intermittent Trace
- Is patient cable fully inserted into monitor receptacle?
- Are electrode wires fully inserted into patient cable?
- Are electrode wires firmly attached to electrodes?
- Are electrode wire connectors loose or worn?
- Have electrodes been applied properly?
- Are electrodes properly located and in firm skin contact?
- Is patient cable damaged?

Wandering or Irregular Baseline
- Is there excessive cable movement? This can be reduced by clipping to patient's clothing.
- Is the power cord on or near the monitor cable?
- Is there excessive movement by the patient? Does he have muscle tremors from anxiety or shivering?
- Is site selection correct?
- Was proper skin prep and application followed?
- Are the electrodes still moist?

Low Amplitude Complexes
- Is size control adjusted properly?
- Were the electrodes applied properly?

- Is there dried gel on the electrodes?
- Change electrode sites. Check 12-lead ECG for lead with highest amplitude and attempt to simulate that lead.
- If none of the above steps remedies the problem, the weak signal may be the patient's normal complex.

Sixty Cycle Interference
- Is the monitor size control set too high?
- Are there nearby electrical devices in use, especially poorly grounded ones?
- Were the electrodes applied properly?
- Is there dried gel on the electrodes?
- Are lead wires or connections damaged?

Excessive Triggering of Heart Rate Alarms
- Is Hi–Low alarm set too close to patient's rate?
- Is monitor sensitivity level set too high or too low?
- Is patient cable securely inserted into monitor receptacle?
- Are lead wires or connections damaged?
- Has the electrode site been properly selected? A site of low amplitude may cause failure of the monitor to sense each QRS.
- Were electrodes applied properly?
- Is the baseline unstable, or is there excessive cable or lead wire movement? Check steps to remedy the problem.

Skin Irritation
- Is there a residue of alcohol or acetone or skin conditioners on the skin under the electrodes?
- Was the skin dry before the electrodes were applied?
- Was skin preparation technique harsh?
- Is the patient sensitive to gels, adhesives, or prep solutions?
- Is there DC leakage from the monitor?

Skin Preparation

Proper skin preparation and application of electrodes are imperative to good monitoring.

1. Select site. Avoid bony protuberances, joints, and folds in skin. Areas where muscle attaches to bone have the least motion artifact.
2. Shave excessive body hair from site.
3. Remove residue from oils, lotion, and so forth used in patient care. Sites must be free of any oil film or residue which could affect electrode adhesion.

It is important to follow the electrode manufacturer's directions for skin preparation because the chemical reaction between alcohol or other skin prep materials and the adhesives used in some electrodes may cause skin irritation or nonadhesion to the skin.

The electrode manufacturer's directions should also be followed in the application of electrodes. Proper application of electrodes will ensure a good monitor trace and comfort for the patient.

SOLVING ECG MONITOR PROBLEMS

Several problems may occur in monitoring ECG, including baseline but no ECG trace, intermittent traces, wandering or irregular baseline, low amplitude complexes, 60 cycle interference, excessive triggering of heart rate alarms, and skin irritation. The steps to take when such problems occur are outlined in the chart titled ECG Monitor Problem Solving.

BIBLIOGRAPHY

Andreoli K et al: Comprehensive Cardiac Care, 4th ed. St. Louis, C. V. Mosby, 1979

Hammond C: Plain talk about cardiac monitoring. RN 42:34–43, 1979

Marriott H, Fogg E: Constant monitoring for cardiac dysrhythmias. Mod Concepts Cardiovasc Dis 39:103–108, 1970

Vinsant MO: Commonsense Approach to Coronary Care. St. Louis, C. V. Mosby, 1981

Whley HN: Present status of monitoring in the coronary care unit. Heart Lung 7:67–68, 1978

Shirley J. Hoffman

ARTIFICIAL CARDIAC PACING*

Electrical stimulation of the heart was tried experimentally as early as 1819. In 1930 Hyman noted that he could inject the right atrium with a diversity of substances and restore a heartbeat. He devised an "ingenious apparatus" that he labeled an *artificial pacemaker,* which delivered a rhythmic charge to the heart. In 1952 Zoll demonstrated that patients with Stokes–Adams syndrome could be sustained by the administration of current directly to the chest wall. Lillehei in 1957 affixed electrodes directly to the ventricles during open-heart surgery. In the period 1958 to 1961, implantable pacemakers for treatment of complete heart block came into use in a rather extensive fashion. Over subsequent years, various improvements and refinements have been and continue to be made for both short-term temporary pacing and long-term permanent pacing.

INDICATIONS FOR ARTIFICIAL PACING

Artificial cardiac pacing is indicated for any condition that results in failure of the heart to initiate or conduct an intrinsic electrical impulse at a rate normally adequate to maintain body perfusion. It may be used prophylactically when certain arrhythmias or conduction defects warn of such failure. Cardiac pacing may also be used to interrupt tachyarrhythmias that are unresponsive to other forms of therapy.

Bradyarrhythmias that may preclude adequate cardiac output include symptomatic sinus bradycardia, sinus arrest, sick sinus syndrome, and symptomatic second and third degree heart

*We wish to acknowledge the contribution of Alva R. Degner, R.N. to the preparation of this section in previous editions of the book.

blocks. The effect on the patient and the underlying cause of each of these rhythms must be evaluated when considering artificial pacing as a mode of therapy or when considering the need for permanent pacing.

Heart Block. Mobitz I (Wenckebach) second degree block following inferior myocardial infarction is most often asymptomatic and transient and usually does not require pacing. Mobitz II second degree block resulting from anterior myocardial infarction is a much less stable rhythm. It may result in sudden third degree block with a slow ventricular rhythm or even ventricular standstill and usually requires pacing. Bifascicular block (right bundle branch block with hemiblock of the left bundle branch) following anterior myocardial infarction is considered an indication for pacing by many physicians, since this can also result in symptomatic third degree block or ventricular standstill.

Third degree (complete) block may or may not be an indication for pacing, depending upon the anatomic site of the block. Complete block in the atrioventricular (AV) node usually results in a junctional escape rhythm with an adequate heart rate. It is usually transient and does not require pacing. Complete block at the level of the bundle branches, however, requires an escape focus in the Purkinje fibers to stimulate the ventricles. If such a focus arises, it will usually depolarize the ventricles at a rate that is too slow to provide adequate cardiac output, and the patient will require artificial pacing.

Sick sinus syndrome is often manifested by alternating tachycardia and bradycardia (tachy-brady syndrome). This requires artificial pacing for the bradycardia and suppressive antiarrhythmic therapy to control the tachyarrhythmia.

Persistent ventricular tachycardia is sometimes successfully suppressed by overdriving with an artificial pacemaker. Pacing is used occasionally to suppress supraventricular tachyarrhythmias.

Rapid atrial pacing may be used to induce atrial fibrillation in the patient whose chronic atrial fibrillation has been converted to sinus rhythm with inadequate rate. Recently, pacing has been used successfully to prevent symptoms of severe bradycardia due to vagal reaction or hypersensitive carotid body.

The critical care nurse should anticipate any of the above arrhythmias in patients who have atherosclerotic heart disease, acute myocardial infarction, or digitalis toxicity. Myocardial fibrosis and cardiomyopathies may cause these arrhythmias; occasionally, heart block may be of congenital origin.

METHODS OF PACING

Various methods of pacing have been used over the years, including external pacing, transthoracic pacing, epicardial pacing, and endocardial pacing.

External pacing, using pacing electrodes on the chest wall and requiring large amounts of electrical energy, is used only in severe emergencies for the unconscious patient. It has been abandoned for use in the conscious patient because of the severe pain and burns associated with this method.

Transthoracic pacing is occasionally used in emergency situations, but it is not suitable for long-term pacing or as prophylaxis against warning arrhythmias. This type of pacing involves introduction of a pacing wire into the heart through a needle in the anterior chest wall.

Epicardial pacing can be accomplished via thoracotomy (or occasionally through a subxyphoid incision) and the placement of pacing electrodes directly on the surface of the heart. This method is often used as a temporary adjunct during and after heart surgery. The pacing wires are sutured to the epicardial surface of the heart, brought outside through the chest incision, and connected to a temporary pacemaker generator. The wires may be removed without reopening the incision after scar tissue has formed over the tips. Permanently implanted epicardial pacemakers are used in patients in whom thoracotomy is warranted, either for surgery or for the specific purpose of pacemaker implantation. Many physicians prefer to use the recently available "screw-in" type electrodes, the tips of which can be rotated into the epicardium (see Fig. 9-3). The main advantage of epicardial pacing is the stability of the electrodes. They have a very low incidence of displacement.

Endocardial pacing using a transvenous pacing catheter is the most common method of pacing. This method can be used for either temporary or permanent pacing. For temporary pacing, the catheter is introduced into a superficial vein with use of local anesthesia. The brachial, femoral,

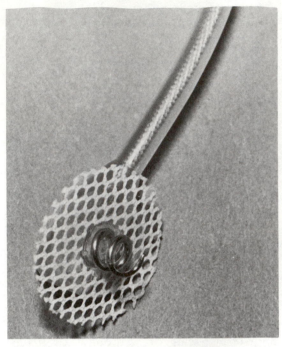

FIGURE 9-3.
Screw-in type electrode for permanent epicardial pacing.

insertion. The balloon is inflated with air in the vena cava and carries the catheter in the direction of blood flow through the right atrium, the tricuspid valve, and into the right ventricle. The balloon is then deflated and lodged against the right ventricular wall.

Some physicians place the tip of the catheter in the pulmonary outflow tract when the right ventricle is enlarged. Since the heart size often decreases after the initiation of effective pacing, this position reduces the risk of perforation of the ventricle relative to positioning in the ventricular apex.

CLASSIFICATION OF PACEMAKERS

Pacemaker Pulse Generators
Pacemaker pulse generators are classified in several ways: temporary, permanent, fixed-rate, or demand.

Temporary generators are those used for short-term pacing. The proximal ends of the pacing catheter are attached to the generator, and the generator is secured to the patient, usually on the

external jugular, or subclavian veins may be used. The subclavian site affords catheter stability and allows for patient mobility; however, pneumothorax may occur as a complication of catheter insertion. The femoral vein affords easy access, but use of this site markedly reduces patient mobility.

The pacing catheter is threaded through the vein, the vena cava, the right atrium, and into the right ventricle. It is lodged between the trabeculae and placed in contact with the endocardial surface of the right ventricle (see Fig. 9-4). The insertion procedure may be done under fluoroscopy. An alternate guide for positioning the catheter is to attach the "V" lead of the ECG machine to the negative (pacing, distal) electrode on the catheter with an alligator clamp (see Fig. 9-5). The distal catheter electrode becomes an "exploring" ECG electrode, and catheter position can be determined by analysis of ECG complex changes as the catheter is advanced. The ECG will reveal a current of injury pattern when the tip of the catheter touches the endocardium.

The experienced clinician can often accomplish "blind" insertion, utilizing only the standard ECG monitor to indicate successful pacing. Many physicians prefer to use the balloon-tipped flow-directed pacing catheter to facilitate

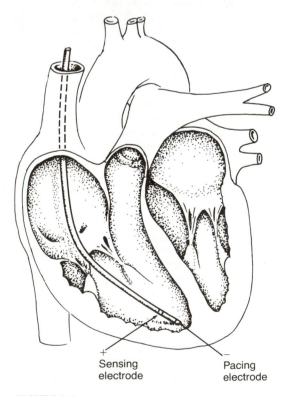

Sensing electrode

Pacing electrode

FIGURE 9-4.
Transvenous pacing catheter in place.

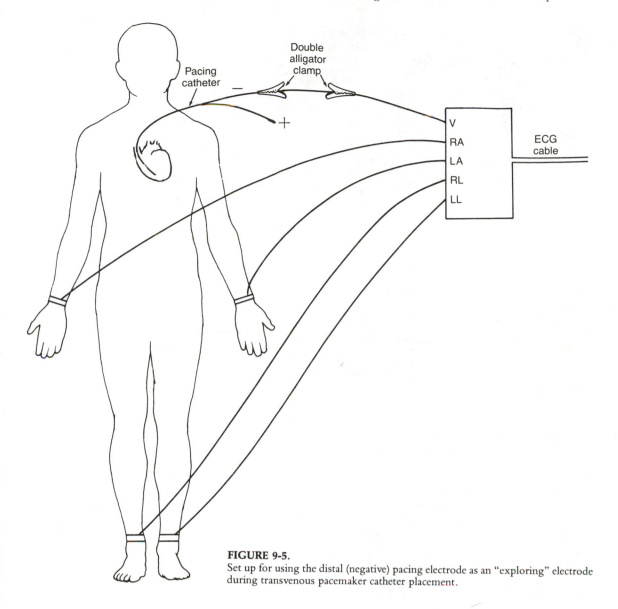

FIGURE 9-5.
Set up for using the distal (negative) pacing electrode as an "exploring" electrode during transvenous pacemaker catheter placement.

arm or abdomen. Once the catheter has been connected to the generator, the nurse must hold the generator until it has been secured to the patient. This will prevent the generator (and the catheter) from being dropped inadvertently to the floor.

Permanent generators, as shown in Figure 9-6, are implanted within the patient, usually in the pectoralis major muscle or overlying the abdomen. The catheter is placed by way of a central vein, and the pacing electrodes are connected subcutaneously to the implanted generator. If the electrodes remain functional at the time of generator battery failure, the electrodes are left intact and only the generator is replaced.

Presently, most permanent pulse generators are powered by lithium batteries that have an expected power life of 7 to 12 years. Although the generators now in use are much smaller in size than those used a few years ago, researchers are continuing their efforts to increase the effective life span and decrease the size of permanent generators.

Pacemaker generators are also classified according to pacing mode. They may be used as fixed-rate pacemakers or in the demand mode.

Fixed-rate (asynchronous) pacemakers discharge an electrical stimulus at a preset interval and function independently of any other electrical activity in the heart. This mode of pacing is

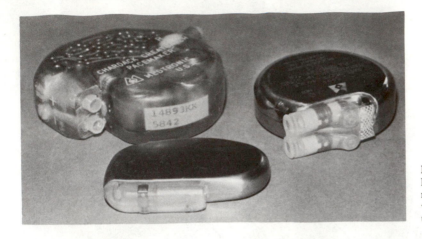

FIGURE 9-6.
Permanent pulse generators, old and new. Note the decrease in size and weight that has been achieved over the years.

used only for patients who are entirely pacemaker dependent (no spontaneous supraventricular impulses reach the ventricles) and free from ventricular depolarization by ectopic beats. If any spontaneous beats are conducted through the ventricles, there is danger of the asynchronous pacemaker initiating a stimulus during the vulnerable period (downstroke) of the T wave and precipitating dangerous ventricular arrhythmias.

Demand (synchronous) pacemakers initiate an impulse only when a preset R-R interval has elapsed without any spontaneous electrical activation of the ventricle. This escape interval is determined by the rate at which the pacemaker is set; that is, if the rate is set at 60 beats per minute, the escape interval is one second. The pacemaker senses and is inhibited by ventricular depolarization. This ability to sense depolarization allows spontaneous ventricular beats to occur without interference from the pacemaker and obviates the risk of pacemaker discharge on the T wave (if the unit is functioning properly). If the patient is

entirely pacemaker dependent, discharge will occur regularly at the preset escape interval. If the patient's spontaneous R-R intervals are shorter than the escape interval of the pacemaker, pacemaker activity is suppressed (see Fig. 9-7).

Occasionally the demand pacemaker will sense high amplitude ventricular repolarizations in addition to depolarizations, thus resetting the escape interval from the T wave on the ECG instead of the QRS (see Fig. 9-8). This situation is not dangerous but results in a pacing rate that is slower than that indicated by the rate setting on the generator. Proper function can be attained by decreasing the sensitivity of the pacemaker until only depolarization is sensed.

Some pacemakers allow for a longer escape interval after a sensed spontaneous beat than the escape interval between subsequent paced beats. This lengthened escape interval, called *rate hysteresis,* provides more opportunity for normal conduction of spontaneous impulses and results in less competition between intrinsic and paced rhythms.

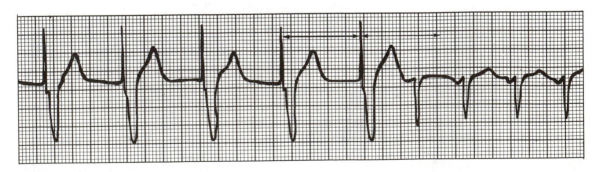

FIGURE 9-7.
Demand pacing. Pacemaker is inhibited by each spontaneous beat that appears at a shorter interval than that indicated on the pacemaker rate settings.

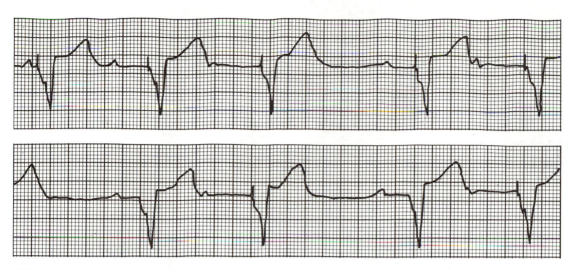

FIGURE 9-8.
Ventricular-inhibited pacemaker sensing T waves.

Variations. Temporary pacemakers can be operated in either the demand or fixed-rate mode. They can be made to discharge at a fixed rate by turning the sensing mechanism off. Permanent demand pacemakers can be converted to fixed-rate by applying a specially manufactured magnet over the implanted generator to turn off the sensing mechanism. This procedure can be used to assess the discharge and capture capabilities of the demand pacemaker (ventricular depolarization by the pacemaker stimulus) that are being inhibited by a spontaneous rhythm.

Many of the newer, permanently implanted pacemakers can be externally programmed. By using a special programmer, changes in rate, energy output, sensitivity, mode, refractory period (period after the QRS during which the pacemaker cannot discharge an impulse), and hysteresis can be accomplished.

A-V Sequential Pacemakers

A-V sequential pacemakers can initiate electrical impulses sequentially in the atria and in the ventricles (see Fig. 9-9). Since atrial contraction contributes 15% to 20% to ventricular stroke volume, patients who have low cardiac reserve will develop hypotension or congestive heart failure without this "atrial kick." When a ventricular pacemaker is used, either A-V dissociation or retrograde atrial conduction results (see Figs. 9-9 and 9-10). In either case, the atria and ventricles do not contract in proper sequence and atrial kick is lost.

The A-V sequential pacemaker has both atrial and ventricular pacing electrodes that pace both chambers in sequence with a preset delay interval (see Fig. 9-11). Both atrial and ventricular impulse discharges are reset by *ventricular* stimuli. The atrial electrode does *not* sense P waves (see Fig. 9-12). It resets its timing from the QRS

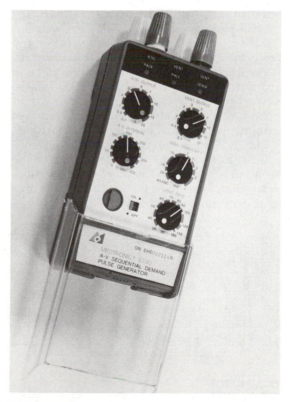

FIGURE 9-9.
A-V sequential temporary pulse generator.

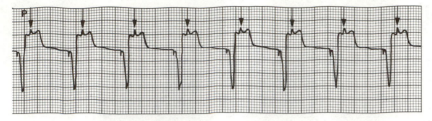

FIGURE 9-10.
(A) Pacing with retrograde conduction. Each pacemaker stimulus is conducted retrograde through the atria as well as antegrade through the ventricles. Retrograde atrial conduction produces a P wave after each paced QRS.

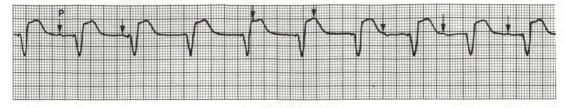

FIGURE 9-10.
(B) Pacing with A-V dissociation. P waves are dissociated from paced QRSs, indicating that pacemaker stimulus is not conducted retrograde to atria.

and stimulates the atria at the preset escape interval after the last QRS. The ventricular electrode senses the same QRS and stimulates the ventricles at an escape interval equal to the atrial escape interval plus the preset A-V delay interval.

If the atrial impulse is conducted to the ventricles before the A-V delay interval has elapsed, the ventricular electrode will sense this impulse and will be inhibited (see Fig. 9-13). These mechanisms allow each ventricular contraction to be preceded by atrial contraction, thus approximating a normal hemodynamic situation.

The A-V sequential pacemaker has come into more common usage with the advent of the tined and J-shaped atrial pacing lead. This catheter has been found to be less easily displaced than those previously available (see Fig. 9-14).

Swan-Ganz catheters with pacing electrodes at various intervals along the catheter for A-V sequential pacing are now being studied. If successful, this would obviate the need for a separate pacing catheter for the patient who also needs hemodynamic pressure monitoring.

OVERDRIVE AND UNDERDRIVE PACING

Occasionally, pacing is used to interrupt tachyarrhythmias that are unresponsive to other forms of therapy. These arrhythmias may be of either ventricular or supraventricular origin. A temporary transvenous pacemaker catheter electrode is placed in the chamber of arrhythmia

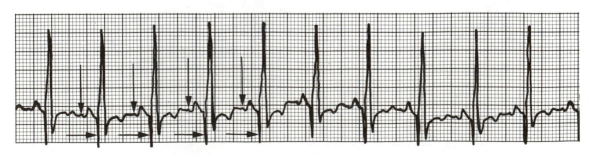

FIGURE 9-11.
A-V sequential pacemaker stimulating both the atria and the ventricles. Vertical arrows indicate atrial pacing spikes; horizontal arrows indicate ventricular pacing spikes.

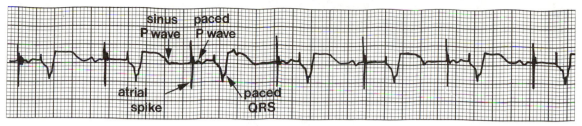

FIGURE 9-12.
A-V sequential pacemaker. Since pacemaker does not sense spontaneous atrial activity, sinus P waves may be found that are unrelated to pacemaker activity. Lack of paced P waves in complexes 2, 5, and 7 results from atrial pacemaker discharging during the atrial refractory period following sinus P waves.

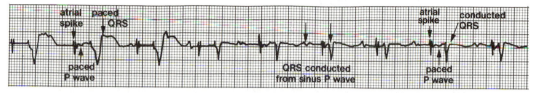

FIGURE 9-13.
A-V sequential pacemaker with QRSs resulting from ventricular pacing, from conduction of sinus impulse, and from conduction of paced P waves.

origin. Since most supraventricular tachycardias are of the reentry type, a pacemaker stimulus is initiated at such time as to render the reentry circuit refractory, thus interrupting completion of the circuit and terminating the arrhythmia.

The same principle can be applied to reentrant ventricular tachycardias. Overdrive pacing may be accomplished by increasing the pacing rate until pacemaker capture occurs during the non-refractory period between spontaneous beats. Once the ectopic focus has been suppressed, the pacing rate can usually be decreased gradually, and the pacing stimulus will continue to maintain control of the ventricles.

When overdrive pacing fails to terminate the ventricular arrhythmia, underdrive pacing may be attempted. The pacing rate is set at less than the ectopic discharge rate in an attempt to accomplish ventricular capture by the pacing stimulus.

The most common cause of ventricular tachyarrhythmias is acute myocardial infarction. Usually the ectopic focus will be inherently suppressed at some point after the infarct has begun to heal. The pacemaker is then no longer needed and can be removed.

TYPES OF PACING CATHETERS
Pacing catheters are either unipolar or bipolar, referring to one electrode or two *within* the catheter. All electrical circuits must have two

electrodes to complete the circuit. The unipolar catheter requires a second electrode outside the catheter itself.

The *bipolar catheter* has a negative pacing electrode at the tip and a positive sensing electrode about one centimeter proximal to the tip (see Fig. 9-15). Virtually all temporary pacemakers

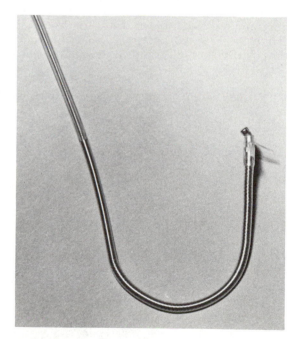

FIGURE 9-14.
J-shaped, tined transvenous atrial pacing lead.

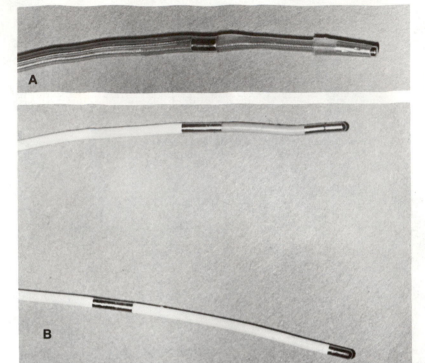

FIGURE 9-15.
(A) Permanent bipolar pacing catheter.

FIGURE 9-15.
(B) Temporary bipolar pacing catheters.

utilize bipolar catheters. The negative distal electrode should be attached to the negative terminal on the generator and the positive proximal electrode to the positive terminal. Occasionally improper sensing can be corrected by reversing the attachment of the catheter tips at the generator terminals (reversed polarity). When reversing the polarity of a bipolar catheter does not correct faulty sensing, conversion to a unipolar system may solve the problem. This is accomplished by disconnecting the bipolar positive electrode from the generator and replacing it with the wire from a monitoring electrode on the anterior chest (see Fig. 9-16). When the chest electrode is used as part of the pacing system, it should be labeled as such so that it will not be confused

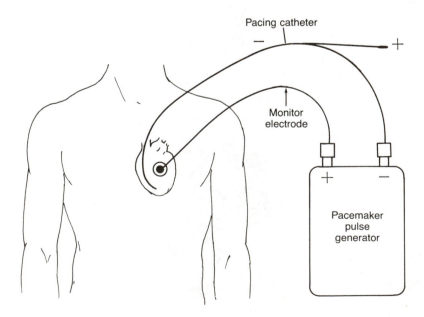

FIGURE 9-16.
Conversion of bipolar pacing system to unipolar. The monitoring electrode on anterior chest is used as positive pole in pacemaker system.

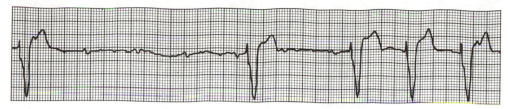

FIGURE 9-17.
Ventricular pacemaker. Failure to discharge is indicated by lack of pacemaker spikes at appropriate intervals.

with other chest electrodes that are being used for monitoring cardiac rhythm.

The *unipolar catheter* has only a negative pacing electrode at its tip. The positive pole is outside the catheter itself. In permanent pacing, the generator case is the positive pole. The majority of permanent pacemakers use the unipolar catheter.

PACING AND SENSING THRESHOLDS

The pacing electrodes should be positioned so that the generator can be set at a relatively small amount of electrical energy and low degree of sensitivity and still allow successful pacing.

The lowest level of electrical energy that is required to initiate consistent ventricular capture at the pacing electrode site is called the *pacing threshold*. This threshold level is determined after successful pacing has been established by decreasing the energy output of the generator until capture ceases, then increasing output until capture is regained. The threshold is expressed as milliamperes (MA) at this level. The generator output is then set at several MA above threshold to allow for the usual increase in threshold level that occurs over a period of a few days after pacing has been initiated. Hypokalemia may cause an increase in pacing threshold, as do β-adrenergic and mineralocorticoid drugs.

Sensing threshold is determined for permanent pacemakers. The amplitude of the intrinsic depolarization wave at the site of the sensing electrode is measured. If the amplitude is insufficient to ensure sensing, the pacing electrode is repositioned.

COMPLICATIONS OF PACING

Failure of proper function in the demand pacemaker can be determined on the cardiac monitor or ECG. The pacemaker may malfunction because of failure to discharge a stimulus, failure to cap-

ture the ventricles, or failure to sense intrinsic depolarizations.

Since stimulus discharge from the pacemaker causes an artifact or "spike" to appear on the ECG, *failure to discharge* results in absence of the artifact (see Fig. 9-17). This failure may be within the generator itself (either mechanism or battery failure), at the site of lead attachment to the generator, or within the lead due to fracture of wires. When failure occurs in the temporary pacemaker, check the connections at the generator terminals, replace the batteries in the generator, or replace the generator. If these efforts do not solve the problem, it must be assumed that wire fracture is the culprit. If only one wire is fractured, conversion to a unipolar system, using a chest electrode to replace the fractured wire, will provide successful pacing. When the permanent pacemaker fails to discharge a stimulus, the problem must be solved operatively. If the situation is emergent, the physician may insert a temporary transvenous pacemaker to support the patient hemodynamically until the permanent pacemaker problem can be corrected.

Failure of the pacing stimulus to capture the ventricles will be noted by the absence of the QRS immediately following the pacemaker artifact on the ECG (see Fig. 9-18). If the pacing threshold has increased, the MA may need to be increased until ventricular capture occurs. Displacement of the pacing electrode may cause failure to capture. It is sometimes possible to regain capture by repositioning the patient, often in the left lateral decubitus position, until the electrode can be repositioned.

Battery failure can also cause failure to capture. If the patient is pacemaker dependent and becomes symptomatic, drug therapy (atropine, isoproterenol) and cardiopulmonary resuscitation may be required until the cause of the problem is found and corrected.

Failure of the pacemaker to sense spontaneous beats results in inappropriately placed pacemaker artifacts on the ECG (see Fig. 9-19). This may be caused by improper electrode placement, bat-

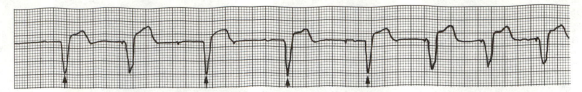

FIGURE 9-18.
Ventricular demand pacemaker. Lack of QRS following each pacemaker spike indicates failure to capture. Complexes 1, 3, 4, and 5 result from a spontaneous ventricular escape focus.

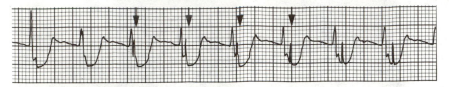

FIGURE 9-19.
Ventricular demand pacemaker. Failure to sense is indicated by pacemaker spikes at inappropriate intervals following spontaneous QRSs.

tery or component failure, or lead wire fracture. Ventricular arrhythmias caused by occurrence of the pacemaker stimulus during the vulnerable phase of the T wave are most likely to occur in the patient who has an acute cardiac disease process, electrolyte imbalance, or drug toxicity but are seldom seen in the patient who is hospitalized for battery replacement rather than acute illness. The most likely cause for sensing failure in the temporary pacemaker is electrode displacement. If nonsensing renders the pacemaker totally ineffective, it may be advantageous to turn the pacemaker off until the electrode can be repositioned.

Ventricular irritability at the site of the endocardial catheter tip is a frequent occurrence after initial catheter insertion. The premature ventricular complexes usually appear similar in configuration to the pacemaker complexes (see Figs. 9-20 and 9-21). Irritability from the catheter as a foreign body usually disappears after 2 or 3 days.

Perforation of the ventricular wall or septum by the transvenous catheter occurs in a small number of patients. This may or may not result in noncapture. It can be suspected on cardiac monitoring if the patient is monitored in a modified V$_1$ lead. Right ventricular pacing should provide a negative QRS in this lead. Often ventricular perforation results in pacing from the left ventricle, and the QRS becomes positive in polarity. Pericardial tamponade, causing a decrease in blood pressure and increase in sinus node discharge rate, must be watched for after ventricular wall perforation.

Tamponade occurs infrequently because of the ability of myocardial fibers to regain their integrity after the catheter has been pulled back into the ventricle; however, anticoagulation therapy should be discontinued after perforation.

Retrograde migration of the right ventricular pacing catheter into the right atrium may result in atrial pacing (pacing artifact followed by P wave) or inhibition of the pacemaker by atrial depolarizations. The effects on the patient depend on the ability of the AV node to conduct atrial impulses and on the ability of a lower escape focus to emerge at an adequate rate.

Abdominal twitching or hiccoughs occur occasionally as a result of electrode placement against a thin right ventricular wall and resultant electri-

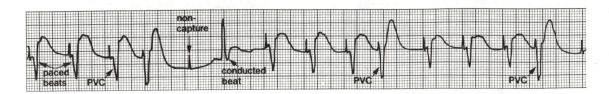

FIGURE 9-20.
Ventricular demand pacemaker with PVCs. This strip also shows one noncaptured pacemaker spike followed by a spontaneous conducted beat.

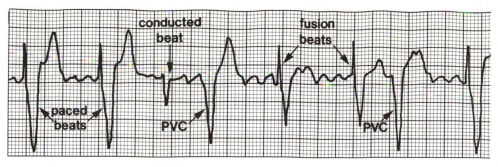

FIGURE 9-21.
Ventricular demand pacemaker with PVCs and with fusion beats that result from ventricular depolarization by both the pacemaker and a spontaneous beat.

cal stimulation of the abdominal muscles or diaphragm. This is usually very uncomfortable for the patient, and the electrode should be repositioned as soon as possible.

Infection and phlebitis can occur at the temporary pacemaker insertion site, and infection or *hematoma* may occur at the site of permanent generator implantation. These sites must be inspected for swelling and inflammation and kept dry. Sterile technique must be used when changing dressings.

Migration of the permanent generator from its initial site of implantation may occur in patients who have very loose connective tissue. This may or may not require reimplantation. *Erosion* at the implantation site occurs rarely.

Defibrillation of the patient while the temporary pacemaker system is intact may affect various components of the generator and cause it to malfunction. The temporary generator should be turned off *and* the catheter wires disconnected from the generator if at all possible before defibrillating.

PACEMAKER SAFETY

Electrical safety precautions must be observed when the patient has a temporary pacemaker. Electrical equipment in the room should be kept at a minimum and must be properly grounded. Use of a nonelectric bed is preferable. If an electric bed is used, it should remain disconnected from AC current. A tap bell should be provided for the patient and the electric call light disconnected. Only battery-operated electric shavers, toothbrushes, or radios may be used. An AC powered television may be used if it is operated by someone who is not in contact with the patient. The nurse should avoid simultaneous contact with the patient and any electrical equipment. The patient's bed must be kept dry at all times. Diathermy and electrocautery equipment should not be used because their waves may be sensed by and inhibit the demand pacemaker.

If an older model temporary pacemaker generator with exposed metal catheter tips or terminals is in use, these metal parts must be insulated. A rubber glove can be cut and taped over the exposed metal to provide insulation from external current sources.

The plastic cover supplied with the temporary generator must be kept in place over the dials to prevent inadvertant change in settings. The generator should be securely attached to the patient's arm or abdomen. The catheter should be securely taped to the patient's skin without direct tension on the catheter. Motion of the extremity nearest the catheter entry site should be minimized, especially if the femoral site has been used.

According to manufacturers of permanent pacemaker generators, there are very few electrical hazards associated with the permanent generators currently in use. These generators are shielded from external electrical sources and are not affected by microwave ovens or small appliances. There have been rare reports of unipolar pacemakers being affected by large electromagnetic fields, such as radio transmitters. Defibrillator paddles should not be placed directly over or adjacent to the implanted generator.

PATIENT TEACHING

A planned and systematic approach to teaching the patient to live with his pacemaker is a vital part of nursing care. A helpful tool in patient teaching is a progress report accessible to the physician and other members of the team, along with written guidelines for the nurse who is

TEACHING THE PATIENT WITH A PACEMAKER

1. Knowledge of condition
- Elicit the patient's previous knowledge of pacemakers and clarify any misconceptions.
- If appropriate, clarify the difference between heart block and heart attack. (A patient may confuse cardiac monitoring with pacing and become very anxious when the monitoring electrodes are removed.)
- Don't assume *anything* about the patient's understanding.
- The anatomy of the heart should be discussed in general terms when explaining the need for pacing and how the pacemaker takes the place of or complements spontaneous rhythm.
- The difference between temporary and permanent pacing should also be discussed.

2. Patient activity
- Passive and active range of motion exercises should be started on the affected arm 48 hours after pacemaker implantation in the pectoralis major muscle to avoid "frozen shoulder."
- The patient should be instructed to repeat these exercises several times daily until the implantation site is completely free of discomfort through all ranges of arm motion.
- Explain that the pacemaker is relatively sturdy and that touching or bathing the implantation site will not damage it.
- The patient's activities of daily living and recreational activities should be discussed *before* permanent pacing to ascertain an appropriate site for implantation; for example, the right pectoralis muscle should not be used in the right-handed rifle hunter.
- Abdominal implantation may be preferable for the avid swimmer because of the strenuous arm activity.
- Activities that may result in high impact or stress at the implantation site should be avoided. This includes all contact sports.
- Instruct the patient to report any activity that may have damaged his pacemaker.
- The patient can return to work at the discretion of his physician.
- Discuss the type of work he will do and what his job entails. He may return to whatever degree of sexual activity he wants or tolerates.
- The patient should be aware that his pacemaker may set off the alarm on metal-detector devices in airports.

3. Signs of pacemaker malfunction
- The symptoms of pacemaker malfunction are those associated with decreased perfusion of the brain, heart, or skeletal muscles.
- The patient should be instructed to report any dizziness, fainting, chest pain, shortness of breath, undue fatigue, or fluid retention.
- Fluid retention should be described in terms of sudden weight gain, "puffy ankles," "tightness of rings," and so forth.
- Patient should be instructed to take his pulse once daily upon awakening. He should report a pulse rate that is more than 5 beats per minute slower than that at which his pacemaker is set.
- Patient should be aware that his pulse may be somewhat irregular if he has a demand pacemaker and has some spontaneous beats as well as paced beats. It must be stressed that this does not signify pacemaker malfunction.

4. Signs of infection
- The patient should report any redness, swelling, drainage, or increase in soreness at the implantation site.

5. Pulse generator replacement
- Instruct the patient regarding the expected life of his pacemaker battery.
- He should know that generator replacement requires hospitalization for about 3 days, and that usually only the generator will need to be replaced.

6. Medications
- The patient should be instructed regarding any medication he will be taking at home.
- He should know the name of the medication, as well as the dose, frequency of administration, side-effects, and use of each medication.

7. Safety measures
- The patient should inform any physician or dentist by whom he is seen of his pacemaker, as well as of the medications that he is taking.
- He should carry a pacemaker identification card with him at all times. This card shows the brand and model of his pacemaker, the date of insertion, and the rate at which it is set.
- It is also advisable to wear a medical alert bracelet or necklace stating that he has a pacemaker.

8. Follow-up care
- The importance of physician or clinic follow-up visits should be stressed.
- The follow-up visit will include an interval history and physical examination and a 12-lead ECG.
- Many pacemaker clinics have specialized equipment available to measure the rate, amplitude, duration, and contours of the pacemaker artifact. This information is very helpful in predicting battery depletion. Some clinics have the capability for obtaining this information by telephone, reducing the necessity for travel to the clinic.

instructing the patient. The patient's family should also be involved in the learning process.

Patient teaching relative to pacemakers begins at the time the decision for pacemaker insertion is made. The patient and his family should be told why the pacemaker is necessary. The insertion procedure should be explained, as well as the immediate postinsertion care that can be expected.

Many booklets and media presentations are available to aid the nurse in teaching the pacemaker patient. It is helpful to have written guidelines for the patient to review after discharge from the hospital.

The depth of teaching that is appropriate and the teaching tools used depend on such variables as the patient's age, intellect, attention span, vision, and interest in learning. An occasional patient will demonstrate difficulty in accepting the prospect of living with a pacemaker. His initial teaching should be confined to the positive aspects of life with a pacemaker. Knowledge of the function and care of the pacemaker are of no interest to him until he is able to accept it as part of his life. Many misconceptions can be negated by asking the patient what he knows or has heard previously about pacemakers and if he has any preconceived expectations relative to his pacemaker.

The teaching areas listed in the accompanying chart should be covered with the patient during the course of his hospitalization.

The nurse who cares for the patient with an artificial pacemaker must have thorough knowledge of the heart, the pacemaker, and the patient as a person. This knowledge must be applied continuously from the time the decision for pacemaker insertion is made until the patient is discharged from the hospital and sometimes beyond, to follow-up care. The nurse plays a vital role in assuring successful pacing and in reassuring the patient, whose well-being depends on successful pacing. Caring for the pacemaker patient is a challenging but most rewarding experience when the nurse is secure in her knowledge of the subject.

BIBLIOGRAPHY

Bognolo D et al: Atrial and atrioventricular sequential pacing rationale and clinical experience. J Fla Med Assoc 66:1028–1033, 1979

Davies H, Nelson WP: Understanding Cardiology. Boston, Butterworth, 1978

Hyman AL: Permanent programmable pacemakers in the management of recurrent tachycardias. Pace 2:28–39, 1979

Lichstein E et al: Indications for pacing in patients with chronic bifascicular block. Pace 1:540–542, 1978

Mangiola S: Self-Assessment in Electrocardiography. Philadelphia, Lippincott, 1977

Mansour KA et al: Further evaluation of the sutureless, screw-in electrode for cardiac pacing. J Thorac Cardiovasc Surg 77, No. 6:858–862, 1979

Parsonnet V et al: Transvenous insertion of double sets of permanent electrodes. JAMA 243, No. 1:62–64, 1980

Preston TA: The use of pacemaking for the treatment of acute arrhythmias. Heart Lung 6, No. 2:249–255, 1977

Proctor D et al: Temporary cardiac pacing: Causes, recognition, and management of failure to pace. Nurs Clin North Am: Cardiac Care 13, No. 3:409–422, 1978

Rossel CL, Alyn IB: Living with a permanent cardiac pacemaker. Heart Lung 6, No. 2:273–279, 1977

Sutton R, Citron P: Electrophysiological and hemodynamic basis for application of new pacemaker technology in sick sinus syndrome and atrioventricular block. Br Heart J 41, No. 5:600–612, 1979

Yashar JJ et al: Atrioventricular sequential pacemakers: Indications, complications, and long-term follow-up. Ann Thorac Surg 29, No. 1:91–98, 1980

Lane D. Craddock

CARDIOPULMONARY RESUSCITATION

DEFINITIONS

Because of the dual nature of resuscitation—that is, availability (ventilation) and transport (circulation) of oxygen—the more appropriate term is *cardiopulmonary resuscitation (CPR)*.

Cardiac arrest is the abrupt cessation of effective cardiac pumping activity resulting in cessation of circulation. There are only two types of cardiac arrest: cardiac standstill (asystole) and ventricular fibrillation (plus other forms of ineffective ventricular contraction, such as ventricular flutter and rarely ventricular tachycardia). The condition referred to as "profound cardiovascular collapse" will not be specifically included because its recognition and definition are nebulous and management less specific. One form, referred to as "cardiogenic shock," is included in Chapter 8.

Resuscitation, liberally interpreted, is the restoration of vital signs by mechanical, physiological, and pharmacological means.

The application of cardiopulmonary resuscitation is made possible by the concept of clinical versus biological death.

Clinical death is defined as the absence of the vital signs, and *biological death* refers to irreversible cellular changes. As determined both experimentally and clinically, the interval between clinical and biological death is approximately 4 minutes.

WHO SHOULD BE RESUSCITATED

It is easier to determine who should *not* be resuscitated than who should be resuscitated. Individuals who should not be resuscitated include persons with known terminal illness and those who have been clinically dead for longer than 5 minutes. Both represent situations in which resuscitation would likely prove impossible and survival would be meaningless.

All others should be regarded as candidates for resuscitation. *Remember* that resuscitation can always be abandoned, but it cannot be instituted after undue delay.

One additional point, the term *the very elderly* is often used to differentiate likely degrees of vitality and therefore of survival probability. On the surface, this is perhaps reasonable, but age alone should rarely, if ever, determine treatment. Bear in mind that, regardless of chronologic age, a person who is alert and able to carry on any sort of thoughtful conversation is a candidate for resuscitation.

RECOGNITION

The recognition of cardiac arrest depends on the finding of signs of absence of circulation such as: (1) unconscious state (preceded, of course, by less profound states of mental obtundation), (2) pulselessness, (3) dilated pupils, and (4) minimal or absent respirations. Two things should be noted. First, the pupils require a certain amount of time to dilate, which has been estimated at approximately 45 seconds but may be longer than 1 minute. It is therefore occasionally a valu-

able sign for pinpointing the time of cardiac arrest. Second, inadequate respiratory excursions may be noted in the early seconds of cardiac arrest, and these should not cause delay in recognition of the other signs.

Pulselessness is best determined by palpation of either the carotid or femoral arteries. Palpation of the carotid is almost always immediately available, whereas palpation of the femoral is not. Brachial or radial pulse palpation is of lesser value. Pulselessness should not be determined by attempting to obtain a blood pressure.

An ideal situation should exist in coronary care units or well-equipped critical care units which includes continuous monitoring, electronic warning signals, automatic conditioned response of a skilled team without the delay of feeling pulses, auscultating over the precordium, and the like.

THE RESUSCITATION TEAM

An organized approach to resuscitation is essential. Resuscitation should be approached by a team made up of trained personnel including nurses, physicians, ECG technicians, inhalation therapy technicians, and individuals to transport special instruments (*e.g.,* defibrillators, pacemakers, and special tray sets).

The team should also include an administrative or secretarial member who can do the legwork, make all necessary phone calls, and perform other miscellaneous duties which are a minor but necessary part of every prolonged resuscitation attempt. A common method of organizing a resuscitation team is to designate specific individuals who will respond to all cardiac emergencies; this works quite well, but it is not the only method nor is it always feasible.

Below is an illustration of a successful method of resuscitation geared to an institution with trained resuscitative personnel. The team includes a nurse who serves as the primary member. The first nurse present becomes the initial captain of the team, who also institutes the resuscitation attempt as outlined.

A single call, preferably by the secretary, should immediately summon the entire team — ECG technicians, inhalation therapy technicians, available physicians including house staff and senior staff members in the area, nurses from the appropriate intensive care unit who will immediately transport the defibrillator, monitor, and pacemaker instrument to the site of the emergency, and the nursing supervisor.

The last but not least member of the team is the switchboard operator, who must immediately alert the entire team in preference to all other duties. A single digit on the telephone dial should be used to alert the switchboard. The switchboard operator will often know where to find key physician members of the team and can summon them individually.

Hospitals with house officers who carry emergency electronic communication equipment are at an obvious advantage and should have the best resuscitation statistics. Many smaller institutions, however, may be just as successful using only nursing personnel and well-trained technicians. Minor variations in approaches may bring the same results.

Two additional factors are crucial to the team's success. The team must have a definite routine which is kept up-to-date by all members. Furthermore, nursing personnel and other key nonphysician members must be sanctioned to act spontaneously.

STEPS IN CPR

There are two settings in which health care personnel may encounter a person in need of CPR: (1) that of a patient whose ECG is being continuously monitored, as in the coronary care unit, and (2) that in an area where the patient is not under continuous monitoring, such as an ordinary hospital room or unit.

For the continuously monitored patient, the arrhythmia sets the alarm, and if it is ventricular fibrillation, the patient is immediately defibrillated (without prior attempts by other means), after which a physician is summoned for evaluation.

In the unmonitored patient, proceed immediately as described below. (For a summary of the following steps see the chart titled Steps in CPR later in this section.)

1. Sharp Blow to the Precordium
A sharp blow to the precordium requires virtually no time and may institute a cardiac rhythm; if so, it may be the only required resuscitation. This is referred to as *thumpversion* and is especially effective in ventricular tachycardia.

2. Call for Help
To call for help simply relay the message "code zero" or "red alert," together with the location of the patient to a second individual who then places the emergency call to bring the team together.

3. Obtain Adequate Airway
Immediately institute artificial ventilation (mouth-to-mouth).

4. External Cardiac Compression
External cardiac compression is a simple technique which is applied by standing at either side of the patient, placing the heel of one hand over the lower half of the sternum and the heel of the other hand over the first. Applying vigorous compresson directly downward, depress the sternum between 1½ and 2 inches, releasing abruptly, and maintaining this rhythm at the rate of 60 to 80 times per minute. To be effective this technique must be learned correctly and applied skillfully. All that is required to learn this technique is a little attention to instructors, two hands, and a lack of timidity.

If a single individual must apply both ventilation and massage, it is best to give two or three quick inflations by mouth-to-mouth or other readily available means of inflating the lungs, followed by 12 to 15 external cardiac compressions. This routine may be maintained until additional members of the team arrive.

The generally accepted theory underlying CPR maintains that the heart functions as a pump, and the valves operate appropriately as one-way passages during external compression. More recent work, using two-dimensional echocardiography during CPR in animals and humans, indicates that different mechanisms may necessitate some minor alterations in the standard CPR procedure. The new studies emphasize that the heart serves primarily as a conduit, not as a pump, and that the properties of veins as capacitors and arteries as conduits influence cerebral and coronary circulation during CPR. Venous beds may act as reservoirs, while some venous circuits function as barriers to retrograde flow owing to the presence of valves. Arteries show less tendency to collapse and therefore should receive more blood during artificial massage. The splanchnic venous bed, however, may form a large static pool that robs the total circulation during CPR. Some advocate abdominal compression to prevent this. Although present techniques should not be changed until more evidence shows these newer techniques to be superior, it is imperative to keep an open mind, since even small improvements could prove salutary.

5. External Countershock

External countershock should be applied as soon as the instrument is available. This should be done without knowing the specific rhythm diagnosis if there is a delay in determining this.

If *cardiac standstill* is present, the countershock will take only moments and will do no harm. If *ventricular fibrillation* is present, the earliest possible countershock delivered is the one most likely to be effective and should be done at a time when the rhythm may more likely be maintained.

A specific *diagnosis* now is required (the word *recognition* has been used up to now, not diagnosis). As mentioned earlier, this will be either cardiac standstill or ventricular fibrillation (continued in Items 9 and 10).

6. Intravenous Infusion

This item is devoted to a very important member of the team—the nurse who is first available after two members are applying ventilation and massage. This individual will be in charge of the emergency cart and therefore responsible for preparing the drugs to be used and an intravenous infusion set (with several types of venipuncture equipment). Moreover, this individual must handle whatever is necessary to see that an intravenous infusion is started, thus paving the way for drug therapy. The importance of this function underlies the continuously available venous cannula maintained in patients in critical care units.

At this point the need for an intravenous infusion is obvious and must be fulfilled by whatever route is feasible. The simplest of all is the insertion of a needle, cannula, or scalp needle into an *arm vein*. Failing this, the *femoral vein* is readily accessible, and a very large cannula can easily be inserted into the largest blood vessel in the body (the *inferior vena cava*) by simple puncture. A cutdown on a branch of the *basilic system* just above the elbow crease on the medial aspect of either arm or on the *external jugular vein* will allow insertion of a large cannula into the *superior vena cava* or right atrium.

The *subclavian venipuncture* is perhaps ideal, being readily available and easily done. In addition, it may be used for rapid infusion or withdrawal and monitoring of central venous pressure (CVP) and O_2 saturation, and it is well tolerated for long periods of time. The *internal jugular route* is also excellent but is less desirable than the subclavian.

The *intracardiac route* should be reserved for situations in which urgency takes precedence over availability of the intravenous route. This should be a rare occurrence.

7. Endotracheal Intubation

Endotracheal intubation is required for the patient whose spontaneous cardiac rhythm and respiration have not resulted from the measures outlined above.

8. Pharmacologic Agents

Pharmacologic agents and appropriate preparations to be made ready immediately include the following:

a. *Sodium bicarbonate* in a 5% solution is given in 50 ml aliquots every 5 to 10 minutes and is the initial drug used. Tromethamine (THAM) can also serve as a buffer, but it has disadvantages and is used much less often than sodium bicarbonate.

   It has been argued that giving sodium bicarbonate intravenously results in a rise in PCO_2 (by the reaction $HCO_3^- + H^+ \rightarrow H_2CO_3 \rightarrow H_2O + CO_2$) and an increase in osmolality. This is often the case, but there is little choice when significant acidosis is present, as is the situation in virtually all instances of cardiopulmonary arrest. Thus, consensus holds that alkalinization is important, even vital, and that increased osmolality is seldom sufficient to be a major factor.

b. *Epinephrine* (Adrenalin) in a 1:1,000 aqueous solution.

c. *Isoproterenol* should be available in an intravenous preparation; 2 mg in 250 ml of appropriate vehicle solution is an adequate routine preparation.

d. *Calcium chloride* 10% solution.

e. *Lidocaine* (Xylocaine) should be prepared in an intravenous solution of varying concentration, but 1 mg/ml is an adequate solution for initial use. This drug is used most frequently by intravenous push in 50-mg doses.

f. A *vasopressor,* preferably a peripheral vasoconstrictor such as methoxamine (Vasoxyl) or phenylephrine (Neo-Synephrine, an alphamimetic) or norepinephrine (both alpha and beta stimulating) should be available in an intravenous infusion of appropriate concentration.

Intravenous Push. The critical emergency drugs given by intravenous push (sodium bicarbonate, epinephrine, calcium chloride, lidocaine) are all supplied in ready-to-use forms and should be readily available.

Other preparations such as procainamide (Pronestyl), quinidine, diuretics such as ethacrynic acid (Edecrin) and furosemide (Lasix), mannitol, dexamethasone (Decadron), and propranolol (Inderal) should be available, though they are not routinely prepared for immediate use.

The inotropic and chronotropic agent *glucagon* has gained use in some situations. Its effects are less predictable, and it should not be considered a routine drug. Its inotropic effect is substantial, though less than that of isoproterenol, and it has the advantage of a lesser chronotropic effect and generally induces less hyperexcitability.

The catecholamine *dopamine* has emerged as perhaps the inotropic agent of choice. Its central inotropic effect is comparable to that of iso-proterenol, but it has the advantage of augmenting renal blood flow. It has largely replaced isoproterenol and norepinephrine for enhancing perfusion pressure (although isoproterenol is still more effective as a temporary medical "pacemaker").

New drugs that have become useful in car-diopulmonary emergencies include bretylium and dobutamine; the class referred to as *calcium antagonists* (for example, verapamil) are not yet fully evaluated but are unlikely to be important except in very special situations (such as recurrent arrhythmias associated with variant angina). Disopyramide (Norpace) is not yet available for parenteral use and probably will have limited value.

The most important new antiarrhythmic is *bretylium* (Bretylol). Its actions are complex and include adrenergic influences that give it a modest inotropic effect (unlike other antiarrhythmics). Its major action is a striking antifibrillatory effect produced by prolongation of both the action potential duration and the effective refractory period. Occasionally it causes defibrillation without use of countershock. This sharp rise in threshold for ventricular fibrillation and ventricular tachycardia makes it extremely effective when these rhythm disturbances are recurrent, and it is becoming the drug of choice in this circumstance. It is given by intravenous bolus, in a usual dose of 500 mg, and it can be repeated one or more times within one hour.

The inotropic drug *dobutamine* has also become useful. A derivative of isoproterenol, it has the advantage of possessing minimal chronotropic effect. When dopamine produces tachycardia, dobutamine may provide potent inotropy without the harmful effects of excess heart rate.

9. Countering Cardiac Standstill
If cardiac standstill is present, epinephrine should be given routinely, usually 1 mg intra-venously, and artificial ventilation and circulation should be continued; if unsuccessful, epinephrine should be repeated and the iso-proterenol drip started. At this point, calcium chloride, 0.5 to 1.0 g, is given intravenously.

If there is no response, continued artificial ventilation and circulation, continued intravenous epinephrine injections, and insertion of a transvenous pacemaker are indicated (less often a percutaneous transthoracic pacemaker is used).

10. In Case of Ventricular Fibrillation
If ventricular fibrillation is present, epinephrine is given intravenously (it is important that the continuous artificial ventilation and circulation are maintained and that interruptions not exceed 5 sec) and external *countershock* is given at the maximum setting of the instrument with immediate resumption of artificial circulation and ventilation. If unsuccessful, the cycle should be repeated.

If ventricular fibrillation persists in spite of the above or if reversion to ventricular fibrillation occurs each time it is applied, intravenous *antiarrhythmics* should be given without delay.

It is here that *bretylium* is probably the drug of choice (dosage as given above) and should be administered before time is wasted going "down-the-line" of other more commonly used agents.

If bretylium is ineffective, *lidocaine* is given by push in 50- to 100-mg aliquots. *Procainamide,* if preferred, may also be given by intravenous push, and either drug may be given by intravenous drip. *Beta blocking drugs* such as pro-pranolol (Inderal) may be effective here. *Quinidine* is preferred by some, but its tendency to lower peripheral blood pressure and reduce myocardial contractility (resulting in a diminished cardiac output should a rhythm be resumed) constitute important disadvantages.

It should also be emphasized that regardless of the initial mechanism (whether it be an irritable or a depressive phenomenon), once cardiac arrest has gained foothold with some duration it must be assumed that the heart is depressed, making the routine use of depressive drugs unwarranted.

Since uneven tissue perfusion, particularly myocardial perfusion, may be a factor in perpetuating the ventricular fibrillation or standstill, a *vasopressor agent* of the peripheral constrictor type may be of value at this point. Digitalis and potassium chloride are rarely indicated in resuscitative attempts, their use being based on knowledge of special preexisting situations.

As indicated above, depressive cardiac mechanisms are often the cause of repetitive ventricular fibrillation and paradoxically, pacing the heart (pharmacologically with isoproterenol or electronically by transvenous pacing catheter) is the treatment of choice in some cases (after resumption of rhythm, of course).

11. *Pericardial Tap*
If the above fail
a. Pericardial tap should be performed, preferably by the subxyphoid route; although an uncommon factor in cardiac arrest, it may result in dramatic recovery.
b. Consider further underlying causes subject to treatment such as pneumothorax (insertion of chest tubes); pulmonary embolism (assisted circulation, surgery); ventricular aneurysm, rupture of papillary muscle or interventricular septum (assisted circulation, surgery); subvalvular muscular aortic stenosis with extreme gradients (propranolol, reserpine, etc.).

12. *Terminating Resuscitation*
Failing these, the decision to terminate resuscitative attempts is imminent, based on central nervous system (CNS) changes or the assumption of a nonviable myocardium.

POSTRESUSCITATIVE CARE
If there is resumption of spontaneous cardiac activity, the situation should be thoroughly evaluated as to the clinical state, underlying causes, and complicating factors in order to determine proper management. A routine as follows has been found successful: intravenous diuretic (*e.g.,* furosemide 80 to 240 mg) a steroid such as dexamethasone for its salutary effect on cerebral edema, and electrical and physiological monitoring in a critical care unit. A portable chest roentgenogram is routine, and arterial blood gases should be obtained as indicated. Continuous oxygen therapy is maintained; an intravenous infusion is of course essential. Routine measurements other than continuous ECG monitoring include frequent blood pressures (ideally done by intra-arterial cannula), hourly urine volumes, frequent bedside estimates of tissue perfusion, and CVP and O_2 saturation measurements.

If CNS damage is evident, hypothermia should be instituted immediately, additional mannitol or intravenous urea should be given, and dexamethasone for cerebral edema should be continued. Monitoring otherwise is continued as outlined above.

If oliguria or anuria is present, massive doses of furosemide should be given immediately. If there is no response to these, management as in acute renal insufficiency should be instituted.

The specific approach in the postresuscitative period will depend not only upon the patient's condition at the time, but on the underlying disease process, the previous condition of the patient, and the events in the immediate postresuscitative period. More patients are being studied by catheter techniques acutely to evaluate them for emergency surgical procedures

---

STEPS IN CPR

1. Deliver a sharp blow to the precordium if patient is unmonitored. If patient is being monitored and ventricular fibrillation has occurred, patient is defibrillated immediately without administering the thump.
2. Call for help—"cor zero" or "red alert." Give code and location to second person who then places emergency call.
3. Establish airway and institute artificial mouth-to-mouth ventilation.
4. Apply external cardiac compression.
5. Apply external countershock as soon as the instrument is available.
6. If cardiac standstill has occurred
   - Give epinephrine routinely—usually 1 mg intravenously.
   - Continue artificial ventilation and circulation.
   If unsuccessful
   - Repeat epinephrine.
   - Start isoproterenol drip.
   - Give calcium chloride, 0.5 to 1.0 g intravenously.
   If no response
   - Continue artificial ventilation and circulation.
   - Continue intravenous epinephrine injections.
   - Insert transvenous pacemaker.
7. If ventricular fibrillation is present
   - Administer epinephrine intravenously.
   - Maintain artificial ventilation and circulation (any interruption not to exceed 5 sec).
   - Give external countershock at maximum setting, followed by immediate resumption of artificial ventilation and circulation.
   - If unsuccessful, repeat the cycle and give intravenous antiarrhythmics without delay.
   - Consider using a vasopressor agent at this point.

such as saphenous bypass grafts. The state of this art is changing rapidly, and it is frequently necessary to transfer the patient to a facility where these procedures are available.

Complications of Resuscitation

Resuscitation has come a very long way; it has changed drastically with time and undoubtedly will continue to do so. It has proved its worth beyond doubt. There are of course complications including (1) injuries to sternum, costal cartilages, ribs, esophagus, stomach, liver, pleura, and lung, any one of which can be serious; (2) the production, fortunately rare, of a live patient with permanent CNS damage, rendering the patient totally dependent; and (3) medical-legal considerations, which originally leaned against the attempt because of the frequency of undignified failures.

This last medical-legal consideration should probably be ignored for the most part, since we are dealing with an earnest and reasonable approach to the treatment of sudden death in reversible situations. Nonetheless it does emphasize that resuscitation should always be applied by well-trained, responsible people. The aim of resuscitation is to reverse the reversible and not to inflict suffering in situations involving the irreversible. The alternative in both, of course, is death. To differentiate between reversible and irreversible requires good judgment which, as someone has said, "is difficult to learn, impossible to teach."

Phillip S. Wolf

COMMONLY USED ANTIARRHYTHMIC AGENTS

PHARMACOLOGIC AGENTS

Features of those agents most commonly used for management of arrhythmias are listed in Table 9–1.

Digitalis Preparations

DIGOXIN

This agent is often the first selected for patients with supraventricular arrhythmias such as paroxysmal atrial tachycardia, atrial fibrillation, or atrial flutter. Digoxin has little effect on multifocal atrial tachycardia. Digitalization often produces reversion to a normal sinus rhythm or, in the case of atrial fibrillation or flutter, slowing of the ventricular rate to a more satisfactory level. Digoxin should not be used to treat sinus tachycardia except when the tachycardia is secondary to congestive heart failure. The reduction in heart rate in such instances results from improved cardiac output.

Table 9–2 lists the chief characteristics of three digitalis preparations. Since digoxin receives the widest use, it merits further discussion.

Seventy percent to 80% of an oral dose of digoxin is absorbed. Digoxin is also absorbed when given intramuscularly, but this route is painful and has few advantages. When given intravenously (preferable for many seriously ill patients) the usual starting dose is 0.5 mg, followed by 0.25 mg every 2 to 4 hours. Total dosage requirements vary widely. As stated previously, some patients will not respond to customary doses of digoxin.

In order to minimize the risks of *digitalis toxicity,* a serious and sometimes lethal complication, the following options should be considered for the patient with a supraventricular tachycardia:

- Stop treatment if the heart rate has reached a satisfactory, although not ideal, level and further doses of digoxin produce no further slowing (an example is atrial fibrillation with a ventricular rate of 100 to 120/min).
- Choose a second drug for control of heart rate such as propranolol.
- Attempt electrical cardioversion.
- Use an agent such as quinidine, procainamide, or disopyramide, which may reestablish normal sinus rhythm.

Alternate forms of digitalis are useful in specific circumstances.

OUABAIN

Given only intravenously, exerts an effect on atrial arrhythmias within minutes. Its chief benefits are for the two following types of patients: those in whom speed of rhythm control is important and those in whom the status of digitalization is uncertain. In each instance small

Table 9–1
Pharmacokinetics of Most Commonly Used Antiarrhythmic Drugs

Drug	Effect on ECG	Dose & interval	Route	Adverse effects	Therapeutic plasma level
Digoxin	Prolongs P-R (±) ST depression	0.5 mg initially; 0.25 mg q 2–4 hr total 1.0–1.5 mg first 24 hr	IV or PO	Nausea; vomiting; abdominal pain; blurred or colored vision; weakness; psychosis; VPCs; heart block	0.8–1.8 ng/ml
Quinidine	Prolongs QRS, QT, & P-R (±)	100–600 mg q 4–6 hr	PO	GI symptoms; cinchonism; thrombocyto-penia; hypoten-sion; heart block; ventricular tachycardia	2.3 μg–5.0 μg/ml
Procaina-mide (Pronestyl)	Prolongs QRS, QT, & P-R (±)	500 mg–1 g; then 2–5 g/day 250–500 mg q 3–6 hr 100 mg q 5 min to 1 g total Maintenance: 2–4 mg/min	PO IM IV	GI symptoms; psy-chosis; hypoten-sion; rash; lupus-like syndrome	4 μg–10 μg/ml
Disopyra-mide (Norpace)	Prolongs QRS, QT, & P-R	Loading: 200–300 mg Maintenance: 100–200 mg q 6 hr	PO	Anticholinergic effects; hypo-tension; heart failure; heart block; tachy-arrhythmias	2 μg–8 μg/ml
Propran-olol (Inderal)	Prolongs P-R, no change QRS, shortens QT	10–80 mg q 6 hr 0.3–5 mg total (not > 1 mg/min)	PO IV	Hypotension; heart failure; heart block; asthma	Not established; 50–100 ng/ml needed for beta blockade

increments of ouabain (0.1 mg IV q ½ hr) may produce either a favorable response or evidence of toxicity such as the development of ventricular premature beats. The latter indicates that safe levels of digitalization have been exceeded. The small, step-wise doses and the shorter half-life make this approach somewhat safer than the use of digoxin for this purpose.

DIGITOXIN
By virtue of its relatively slow excretion, is especially useful in some patients with chronic atrial fibrillation or atrial flutter who continue to exhibit rapid ventricular rates. The vagotonic action of digitoxin on the AV node is more consistent than that of digoxin, leading to more dependable rate control.

Table 9–2
Digitalis Preparations

Agent	Onset of action in minutes	Peak effect in hours	Average half-life	Principal excretory path	Average digitalizing dose		Usual daily oral maintenance dose
					oral	IV	
Ouabain	5–10	½–2	21 hr	renal; some gastrointes-tinal	—	0.3–0.5 mg	—
Digoxin	15–30	1–2	33 hr	renal	1.25–1.5 mg	0.75–1.0 mg	0.25–0.5 mg
Digitoxin	25–120	4–12	4–6 days	hepatic	0.7–1.2 mg	1.0 mg	0.1 mg

DIGITALIS TOXICITY

All digitalis glycosides should be used with great caution in patients with Wolff-Parkinson-White (WPW) syndrome who develop atrial fibrillation or flutter. Digitalis reduces the refractory period of the accessory pathway. This action leads to transmission of potentially very rapid atrial rates to the ventricle. Ventricular fibrillation may result.

Excessive doses of digitalis can be avoided by considering some principles of its metabolism. When renal function is normal, one-third of the digoxin stored in the body is excreted daily. The renal clearance of digoxin directly relates to the creatinine clearance. When serum creatinine is elevated to 2 to 5 mg/dl, the maintenance dose of digoxin should be reduced by at least one-half. More severe levels of renal failure require an even further reduction of dosage. Because creatinine levels rise only after considerable loss of renal function, a normal serum creatinine does not assure a normal clearance of digoxin.

It is prudent to reduce the maintenance dose of digoxin in the elderly patient. Creatinine clearance declines with age. A second factor that favors accumulation of digoxin in this age group is the age-related decrease in muscle mass. Skeletal muscle is the major body depository for digoxin. A decrease in muscle mass is reflected in increased glycoside concentration in the serum and in the heart. Features of digitalis toxicity are listed in the accompanying chart.

Other conditions which may lead to digitalis toxicity include hypokalemia, hypomagnesemia, hypothyroidism, pulmonary hypertension, and severe heart disease of any etiology. Concomitant therapy with quinidine is also known to increase the serum digoxin level. Certain of these states, such as severe heart failure, are themselves associated with atrial arrhythmias. The utmost care is required in choosing the dose of digitalis for these patients.

Measurements of serum digoxin levels have assisted in many cases in arrhythmia management. The normal range is 0.8 to 1.8 ng/ml (Table 9-1). It cannot be stressed too strongly that the serum level is only a guide and not an absolute indicator of the adequacy of digitalization. The clinical status of the patient, in particular the adequacy of rate control, often provides more useful information about the status of digitalization than absolute serum levels. As a common clinical example, a patient with chronic atrial fibrillation may require larger than customary doses of digoxin for maintenance of a satisfactory ventricular rate. A serum level above

MANIFESTATIONS OF DIGITALIS TOXICITY	
Gastrointestinal	Anorexia Vomiting Abdominal pain Diarrhea Unexplained weight loss
Neurologic	Weakness Blurred or colored vision Psychosis
Cardiac (entirely manifest as arrhythmias)	Atrial tachycardia, commonly with AV block Junctional tachycardia Ventricular ectopic rhythm SA node depression AV block Bidirectional tachycardia

the "therapeutic range" in this instance may be misleading as an indicator of toxicity.

Quinidine

Quinidine is highly effective in the management of atrial and ventricular ectopic rhythms. These include supraventricular tachycardia, atrial fibrillation, atrial flutter, multifocal atrial tachycardia, ventricular premature contractions, and ventricular tachycardia. Quinidine has been found superior to placebo treatment in maintaining sinus rhythm after cardioversion from atrial fibrillation or flutter.

Quinidine has two modes of action. It is vagolytic and by this mechanism enhances conduction through the AV node. This action tends to speed the ventricular rate in atrial fibrillation or flutter; prior digitalization prevents this undesirable effect. Second, quinidine exerts a direct myocardial effect that prolongs AV conduction, His-Purkinje conduction times, and the duration of repolarization (the QT interval on the ECG).

Quinidine sulfate is well absorbed orally and reaches a peak serum level at about 1.5 hours. In contrast, quinidine gluconate absorbs more slowly with a peak level occurring at about 4 hours. It would be expected that quinidine gluconate could be given less frequently (every 8 to 12 hr) than the sulfate compound (every 6 to 8 hr) because of the more prolonged absorption of the gluconate salt, which also results in lower peak levels. The effective dose in any given patient will vary quite widely as a result of patient variation, the disease state, the presence of other drugs, and differences in composition of other products. An initial total dose of 600 to 900 mg daily is usually given. The dose should be gradually increased as needed with attention directed to ECG signs of toxicity (prolonged QRS and QT intervals).

Blood levels offer a guideline for management and should be obtained after the first 6 to 8 doses. With current techniques the therapeutic levels range from 2.3 μg to 5.0 μg/ml. An occasional patient may show signs of toxicity with "therapeutic" serum levels. In some of these patients, the QT interval may show considerable prolongation over the pretreatment ECG and warn of impending toxicity. Excessive serum levels are associated with a high frequency of toxicity. Conversely, some patients may be controlled at "subtherapeutic" blood levels. The dosage of the drug should not be raised further in this situation.

Quinidine should not be given intramuscularly because of erratic absorption and the tendency to produce pain at the injection site. The intravenous route is hazardous because quinidine produces vasodilatation and sometimes circulatory collapse. Intravenous quinidine, given by slow drip, should be reserved for patients with serious rhythm disorders that have not responded to other modes of therapy.

QUINIDINE TOXICITY

About 30% of the patients on quinidine cannot tolerate the drug because of troublesome side-effects. Diarrhea is the most common, is unrelated to plasma concentrations, and is often associated with nausea and vomiting. Cinchonism (headache, visual, auditory, and vestibular symptoms) occurs with increased plasma concentrations. Arrhythmias, especially ventricular ectopic rhythms, occur more frequently in patients with advanced cardiac failure. A very slow ventricular rate in patients with atrial fibrillation or flutter also predisposes to ventricular arrhythmias. Transient ventricular flutter or fibrillation may produce the entity known as "quinidine syncope."

Sudden death occurs in a small percentage of patients on maintenance quinidine. A retrospective look at patients with quinidine syncope reveals a prolonged QT interval in many cases. Other patients may show AV block. Finally, idiosyncratic reactions occur in some patients; these include fever, rash, thrombocytopenia, hemolytic anemia, and hepatic dysfunction.

As a rule, the maintenance dose of quinidine should be reduced to 70% in the presence of congestive failure and to 50% with renal failure. The blood level should be checked at the peak serum concentration (1.5 hr after oral use) and at the trough (1 hr before the next dose).

Procainamide (Pronestyl)

Procainamide is highly effective for atrial and ventricular ectopic rhythms whether given orally, intramuscularly, or intravenously. Like quinidine, procainamide has a mild vagolytic effect on the AV node, which in some patients will prove deleterious by increasing the ventricular rate. Procainamide has the potential for myocardial depression. It decreases conduction throughout the heart and can prolong the QRS and QT intervals. A reduced cardiac output and hypotension may occur after rapid intravenous use or when the oral dose accumulates as a result of renal failure.

A metabolite of procainamide, N-acetylprocainamide (NAPA), also has antiarrhythmic activity. NAPA has a longer serum half-life than procainamide. Renal failure produces a toxic level of NAPA that is not detected by the usual serum measurements. Patients with renal failure should therefore be treated with lower doses of procainamide and followed closely to detect QRS prolongation.

Procainamide is well absorbed orally, reaching a peak level at one hour. The usual dose ranges from 250 to 500 mg every 3 to 6 hours. Therapeutic plasma levels range between 4μg to 10μg/ml. Earlier investigations indicated that the serum level fell to subtherapeutic levels after 3 to 4 hours. Many patients, however, exhibit a continued response for longer periods. This effect probably results from the more prolonged antiarrhythmic action of NAPA.

Procainamide is given intravenously in initial doses of 100 mg by slow infusion and repeated every 5 minutes until either a therapeutic effect is obtained or toxicity (hypotension or widening of the QRS complex) is noted. The total intravenous dose should not exceed 1 g. The loading dose is followed by a maintenance infusion of 2 to 4 mg/minute. The dose should be reduced in patients with heart failure or hepatic or renal insufficiency.

PROCAINAMIDE TOXICITY

Commonly encountered side-effects of procainamide include nausea, vomiting, and diarrhea with the oral route. Rash, fever, agranulocytosis, and frank psychosis are occasionally seen. Long-term use leads to a very high incidence (80%) of antinuclear antibodies (ANA). Thirty percent of patients develop a lupuslike syndrome characterized by high ANA titer, fever, pleuropericarditis, and arthritis. Discontinuing the drug usually reverses these findings.

Lidocaine (Xylocaine)

This drug is of great value in the management of ventricular ectopic rhythms in the critically ill. Lidocaine has the advantages of rapid effectiveness and minimal effect on cardiac contractility.

An initial intravenous bolus of 50 to 100 mg will usually suppress ectopic activity for approximately 20 minutes. Recurrence of ventricular premature contractions (VPCs) calls for a repeat intravenous bolus followed by a sustained intravenous infusion of 1 to 4 mg/minute. The dosage is adjusted to control ventricular ectopic beats. Care is taken to avoid excessive doses which produce agitation or seizures. As a rule, lidocaine is not helpful in the management of supraventricular arrhythmias.

Since lidocaine is metabolized by the liver, the dose should be reduced when hepatic blood flow is decreased, as in congestive heart failure. AV block with a slow junctional or ventricular focus is also a contraindication to the use of lidocaine.

Phenytoin (Dilantin)

This drug is usually ineffective for atrial arrhythmias. It is largely reserved for digitalis-toxic rhythms, in which it has moderate success. Such rhythms include atrial tachycardia, with or without block, and atrial fibrillation or flutter with a very slow ventricular rate and multiple VPCs. In this setting phenytoin may increase the ventricular rate to a more normal range and abolish the ventricular ectopic activity.

Phenytoin should be given slowly and intravenously undiluted from the vial. The rate of administration should not exceed 50 to 100 mg every 5 minutes. The drug should be given until the arrhythmia is controlled or a maximal dose of 1g is given. Phenytoin is seldom used in maintenance by the oral route.

Beta Adrenergic Blocking Agents

Propranolol (Inderal), currently the only beta blocking agent authorized for treatment of arrhythmias in this country, is useful for a variety of atrial and ventricular tachyarrhythmias. Propranolol increases the degree of block at the AV node and reduces the heart rate in patients with atrial fibrillation or flutter. In some, these

rhythms may revert to a sinus rhythm. Propranolol may be useful alone or as an adjunct to digitalis or quinidine. Beta blockade is especially helpful in some patients with chronic atrial fibrillation or flutter in whom digitalization is insufficient to control the ventricular rate. Propranolol is the agent of choice for rapid atrial arrhythmias due to hyperthyroidism.

The oral dose of propranolol varies over a wide range due to differences in the rate of removal by the liver. The usual dose is between 80 and 320 mg daily given in three or four divided doses. On occasion, however, even low doses of propranolol (10 to 20 mg daily) increase the degree of block at the AV node and provide satisfactory control of the heart rate. The dose in each situation must be "titrated," beginning with small amounts of the drug and adjusting further doses according to the degree of response. Therapeutic serum level measurements have not been established. Beta blockade is usually present at 50 to 100 ng/ml.

The intravenous use of propranolol requires great caution. Hypotension, acute pulmonary edema, and cardiovascular collapse may occur with intravenous doses as low as 1 mg. Doses of 0.3 to 0.5 mg IV should be used initially with close ECG and blood pressure monitoring. The dose should be repeated every 1 to 2 minutes and increased slowly as needed. The total intravenous dose should not exceed 7 to 10 mg in the first 2 to 3 hours.

PROPRANOLOL TOXICITY

Side-effects are common. Sinus bradycardia, usually well-tolerated, need *not* be regarded as a complication. Fatigue, depression, nausea, diarrhea, alopecia, impotence, increased peripheral vascular insufficiency, and hypoglycemia have been noted.

Propranolol depresses cardiac output in patients with preexisting congestive heart failure and therefore is contraindicated in such patients. An exception to this statement is the patient with heart failure due to atrial fibrillation or flutter with a very rapid ventricular response. Reduction of the ventricular rate in this instance may improve cardiac output and offset the depressant action of propranolol on the heart.

The drug should be used with great caution in patients with asthma, in whom it may induce irreversible and fatal bronchospasm. Finally, in the insulin-dependent diabetic patient, propranolol may mask the symptoms of hypoglycemia; thus the drug should be given with great care.

Disopyramide (Norpace)

Disopyramide is effective for both atrial and ventricular arrhythmias. By prolonging the refractory period of the accessory pathway, disopyramide may be especially effective in patients with WPW syndrome who develop supraventricular tachyarrhythmias.

Disopyramide is well absorbed by the oral route. Peak plasma levels occur in 2 hours; plasma half-life approximates 6 hours. Excretion occurs mainly by the renal route. Oral doses range from 100 to 300 mg every 6 hours. Effective plasma levels occur at about $2\mu g$ to $8\mu g$/ml. The intravenous route has not been approved for general use.

DISOPYRAMIDE TOXICITY

Disopyramide causes a slight to moderate decrease in cardiac output. It may precipitate overt cardiac failure in patients with limited myocardial reserve. The drug should be avoided in patients with advanced heart block. The most frequent side-effects of this drug are anticholinergic, namely, dry mouth, blurred vision, and, especially in males with prostatic enlargement, urinary retention.

Disopyramide, similar to quinidine and procainamide, can prolong the QT interval. Patients with marked prolongation of this interval appear especially susceptible to malignant ventricular rhythms and sudden death.

Atropine

Given intravenously, atropine blocks those arrhythmias related to excessive vagal activity. These include severe sinus bradycardia, SA block, and AV block. Atropine is ineffective in high grades of AV block due to extensive destruction of the conduction system. In low doses, atropine may exert a paradoxical effect and cause bradycardia and decreased AV conduction. If these occur, a larger intravenous dose (usually 0.5 to 1.5 mg) will usually produce the desired increase in heart rate.

Other Agents

Three agents have received extensive experimental study but have not yet been released for clinical use in this country. A brief mention of each drug follows.

Verapamil is an effective agent for supraventricular tachyarrhythmias. It depresses myocardial contractility and induces heart block and asystole in some individuals.

Amiodarone is a highly effective agent for supraventricular and ventricular arrhythmias. Corneal microdeposits occur nearly universally. Heart block develops in some patients with pre-existing conduction disturbances.

Aprindine is useful for supraventricular and ventricular arrhythmias, but troublesome side-effects, both neurologic and cardiac (depression in contractility and AV conduction) may limit its usefulness.

CARDIOVERSION

Direct current (DC) cardioversion has become the treatment of choice for many patients with supraventricular arrhythmias, including atrial fibrillation and atrial flutter, and ventricular tachycardia. Only a brief discussion of the technique follows. The reader is referred to Lown's classic review for more comprehensive information.[1]

1. It is helpful to begin the patient on quinidine, 0.2 g every 6 to 8 hr for 24 hr prior to conversion, which will produce reversion to sinus rhythm in up to 15% of such patients.
2. The patient is maintained in a fasting state for 8 hr before cardioversion.
3. An intravenous infusion is begun with the patient on a monitor and with all necessary resuscitation apparatus readily available.
4. Ideally, digitalis should be withheld for 24 hr prior to cardioversion, although cardioversion may be attempted in an emergency situation without this precaution.
5. Sedation is induced with the use of intravenous diazepam (Valium) in graduated doses of 5 to 10 mg.
6. Care should be taken to synchronize the electrical impulse with the apex of the R wave of the monitored lead.
7. Two paddles are then placed, one at the upper right sternal area and the other behind the left scapula or over the cardiac apex. A generous amount of electrode jelly is used to prevent skin burns and to decrease electrical resistance; firm pressure is exerted. One should avoid contact with the patient or the bed.
8. Initially, begin with 25 to 50 watt/sec (J) and increase until either reversion is achieved or a single shock level of 400 watt/sec is delivered.
9. Following the procedure, the patient should be observed closely for changes in rhythm, blood pressure, and respirations.

REFERENCES

1. Lown B: Electrical reversion of cardiac arrhythmias. Br Heart J 29:469, 1967

BIBLIOGRAPHY

Anderson JL, Harrison DC, Meffin PJ, Winkle RA: Antiarrhythmic drugs: Clinical pharmacology and therapeutic uses. Drugs 15:271, 1978

Ayres SM, Grace WJ: Inappropriate ventilation and hypoxemia as causes of cardiac arrhythmias. Am J Med 46:495, 1969

Danahy DT, Aronow WS: Lidocaine-induced cardiac rate changes in atrial fibrillation and atrial flutter. Am Heart J 95:474, 1978

Gaughan CE, Lown B, Lanigan J, Voukydis P, Besser HW: Acute oral testing for determining antiarrhythmic drug efficacy: I. Quinidine. Am J Cardiol 38:677, 1976

Josephson ME, Caracta AR, Ricciutti MA, Lau SH, Damato AN: Electrophysiologic properties of procainamide in man. Am J Cardiol 33:596, 1974

Marcus FI: Digitalis pharmacokinetics and metabolism. Am J Med 58:452, 1975

Niarchos AP: Disopyramide: Serum level and antiarrhythmic conversion. Am Heart J 92:57, 1976

Nies AS, Shand DG: Clinical pharmacology of propranolol. Circulation 52:6, 1975

Reynolds EW, Vander Ark CR: Quinidine syncope and the delayed repolarization syndromes. Mod Concepts Cardiovasc Dis 45:117, 1976

Smith TW, Haber E: Digitalis: medical progress. N Engl J Med 289:945, 1973

Wolf PS: Arrhythmias in chronic pulmonary disease. Angiology 30:676, 1979

Zipes DP, Troup PJ: New antiarrhythmic agents. Am J Cardiol 41:1005, 1978

Julie A. Shinn

INTRA-AORTIC BALLOON PUMP COUNTERPULSATION

Prior to the advent of critical care units, cardiac patients frequently died as a result of arrhythmias following acute myocardial infarction. Critical care units, offering continuous ECG monitoring, effectively reduced mortality due to arrhythmias by early detection and treatment. Acute left ventricular power failure, resulting in cardiogenic shock, emerged as a major cause of death following myocardial infarction. Over the last 2 decades, research emphasis and clinical therapy have been directed toward minimizing or preventing myocardial infarct extension and acute left ventricular power failure. Mortality rates ranged from 80% to 100% in patients suffering from cardiogenic shock. Invasive hemodynamic monitoring, diuretic agents, and vasoactive and inotropic drugs offered little assistance in decreasing mortality. Similar problems were encountered as cardiac surgery became more sophisticated and more complex surgery was performed. Among its complications was the development of acute left ventricular power failure, resulting in an inability to wean patients from cardiopulmonary bypass.

Therapeutic goals were directed toward (1) increasing oxygen supply to the myocardium, (2) decreasing left ventricular work, and (3) improving cardiac output. Prior to intra-aortic balloon pumping (IABP), no one therapeutic agent was capable of meeting these three goals.

IABP counterpulsation was designed to increase coronary artery perfusion pressure and blood flow during the diastolic phase of the cardiac cycle by inflation of a balloon in the thoracic aorta. Deflation of the balloon, just prior to systolic ejection, was designed to decrease the impedance to ejection and thus, left ventricular work. Inflation and deflation counterpulsated each heart beat. With improved blood flow and effective reduction in left ventricular work, the hopeful result was to improve myocardial pump function and increase cardiac output.

IABP was first introduced clinically by Kantrowitz and associates in 1967. This therapeutic approach was instituted for treatment of two patients with left ventricular power failure following acute myocardial infarction. Since that time, IABP has become a standard treatment for medical and surgical patients with acute left ventricular power failure that is unresponsive to pharmacologic and volume therapy.

DESCRIPTION

The intra-aortic balloon catheter is constructed of a biocompatible polyurethane material. Polyurethane is also used to make the balloon which is mounted on the end of the catheter. Filling of the balloon is achieved with pressurized gas that enters through small perforations in the cathe-

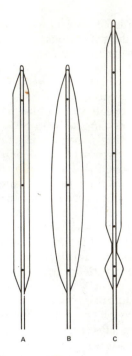

FIGURE 9-22.
Balloon configurations include *(A)* cylindrical shape, *(B)* fusiform shape, and *(C)* dual chamber.

ter. There are several configurations of balloons available, one model having two chambers and the others having single chambers (see Fig. 9-22). Inflation patterns differ in that some inflate from one end to the other while some inflate from the center. Types of balloons used are determined by physician preference and the type of equipment used to drive the balloon pump catheter. It is felt that configuration of the balloon may affect performance characteristics. However, it is not the purpose of this text to advocate any one particular model.

Proper position of the balloon is in the thoracic aorta just distal to the left subclavian artery and proximal to the renal arteries (see Fig. 9-23). Insertion of the catheter is achieved through a dacron graft which has been anastomosed to either a femoral or iliac artery. The catheter is advanced until proper position has been achieved. End-to-side anastomosis of the graft to the artery allows for proper securing of the catheter without obliteration of blood flow to the extremity. Suture is used around the graft to secure the catheter in position so that it will not slip out of the artery. Saphenous vein may also be used for the graft. In some selected patients with healthy vascular tissue, a purse string suture may be run through the adventicial layer of the artery

to secure the catheter. In this situation, a graft is not necessary. A new catheter is available on the market which allows for percutaneous insertion using a Seldinger technique. Currently, the majority of physicians use a temporary graft for insertion. Other approaches have been described. The most common alternative used is direct insertion into the thoracic aorta. Since this requires a thoracotomy incision, it is essentially restricted to use in cardiac surgery patients.

Once in place, the catheter is attached to a machine console that has three basic components: (1) a monitoring system, (2) an electronic trigger mechanism, and (3) a drive system which moves gas in and out of the balloon. Monitoring systems have the capability of displaying the patient's ECG, an arterial waveform showing the effect of balloon inflation/deflation, and a balloon waveform which illustrates the inflation and deflation of the balloon itself. The standard trigger mechanism for the balloon pump is the R wave that is sensed from the patient's ECG. This trigger will cause the balloon to inflate with each cardiac cycle. Adjustment of exact timing is controlled on the console of the machine. Precise timing will be discussed later. The drive system

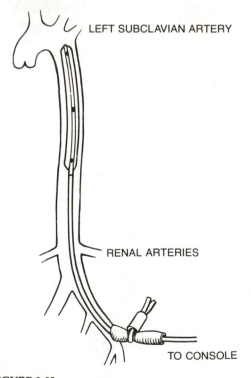

FIGURE 9-23.
Proper position of the balloon catheter illustrating exit site through a dacron graft.

is the actual mechanism which drives gas into and out of the balloon by alternating pressure and vacuum. Each machine must have pressurized tanks of either helium or carbon dioxide to drive the balloon.

Prior to discussing the actual timing of balloon inflation and deflation, it is important to understand the physiologic principles of IABP.

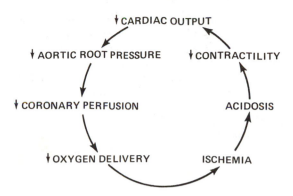

FIGURE 9-24.
Cycle leading to cardiogenic shock.

PHYSIOLOGIC PRINCIPLES

In the failing heart, greater work is required to maintain cardiac output. With this added work requirement, oxygen demand increases. This may occur at a time when the myocardium is already ischemic and coronary artery perfusion is unable to meet the oxygen demands. As a result, left ventricular performance diminishes even further, resulting in decreased cardiac output. A vicious cycle ensues that is difficult to interrupt (see Fig. 9-24). Without interruption of the cycle, cardiogenic shock may be imminent. This cycle can be broken with IABP by increasing aortic root pressure during diastole through inflation of the balloon. With increased aortic root pressure, the perfusion pressure of the coronary arteries will be increased.

Effective therapy for the patient in left ventricular power failure also involves decreasing myocardial oxygen demand. Four major determinants of myocardial oxygen demand are (1) afterload, (2) preload, (3) contractility, and (4) heart rate. IABP can have an effect on all of these factors. It will directly decrease afterload and will indirectly affect the other three determinants as cardiac function improves.

Afterload is the amount of wall tension that must be generated by the ventricle to raise intraventricular pressure, allowing the ventricle to overcome impedance to ejection. When adequate intraventricular pressure is reached, the semilunar valve is forced open and ejection occurs. This occurs in either ventricle. Since IABP assists the left heart, only the left ventricle will be discussed. Impedance to ejection is a result of the aortic valve, aortic end–diastolic pressure, and vascular resistance. With greater impedance, afterload increases, and thus, more oxygen is demanded by the ventricle for energy. The aortic valve is a factor that does not change unless stenosis, which increases afterload, is present. Greater aortic end–diastolic pressures require higher afterload to overcome this impedance to ejection. Vascular resistance will increase im-

pedance when vessels become vasoconstricted. Vasodilation or lower vascular resistance will decrease impedance to ejection and thus, afterload decreases.

Deflation of the balloon in the aorta, just prior to ventricular systole, lowers aortic end–diastolic pressure, which decreases impedance. The greatest amount of oxygen required during the cardiac cycle is for the development of afterload. With decreased impedance, the workload of the ventricle also decreases. In this way, IABP can effectively decrease the oxygen demand of the heart.

Preload is the volume or pressure in the ventricle at end diastole. Volume in a chamber creates pressure. An individual in acute left ventricular power failure has increased volume in the ventricle at end diastole due to the heart's inability to pump effectively. This excessive increase in preload also increases the workload of the heart. Clinically, preload of the right heart is measured by central venous pressure or right atrial pressure, and preload of the left heart is measured with the pulmonary capillary wedge pressure or left atrial pressure. These pressures increase when the ventricles are in failure.

IABP helps to decrease excessive preload in the left ventricle by decreasing impedance to ejection. With decreased impedance, there is a more effective forward flow of blood. Preload is decreased, with more efficient emptying of the left ventricle during systole.

Contractility refers to the velocity of contraction during systole. With greater velocity, the workload of the heart is increased. Although contractility requires oxygen, good contractility is a benefit to cardiac function. Good contractility ensures good, efficient pumping, which serves to increase cardiac output. In failure, contractility is depressed. The biochemical status of the myocardium directly affects contractility. Contractility is depressed when calcium levels are low, when catecholamine levels are low, and when ischemia is present with resultant acidosis.

IABP can serve to increase oxygen supply, thereby decreasing ischemia and acidosis. In this way, IABP contributes to improve contractility and better cardiac function (refer to Fig. 9-24).

Heart rate is a major determinant of oxygen demand because the rate determines the number of times per minute the high pressures must be generated during systole. Normally, myocardial perfusion takes place during diastole. Coronary artery perfusion pressure is determined by the gradient between aortic diastolic pressure and myocardial wall tension. It can be expressed by the following equation:

coronary perfusion pressure =
aortic diastolic − myocardial wall
pressure   tension

Tension in the muscle retards blood flow, which is why approximately 80% of coronary artery perfusion occurs during diastole. With faster heart rates, diastolic time becomes shortened, with very little change occurring in systolic time. A rapid heart rate not only increases oxygen demand, but also decreases the time available for delivery of oxygen. In acute ventricular power failure, an individual may not be able to maintain cardiac output by increasing the volume of blood pumped with each beat (stroke volume) because contractility is likely to be depressed. Cardiac output is a function of both stroke volume and heart rate.

cardiac output = stroke volume × heart rate

If stroke volume cannot be increased, heart rate must increase to maintain cardiac output. This is very costly in terms of oxygen demand.

By improving contractility, IABP contributes to improve myocardial pumping and the ability to increase stroke volume. Decreasing afterload also improves pumping efficiency. With improved myocardial function, heart rate will decrease. IABP will also serve to increase coronary artery perfusion pressure by increasing aortic diastolic pressure during inflation of the balloon, resulting in improved blood flow and oxygen delivery to the myocardium.

Physiologic effects of IABP are summarized in the chart that follows. Proper inflation of the balloon will serve to increase oxygen supply, and proper deflation of the balloon will decrease oxygen demand. Timing of inflation and deflation is crucial and must coincide with the cardiac cycle.

DIRECT PHYSIOLOGIC EFFECTS OF INTRA-AORTIC BALLOON PUMP (IABP)

Inflation:
1. ↑ aortic diastolic pressure
2. ↑ aortic root pressure
3. ↑ coronary perfusion pressure
4. ↑ oxygen supply

Deflation:
1. ↓ aortic end-diastolic pressure
2. ↓ impedance to ejection
3. ↓ afterload
4. ↓ oxygen demand

TIMING

Systole and diastole are the two major components of the cardiac cycle.

The first step to proper timing of the balloon pump is the identification of the beginning of systole and diastole on the arterial waveform. Every patient must have an arterial catheter in place to monitor timing. The cycle of the left heart will be used to describe the events of the cardiac cycle. Systole begins when left ventricular pressure exceeds left atrial pressure, forcing the mitral valve closed.

There are two phases to systole: (1) isovolumic contraction and (2) ejection. Once the mitral valve is closed, isovolumic contraction begins and continues until enough pressure is generated to overcome impedance to ejection. When ventricular pressure exceeds aortic pressure, the aortic valve is forced open, initiating ejection or phase two. Ejection continues until pressure in the left ventricle falls below pressure in the aorta. At this point the aortic valve closes and diastole begins.

Closing of the valve creates an artifact on the arterial waveform that is called the *dicrotic notch*. The dicrotic notch is used as a timing reference to determine when balloon inflation should occur. Inflation should not occur before the notch because systole has not been completed.

After aortic valve closure, two phases of diastole begin: (1) isovolumic relaxation and (2) ventricular filling. Following aortic valve closure, there is a period of time in which neither the aortic nor mitral valve is open. The mitral valve remains closed because left ventricular pressure is still higher than left atrial pressure. This phase is isovolumic relaxation. When left ventricular pressure falls below left atrial pressure, the mitral valve is forced open by the higher pressure in the left atrium. This begins the filling phase of diastole. Balloon inflation should continue throughout diastole. Deflation should be timed to occur at end diastole, just prior to the next sharp systolic upstroke on the arterial waveform.

Figure 9–25 illustrates the cardiac cycle with left atrial, left ventricular, and aortic pressure superimposed on one another. Note the systolic upstroke seen on the aortic tracing and the appearance of the dicrotic notch.

Figure 9–26 illustrates a radial artery waveform with the beginning of systole and diastole marked. The amount of time balloon inflation should last can be estimated by knowing the patient's heart rate. Systole is roughly one-third of the cardiac cycle and diastole is approximately two-thirds. Each R to R interval on the ECG represents one cardiac cycle. Heart rate per minute is actually the number of cardiac cycles per minute. With each minute equaling 60,000 msec, dividing 60,000 msec by heart rate equals the total milliseconds in each cardiac cycle or R to R interval. Approximately one-third of the R to R interval will be systole or the number of milliseconds the balloon is deflated, and two-thirds will be diastole or the balloon inflation interval. It is wise to add extra time to the deflation period until fine adjustment of the waveform can be made.

The accompanying chart outlines the steps taken to determine inflation and deflation time for a patient with a heart rate of 60. This method can be used as a guide for initial establishment of balloon pumping.

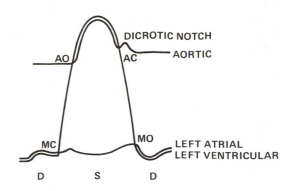

FIGURE 9-25.
Cardiac cycle of the left heart with aortic, left ventricular, and left atrial pressure waveforms. *(AO)* aortic valve opening; *(AC)* aortic valve closure; *(D)* diastole; *(MO)* mitral valve opening; *(MC)* mitral valve closure; *(S)* systole.

CONTRAINDICATIONS
Now that the principles of IABP have been outlined, it will be clear why IABP is advantageous in a variety of patients. Few contraindications exist to its use.

A competent aortic valve is necessary if the patient is to benefit from IABP. With *aortic insufficiency,* balloon inflation would only increase aortic regurgitation and offer little, if any, augmentation of coronary artery perfusion pressure.

Severe peripheral vascular occlusive disease is also a contraindication to use of IABP. Occlusive disease would make insertion of the catheter quite difficult and possibly interrupt plaque formation along the vessel wall. In patients who absolutely require IABP, insertion can be achieved by way of the thoracic aorta, thus bypassing diseased peripheral vessels.

CALCULATION OF INFLATION AND DEFLATION TIME FOR A HEART RATE OF 60

$$\frac{\text{msec in one}}{\text{R to R interval}} = \frac{60{,}000 \text{ msec/min}}{\text{patient's heart rate (60 beats/min)}}$$

one R to R interval = 1000 msec
systole (⅓) ∼ 400 msec
diastole (⅔) ∼ 600 msec

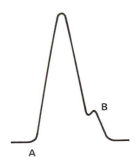

FIGURE 9-26.
Arterial waveform with *A* representing the point of balloon deflation prior to the systolic upstroke and *B* representing balloon inflation at the dicrotic notch.

Any previous aortofemoral or aortoiliac *bypass graft* would also contraindicate femoral artery insertion.

The presence of an *aortic aneurysm* is also a contraindication to the use of IABP. A pulsating balloon against an aneurysm may predispose the patient to dislodgement of aneurysmal debris with resultant emboli. A more serious complication would be rupture of the aneurysm. The chart that follows lists the contraindications to IABP.

CONTRAINDICATIONS TO IABP
- Aortic valve incompetence
- Severe peripheral vascular occlusive disease
- Previous aortofemoral or aortoiliac bypass grafts
- Aortic aneurysm

INDICATIONS

Two major applications of IABP currently employed are for treatment of cardiogenic shock following myocardial infarction and for acute left ventricular power failure following cardiac surgery. In addition, other applications have been made for other types of patients with cardiac pathophysiology (see accompanying chart). Successful support of the septic shock patient and the cardiovascular patient undergoing general surgery has also been reported.

INDICATIONS FOR IABP
- Cardiogenic shock following acute infarction
- Left ventricular power failure in the postoperative cardiac surgery patient
- Severe unstable angina
- Postinfarction angina
- Postinfarction ventricular septal defect or mitral regurgitation
- Refractory ventricular tachyarrhythmias
- Septic shock
- General surgery for the patient with cardiovascular disease

---

Cardiogenic Shock

Treatment of cardiogenic shock is complicated and the mortality remains high. Approximately 15% of patients with myocardial infarction will develop cardiogenic shock. The presence of car-

diogenic shock is confirmed by the following accepted criteria:

- Low cardiac output syndrome
- Cardiac index of 2.0 liters/min/M^2 or less
- Systolic blood pressure < 80 torr or < 100 torr in a formerly hypertensive patient
- Urine output < 20 ml/hr

Patients will first be given a short period of treatment with various inotropic drugs, vasopressors, and volume. A lack of or minimal response in arterial pressure, urine output, and mental status following this therapy will indicate a need for assisted circulation with IABP. Once hypotension is present, the self-perpetuating process of injury will be in effect. Control of further injury and improvement in survival require early reversal of the shock state.

Most research centers agree that patients who hemodynamically exhibit left ventricular end-diastolic pressures or pulmonary capillary wedge pressures of > 18 torr with cardiac indexes of < 2.0 to 2.2 liter/minute/meter^2 carry high mortality and should be considered for IABP if they are unresponsive to a short period of pharmacologic therapy.

RESPONSE PATTERNS

Once IABP is instituted, improvement should be seen in 1 to 2 hours. At this time steady improvement should be seen in cardiac output, peripheral perfusion, urine output, mental status, and pulmonary congestion. With improved cardiac function, one should also see a decrease in CVP and pulmonary capillary wedge pressure. Average peak effect should be achieved within 24 hours.

There are three general responses to IABP therapy. One group of patients will achieve hemodynamic stabilization and survive with the support of medical therapy and IABP. A second group of patients will continue to deteriorate with the support of IABP and will die from irreversible cardiogenic shock. A third group of patients will become dependent on IABP for circulatory support. Attempted withdrawal of IABP in this group results in hemodynamic deterioration. Some of the patients in this group may achieve some benefit from cardiac surgical intervention. There are centers that advocate early resection of infarcted tissue or coronary artery bypass grafting for this group of patients. Surgery on patients in cardiogenic shock will carry extremely high risk. Many of the nonoperated patients will die from complications of their illness.

Postoperative Left Ventricular Power Failure

Successful reduction in mortality has been achieved by utilizing IABP for patients with acute left ventricular power failure or cardiogenic shock following cardiac surgery. There are two major conditions which might lead to postoperative pump failure. These are severe preoperative left ventricular dysfunction and intraoperative myocardial infarction.

IABP can be used to wean patients from cardiopulmonary bypass and to provide postoperative circulatory assistance until left ventricular recovery occurs. In these situations, early recognition of failure is evidenced by the heart's inability to support circulation following cardiopulmonary bypass.

Early recognition and treatment is crucial if left ventricular power failure is to be reversed. Later development and recognition of failure following cardiac surgery results in much higher mortality, even with the assistance of IABP.

High-Risk Cardiac Surgery Patients

IABP has also been used in the high-risk cardiac surgery patient for safer induction of anesthesia. Patients who develop signs of acute cardiac ischemia unresponsive to pharmacologic therapy may benefit from IABP during *anesthesia induction* and for support prior to *cardiopulmonary bypass*.

IABP may also be employed during *cardiac catheterization* for this same group of high-risk patients. In this situation, cardiac catheterization studies are generally followed by emergency cardiac surgery. In this category would be patients with unstable angina, postinfarction angina and postinfarction ventricular septal defects, or mitral regurgitation with resultant cardiac failure. IABP has been successfully used to abolish or markedly decrease the incidence of angina attacks in patients in whom previous medical therapy has failed. The use of IABP for patients with cardiac failure following ventricular septal rupture or mitral valve incompetence will aid in the promotion of forward blood flow. This will decrease shunting through the septal defect and decrease the amount of mitral regurgitation.

Postoperative Complications

Complications in the postoperative period, related to ventricular performance, might also indicate the use of IABP. Limited use of IABP in the pulmonary artery for right ventricular afterload reduction has been reported following right ventricular infarction resulting in severe failure following cardiac surgery. A small number of patients with refractory ventricular tachyarrhythmias may benefit from the physiological effects of IABP. This group is comprised of patients with myocardial ischemia, infarction, or ventricular aneurysms. IABP is instituted when pharmacologic management fails to suppress irritable foci. In these situations, IABP is used as support until blood flow can be restored by surgical revascularization or by resection of irritable foci, the ventricular aneurysm, or the area of infarction.

Septic Shock

A newer application of IABP has been for the support of patients in septic shock. Patients in septic shock have very low systemic vascular resistance due to vasodilatation caused by the endotoxin. To review, mean arterial blood pressure is a function of cardiac output and systemic vascular resistance. In order to maintain adequate perfusion pressure to vital organs, the patient in septic shock must maintain a very high cardiac output. IABP has been used when traditional vasopressor support fails to maintain adequate mean arterial pressure. Prolonged, inadequate perfusion pressure will result in possible renal failure or myocardial infarction. IABP is advocated by some clinicians to assist blood pressure maintenance and increase coronary perfusion when traditional support fails.

General Surgery for High-Risk Patient

Another newer application of IABP is for the high-risk cardiovascular patient undergoing a general surgical operation. Any patient with ischemic heart disease will be a higher risk for general anesthesia and the surgical procedure. IABP is used to ensure adequate coronary artery perfusion pressure during the procedure.

PATIENT MANAGEMENT

Patients requiring IABP are managed much like any other critically ill patient in cardiogenic shock or acute left ventricular power failure. Nursing assessment and management of these conditions are discussed elsewhere in the text. There are additional nursing skills and assessment considerations specific to IABP therapy that must be included in the care of these patients.

Cardiovascular System

Monitoring the cardiovascular system is extremely important to determine the effectiveness of balloon pump therapy. The basis for this assessment should include vital signs, cardiac output, heart rhythm and regularity, urine output, color, perfusion, and mentation.

VITAL SIGNS

Three important vital signs with respect to IABP are heart rate, mean arterial blood pressure (MAP), and pulmonary capillary wedge pressure.

Since timing of the balloon pump is based on *heart rate*, any variation of heart rate may significantly affect the performance of the balloon pump. Any variation in heart rate of 10 beats or greater necessitates an evaluation and possible readjustment of inflation and deflation timing. Large variations in heart rate may also indicate a change in the patient's overall clinical status.

MAP should improve with effective IABP. An acute change in MAP may require a quick evaluation of timing and then a further assessment of other vital signs. These patients tolerate very little change in volume status, and an acute drop in MAP may also indicate volume depletion.

The *pulmonary capillary wedge pressure* is an important parameter for monitoring volume status. It will provide an early indication of volume depletion or volume overload.

Blood pressure readings require special consideration. Because the balloon inflates during diastole, peak–diastolic pressure may be higher than peak–systolic pressure. It is important to remember that monitoring equipment cannot distinguish systole from diastole but only peak pressures from low–point pressures. For this reason, a monitor digital display of systolic pressure may actually represent peak-diastolic pressure. It is advisable to record blood pressure as systolic, peak diastolic, and end diastolic; that is, 100/110/60. These pressures can be read from a strip recording of the arterial waveform.

To determine the effect of the balloon pump, pressures (systolic, diastolic, and MAP) can also be recorded with the pump on as well as with the pump off.

HEART RHYTHM AND REGULARITY

Heart rhythm and regularity are also important considerations. Early recognition and treatment of *arrhythmias* are crucial not only for patient safety but also for effective IABP. Irregular arrhythmias may inhibit efficient IABP because timing is set by the patient's regular R to R interval on the ECG. A safety feature of all balloon pump consoles is automatic deflation of the balloon for premature QRS complexes. Any patient who develops a bigeminal rhythm will then lose 50% of the balloon assistance. If the arrhythmia persists, another alternative might be use of the systolic peak on the arterial waveform as the trigger mechanism for balloon inflation.

OTHER OBSERVATIONS

Urine output, color, perfusion, and *mentation* are all important assessment parameters to determine the adequacy of cardiac output. Any deterioration in these signs might also indicate a fall in cardiac output. If the patient is responding to IABP, these signs should also show improvement. Cardiac output measurement with a pulmonary artery catheter is indicated when deterioration is evident or when a major change in volume or pharmacologic therapy has been instituted. Monitoring the patient's ability to maintain cardiac output is also important during weaning procedures from IABP.

Special attention should be given to the *left radial pulse*. A decrease or absence of the left radial pulse may indicate that the balloon has advanced up the aorta and may be partially or totally obstructing the left subclavian artery.

The presence of the balloon catheter in the femoral or iliac artery predisposes the patient to impaired circulation of the involved extremity. The extremity with the catheter in place will also be relatively immobile. Any flexion of the hip may kink the catheter and impair balloon pumping. Extremities should be checked hourly for pulses, color, and sensation. Any deterioration in the affected extremity should be reported to the physician. Severe vascular insufficiency will necessitate the removal of the catheter. Patients should be encouraged to flex their feet frequently every hour to avoid venous stasis. If unable to do this, the nurse can do this for them.

Some physicians advocate the use of heparin therapy to prevent possible thrombus formation around the catheter and vascular insufficiency. Each physician will determine whether the risks of anticoagulation outweigh the benefits for the individual patient. If anticoagulation is used, it is advisable to perform a guaiac test periodically on nasogastric drainage and stools for the presence of blood. Observation of *urine* for hematuria, *skin* for petechiae, and any *incisions* for oozing of blood should also be part of patient assessment.

If any of these are noted, the physician should be alerted. Heparin therapy may require adjustment or possible reversal with protamine sulfate.

Pulmonary System

The majority of patients on IABP will require intubation and ventilatory assistance. Many will have suffered respiratory insufficiency due to the fluid overload associated with cardiac failure. Any intubated patient has an increased risk of *respiratory tract infection*. This risk increases greatly in the debilitated patient. Invasive hemodynamic monitoring catheters and the balloon catheter will also restrict the patient's mobility, requiring modification in turning. This may increase the risk of *atelectasis*. Turning is appropriate as long as the extremity with the balloon catheter is kept straight. It may be helpful to use a soft restraint around the ankle of the affected extremity to remind the patient to avoid flexion of the hip. For the same reason, the head of the bed cannot be elevated more than 30°. In addition, elevation may cause the catheter to advance up the aorta.

Some patients might require horizontal lifting for placement of chest x-ray film when portable roentgenograms are taken. Daily chest roentgenograms are needed to follow pulmonary status and to inspect intravenous catheter placement. The position of the balloon catheter can also be determined in this manner.

Renal System

Patients in cardiogenic shock are at risk for the development of acute renal failure. Urine output and quality should be monitored closely. Serum levels of blood urea nitrogen and creatine should be included in daily laboratory studies to monitor renal function. It is advisable to study creatine clearance in addition to serum creatine. Creatine clearance will indicate renal dysfunction and possible failure much earlier than serum creatine. Serum creatine does not rise until significant renal function is lost. Also, any acute, dramatic drop in urine output might be an indication that the catheter has slipped down the aorta and is obstructing the renal arteries. A portable roentgenogram can confirm this suspicion. Predisposition to urinary tract infection is also present in patients with indwelling Foley catheters. Good catheter hygiene and maintenance of an acidic urine will help prevent infection.

Psychosocial Considerations

Balloon insertion is usually an unplanned, emergent procedure for patients with deteriorating conditions. Abundant monitoring is frightening for both the patient and family. Every effort should be made to explain surroundings and procedures to patients. The goal is to make them feel more secure in their environment and to alleviate anxiety.

Family members need to be prepared for the first visit after balloon insertion. Good preparation helps them to deal with the stress of the situation and also to be more supportive for the patient. Honest communication with the family is very important. This helps them to interpret the situation realistically and to view changes in the patient's condition with appropriate significance. Families will also be carrying the responsibility of making decisions regarding the patient's care. It is often helpful to provide contact with another nonmedical personnel member such as a social worker or clergyman. These individuals can provide additional support to the family. Sometimes it is easier to express feelings of hopelessness or fear of the patient's death when dealing with an individual who is not directly involved in the patient's care.

Critically ill patients often suffer from sleep deprivation and disorientation. Immobility and unfamiliar noises and machinery also serve to increase stress and anxiety in the patient. Frequent orientation by staff and family visits can help to alleviate some of this stress. Good care planning can help to organize procedures such as suctioning, turning, and dressing changes so that patients receive longer periods of uninterrupted rest.

Other Considerations

Nutrition should be an early consideration to promote healing and strength. Hyperalimentation can be instituted to provide nutrients and essential vitamins. Tube feedings might also be considered in patients who are able to tolerate them.

Infection is a major problem in the debilitated patient. Thus it is extremely important to maintain sterile technique, particularly in relation to the dressing over the balloon catheter exit site. Many of these patients will have a dacron graft lying beneath subcutaneous tissue. The presence of the graft increases the risk for wound infection. Once bacteria lodge in the graft, infection is relatively impossible to treat. Intravenous antibiotics have little effect; because the graft has no blood supply, it does not receive any benefit from the antibiotics. Once the wound is infected, the graft must be removed for successful treatment. For that reason, dressings should be changed with sterile gloves and ideally, a sterile mask. Dressings should be kept clean and dry. Some institutions use sterile, occlusive dressings for this type of wound care.

WAVEFORM ASSESSMENT

An important nursing function in the care of patients on IABP is the analysis of the arterial pressure waveform and the effectiveness of IABP. Nurses must be able to recognize and correct problems in balloon-pump timing.

Step 1. The first step in timing assessment is the ability to recognize the beginnings of systole and diastole on the arterial waveform (see Fig. 9–26). Systole begins at point *A* on Figure 9–26 where the sharp upstroke begins. Point *B* marks the dicrotic notch, which represents aortic valve closure. It is at this point that diastole begins and the balloon should be inflated. Balloon deflation occurs just prior to point *A*, at end diastole.

The chart that follows lists five criteria that can be used to measure the effectiveness of IABP on the arterial pressure waveform. To effectively evaluate the waveform, it is necessary to view the patient's unassisted pressure tracing alongside the assisted pressure tracing. To do this, the machine can be adjusted so that the balloon inflates and deflates on every other beat; that is, a 1:2 assist ratio. Most patients will tolerate this well for a brief period of time. Many machine consoles are capable of freezing the waveform on the console monitor so that it would only be necessary to assist 1:2 for one screen. The machine can then return to 1:1 assistance while the nurse assesses the tracing. Another alternative would be to obtain a strip

recording of the 1:2 assistance for analysis. These two approaches might be necessary if the patient's MAP drops significantly on 1:2 assistance.

Step 2. Using the first criterion, the patient's dicrotic notch should be identified. Comparison is then made with the assisted tracing to see that inflation occurs at the point of the dicrotic notch. Inflation before the dicrotic notch will abruptly shorten the patient's systole and increase ventricular volume as ejection is interrupted. Late inflation, past the dicrotic notch, will not raise coronary artery perfusion pressure as effectively. The peak diastolic pressure may not be as high as it would be with proper timing. Also, the duration of assistance during diastole will be unnecessarily shortened.

Step 3. Next, the slopes of systolic upstroke and diastolic augmentation should be compared. The diastolic slope should be sharp and parallel the systolic upstroke. A diastolic slope that reaches its peak slowly indicates that the increase in aortic root pressure rises slowly and is not as effective in immediately increasing coronary perfusion pressure. The greater the peak in diastolic pressure, the greater increase there will be in aortic root pressure. For that reason, balloon assistance should be adjusted until the highest peak possible is achieved. The method of doing this will vary with different brands of consoles. The nurse should be familiar with the particular console used by the institution.

Step 4. Deflation should occur just prior to systole, causing an acute drop in aortic end-diastolic pressure. This quick deflation displaces between 20 to 40 ml of volume, depending on the size of the balloon. This displacement of volume causes a drop in pressure because the volume was contributing to pressure. The result is an end-diastolic dip in pressure that reduces the impedance to the next systolic ejection. The end-diastolic pressure without the balloon assistance should be compared with the end-diastolic pressure with the dip created by balloon deflation. Optimally, a pressure difference of at least 10 torr should be obtained. Better afterload reduction is achieved with the lowest possible end-diastolic dip.

The point of deflation is also crucial. Deflation that is too early will allow pressure to rise to normal end-diastolic levels preceding systole. In this situation, there will be no decrease in afterload. Early deflation may actually have a "sink-like" effect on the aortic root, impairing

---

CRITERIA FOR ASSESSMENT OF EFFECTIVE IABP ON THE ARTERIAL PRESSURE WAVEFORM
- Inflation occurs at the dicrotic notch.
- Inflation slope is parallel to the systolic upstroke.
- Diastolic augmentation peak is greater than or equal to the preceding systolic peak.
- An end-diastolic dip in pressure is created with balloon deflation.
- The following systolic peak (assisted systole) is lower than the preceding systole (unassisted systole).

coronary perfusion because blood is distracted to the area of the pressure drop. Late deflation will encroach upon the next systole and actually increase afterload owing to greater impedance to ejection.

Step 5. Finally, if afterload has been reduced, the next systolic pressure peak should be lower than the unassisted systolic pressure peak. This implies that the ventricle did not have to generate as great a pressure to overcome impedance to ejection. This may not always be seen because the systolic pressure peak also represents the compliance of the vasculature. If the vasculature is noncomplaint due to atherosclerotic disease, the systolic peak may not change very much. Figure 9-27 illustrates the five points which must be assessed on the waveform. Figure 9-28 demonstrates possible errors in timing.

Balloon fit. The fit of the balloon to any particular patient's aorta will determine how well each of these criteria are met. Ideally, approximately 80% to 90% of the aorta should be occluded with balloon inflation. Any occlusion greater than this may damage aortic tissue. Occasionally, the larger balloon cannot be threaded through the femoral or iliac arteries, so a smaller balloon must be used. In this situation, the effect of inflation and deflation will not be as dramatic on the waveform. In a patient who is hypotensive or hypovolemic, the balloon will not have as pronounced an effect on the waveform because

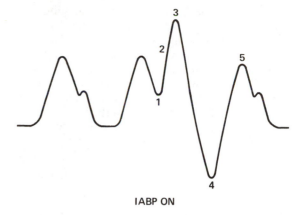

IABP ON

FIGURE 9-27.
Inspection of the arterial waveform with intra-aortic balloon assistance should include observation of *(1)* inflation point; *(2)* slopes; *(3)* diastolic peak pressure; *(4)* end–diastolic dip; *(5)* next systolic peak.

there is less volume displacement as the balloon inflates or deflates.

TROUBLESHOOTING

Conduction Problems
Some console units require a separate set of ECG leads for input into the trigger mechanism. Some units can be jacked into the primary monitor, requiring only one set of ECG leads. The

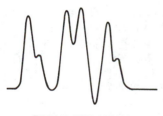

EARLY INFLATION

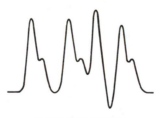

LATE INFLATION

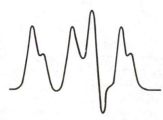

EARLY DEFLATION

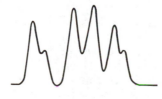

LATE DEFLATION

FIGURE 9-28.
Illustration of possible errors occurring with timing.

nurse should be familiar with the capabilities of the particular console. Maintenance of good conduction through the skin is important.

Any ECG artifact will interfere with the console's ability to recognize the trigger, or R wave, and will result in ineffective assistance. Any interference will cause an automatic deflation of the balloon. If the amplitude of the R wave is too low to trigger effectively, this can be corrected by changing lead placement. Any pacemaker artifact may also be interpreted as a trigger. This is generally not a problem with ventricular pacemakers. Atrial pacing artifact occurs just before atrial contraction during diastole. Since it is not desirable for balloon deflation to occur before end diastole, adjustments must be made. Inflation time can be delayed until the dicrotic notch is seen on the arterial waveform. This delay time will be longer than the normal delay set before inflation occurs.

A cardiac arrest due to ventricular fibrillation or asystole will not provide a trigger for IABP. In this situation, the machine can be turned off. It should not be left off for more than 5 minutes because this will likely result in platelet aggregation around the balloon. It should be inflated periodically to avoid this problem. Some consoles are capable of pumping at a preset rate regardless of the patient's ECG pattern. Cardioversion or defibrillation can be performed while the machine remains on. The machines are insulated so that this electric current will not damage the internal mechanisms. Tachycardias may also impair pumping ability. Often, switching the machine to a 1:2 assist will increase its ability to follow the rapid rate with increased effectiveness.

Balloon Problems

A small amount of gas will normally diffuse out of the balloon. This necessitates that the balloon be evacuated and filled periodically. Normally, this is required approximately every 3 to 4 hours. Some consoles do this automatically and some require manual refilling by the nurse. Loss of balloon volume will be evident when the diastolic pressure peak and end-diastolic dip begin to decrease. Any increase in frequency required for refilling might suggest a leak in catheter connection. Normal diffusion of gas should be only 1 to 2 ml/hour. Rarely, a balloon may develop a leak. Initially a loss in balloon effectiveness will be noted. With refilling, a greater loss of volume will be noted. Eventually, blood will back up into the catheter. The physi-

cian should be notified immediately because the faulty balloon will have to be removed to avoid the possibility of gas embolus. Because carbon dioxide is highly soluble in blood, a small leak is rarely a serious problem. Helium does not have this characteristic, and a leak is therefore more serious, even a small one. In this situation, it is important to keep the balloon moving slightly while decreasing its volume. The frequency of inflation should be decreased to the absolute minimum.

Vacuum Problems

Each machine will have an alarm system that will alert the nurse to any loss of vacuum. The vacuum will be responsible for deflation of the balloon. Any decrease in vacuum will interfere with the balloon's ability to deflate. On the other hand, a loss of pressure from the compressor pump will interfere with effective inflation. Any fault in the drive system (the vacuum or compressor) requires that the console be changed. The malfunctioning console should then be inspected by a biomedical engineer or the service representative from the particular company.

WEANING

Indications

Weaning patients generally can begin 12 to 24 hours after insertion. Some patients will require longer periods of support. Weaning can begin when a patient shows evidence of *hemodynamic stability*. A patient should not require excessive vasopressor support to maintain hemodynamic stability. Ideally, vasopressor support should be minimal when weaning begins. After the balloon is removed, it is much easier to increase vasopressor support than it is to reinsert a balloon catheter for hemodynamic support. Each physician will determine his own criteria for hemodynamic stability. General guidelines might include a cardiac index > 2 liters per minute, a pulmonary wedge pressure < 20 torr, and a systolic blood pressure > 100 torr.

The patient should also exhibit signs of *adequate cardiac function* evidenced by good peripheral pulses, adequate urine output, absence of pulmonary edema, and improved mentation. *Good coronary artery perfusion* will be evidenced by an absence of life-threatening arrhythmias and no evidence of ischemia or injury on the ECG.

Complications may also require abrupt cessation of IABP. This may or may not result in a reinsertion of another balloon catheter. Severe vascular insufficiency evidenced by a loss of pulses in the distal extremity, pain, and pallor is definitely an indication to remove the balloon catheter from that particular insertion site. Any balloon that develops a leak also requires removal for obvious reasons. The physician may choose to reinsert the balloon catheter in another extremity or to replace the faulty balloon if the patient is hemodynamically unstable. Depending upon the philosophy of the institution and physician, a deteriorating, irreversible situation might also be an indication for weaning or discontinuing balloon pump support. The accompanying chart lists major indications for weaning the patient from IABP.

INDICATIONS FOR WEANING FROM IABP
- Hemodynamic stability
    Cardiac index > 2 liters/min
    Pulmonary capillary wedge pressure < 20 torr
    Systolic blood pressure > 100 torr
- Minimal requirements for vasopressor support
- Evidence of adequate cardiac function
    Good peripheral pulses
    Adequate urine output
    Absence of pulmonary edema
    Improved mentation
- Evidence of good coronary perfusion
    Absence of life-threatening arrhythmias
    Absence of ischemia on the ECG
- Severe vascular insufficiency
- Balloon leakage
- Deteriorating, irreversible condition

Approaches

Weaning may be achieved by any combination of the approaches listed in the chart that follows. The first likely step would be to decrease the assist ratio from 1:1 to 1:2, and so on until the minimum assist ratio is achieved on any particular console. A patient might be assisted at the first decrease for up to 4 to 6 hours. A minimum amount of time should be 30 minutes. During this time, the patient must be assessed for any change in hemodynamic status. An increasing heart rate with decreasing blood pressure indicates a deterioration in hemodynamic status. Cardiac output should also be assessed at this time. A decrease in cardiac output or any evidence listed previously indicates the patient is not tolerating the weaning. Weaning should be temporarily discontinued. Therapy may be ad-

justed for the patient prior to another weaning attempt. If the first decrease in assist ratio is tolerated, the assist ratio is decreased to minimum with 1 to 4 hours allowed for each new assist ratio. Again, the patient must be continually assessed for any indications of intolerance to the process.

APPROACHES TO WEANING FROM IABP
- Gradual decrease of assist ratio
- Decrease diastolic augmentation
- Decrease balloon volume

Another approach, which might be utilized in conjunction with decreasing assist ratio, is decreasing the diastolic augmentation. This will result in decreased aortic root pressure, which should be tolerated by the patient who is ready for weaning. At this time, and also during decreasing assist ratio, the patient's ECG should be monitored for any ST segment changes. In addition, a return of angina is an indication that this procedure is not being tolerated.

The preceding steps may be all that are required to assess the patient's ability to maintain hemodynamic stability without IABP. Some physicians might also choose to decrease balloon volume so that the balloon merely quivers at the lowest assist ratio. It is important to maintain movement of the balloon to avoid platelet aggregation around the balloon. By maintaining a quiverlike state, the balloon never completely inflates. At this point, IABP has essentially been discontinued because the patient receives no hemodynamic benefit from balloon inflation.

Removal of the Balloon Catheter

Removal is a surgical procedure; hence, the patient will most often return to the operating room after weaning is complete. Prior to removal, the patient is heparinized. After the balloon catheter has been removed, a Fogarty catheter is passed proximally to the aortic bifurcation and distally to the popliteal artery. The purpose of this procedure is to remove any clot formation that may be present and to prevent thromboembolic complications. The graft is then removed, and the arteriotomy is closed with either a dacron or saphenous vein patch. The patch secures hemostasis and decreases the potential for late femoral artery or iliac artery stenosis. Upon return to the intensive care unit, the patient will require frequent assessment of perfusion to the distal extremity.

COMPLICATIONS

Insertion of the catheter in a patient with severe atherosclerotic vascular disease might result in arterial perforation or occlusion. Iatrogenic dissection of the aorta is rare but has been reported. Vascular insufficiency is the most common complication of IABP. Vascular insufficiency may be permanent, or it may possibly be relieved by aortofemoral or ileofemoral bypass grafting. Neuropathy in the catheterized extremity is another reported complication.

Decreased circulating platelets in the first 24 hours of IABP and a minimal decrease in red blood cell count have been reported; however, they are not thought to be significant problems. There is a low incidence of balloon leakage or rupture. This might result from balloon inflation against a calcific, atherosclerotic plaque in the aorta. This disruption in the balloon surface may be as small as a pinhole or may be a large tear. The danger associated with this is gas embolism. There is some safety advantage in using carbon dioxide when leaks are small; however, either carbon dioxide or helium would be dangerous if a patient received a large bolus of gas through a large tear.

Finally, a complication of any catheter insertion is the possibility of infection at the insertion site. This can be a considerable problem in the unstable, critically ill patient because of the necessity of catheter removal. However, the advantages of IABP clearly outweigh the risks associated with its use for appropriately selected patients.

BIBLIOGRAPHY

Bolooki H: Clinical Application of Intra-Aortic Balloon Pump. Mount Kisco, Futura, 1977

Bregman D: Clinical experience with the dual-chambered intra-aortic balloon and system 80. J Thorac Cardiovasc Surg 15, No. 2:193–201, 1974

Bregman D, Goetz RH: Clinical experience with a new cardiac assist device: The dual-chambered intra-aortic balloon assist. J Thorac Cardiovasc Surg 62, No. 4:577–591, 1971

Bregman D et al: Unidirectional intra-aortic balloon pumping (IABP) and open heart surgery. Transplant Proc 8, No. 1:79–81, 1976

Cleveland JC et al: The role of intra-aortic balloon counterpulsation in patients undergoing cardiac operations. Ann Thorac Surg 20, No. 6:652–660, 1975

Cohn LH: Intra-aortic balloon counterpulsation in low cardiac output states. Surg Clin North Am 55, No. 3:545–558, 1975

DeWood MA et al: Intra-aortic balloon counterpulsation with and without reperfusion for myocardial infarction shock. Circulation 61, No. 6:1105–1112, 1980

Dorr KS: The intra-aortic balloon pump. Am J Nurs 75, No. 1:52–55, 1975

Frazee S, Nail L: New challenge in cardiac nursing: The intra-aortic balloon. Heart Lung 2, No. 4:526–532, 1973

Gold HK et al: Intra-aortic balloon pumping for control of recurrent myocardial ischemia. Circulation 47:1197–1203, 1973

Gold HK et al: Intra-aortic balloon pumping for ventricular septal defect or mitral regurgitation complicating acute myocardial infarction. Circulation 47:1191–1196, 1973

Kantrowitz A et al: Initial clinical experience with intra-aortic balloon pumping. Trans Am Soc Artif Intern Organs 15:400, 1969

Kerber RE et al: Effect of intra-aortic balloon counterpulsation on the motion and perfusion of acutely ischemic myocardium: An experimental echocardiographic study. Circulation 54, No. 5:853–859, 1976

Lamberti JJ et al: Intra-aortic balloon counterpulsation: Indications and long term results in postoperative left ventricular power failure. Arch Surg 109:766–771, 1974

Miller DC et al: Pulmonary artery balloon counterpulsation for acute right ventricular power failure. J Thorac Cardiovasc Surg (Nov) 80:760–763, 1980

O'Rourke MF, Sammel N, Chang VP: Arterial counterpulsation in severe refractory heart failure complicating acute myocardial infarction. Br Heart J 41:308–316, 1979

Reed EA: Intra-aortic balloon pump. AORN J 23, No. 6:995–1001, 1976

Saini VK et al: Nutrient myocardial blood flow in experimental myocardial ischemia: Effects of intra-aortic balloon counterpulsation and coronary reperfusion. Circulation 52:1086–1090, 1975

Sanders CA et al: Mechanical circulatory assist: Current status and experience with combining circulatory assistance, emergency coronary angiography, and acute myocardial revascularization. Circulation 45:1292–1312, 1972

Siska K et al: Effect of intra-aortic balloon counterpulsation in experimental myocardial injury following acute coronary occlusion: Biochemical, ultrastructural, and physiological aspects. Cardiovasc Res 8:404–417, 1974

Spotnitz HM et al: Left ventricular mechanics and oxygen consumption during arterial counterpulsation. Am J Physiol 217, No. 5:1352–1358, 1969

Stewart S, Biddle T, DeWeese J: Support of the myocardium with intra-aortic balloon counterpulsation following cardiopulmonary bypass. J Thorac Cardiovasc Surg 72, No. 1:109–114, 1976

Swank M et al: Effect of intra-aortic balloon pumping on nutrient coronary flow in normal and ischemic myocardium. J Thorac Cardiovasc Surg 76, No. 4:538–544, 1978

Weber KT, Janicki JS: Coronary collateral flow and intra-aortic balloon counterpulsation. Trans Am Soc Artif Intern Organs 19:395–401, 1973

Weber KT, Janicki JS: Intra-aortic balloon counterpulsation: A review of physiological principles, clinical results, and device safety. Ann Thorac Surg 17, No. 6:602–636, 1974

Weber KT, Janicki JS, Walker AA: Intra-aortic balloon pumping: An analysis of several variables affecting balloon performance. Trans Am Soc Artif Intern Organs 18:486–492, 1972

Whitman G: Intra-aortic balloon pumping and cardiac mechanics: A programmed lesson. Heart Lung 7, No. 6:1034–1050, 1978

Assessment Skills for the Nurse: Cardiovascular System

10

Phillip S. Wolf

ARRHYTHMIAS AND CONDUCTION DISTURBANCES

Disorders of the heartbeat occur in the majority of patients with acute myocardial infarction. Acute respiratory failure is a frequent cause of arrhythmias as well. The importance of rhythm disturbances in these situations differs; some lack clinical significance while others are lethal.

Arrhythmias commonly encountered in monitored patients can be recognized with a little practice. The types that occur most frequently are discussed in the following section. In dealing with these disturbances of rhythm, the nurse must appraise the patient's total clinical situation.

Understanding of arrhythmias is helped by knowledge of the conduction system. Before beginning your study of this section, you might find it helpful to review the conduction system (pp. 53–58) and the principles of electrocardiography. (See also Figs. 10-1 and 10-2.)

ECG TERMS ASSOCIATED WITH ARRHYTHMIAS

TACHYCARDIA — A heart rate in excess of 100/min.

BRADYCARDIA — A heart rate under 60/min.

ISOELECTRIC LINE — The straight line seen when no electrical activity is occurring. The baseline of the tracing.

P WAVE — A deflection from the baseline produced by *depolarization* of the atria.

P-R INTERVAL — The time required for the impulse to travel through the atria into the first portion of the conduction system, the AV junction. Normal limits are 0.12 to 0.2 sec. The interval is measured from the beginning of the P wave to the start of the QRS complex.

QRS COMPLEX — A deflection from the baseline produced by depolarization of the ventricles. Normal duration is 0.06 to 0.08 sec.

ST SEGMENT — The segment between the *end* of the QRS complex and the *beginning* of the T wave.

Q-T INTERVAL — The time required for the ventricles to depolarize and repolarize. Usual duration is 0.32 to 0.40 sec. The interval is from the *beginning* of the QRS complex to the *end* of the T wave.

T WAVE — A deflection from the baseline produced by ventricular *repolarization* and normally of the same deflection as the QRS complex.

U WAVE — A small, usually positive deflection following the T wave. Its significance is uncertain, but it is typically seen with hypokalemia.

An arrhythmia will result when any of the following three situations exists:

- The *rate* is too slow or too fast (the rhythm may be regular or irregular).
- The *site* of impulse formation is abnormal (atrial fibers, fibers of the AV junction, the His bundle or its branches, or the Purkinje fibers).
- The *conduction* of impulses is abnormal at any point within the conduction system.

In analyzing arrhythmias, it is essential to understand some of the terms commonly used. A partial list of definitions can be found in the accompanying chart.

Sinus Tachycardia

Definition: A rapid heart rate (100 to 180 beats/min). The rhythm is regular but usually

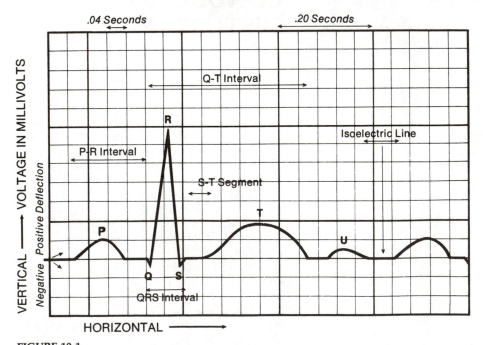

FIGURE 10-1.
Schematic representation of the electrical impulse as it traverses the conduction system, resulting in depolarization and repolarization of the myocardium.

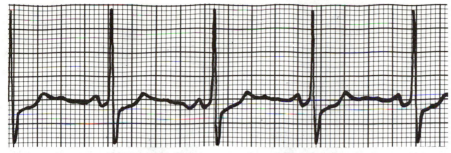

FIGURE 10-2.
Normal sinus rhythm. (Rate = 60 to 100 beats per minute.)

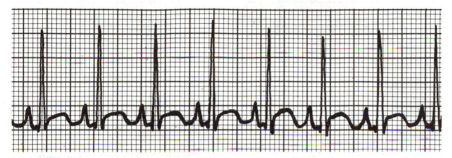

FIGURE 10-3.
Sinus tachycardia.

varies from minute to minute. The rapid rate decreases diastole more than systole (see Fig. 10-3).

Etiology: Sinus tachycardia may be a physiological response to any form of stress and is found in all age groups. It occurs in such diverse conditions as excitement, physical exertion, fever, anemia, hyperthyroidism, and hypoxia, and with the administration of some drugs, such as atropine, isoproterenol, and epinephrine. Sinus tachycardia may also occur with heart disease and is often present with congestive heart failure.

Sinus tachycardia results from decreased vagal tone or increased sympathetic nervous system activity and the release of catecholamines (epinephrine and norepinephrine) by the adrenal medulla and from nerve endings in the heart.

Symptoms: Ordinarily the only symptom described is a sense of "racing of the heart." The cause of sinus tachycardia determines its prognosis, not the duration of the arrhythmia, which in and of itself is usually harmless. In persons who already have depleted cardiac reserve, ischemia, or congestive heart failure, the persistence of a fast rate may worsen the underlying condition.

Treatment: Specific measures may include sedation, digitalis (only if heart failure is present), or propranolol, if the tachycardia is due to thyrotoxicosis.

Sinus Bradycardia

Definitions: A heart rate of fewer than 60 beats per minute with impulses originating in the SA node. Rhythm is regular but may vary from minute to minute. The duration of diastole is lengthened (see Fig. 10-4).

Etiology: Sinus bradycardia is common among all age groups and is present in both normal and diseased hearts. It is also seen in highly trained athletes, patients with severe pain, myxedema, or acute myocardial infarction, and as the result of medication (digitalis or reserpine).

Sinus bradycardia results from excessive parasympathetic activity. Slow rates are tolerated well in persons with healthy hearts. With severe heart disease, however, the heart may not be able to compensate for a slow rate by increasing the volume of blood ejected per beat as is true of the healthy heart. In this situation, sinus bradycardia will lead to a low cardiac output. This in turn may lead to weakness (due to inadequate blood

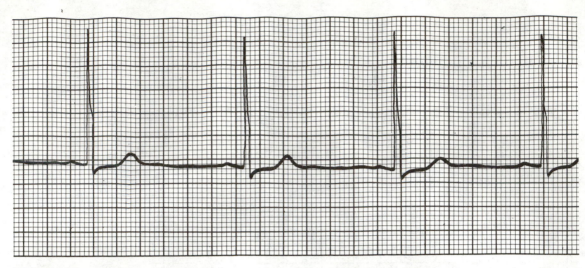

FIGURE 10-4.
Sinus bradycardia.

flow to the muscles), congestive heart failure, or serious ventricular arrhythmias.

Treatment: None is usually indicated unless symptoms are present. If the pulse is very slow and symptoms are present, appropriate measures include atropine to block the vagal effect, isoproterenol, or transvenous pacing.

Sinus Arrhythmia

Definition: All impulses originate in the SA node, but the rate of discharge varies. Some occur prematurely while others are delayed, which causes the rate to alternately increase and decrease. In young persons, the heart rate usually varies with respiration, increasing with inspiration and slowing with expiration (see Fig. 10-5).

Etiology: Sinus arrhythmia is usually a physiological variation in young people. It may indicate disease of the SA node in the elderly (see section on Sick Sinus Syndrome).

Treatment: Usually none is necessary.
May have episodes of CNS disturbance confusion, syncope. May need pace maker

Atrial Premature Contraction (APC)

Definition: During the normal cardiac rhythm, a contraction occurs earlier than expected. The stimulus for this contraction arises from elsewhere in the atrium rather than from the SA node. The P wave is usually visible and typically has a somewhat different form than the P wave of the sinus impulse. The QRS complex is usually of normal configuration but may appear distorted when the APC is conducted aberrantly, or the QRS may not occur at all (APC is

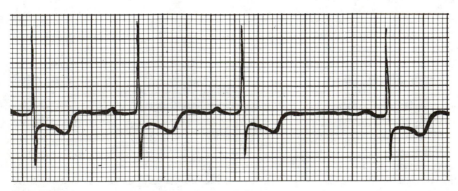

FIGURE 10-5.
Sinus arrhythmia.

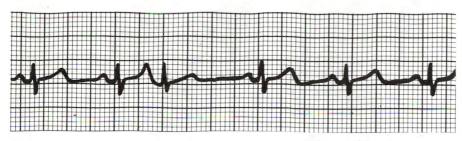

FIGURE 10-6.
Atrial premature contraction.

blocked). A short pause, usually less than "compensatory," is present (see definition of VPC below) (see Fig. 10-6).

Etiology: This is a common arrhythmia seen in all groups. It may occur in normal individuals and in patients with rheumatic heart disease, ischemic heart disease, or hyperthyroidism.

An impulse arises in the atrial musculature from an ectopic focus, producing an atrial contraction. Usually the stimulus travels through the AV junction and continues its normal course through the ventricles. If an APC occurs too early, it may be blocked because the AV junction is refractory from the previous stimulus and is unable to receive the current one. In most instances, the atrial ectopic beat is followed by an incomplete compensatory pause. The patient may have the sensation of a "pause" or "skip" in rhythm.

Treatment: In many cases, no treatment is necessary. Mild sedation or removal of the exciting cause is indicated if the APCs are symptomatic. If they occur as a result of underlying heart disease, specific drugs such as quinidine, digitalis, or propranolol may be in order.

Supraventricular Tachycardia

Definition: These tachycardias are rapid, regular rhythms. They may originate in an ectopic atrial focus (paroxysmal atrial tachycardia) or in the AV junction (paroxysmal nodal tachycardia). These ectopic rhythms are similar in all respects except their site of origin. In almost all instances recorded, the tachycardia begins with a premature atrial or junctional beat (as in Fig. 10-7).

Significant ECG Changes:

Rate: Range, 140 to 220 beats per minute. The rhythm is regular and the paroxysms may last from a few seconds to several hours or even days.

P waves: Usually upright with atrial tachycardia and may be inverted in leads II, III and aVF when the tachycardia is of junctional origin. If the rate is very rapid, the P wave may merge with the QRS complex superimposed on the T wave (see Fig. 10-8).

P-R interval: If seen, the P-R interval is usually shortened with junctional tachycardia and nor-

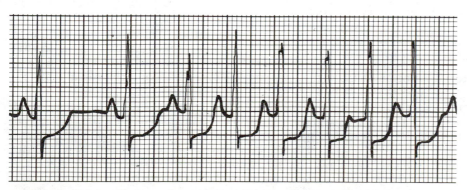

FIGURE 10-7.
Supraventricular tachycardia.

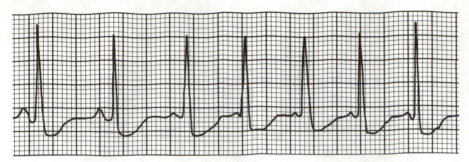

FIGURE 10-8.
A-V junctional tachycardia.

mal, shortened, or, rarely, lengthened with atrial tachycardia.

QRS complex: This is usually of normal configuration, but may be distorted if aberrant conduction is present.

Etiology: These arrhythmias occur often in adults with normal hearts and for the same reasons as APCs. When heart disease is present, such abnormalities as rheumatic heart disease, acute myocardial infarction, or digitalis intoxication may serve as the background for these arrhythmias.

Atrial tachycardia is typically preceded by an APC. The ectopic pacemaker discharges impulses to which the atrium or AV junction responds, firing so rapidly that the SA node is suppressed. Extreme regularity (in a given person the rate stays constant) is one of the hallmarks.

Symptoms: Early symptoms are palpitations and light-headedness. With underlying heart disease, dyspnea, angina pectoris, and congestive heart failure may occur.

Differential Diagnosis: A supraventricular tachycardia must be differentiated from sinus tachycardia. The following points favor the diagnosis of ectopic atrial tachycardia:

- An atrial premature beat often initiates the rhythm.
- It begins and terminates abruptly.
- The rate is often faster than a sinus tachycardia and tends to be more regular from minute to minute.
- In response to a vagal maneuver, such as carotid sinus massage, the ectopic tachycardia will either be unaffected or revert to a normal sinus rhythm. Sinus tachycardia, on the other

hand, will slow slightly in response to increased vagal tone.

Treatment: Stimulation of the vagal reflex will often terminate the paroxysms. This reflex may be elicited by brief massage on the carotid sinus (unilaterally), the Valsalva maneuver, or agents that raise the blood pressure such as phenylephrine, 1 mg intravenously, or methoxamine, 5 to 15 mg intravenously. If these measures are unsuccessful, antiarrhythmic drugs including digitalis, quinidine, or propranolol are used. If the attack persists or if complications occur that demand more immediate action, countershock is indicated.

Atrial Flutter

Definition: An ectopic atrial rhythm occurring at a rate of 250 to 350 beats per minute. The ventricular rate is usually one-half the atrial rate at the beginning of the attack. With treatment, the degree of AV block increases and the ventricular rate slows further. The rapid and regular atrial rate produces a "saw tooth" or "picket fence" appearance on the ECG. It is usual for a flutter wave to be partially concealed within the QRS complex or T wave. The QRS complex exhibits a normal configuration except when aberrant conduction is present. The QRS complexes do not follow each flutter wave since the ventricles cannot respond this rapidly (see Fig. 10-9).

Etiology: In the patient with atrial flutter, underlying cardiac disease is usually present, including coronary artery disease, cor pulmonale, or rheumatic heart disease. The ectopic focus becomes the dominant pacemaker and is conducted through the AV junction into the ventricles in normal fashion. Two theories are

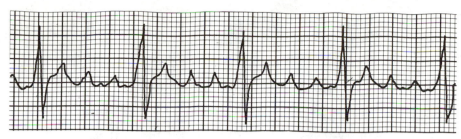

FIGURE 10-9.
Atrial flutter.

currently favored as to the mechanism of atrial flutter. (1) A continuous impulse travels through the atrium, causing a "circus" movement at a very rapid but coordinated rate, and (2) a single ectopic focus discharges rapidly. At the onset of the arrhythmia, the ventricles respond once to every two atrial impulses. Further AV block may develop if the arrhythmia persists, and the ventricles usually respond irregularly every two to six beats. If the ventricular rate is within normal limits, the cardiac output will remain adequate. If the rate is so rapid that the chambers cannot fill adequately, hemodynamic changes occur as described in the section on supraventricular tachycardia.

When the ventricular rate is rapid, the diagnosis of atrial flutter may be difficult. Vagal maneuvers such as carotid sinus massage will often increase the degree of AV block and allow recognition of flutter waves.

Treatment: If flutter is associated with a high degree of AV block so that the ventricular rate remains within normal limits, no treatment is necessary. When the ventricular rate is rapid, prompt treatment to control the rate or revert the rhythm to a sinus mechanism is indicated. Digitalis is the initial drug of choice. It increases the degree of AV block and thus controls the ventricular rate, or it may produce atrial fibrillation. Reversion to a sinus mechanism often follows. If complications occur suddenly and more

immediate action is required, countershock is indicated.

Atrial Fibrillation

Definition: An atrial arrhythmia occurring at an extremely rapid atrial rate (400 to 600/min), lacking coordinated activity. The AV junction is able to respond only partially to the rapid rate of discharge from the atria; hence, the ventricular rate is slower, irregular, and usually 140 to 170 beats per minute at the onset of the arrhythmia.

Significant ECG Changes: (see Fig. 10-10).

P waves: Absent; irregular "fibrillary" waves (an uneven pattern in the baseline of the tracing) are usually seen.

QRS complex: Complexes may appear normal or show aberrant conduction.

Etiology: Although atrial fibrillation may occur as a transient arrhythmia in healthy young people, the presence of permanent atrial fibrillation is almost always associated with underlying heart disease. One or both of the following are present in patients with permanent atrial fibrillation: atrial muscle disease and atrial distention together with disease of the SA node. Atrial

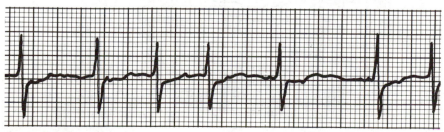

FIGURE 10-10.
Atrial fibrillation.

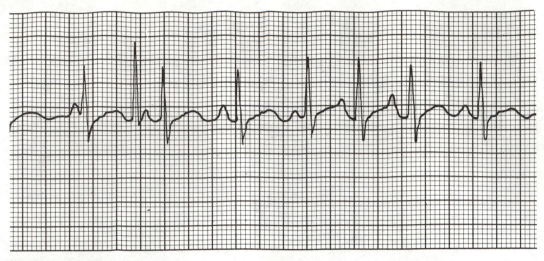

FIGURE 10-11.
Multifocal atrial tachycardia.

fibrillation is usually initiated by APCs. Once established, it is sustained by multiple small circulating wave fronts within the atrium. This is also known as micro reentry.

In patients with heart disease, atrial fibrillation causes the cardiac output to fall because of (1) a rapid rate allowing less time for the ventricles to fill and (2) loss of effective atrial contractions. Signs of another complication may arise from atrial fibrillation, that of peripheral arterial emboli. Due to the passive dilated state of the atria, thrombi can form on the atrial wall and dislodge, producing embolization. The incidence of embolization can be reduced by anticoagulation.

The nurse will note a pulse deficit with atrial fibrillation. The radial pulse is slower than the apical pulse because some systolic contractions are feeble and not palpable in the peripheral arteries.

Treatment: If complications develop rapidly, countershock is indicated immediately. If cardiac output remains sufficient, and the patient is not hypotensive or in significant heart failure, drug therapy is usually tried first. Digitalis is specifically useful because it increases AV block and allows more time for diastolic filling of the ventricles. This produces more volume per stroke. The rhythm may also convert with digi-

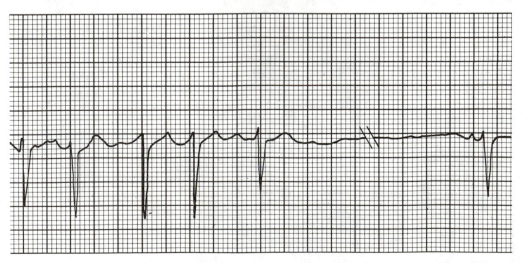

FIGURE 10-12.
Sick sinus syndrome. Atrial fibrillation is followed by atrial standstill. A sinus escape beat is seen at the end of the strip.

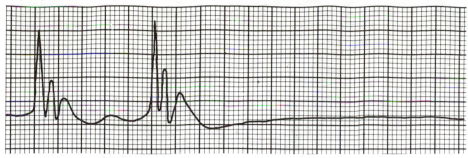

FIGURE 10-13.
Atrial standstill (lower pacemaker does not take over).

talis to a normal sinus mechanism. Quinidine aids in maintenance of normal sinus rhythm.

Multifocal Atrial Tachycardia

Definition: This rhythm characteristically occurs in patients with severe pulmonary disease. Often such patients exhibit hypoxemia, hypokalemia, alterations in serum pH, or pulmonary hypertension. In the example shown in Figure 10-11, note the rapid rate and the variable morphology of the P waves.

Sick Sinus Syndrome

Definition: The term refers to patients exhibiting severe degrees of sinus node depression including marked sinus bradycardia, SA block, and SA node arrest. Often rapid atrial arrhythmias coexist, such as atrial flutter or fibrillation (the "tachycardia-bradycardia syndrome"), which alternate with periods of sinus node depression (see Fig. 10-12).

Treatment: Management of this condition requires control of the rapid atrial arrhythmias with drug therapy and, in selected cases, control of very slow heart rates as well (a permanent transvenous pacemaker).

Atrial Standstill

Definition: Complete cessation of the SA node occurs. The pacemaker shifts to a lower focus, either in the atrium, in the AV junction, or within the Purkinje system (see Fig. 10-13).

Etiology: As with sick sinus syndrome, the sinus arrhythmia may occur in the elderly patient with disease of the SA node. It is also the result of intoxication from quinidine, digitalis, or potassium. Acute myocardial infarction may also produce atrial standstill.

Symptoms: Light-headedness or fainting will occur depending on the duration of standstill. Sudden death, of course, is inevitable if a lower pacemaker does not take over.

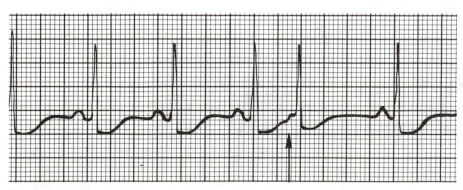

FIGURE 10-14.
A-V junctional premature beats.

Treatment: Intravenous atropine or isoproterenol is sometimes of value. Drugs that depress SA node function such as digitalis and quinidine should be discontinued, and hyperkalemia, if present, should be managed with intravenous sodium bicarbonate or glucose and insulin mixtures. If the arrhythmia is recurrent, an artificial pacemaker is the preferred management.

AV Junctional Premature Beats

Definition: An impulse from an ectopic focus in the AV junction or His bundle occurring earlier than the normal sinus impulse. The P waves are inverted in leads II, III and aVF and may occur before, during, or after the QRS complex (see Fig. 10-14).

Etiology: As with APCs, junctional premature beats may occur in normal persons or in those with underlying heart disease. The AV junction or His bundle acts as pacemaker. The impulses pass normally through the conduction system into the ventricles, producing a normal QRS. Aberrant conduction, however, may occur and lead to confusion with a ventricular premature contraction (VPC). It is helpful to obtain a long rhythm strip to find prematurities that are normally conducted. This may establish that the abnormal-appearing beats with wide QRS complexes are atrial with aberrant conduction.

An inverted P wave is produced when the AV junction stimulates the atria and causes the impulse to travel upward through the atrial fibers in retrograde fashion.

Treatment: Identical to the management of APCs.

Ventricular Premature Contraction (VPC)

Definition: A ventricular contraction originating from an ectopic focus in the Purkinje network of the ventricles, occurring earlier than the expected sinus beat. In contrast to an APC with aberrant conduction, there is no P wave before the QRS complex. An inverted P wave may follow the VPC due to retrograde depolarization of the atria (see Fig. 10-15).

The QRS complex cannot be missed. It is not only premature, but it is bizarre, widened, and notched, and it may be of greater amplitude. The T wave of the VPC is opposite in deflection to the QRS complex. A compensatory pause often follows the premature beat as the heart awaits the next stimulus from the SA node. The pause is considered fully compensatory if the cycles of the normal and premature beats equal the time of two normal heart cycles.

Etiology: VPCs are the most common of all arrhythmias and can occur in any age group, with or without heart disease. They are especially common in a person with myocardial disease (ischemia, myocardial infarction, or following cardiac surgery) or with myocardial irritability (hypokalemia or digitalis intoxication).

If VPCs occur after each sinus beat, a bigeminal rhythm is present (see Fig. 10-16). Trigeminy is a VPC occurring after two consecutive sinus beats. When VPCs originate from

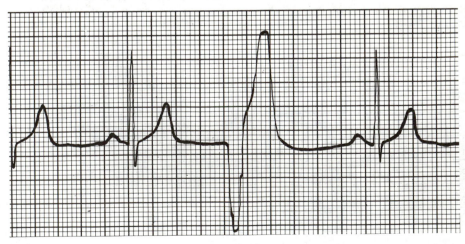

FIGURE 10-15.
Ventricular premature contraction.

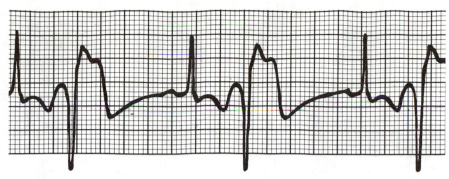

FIGURE 10-16.
Bigeminal rhythm.

different ectopic foci, they are known as *multifocal*.

Symptoms: Often VPCs are asymptomatic, but some people may experience a "thump" or "skipping" sensation. VPCs may be the earliest sign of heart disease, and when they are especially frequent or approach the apex of the T wave, they may be the forerunner of more serious arrhythmias such as ventricular tachycardia or fibrillation.

Treatment: If infrequent, isolated VPCs require no treatment. Multiple, "back to back" VPCs or VPCs falling on the apex of the T wave of the previous beat, are managed with antiarrhythmic agents, including lidocaine, procainamide, quinidine, and propranolol. If the serum potassium is low, potassium replacement may correct the arrhythmia. If the arrhythmia is due to digitalis toxicity, withdrawal of the drug may correct it.

Ventricular Tachycardia

Definition: The ventricular ectopic focus emits a series of rapid and regular impulses, and the ventricular contractions are dissociated from the atrial contractions.

The ventricular rate ranges from 100 to 220 beats per minute. P waves are rarely seen to superimpose on the rapid, bizarre QRS–T complexes. The QRS complex resembles that of VPCs, and the T wave, when visible, is opposite in deflection to the QRS complex. In the example shown, ventricular tachycardia terminates spontaneously, resulting in sinus rhythm. An "R on T" VPC is present in the next to last beat (see Fig. 10-17).

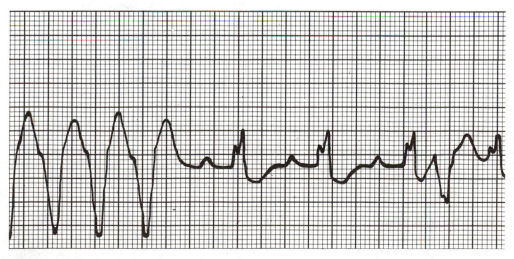

FIGURE 10-17.
Ventricular tachycardia.

Idioventricular rhythm

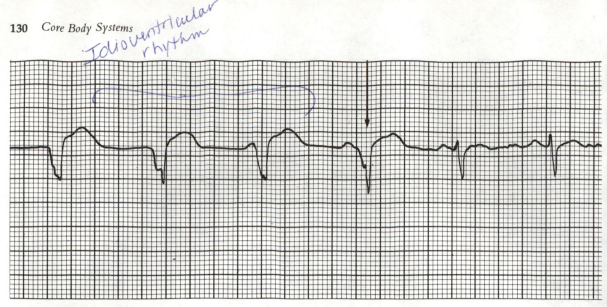

FIGURE 10-18.
Accelerated ventricular rhythm. The first three beats are of ventricular origin. The fourth beat *(arrow)* represents a fusion beat. The subsequent two beats are of sinus origin.

Etiology: Ventricular tachycardia is rare in adults with normal hearts but is common (20% to 30%) as a complication of myocardial infarction or digitalis intoxication.

Ventricular tachycardia is thought to arise within the Purkinje network. A reentrant mechanism is usually present, causing a circulating wave front. Each completion of the wave front causes a ventricular contraction appearing as a series of VPCs. The atria continue to respond to the SA node, but the atria and ventricles beat independently. The rapid rate without a properly timed atrial contraction leads to decreased cardiac output.

Symptoms: Palpitations, angina pectoris, weakness, and fainting are frequent symptoms. Hypotension or congestive heart failure may follow due to decreased stroke volume.

Treatment: Lidocaine, procainamide, propranolol, quinidine or disopyromide, and occasionally potassium chloride may terminate the arrhythmia. Electrical countershock is almost always effective. If the arrhythmia is due to digitalis intoxication, digitalis should be stopped and potassium given.

Accelerated Ventricular Rhythm

Definition: This ectopic ventricular rhythm resembles ventricular tachycardia except that the rate is slower. The ventricular rate is between 60 and 100 beats per minute, and the characteristically wide QRS complexes are identified as being of ventricular origin. Often the ventricular rate closely parallels the sinus rate (see Fig. 10-18).

Etiology: Typically this rhythm occurs in patients with acute myocardial infarction. Less commonly it may occur as a result of ischemia or digitalis intoxication.

Treatment: In most cases, no treatment is necessary because the arrhythmia terminates spontaneously in less than 30 seconds.

Ventricular Fibrillation

Definition: Rapid irregular and ineffectual contractions of the ventricle. The ECG shows a wavering baseline and bizarre waveforms.

Etiology: Ventricular fibrillation is favored by several causes. These include myocardial infarction, VPCs occurring at the apex of the preceding T wave, and drugs such as digitalis or quinidine in toxic doses (see Fig. 10-19).

Symptoms: With ventricular fibrillation, the ventricles immediately cease to expel blood, and death will occur rapidly in untreated cases. Loss of consciousness occurs within 8 to 10 seconds, and a seizure may occur. No pulse is elicited and the pupils become dilated. Clinical death is pres-

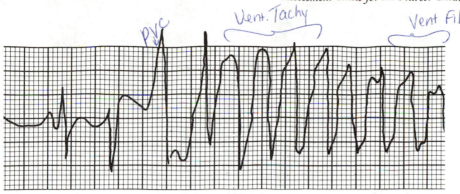

FIGURE 10-19.
Ventricular fibrillation.

ent, and biologic death follows in a few moments. Ventricular fibrillation is the most common basis of sudden death and is nearly always fatal if resuscitation is not immediately instituted. Rarely, ventricular fibrillation will terminate spontaneously within seconds.

Treatment: The best treatment is prevention. In monitored patients with multiple, consecutive, or encroaching VPCs, immediate treatment with lidocaine or procainamide will often prevent more serious ventricular rhythms. If fibrillation occurs, rapid defibrillation with DC countershock performed by the nurse in attendance is the management of choice (see the discussion of cardiopulmonary resuscitation in Chapter 9).

First Degree AV Block

Definition: A delay in conduction through the AV junction. The P-R interval exceeds the upper limit of 0.20 second in duration. In the example shown, the P-R interval is 0.30 second (see Fig. 10-20).

Etiology: This finding occurs in all ages and in both normal and diseased hearts. Drugs such as digitalis, quinidine, and procainamide may prolong the P-R interval into the abnormal range.

The impulse originates normally in the SA node and travels through the atria in normal sequence. The AV junction delays the conduction for a longer than normal interval. When the impulse does pass through the AV junction, the ventricles respond normally. This conduction disturbance is of no significance except when it is a precursor of second or third degree AV block.

Treatment: None needed.

Second Degree Block—Mobitz I (Wenckebach)

Definition: With each beat, the delay of conduction through the AV junction is progressively increased. Eventually, the sinus impulse is completely blocked and no QRS complex occurs.

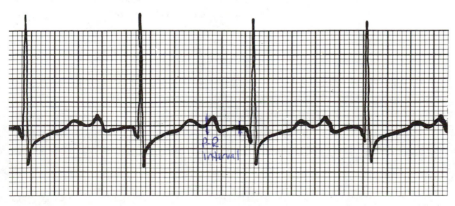

FIGURE 10-20.
First degree A-V block.

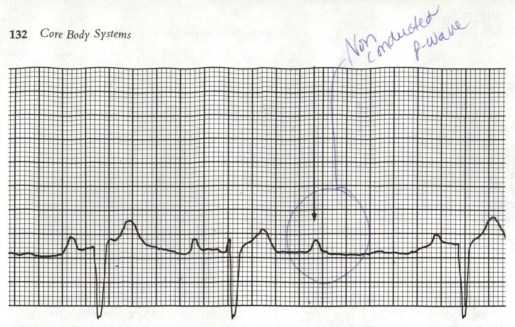

Non conducted p-wave

FIGURE 10-21.
Second degree block—Mobitz I (Wenckebach). The arrow indicates the nonconducted P wave in this sequence.

Significant ECG Changes   (See Fig. 10-21.)

P-R interval: Progressively lengthens with each beat.

QRS complex: Normal configuration, but progressively delayed after each P wave until one is dropped. The interval between successive QRS complexes shortens until a dropped beat occurs.

Etiology: Of the two types of second degree block, the Wenckebach phenomenon is the more common. Inferior myocardial infarction and digitalis toxicity may cause this type of second degree block.

Treatment: No treatment is required except to discontinue digitalis when it is the offending agent.

Second Degree Block—Mobitz II

Definition: With this rhythm, some sinus impulses are conducted through the AV junction with a constant P-R interval. Other sinus impulses are blocked completely. The ventricular rate is a fraction (1:2, 1:3, 1:4, etc.) of the atrial rate. In the strip shown, note the blocked P wave *(arrow).* (See Fig. 10-22.)

Etiology: Mobitz II AV block indicates more severe impairment of AV conduction. It is seen, for example, with acute anterior myocardial infarction, and its presence implies extensive destruction of the ventricular septum. Digitalis toxicity is not a cause.

Atrial contractions result from regular SA impulses. Only those impulses which penetrate the AV junction cause ventricular contractions. No

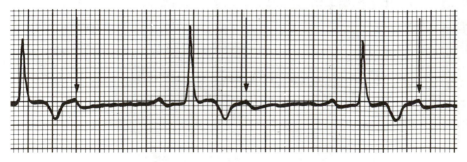

FIGURE 10-22.
Second degree block—Mobitz II. Arrows denote blocked P waves.

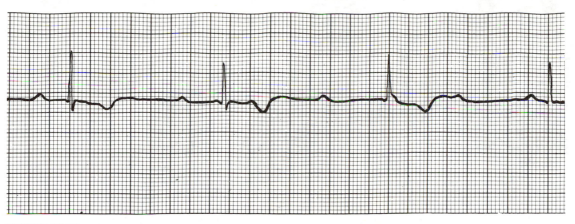

FIGURE 10-23.
Third degree block (complete A-V block).

symptoms occur unless the ventricular rate is so slow that cardiac output falls. This type of arrhythmia is potentially dangerous because it may progress to third degree block or ventricular standstill.

Treatment: Constant monitoring and observation for progressive degrees of AV block are required. Medications used include isoproterenol and epinephrine. Transvenous pacing is often indicated.

Third Degree Block (Complete AV Block)

Definition: None of the sinus impulses are conducted through the AV junction. The atrial rate is faster than the ventricular rate. The atrial rate is usually normal and regular. The ventricular rate is regular but slower, averaging 30 to 45 beats per minute. The P-R interval is variable as in the example shown. The QRS complex is of normal configuration if it originates in the His bundle and becomes widened if it originates from below this point (see Fig. 10-23).

Etiology: Occasionally complete heart block is congenital. In acquired cases, causes include degeneration of the conduction system due to advanced age, acute myocardial infarction, myocarditis, cardiac surgery, and digitalis intoxication.

With complete AV block, the SA node continues to pace in normal fashion, but the impulse is blocked at the AV junction. A lower cardiac pacemaker initiates the rhythm from a point distal to the AV junction.

Symptoms: If the ventricular rate is adequate to allow a normal cardiac output, the person is asymptomatic. When the rate is slow and cardiac contraction impaired from underlying heart disease, the cardiac output will fall. In the latter instance, heart failure may result and the patient may develop Adams-Stokes seizures (episodes of ventricular tachycardia, fibrillation, or cardiac standstill resulting in syncope, hypoxic seizures, coma, or death). Untreated cases with symptoms carry a poor prognosis, and many such patients die within the year.

Treatment: Isoproterenol is the drug of choice. Temporary or permanent pacing is usually indicated. The nurse should familiarize herself with the benefits and hazards of electrical pacing (see Chapter 9).

Bundle Branch Block (BBB)

Definition: A delay of conduction through the right or left bundle.

Significant ECG Changes:

QRS complex: Prolonged to 0.12 second or longer. Typically, the QRS complex is notched or slurred with a widening of the QRS complex. With right BBB, the S wave in lead I is broadened and an R^1 is present in V_1. Left BBB produces a positive broad deflection in lead I and a broad negative deflection in lead V_1. The T wave is wide and of opposite direction to the QRS complex (see Fig. 10-24).

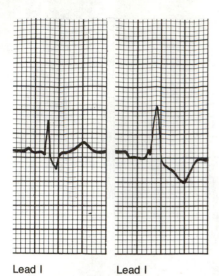

Lead I   Lead I

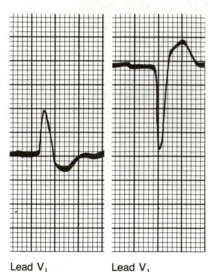

Lead V₁   Lead V₁
RBBB   LBBB

FIGURE 10-24.
Bundle branch block.

Etiology: The most common causes of BBB are myocardial infarction, hypertension, and cardiomyopathy. It may also result from medications including procainamide and quinidine, or from hyperkalemia.

When conduction through one bundle is blocked, the impulse travels along the unaffected bundle and eventually reaches the other blocked area by way of the ventricular musculature. Transmission by this route is slower, and right and left ventricular contractions do not occur simultaneously. The abnormal contraction produces a wide QRS complex.

Symptoms: Cardiac output is not decreased, and thus the arrhythmia itself does not produce symptoms.

Treatment: The underlying heart disease determines treatment and prognosis.

Shirley J. Hoffman

SERUM ELECTROLYTE ABNORMALITIES AND THE ELECTRO-CARDIOGRAM

The maintenance of adequate fluid and electrolyte balance assumes high priority in the care of patients in any medical, surgical, or coronary intensive care unit. Patients being treated for renal or cardiovascular diseases are especially vulnerable to electrolyte imbalances. The cure may well be worse than the disease if electrolyte abnormalities go undetected or ignored, since they frequently are caused by the treatment rather than by the disease itself.

Dialysis can very quickly cause major shifts in electrolyes. Certainly the often insidious drop of serum potassium levels in the digitalized cardiac patient who receives diuretics is well known. Diuretics are also frequently used as part of the medical regimen for the control of hypertension. Any addition, deletion, or change in diuretic therapy warrants close following of serum electrolytes.

A history of any of the above-mentioned problems should alert the nurse to check the patient's serum electrolytes on an ongoing basis.

Potassium and calcium are probably the two most important electrolytes that are concerned with proper function of the heart. They help produce normal contraction of cardiac muscle. They are also important in the propagation of the electrical impulse in the heart. Because of the latter function, excess or insufficiency of either electrolyte frequently causes changes in the

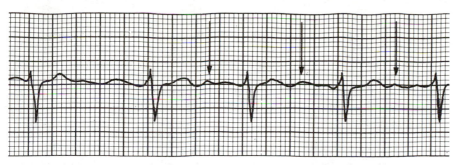

FIGURE 10-25.
Presence of U waves (hypokalemia).

ECG. The nurse who is aware of and is able to recognize these changes may well suspect electrolyte abnormalities before clinical symptoms appear or hazardous arrhythmias occur.

Potassium

Hypokalemia (hypopotassemia) is probably the most frequently encountered electrolyte abnormality. It is commonly associated with vomiting, diarrhea, prolonged digitalis and diuretic therapy, and prolonged nasogastric suctioning. The alkalotic patient may also be hypokalemic. Hypokalemia may also accompany excessive steroid administration.

In general, a rise of 0.1 in the pH will account for a fall of 0.5 mEq per liter in serum potassium. In most laboratories, normal serum potassium levels are about 3.5 to 5.0 mEq per liter. The ECG that exhibits U waves should immediately alert the nurse to the possibility of hypokalemia in that patient (see Fig. 10-25). Although the *U wave* is normal for many people, it is worthwhile to obtain a serum potassium level because it may be an early sign of hypokalemia. The normal U wave is often seen best in lead V_3. It is usually easily recognized, but it may encroach on the preceding T wave and go unnoticed (see Fig. 10-26). The T wave may look notched or prolonged when it is hiding the U wave, giving the appearance of a prolonged Q-T interval.

As potassium depletion increases, the U wave may become more prominent as the T wave becomes less so. The T wave becomes flattened and may even invert. The S-T segment tends to become depressed, somewhat resembling the effects of digitalis on the ECG. These ECG changes are not particularly well correlated with the severity of hypokalemia; however, they are good indicators of this abnormality and can be recognized by the nurse who has basic knowledge of ECG complexes.

Untreated hypokalemia can produce ventricular premature contractions (VPCs), atrial or junctional tachycardias, and eventually ventricular tachycardia, ventricular fibrillation, and death. The severity of the arrhythmias resulting from hypokalemia certainly points out the need for early recognition of this problem.

The U wave may also be accentuated in association with digitalis, quinidine, epinephrine, hypercalcemia, thyrotoxicosis, and exercise. The normal U wave should be upright in all leads that have upright T waves, and its polarity may be reversed in the presence of myocardial ischemia and left ventricular strain.

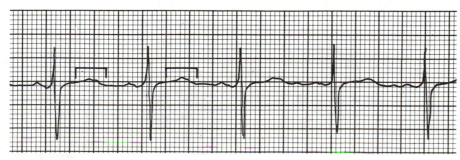

FIGURE 10-26.
Fusion of T and U waves (hypokalemia).

Hyperkalemia (hyperpotassemia) is often the result of overenthusiastic or poorly supervised treatment of hypokalemia. Sometimes early detection of hypokalemia is accomplished, treatment is instituted, and the problem is considered solved. However, if potassium supplements are not stopped or reduced when normal serum potassium levels are reached, hyperkalemia will result.

Other causes of hyperkalemia include Addison's disease, acute renal failure, and acidosis. Tissue breakdown following trauma may cause the release of large amounts of potassium into the bloodstream.

Another not infrequently seen cause of high potassium levels is the use of potassium-sparing diuretics. Triamterene (Dyrenium) is an example of this type of drug that is currently in common usage as an adjunct to the more potent diuretics. It must be remembered that these drugs not only spare potassium but may increase the potassium level of the serum.

The earliest sign of hyperkalemia on the ECG is a change in the T wave. It is usually described as tall, narrow, and "peaked" or "tenting" in appearance (see Fig. 10-27). The T wave height is normally not more than 5 mm in any standard lead and not more than 10 mm in any precordial lead. T waves may be abnormally tall in myocardial infarction and may also be found in ventricular overloading and in patients with cerebrovascular accidents.

As potassium levels rise, changes occur first in the atrial portion of the ECG complex, then in the ventricular portion. The P wave flattens and becomes wider as the result of intra-atrial block. Further potassium elevation causes progression to AV nodal block and a prolonged P-R interval.

The P wave may disappear entirely. With even higher potassium levels, the QRS begins to widen, indicating intraventricular block.

If untreated, severe hyperkalemia will progress to increased widening of the QRS until ventricular fibrillation occurs at serum potassium levels of 8 to 10 mEq per liter. In terms of arrhythmias, the patient may progress from sinus bradycardia to first degree block, through junctional rhythm, idioventricular rhythm, and ventricular tachycardia and fibrillation. Hyperkalemic changes on ECG correlate well with serum potassium levels. The T-wave changes described begin to appear at serum levels of 6 to 7 mEq per liter; the QRS widens at 8 to 9 mEq per liter. Vigorous treatment must be instituted to reverse the condition at this point, as sudden death may occur at any time after these levels are reached.

Calcium

Calcium is the second electrolyte important to normal functioning of the heart. It is thought to have an effect on linking the electrical impulse to myocardial contraction. Calcium increases cardiac contractility and is often administered intravenously to the patient who has sustained cardiac arrest in an attempt to increase the force of cardiac contraction.

Hypercalcemia. Normal serum calcium is about 9 to 11 mg/dl. Hypercalcemia is often seen in patients with hyperparathyroidism, neoplastic diseases, and acute osteoporosis. It may also be seen in patients with sarcoidosis, hyperthyroidism, adrenal insufficiency, acute immobilization, and chlorothiazide therapy.

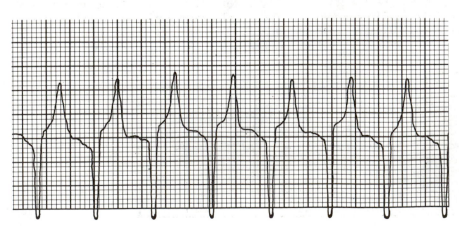

FIGURE 10-27.
Hyperkalemia.

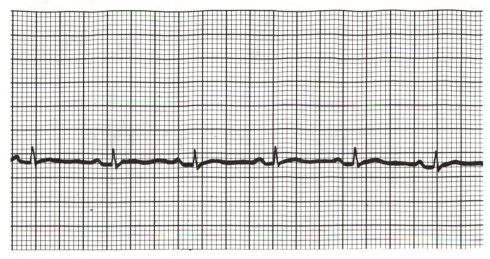

FIGURE 10-28.
Shortened Q-T interval (hypercalcemia). The normal Q-T interval for the above heart rate of 88 beats/minute is 0.28 second to 0.36 second. This patient's serum calcium level was 12.1 mg/dl and the Q-T interval measures 0.24 second.

Clinical symptoms relative to hypercalcemia are mainly neurologic. These may include somnolence or irritability, muscle weakness, or peripheral neuropathies. The patient may also exhibit gastrointestinal symptoms such as anorexia, constipation, nausea, and vomiting. Other hypercalcemic patients may be totally asymptomatic.

Hypocalcemia may occur in patients with renal failure, hypoparathyroidism, and malabsorption syndromes.

Tetany is the most obvious manifestation of hypocalcemia, beginning with numbness and tingling of the mouth and extremities and progressing to muscle spasm and seizure. The patient with mild hypocalcemia may be asymptomatic; however, neurologic testing (Chvostek's sign and Trousseau's sign) may indicate calcium deficit.

ECG Indicators. The Q-T interval length is the most frequent ECG indicator of excess or insufficient calcium. It is somewhat shortened in hypercalcemia and lengthened in hypocalcemia (see Figs. 10–28 and 10–29). In the hypercalcemic patient, the shortening of the Q-T interval takes place especially in the portion from the beginning of the QRS to the apex of the T wave, making the beginning of the T wave an abrupt slope. If this portion of the complex is less than 0.23 to 0.29 second, hypercalcemia may be suspected. U waves may also develop or be accentuated in the hypercalcemic patient. Hypocalcemia may also cause lowering and inversion of the T wave.

The Q-T interval is measured from the beginning of the QRS to the end of the T wave. The normal length of this interval varies with heart rate, sex, and age and can be determined by consulting the chart of calculated normal Q-T

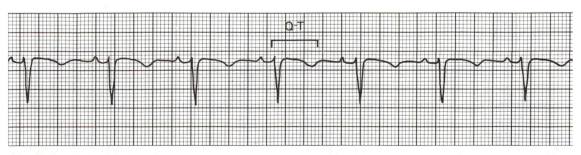

FIGURE 10-29.
Prolonged Q-T interval (hypocalcemia). For this heart rate of 70 beats per minute, the Q-T interval should be between 0.31 and 0.38 seconds. This patient's Q-T interval measures 0.50 seconds because his serum calcium level is 5.4 mg/dl. (Normal serum calcium is 8.5 to 10.5 mg/dl.)

intervals found in most texts on electrocardiography. A general guideline that can be used in clinical situations is that the Q-T interval should be less than half the preceding R-R interval when the heart rate is 65 to 90 beats per minute. The interval will normally shorten during tachycardia and lengthen during bradycardia.

Calcium abnormalities are not often seen in the cardiac patient unless there is an associated noncardiac disease. The more frequent cause of Q-T interval shortening or prolongation in the cardiac patient is the administration of cardiac drugs. Digitalis may cause a *shortened* Q-T interval. Quinidine and procainamide frequently cause *prolongation* of the Q-T interval. Drugs should always be considered when the ECG is evaluated for electrolyte abnormalities.

Arrhythmias are not commonly associated with either calcium excess or calcium insufficiency; however, too rapid intravenous infusion of calcium salts may result in ventricular fibrillation and sudden death. The digitalized patient who receives calcium salts seems especially prone to this reaction for reasons not known.

Summary

Just as the patient who sustains myocardial infarction may not have chest pain, the patient who has electrolyte abnormalities may not exhibit any of the ECG changes described. Conversely, a patient with normal serum electrolytes may show some of these ECG changes for other reasons. None of the ECG manifestations described here even approach being diagnostic. They are of value primarily in alerting one to suspect electrolyte abnormalities. It is appropriate for the nurse, especially one who cares for the critically ill patient, to be alert to ECG changes and to interpret what is seen in the context of what is already known about that patient.

BIBLIOGRAPHY

Arbeit SR et al: Differential Diagnosis of the Electrocardiogram, 2nd ed. Philadelphia, F. A. Davis, 1975
Fisch C: Electrophysiologic basis of clinical arrhythmias. Heart Lung 3:51–56, 1974
Friedman HH: Diagnostic Electrocardiography & Vectorcardiography, 2nd ed. New York, McGraw-Hill, 1976
Goldman MJ: Principles of Clinical Electrocardiography, 10th ed. Los Altos, Lange, 1979
Mangiola S: Self-Assessment in Electrocardiography. Philadelphia, J. B. Lippincott, 1977
Marriott HJ: Practical Electrocardiography, 6th ed. Baltimore, Williams & Wilkins, 1977
Ritota MC: Diagnostic Electrocardiography, 2nd ed. Philadelphia, J. B. Lippincott, 1977

Shirley J. Hoffman

SERUM ENZYME STUDIES

As the role of the nurse has expanded, there is a need for more knowledge on which to base the judgments necessary to assume new responsibilities. Knowledge of the purpose, functions, and significance of laboratory values in relation to the diagnosis and prognosis of acute myocardial infarction can enhance the quality of nursing care available to patients. Armed with a basic understanding of serum enzyme determinations, the nurse can exercise judgment in interpreting them in relation to other information known about the patient. The ability to exercise this kind of judgment may well affect the clinical course or prognosis of the patient. It is certainly as important to the physical and mental well-being of these patients to rule out the presence of acute myocardial infarction as it is to confirm its existence.

Enzyme Function

Enzymes are proteins that are found in all living cells. Different enzymes are found in different kinds of cells and in varying concentrations. The function of enzymes is to serve as accelerating agents or catalysts for chemical reactions. They temporarily combine with one substance to form an enzyme substrate complex, which then breaks down to form the end products of the chemical reaction. When the enzyme has completed this task, it is liberated, unchanged, to continue functioning as a chemical catalyst.

Enzymes are produced in the cells and are released into the plasma. Overactive, diseased, or injured cells increase the release of their particular enzymes into the serum. The difference in composition and concentration of various enzymes from one kind of tissue to another (cardiac, liver, skeletal muscle, and the like) determines which serum enzyme elevations reflect damage to specific tissues. Thus, serum enzyme determinations can be used to detect cell damage and to suggest where the damage has occurred.

Serum Enzyme Determinations

Many studies have been done in relation to the diagnostic value of serum enzyme determinations. As sometimes happens in research, the results vary and are debated by clinical diagnosticians and pathologists alike. To further cloud the issue, enzymes are evaluated by a variety of laboratory methods, and the determinations are reported in different quantitative units. This results in different "normal" ranges, which vary according to the procedures used by the particular laboratory. The nurse must become familiar with the range of normals for each enzyme as it is reported by the laboratory where she works.

Serum enzyme determinations have been helpful in the diagnosis of cardiac, hepatic, pancreatic, muscular, bone, and malignant diseases. Each of these kinds of tissue releases a particular enzyme or enzymes when diseased or damaged. Since each kind of cell contains and releases more than one enzyme, there is overlapping of enzymes from one tissue source to another. For this reason there is no one serum enzyme elevation that is diagnostic of any one disease.

Cardiac Enzymes

The term *cardiac enzyme* is used in reference to those enzymes that occur in and are released in proportionately larger amounts from cardiac tissue. These include creatine kinase or CK (formerly creatine phosphokinase or CPK), hydroxybutyric dehydrogenase (HBD), serum glutamic-oxalacetic transaminase (SGOT), and lactic dehydrogenase (LDH). Serum glutamic-pyruvic transaminase (SGPT) may show a slight increase in the presence of massive myocardial infarction, but it is more specific for liver disease.

Each of these enzymes varies in its degree of specificity for myocardial disease. The relationship between acute myocardial infarction and elevated SGOT and LDH was established in the mid-1950s. CK was added to the list of diagnostic aids in the mid-1960s. Controversy regarding their usefulness continues.

LDH

Total LDH is probably the least specific for cardiac disease of the cardiac enzymes. It is abundant in kidney, cardiac, liver, and muscle tissues and in red cells (see Table 10-1). The onset of LDH elevation occurs 12 to 24 hours after tissue damage, and peak elevation, averaging about three times upper normal, is at 72 hours. Return to normal is not complete for 7 to 11 days. The fact that LDH elevation is prolonged for a week or more after myocardial infarction is often helpful in late diagnosis. Some patients do not come to the hospital until several days after their initial symptoms, so early blood specimens cannot be obtained.

LDH Isoenzymes. Because LDH has widespread distribution in body tissues, its serum level is elevated in a variety of diseases. In 1957 it was found that LDH could be subjected to cer-

Table 10–1
Enzyme Distribution in Cells

	SGOT	CK	LDH (Isoenzymes)
Fast-acting	Heart Kidney Red cells Brain	Brain	Heart Kidney Red cells Brain
Intermediate	Lung Pancreas	Heart	Lymph nodes Spleen Leukocytes Pancreas Lung
Slow-acting	Liver Skeletal muscle	Skeletal muscle	Liver Skeletal muscle Skin

tain procedures that separate the enzyme into five components or isoenzymes that demonstrate five zones of activity of the enzyme. Since enzyme activity is measured by its rate of acceleration of chemical reactions, these five zones range from fastest-acting to slowest-acting.

The two fastest-acting isoenzymes are found in cardiac muscle, the renal cortex, erythrocytes, and the cerebrum and reflect disease or damage in these tissues. Thus, if these isoenzymes are elevated in the serum of a patient who presents with chest pain but who has no evidence of renal, hemolytic, or cerebral disease, myocardial infarction is the likely diagnosis.

The two slowest-acting LDH isoenzymes are found in the liver, skeletal muscle, and skin. These reflect acute liver disease or hepatic congestion, muscle injuries, or dermatologic disease or trauma. The intermediate isoenzyme is found in lymph nodes, spleen, leukocytes, pancreas, and lung tissue. It in turn reflects disease or damage to these tissues.

These five isoenzymes, also called *fractions* of LDH, are numbered 1 through 5. Many laboratories report LDH_1 and LDH_2 as the faster isoenzymes and LDH_4 and LDH_5 as the slower, while others report them in reverse order. Care must be taken in reading the literature on serum enzymes to avoid the confusion caused by various methods of reporting. LDH_1 will henceforth be referred to as fastest-acting and LDH_5 as slowest-acting. Here again the nurse must be aware of how LDH isoenzymes are reported in her hospital laboratory.

The introduction of isoenzyme separation has made determination of the LDH isoenzymes one of the most specific tests for the diagnosis of myocardial infarction. Most diagnosticians consider myocardial infarction the problem when LDH_1 activity is greater than LDH_2. If LDH_2 is greater than LDH_1, the patient may have experienced a severe ischemic episode or only minimal heart damage. Both these isoenzymes have been found in the serum up to 2 weeks or more after infarction even though total LDH has returned to normal.

When blood specimens for LDH determinations are collected, it is essential to avoid hemolysis of the sample. Since LDH is found in erythrocytes, even slightly hemolyzed blood will show an elevation of the serum LDH. It is for this same reason that hemolysis caused by an artificial valve or by use of the cardiopulmonary bypass pump results in elevation of serum LDH. When LDH_1 is greater than LDH_2 on admission and the cardiac isoenzyme CK is not present, a serum haptoglobin level should be determined to exclude hemolysis.

HBD

The enzyme HBD may possibly be the same as the fast-moving cardiac isoenzyme of LDH. It correlates with the LDH fractions and therefore is frequently omitted from the commonly used series of enzymes. HBD activity is always associated with LDH activity. The serum evaluation of both enzymes after myocardial infarction is about the same, both in quantity and in duration of elevation, with only a slight time lag in HBD. In laboratories that do not have the necessary equipment for fractionating LDH isoenzymes, HBD determination can serve as an alternate for this study, although it is felt to be less specific.

CK

CK is the fastest-rising and fastest-falling of all the cardiac enzymes. Onset of serum elevation is about 4 to 6 hours after infarction, with a peak elevation of five to twelve times normal, or more, by 12 to 20 hours. Serum levels may return to normal by the second or third day. This transient nature of CK elevation following myocardial infarction can be a distinct aid to diagnosis if the patient is reached early in the acute episode. However, this frequently is not the case; the CK rise may be missed entirely by the time the patient enters the hospital and is seen by a physician and a tentative diagnosis made. About 90% of patients with myocardial infarction show the early rise in serum CK.

The CK enzyme is second only to LDH isoenzymes in specificity for cardiac damage. CK is found in skeletal and cardiac muscle and in brain tissue. Since red cells contain almost no CK, slight hemolysis does not interfere with the accuracy of its determination. It is of particular value in diagnosing cardiac disease because it is not found in liver tissue as are LDH and SGOT. Hepatic congestion or disease, which frequently accompanies cardiac disease, will therefore not affect CK values. CK determination is also helpful in differentiating myocardial infarction from pulmonary embolism, which often present very similar clinical pictures. Because of the proportionately smaller amount of CK in lung tissue, any rise with pulmonary embolism will be much smaller than the very high elevation associated with myocardial infarction. CK values are normal in pericarditis, but an elevation occurs in myocarditis because of the cardiac muscle involvement.

Recall that overactivity as well as disease or

damage of tissue cells will cause release of enzymes into the serum. This should be kept in mind when CK elevation is found in the patient who collapsed on the golf course or while skiing. Severe or prolonged exercise of the untrained "social athlete" can result in CK elevation for up to 48 hours.

Other conditions causing a rise in CK levels include acute cerebrovascular disease, muscular dystrophy, and other muscle trauma. Elevations are sometimes found following peripheral arterial embolism, repeated intramuscular injections, and operative procedures. Even minor trauma to muscle cells near the sampling site may distort the results. It has been reported that morphine sulfate injected intramuscularly causes a significant increase in CK values in 25% of patients. High concentrations of barbiturates, Valium, morphine sulfate, and anesthetic agents have been shown to decrease the disappearance of CK from the circulation in experimental animals.

CK Isoenzymes. The discovery that CK can be fractionated into isoenzymes is seen by many to be a great boon to the diagnosis of myocardial infarction. CK isoenzymes are again measured by their rate of chemical reaction acceleration. They are designated as BB, the slow-acting isoenzyme found in brain tissue; MB, the intermediate-acting myocardial isoenzyme; and MM, the fast-acting isoenzyme found in skeletal muscle.

Since there are so many causes for total CK release, especially from injured skeletal muscle tissue, the ability to differentiate muscle, myocardial, or brain tissue as the source of the CK elevation can be extremely helpful. CK-MB is reported to be up to 94% sensitive and 100% specific for myocardial infarction. CK-MB may be elevated after acute myocardial infarction even though total CK is not.

The CK-MB isoenzyme is elevated in the serum for only 24 to 72 hours after its initial appearance. It is obvious that proper timing of the blood specimen is extremely important. The peak rise of CK-MB is 12 to 20 hours after initial elevation. If the patient is not seen until 24 to 48 hours after the onset of symptoms of myocardial injury, one must rely more on the LDH isoenzymes.

The rapid appearance and disappearance of the CK-MB isoenzyme may be a positive factor in its usefulness in diagnosing the extension of an acute myocardial infarction. This can be a very difficult diagnosis to make when the resolved chest pain of myocardial infarction recurs and the initial total enzyme elevations have not yet returned to normal. Determination of CK-MB may be especially helpful in the coronary care unit patient when there are additional causes for total enzyme elevations such as cardioversion or defibrillation, multiple intramuscular injections for pain or vomiting, trauma due to falls secondary to arrhythmias, prolonged use of rotating tourniquets, or hypotension.

CK-MB may also be helpful in diagnosing acute myocardial infarction in the postoperative patient. The muscle trauma incurred during surgical procedures will cause all three of the total cardiac enzymes to rise. In these patients, one should be able to determine whether total CK elevation is entirely due to surgical trauma or partially due to myocardial infarction by employing CK isoenzymes as a specific test. Unfortunately, CK isoenzymes are not very helpful in diagnosing myocardial infarction in the postoperative cardiac patient. Some rise in CK-MB will occur after open heart surgery due to cardiac manipulation and cannulation.

SGOT

SGOT is the last of the cardiac enzymes to be discussed. Its tissue distribution is quite widespread, with large SGOT concentrations in red cells and cardiac, liver, skeletal muscle, and renal tissue. Lesser amounts are found in brain, pancreas, and lung tissue. Because SGOT is prevalent in so many kinds of tissue and because of the current capabilities to fractionate LDH and CK, many physicians no longer feel the need to include SGOT as a routine cardiac enzyme determination. Its widespread distribution makes it one of the least specific enzymes, second only to total LDH. Over 95% of patients with myocardial infarction have SGOT elevation; an infarction as little as 5% can cause a serum rise.

SGOT falls between CK and LDH in both degree and duration of elevation. SGOT rise begins about 6 to 8 hours after onset of an acute myocardial episode, reaches its peak in 18 to 36 hours, and returns to normal at the end of 4 to 6 days. Average elevation following myocardial infarction is five times normal but may go much higher with an extensive infarct.

SGOT may become elevated with tachyarrhythmias with or without myocardial infarction, probably reflecting liver decompensation due to decreased perfusion. Liver damage resulting from congestive heart failure or shock due to myocardial infarction can also cause an increase in SGOT. It has been reported that about 25% of

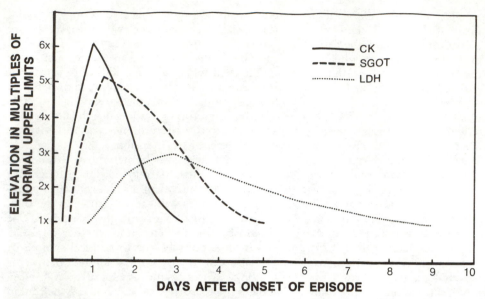

FIGURE 10-30.
Peak elevation and duration of serum enzymes after myocardial injury.

cardioverted patients have elevation of SGOT up to three times normal, probably due to muscle release of the enzyme.

Other causes of SGOT elevation include acute liver damage after alcohol ingestion, tachyarrhythmias with a ventricular rate of over 160 per minute, shock, pericarditis, dissecting aortic aneurysm, unaccustomed vigorous exercise, trauma, cerebral infarction, acute cholecystitis, pancreatitis, and certain drugs such as narcotics and anticoagulants. SGOT rises several days after pulmonary infarction. This may help to differentiate this problem from acute myocardial infarction when the time of onset of symptoms of pulmonary infarction can be determined.

SGPT

As mentioned previously, the SGPT enzyme is more specific for liver disease and does not usually rise with cardiac damage. However, both SGOT and SGPT will rise if myocardial infarction is accompanied by prolonged or profound shock or severe congestive heart failure that results in liver congestion or damage. SGOT evaluation may be of particular value in the early diagnosis of reinfarction. A second infarction often cannot be read on ECG because of the changes already incurred by the first infarction. A rise in SGOT within 6 to 8 hours after an episode of chest pain will help to make the diagnosis.

Comparative Enzyme Peak and Duration

One can almost always be assured that myocardial infarction has not occurred if serum enzyme levels remain normal for 24 hours after onset of symptoms. Transfer from the coronary care unit at this time can be justified as there is only a remote possibility of missing myocardial injury. If infarct has occurred, all the enzymes should be elevated by 24 hours after symptom occurrence (see Fig. 10-30). In comparing enzyme elevations, CK rises first and highest and falls to normal first, followed by SGOT, with LDH rising last. LDH elevation is the lowest but the most prolonged. In comparing the specificity of each enzyme as an indicator of myocardial necrosis, CK isoenzymes are most specific, followed by LDH isoenzymes, total CK, SGOT, and total LDH (least specific).

In general it can be said that the size of a myocardial infarction correlates fairly well with the height of the enzyme peaks and the duration of enzyme elevation, as well as with patient mortality. Some studies show that CK elevation of ten times normal is accompanied by 50% mortality, while a mortality rate of 6% is shown with CK rises of less than five times normal. It has been reported that (1) 81% of ventricular arrhythmias occur in patients whose enzyme levels are more than four times normal; (2) the incidence of congestive heart failure is significantly increased in those with enzyme levels of four to five times normal; (3) patients with cardiogenic shock have enzyme increases of more than five times normal. Research is being done in an effort to use CK-MB to estimate infarct size in terms of grams of necrotic tissue. Currently it is not of sufficient reliability and accuracy to be of clinical use.

If enzyme peak levels do indeed correlate with infarct size, they should be helpful to the nurse in anticipating those complications that are related to infarct size, as well as prognosis and ultimate rehabilitation.

INTERFERING FACTORS

There are a number of "red herrings" to be kept in mind when elevated serum enzymes are evaluated. Severe or *prolonged exercise* has been mentioned. *Defibrillation* with large amounts of voltage or repeated defibrillation may cause enzymes to rise because of the sudden severe contraction of all muscle tissues. Even one defibrillation with 400 watt-seconds may result in enzyme rise sufficient to mimic myocardial infarction. HBD, which is thought to be much like the cardiac isoenzymes of LDH and CK, sometimes rises with *liver disease*.

The extent of *surgical trauma* during operative procedures should be considered when enzyme elevations are evaluated postoperatively. Tissue damage from frequent *intramuscular injections* must also be remembered as a source of enzyme rises. CK elevations of more than eight times normal have been seen after frequent injections. It is also possible to produce elevation of SGOT and SGPT with administration of salicylates, sodium warfarin (Coumadin), and other *drugs* that are detoxified in the liver.

There may be minimal enzyme elevations after *cardiac catheterization* and coronary *angiography,* but these are mainly caused by the injection of intramuscular premedications. The introduction of catheters by arteriotomy or percutaneous routes alone does not cause significant rise of enzymes.

Diagnostic Limitations

It is apparent from the discussion of these four enzyme studies used in diagnosing myocardial infarction that none are actually diagnostic. Many areas still remain unclear or unknown. No enzyme or enzyme fraction has yet been found to exist in cardiac muscle alone. There is much disagreement about the normal range of CK activity. Some studies indicate that the upper limit of normal in females is about two-thirds

that of males, and that blacks may have higher normals that whites. Other enzymes have been found to rise with myocardial necrosis, but they are either no more specific than the ones currently used or are technically difficult and time-consuming to measure.

As yet, enzyme determinations can serve only as an adjunct to diagnosis by ECG and the patient's clinical picture. In order to be of most value they should be ordered with discretion. Consideration must be given to the length of time that has passed since the onset of symptoms, as each enzyme rises and returns to normal at different time intervals. One often finds an order for "stat" enzymes upon admission of the patient with suspected myocardial infarction to the critical care unit. The results will be useless if only an hour or two has passed since the onset of symptoms. If the patient suffered only moderate symptoms and did not come to the hospital until several days later, CK determination is useless because the enzyme will already have returned to normal. Usually two enzyme determinations are considered more valid than one, but the gamut of enzyme tests may not be necessary.

Enzyme determinations have been of greatest value in the patient whose ECG and clinical picture are equivocal for diagnosis of myocardial infarction. Enzyme elevation may well confirm a suspected diagnosis in this case. Sometimes it is difficult or impossible to interpret infarction on ECG because of previous infarction changes, the effects of certain drugs or electrolyte imbalances, conduction defects such as bundle branch block or Wolff-Parkinson-White syndrome, arrhythmias, or a functioning pacemaker. Enzyme determination may be a distinct advantage here. If a definite diagnosis can be made by ECG, there may be no need for enzyme tests, except for academic interest.

It must be stressed that serum elevations are nonspecific in the diagnosis of myocardial infarction, and they must be considered in view of the total clinical picture. We are in a highly technical age of nursing and must not forget to look at and listen to the patient before making judgments and decisions.

BIBLIOGRAPHY

Baillie EE: CK Isoenzymes: Part I. Clinical aspects. Lab Med 10:267–270, 1979

Baillie EE: CK isoenzymes: Part II. Technical aspects. Lab Med 10:339–340, 1979

Galen RS, Reiffel JA, Gambino SR: Diagnosis of acute myocardial infarction: Relative efficiency of serum enzymes and isoenzyme measurements. JAMA 232:145–147, 1975

Roberts R: Can we clinically measure infarction size? JAMA 242:183–185, 1979

Roberts R, Sobel BE: Creatine kinase isoenzymes in the assessment of heart disease. Am Heart J 95:521–528, 1978

Roe CR: Guest Editorial: Validity of estimating myocardial infarct size from serial measurements of enzyme activity in the serum. Clin Chem 23:1807–1812, 1977

Seager, SB: Cardiac enzymes in the evaluation of chest pain. Ann Emergency Med 9, No. 7:346–349, 1980

Sobel BE et al: Factors influencing enzymatic estimates of infarct size. Am J Cardiol 39:130–132, 1977

Thompson PL et al: Enzymatic indices of myocardial necrosis: Influence on short- and long-term prognosis after myocardial infarction. Circulation 59, No. 1:113–119, 1979

Varat MA, Mercer DW: Cardiac-specific creatine phosphokinase isoenzyme in the diagnosis of acute myocardial infarction. Circulation 51:855–859, 1975

Vijayan VK et al: Correlation of ST-segment elevation in 12-lead electrocardiogram with serum CPK in acute myocardial infarction. Ind Heart J 31, No. 1:31–33, 1979

Joan Mersch

AUSCULTATION OF THE HEART

Nurses throughout the country have played an instrumental role in terminating and preventing lethal arrhythmias. With the development of ECG monitoring and the education of nurses in interpreting arrhythmias and initiating emergency treatment, the mortality incidence among patients with myocardial infarction has decreased. However, nurses need to improve their care of patients who develop heart failure. Of the patients who develop blatantly obvious left ventricular failure, many still die.

One of the earliest and frequently the only cardiac sign of congestive heart failure in the adult is the development of a third heart sound. By detecting the third heart sound and realizing its clinical significance, nurses help decrease the incidence of heart failure in patients.

The Characteristics of Sound
Sound is a series of disturbances in matter to which the human ear is sensitive. Sound is a wave motion which has four characteristics — intensity, pitch, duration, and timbre.

Intensity is the force of the amplitude of the vibrations. It is a physical aspect of sound, whereas loudness is a subjective aspect dependent upon (1) intensity of the sound and (2) sensitivity of the ear.

Pitch is the frequency of the fibrations per unit of time. The human ear is most sensitive to vibrations of 500 to 5,000 per second. Vibrations of less than 20 per second or greater than 20,000 per second cannot be heard by the human ear.

Duration is the length of time that the sound persists.

Timbre is a quality dependent upon overtones that accompany the fundamental tone. In other words, most fundamental vibrations have higher frequency vibrations called *overtones*. Overtones account for the difference in sound between the same note played on a piano and on a flute.

Heart Sounds. Sound waves are initiated by vibrations. The heart sounds are produced by vascular walls, flowing blood, heart muscle, and heart valves. Sudden changes in intra-arterial pressures cause the vascular walls to vibrate, resulting in sound production. Turbulence of blood flow is produced when rapidly moving blood passes through chambers of irregular size, such as the chambers of the heart and the great vessels. When the heart muscles contract, sound waves are initiated by the contracting fibers. Sound waves are produced when the heart valves open as the blood flows through or when they close, especially with a sudden snapping of the chordae tendineae. Of the previously mentioned causes of heart sounds, the closing of the heart valves accounts for most of the sound production.

Systole is defined as the time during which the ventricles contract. Systole begins with the beginning of the first heart sound and ends with the beginning of the second heart sound.

Diastole is defined as the time during which the ventricles relax. Diastole begins with the beginning of the second heart sound and ends with the beginning of the next first heart sound. The cardiac cycle is determined by the cycle of the ventricles. In other words, cardiac systole and ventricular systole are synonymous.

Transmission of Heart Sounds. The transmission of the heart sounds is dependent upon the position of the heart, the nature of the surrounding structures, and the position of the stethoscope in relation to the origin of the sound. The stethoscope is a tool used to transmit sounds produced by the body to the ear. Sound waves that travel a shorter distance are of greater intensity; likewise, the shorter the distance the less the possibility for distortion to occur. It then follows that the shorter the tube of the stethoscope the better the transmission of sound. Convenience and comfort as well as maximum sound production must be considered.

In order to facilitate accurate auscultation, the patient should be comfortable, in a quiet room, and in a recumbent position. The bell of the stethoscope transmits low-pitched sounds best when there is an airtight seal and when the instrument is applied lightly to the chest wall. An airtight seal helps to occlude extraneous sounds. The diaphragm of the stethoscope best transmits the high-pitched sounds when it is applied with firm pressure to the chest wall.

CLASSIFICATION OF HEART SOUNDS

The First Heart Sound

The first heart sound is produced by the asynchronous closure of the mitral and tricuspid valves. Mitral closure precedes tricuspid closure by 0.02 to 0.03 second. Such narrow splitting is generally not audible.

The first heart sound is therefore composed of two separate components. The first component of the first heart sound is the closure of the mitral valve. The second component of the first heart sound is the closure of the tricuspid valve.

The first heart sound is generally best heard at the apex. It represents the beginning of ventricular systole.

The Second Heart Sound

The second heart sound is produced by the vibrations initiated by the closure of the aortic and pulmonic semilunar valves.

The second heart sound, like the first heart sound, is composed of two separate components. The first component of the second heart sound is closure of the aortic valve. The second component of the second heart sound is the closure of the pulmonic valve.

With inspiration, systole of the right ventricle is slightly prolonged due to increased filling of the right ventricle. With increased right ventricular filling, the pulmonary valve closes later than the aortic valve.

Aortic valve sounds are generally best heard in the second intercostal space to the right of the sternum, whereas the sound produced by the pulmonic valve is generally best heard in the second left intercostal space.

Splitting of the second heart sound is best heard upon inspiration with the stethoscope placed in the second intercostal space to the left of the sternum. The second heart sound represents the beginning of ventricular diastole. See Figure 10-31 for a graphic representation of the normal first and second heart sounds.

Comparison of ECG and Phonocardiogram

To facilitate understanding of the phonocardiogram, it will be compared with the ECG. The ECG is a graphic representation of the electrical activity of the heart, whereas the phonocardiogram is a recording of the sound vibrations produced by the heart.

When the sinoatrial (SA) node fires, the electrical current travels through the atrial muscle to the atrioventricular (AV) node. The P wave is then written on the ECG. The electrical current then travels down the common bundle of His, right and left bundle branches, Purkinje fibers, and throughout the ventricular muscle. Following electrical stimulation of the ventricles, the latter contract. Early in ventricular systole the mitral and tricuspid valves close. This is the reason the first heart sound occurs during or following ventricular depolarization, which is

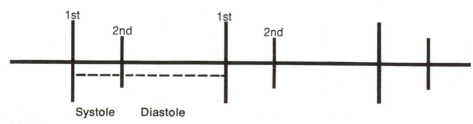

FIGURE 10-31.
Normal heart sounds.

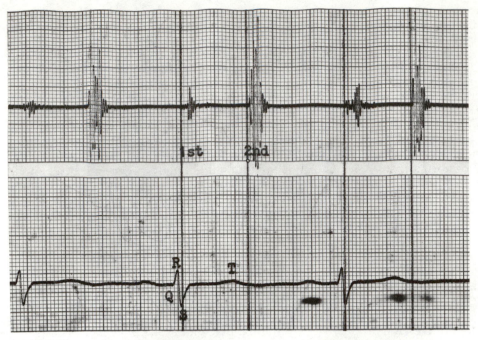

FIGURE 10-32.
Simultaneous recording of a phonocardiogram and an electrocardiogram.

represented on the ECG by the QRS complex (see Fig. 10-32).

During ventricular systole, the blood is forced from the right and left ventricles into the pulmonic and aortic arteries. When the ventricles relax, the aortic and pulmonic semilunar valves close. The second heart sound represents the beginning of ventricular diastole. The second heart sound occurs after the repolarization of the ventricular muscle, which is represented by the T wave on the ECG.

The Third Heart Sound

A third heart sound represents pathology in the adult. The third heart sound is believed to be produced by the rapid inrush of blood into a nonpliable ventricle. During ventricular diastole, the apex extends downward and the mitral valve extends upward. As the ventricle fills, the chordae tendineae become tense and partially close the mitral valve. This, along with the increasing resistance of diastole, causes a sudden decrease in blood flow. The cardiac muscle, chordae tendineae, heart valves, and blood are set into motion and are responsible for the production of sound.

The third heart sound is heard after the closure of the semilunar valves, early in diastole, and best at the apex. Most third heart sounds are of relatively low pitch, between 25 and 35 vibrations per second. They are best heard with the bell of the stethoscope applied lightly to the chest wall (see Fig. 10-33).

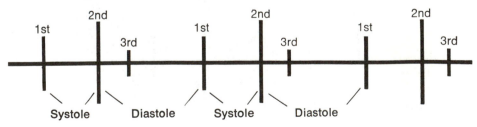

FIGURE 10-33.
Third heart sound.

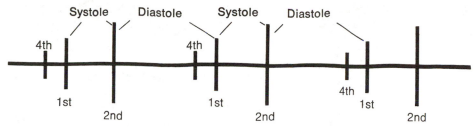

FIGURE 10-34.
Fourth heart sound.

The Fourth Heart Sound

The fourth heart sound, also called an atrial sound, is believed to be produced by atrial contraction that is more forceful than normal. At the end of atrial contraction, more blood is forced from the atria into the ventricle, which causes a sudden increase in ventricular pressure. This increased pressure produces vibrations that cause the fourth heart sound. The fourth heart sound is therefore believed to be produced by atrial contraction and the consequent impact of the rapid inflow of blood on the ventricle.

The fourth heart sound is of low pitch, heard best at the lower end of the sternum and sometimes at the apex. It has a short duration and a low frequency. It is best heard with the bell of the stethoscope. Figure 10-34 shows the timing of the fourth heart sound.

Gallop Rhythms

Gallop rhythm is the name given to the heart sounds when they are grouped so as to mimic the cadence of galloping horses. There are three types of gallop rhythms: the ventricular gallop, the atrial gallop, and the summation gallop.

The protodiastolic or early diastolic gallop rhythm, also known as the *ventricular gallop rhythm,* is believed to be due to an exaggerated third heart sound. This rhythm is commonly heard in congestive heart failure. It is frequently the earliest sign of heart failure. Controversy still exists regarding the significance of the third sound.

The ventricular gallop is generally believed to result from the rapid inflow of blood into a dilated ventricle early in diastole. The third heart sound occurs between 0.12 and 0.18 second after the second heart sound. It is of low pitch and heard best at the apex with the bell of the stethoscope.

A *presystolic gallop* rhythm exists when the gallop sound occurs late in diastole or immediately preceding systole. The sound occurs with atrial systole and is believed to represent an accentuated atrial sound. It occurs with systolic overloading notably in hypertension, myocardial infarction, aortic stenosis, pulmonary hypertension, pulmonary stenosis, and various cardiomyopathies. It is often unaccompanied by heart failure. The presystolic or atrial gallop rhythm is low-pitched and is heard best with the bell of the stethoscope. A left atrial sound is heard best on expiration at the apex, whereas a right atrial sound is best heard on inspiration at the left border of the sternum.

A *summation gallop* occurs because of a tachycardia so rapid that the third and fourth heart sounds combine and are heard as one (see Fig. 10-35).

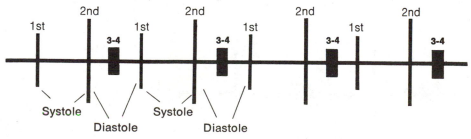

FIGURE 10-35.
Summation gallop.

HEART MURMURS

Mechanisms

In order to understand the heart murmurs, it is vital to understand the mechanism responsible for the sound production and to understand the principles of *turbulence of blood flow*. Blood flows most rapidly in the center of a vessel, less rapidly nearer the wall, and least rapidly immediately along the internal surface of the vessel. In other words, as blood flows through a vessel the friction along the wall of the vessel tends to slow the rate of blood flow nearest the wall. The smoother the internal surface of the vessel, the less turbulence in blood flow. The slower the rate of blood flow, the less chance there is for turbulence.

Any irregularity in the inner surface of the vessel or change in the size of the lumen results in turbulence of blood flow and sound production. The narrower the opening, the more rapid the rate of blood flow and the greater the possibility for turbulence and murmur formation.

The murmurs of mitral stenosis, mitral insufficiency, aortic stenosis, and aortic insufficiency will be discussed. With the knowledge of the mechanisms which produce these murmurs, we can deduce the mechanisms responsible for the other murmurs not discussed.

The mechanisms responsible for the murmurs of mitral stenosis and mitral insufficiency are also responsible for the murmurs of tricuspid stenosis and tricuspid insufficiency. The only difference is that the latter murmurs occur on the right side of the heart. Likewise, the mechanisms responsible for the murmurs of aortic stenosis and aortic insufficiency are also responsible for the murmurs of pulmonary stenosis and pulmonary insufficiency. The difference is that the latter murmurs occur on the right side of the heart.

While it might not be necessary to distinguish the specific heart murmur, it is important to recognize the difference between the extra heart sounds and the murmurs. The key diagnostic sign of early congestive heart failure is the development of the third heart sound.

The Murmur of Mitral Stenosis

In mitral stenosis, the mitral orifice can be narrowed by inflammation or fibrosis of the mitral valve because of rheumatic heart disease or arteriosclerosis. A stenotic mitral valve causes an increased left atrial pressure during ventricular diastole. In ventricular diastole the left atrium contracts, forcing blood through the narrowed opening. This produces turbulence of blood flow and a diastolic murmur. The murmur is low-pitched and rumbling.

The murmur of mitral stenosis may be a crescendo or decrescendo in configuration. It may be a crescendo in shape because the left atrium contracts progressively, the rate of blood flow increases, and the mitral valve becomes narrower. It may be a decrescendo in shape because as the ventricle fills, the left atrium empties, and the amount of blood passing through the stenotic valve decreases. The murmur therefore decreases in intensity and is a decrescendo in shape (see Fig. 10-36).

The Murmur of Mitral Insufficiency

The murmur of mitral insufficiency is heard in systole. Mitral insufficiency occurs when the mitral valve is incompetent, and the valve leaflets fail to approximate. During ventricular systole, intraventricular pressure exceeds intraatrial pressure. With an incompetent mitral valve, the blood regurgitates through the valve opening into the left atrium. This results in turbulence of blood flow and a high-pitched, blowing murmur. The murmur is systolic, heard best at the apex, and is transmitted laterally to the axillary line when the heart is enlarged. As a rule, a murmur is transmitted in the direction of the blood flow that is responsible for the turbulence. The murmur of mitral insufficiency is

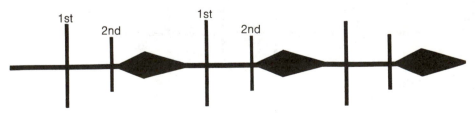

FIGURE 10-36.
Murmur of mitral stenosis.

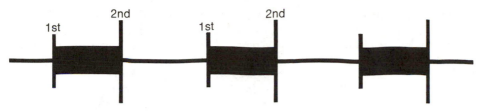

FIGURE 10-37.
Murmur of mitral insufficiency.

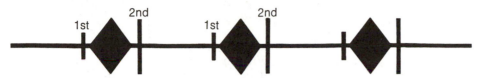

FIGURE 10-38.
Murmur of aortic stenosis.

generally pansystolic or holosystolic (lasting all of systole) (see Fig. 10-37).

The murmur of mitral insufficiency is the murmur of myocardial infarction. In myocardial infarction, dilatation of the left ventricle occurs because of ischemia or necrosis. When the left ventricle is dilated, the papillary muscle tends to move away from the valve leaflets. The chordae tendineae are unable to lengthen, and the mitral leaflets are held open, preventing complete approximation. With dilatation of the left ventricle, the mitral ring dilates. The leaflets remain the same size and are unable to close the enlarged opening. When the left ventricle dilates, it loses its ability to contract and there is an associated papillary muscle dysfunction.

The Murmur of Aortic Stenosis

The murmur of aortic stenosis is heard during systole. Aortic stenosis is the result of narrowing of the aortic cusps. During ventricular systole, the pressure within the ventricle exceeds the pressure of the aorta, and the blood flows out of the ventricle into the aorta. If there is thickening of the aortic cusps or narrowing of the aortic valve, the rapidly flowing blood passes through the constricted valve and causes turbulence of blood flow.

The murmur is of medium pitch and has a rough or harsh sound. It is heard best over the aortic valve area, the second right intercostal space. The murmur of aortic stenosis is transmitted into the arteries of the neck because the blood flow responsible for the turbulence is moving in that direction. It can also be transmitted to the apex, where it may be confused with the murmur of mitral insufficiency — also a systolic murmur. The murmur of aortic stenosis occurs in systole, and it is a diamond shape. It is composed of a crescendo and a decrescendo (see Fig. 10-38).

The Murmur of Aortic Insufficiency

The murmur of aortic insufficiency is diastolic in time. In ventricular diastole, the intraventricular pressure is lower than the intra-aortic pressure. The aortic cusps fail to support the blood and it regurgitates into the ventricle. Turbulence of blood flow results in the formation of a high-pitched, blowing murmur. It is usually best

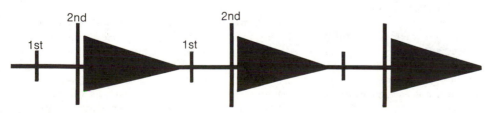

FIGURE 10-39.
Murmur of aortic insufficiency.

heard in the third left intercostal space. As the pressure in the ventricle increases and the aortic pressure decreases, the turbulence of blood flow decreases. The murmur is therefore a decrescendo in shape (see Fig. 10-39).

BIBLIOGRAPHY

Braunwald E: Determinants and assessment of cardiac function. N Engl J Med 296:86–89, 1977

DeGourin EL, DeGourin RL: Bedside Diagnostic Examination, 3rd ed. New York, Macmillan, 1977

Hurst J, Schlant R: Auscultation of the heart. In Hurst J, Logue R (eds): The Heart, 4th ed. New York, McGraw-Hill, 1978

Mason DT (ed): Advances in Heart Disease. New York, Grune & Stratton, 1977

Prior JA, Silberstein JS: Physical Diagnosis: The History and Examination of the Patient, 5th ed. St. Louis, C. V. Mosby, 1977

Thorn GW et al (eds): Harrison's Principles of Internal Medicine, 8th ed. New York, McGraw-Hill, 1977

Carolyn M. Hudak

CENTRAL VENOUS PRESSURE

Central venous pressure (CVP) refers to the pressure of blood in the right atrium or vena cava. It actually provides information about three parameters—blood volume, the effectiveness of the heart as a pump, and vascular tone. CVP is to be differentiated from a peripheral venous pressure, which may reflect only a local pressure.

CVP is measured in centimeters or millimeters of water pressure, and considerable variation exists in the range of normal values cited. Usually pressure in the right atrium is 0 to 4 cm H_2O, while pressure in the vena cava is approximately 6 to 12 cm H_2O.

More important, it is the trend of the readings that is most significant regardless of the baseline value. The upward or downward trend of the CVP, combined with clinical assessment of the patient, will determine appropriate interventions.

For example, a patient's CVP may gradually rise from 6 cm H_2O to 8 cm and then to 10 cm. While this may still be in the range of "normal," other parameters may indicate ensuing complications. Auscultation of breath sounds may reveal basilar rales, a third heart sound may be audible, or the pulse and respiratory rate may be increasing insidiously. In this context the trend of a gradual rise in CVP is more significant than the actual isolated value.

When interpreting CVP data in conjunction with other clinical observations, the nurse has a better understanding of their significance for that particular patient and recognizes the outcome to which nursing interventions must be geared. In this instance the nurse is aware that too much fluid administration would further compromise the patient's circulatory status, and she would act accordingly to reduce this risk.

Sometimes rate of fluid administration is titrated according to the patient's CVP and urinary output. So long as the urinary output remains adequate and the CVP does not change significantly, this is an indication that the heart can accommodate the amount of fluid being administered. If the CVP begins to rise and the urine output drops, indicating a decreased cardiac output to perfuse the kidneys, circulatory overload must be suspected and either ruled out or validated in view of other clinical symptomatology.

The patient who is started on a vasopressor agent will show a rise in CVP due to the vasoconstriction produced. In this situation the blood volume is unchanged, but the vascular bed has become smaller. Again, this change must be interpreted in conjunction with other information the nurse assesses about the patient. Alone, a CVP value can be meaningless, but used in conjunction with other clinical data, it is a valuable aid in managing and predicting the patient's clinical course.

CVP Measurement. For CVP recordings, a long intravenous catheter is inserted into an arm or a leg vein or the subclavian vein and threaded into position in the vena cava close to the right atrium. Occasionally the catheter may be advanced into the right atrium as indicated by rhythmic fluctuations in the pressure manometer corresponding to the patient's heartbeat. In this situation the catheter may simply be with-

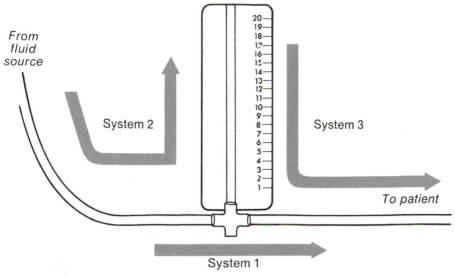

FIGURE 10-40.
Central venous pressure setup. (See text for description.)

drawn to the point at which the pulsations cease.

Figure 10-40 illustrates a typical setup for measuring the CVP. A manometer with a three-way stopcock is introduced between the fluid source and the patient's intravenous catheter. In this way three separate systems can be created by manipulating the stopcock.

System 1 connects the fluid source with the patient and can be used for routine administration of intravenous fluids or as an avenue to keep the system patent.

System 2 runs from the fluid source to the CVP manometer and is opened in order to raise the fluid column in the manometer prior to measuring the venous pressure.

System 3 connects the patient's intravenous catheter with the manometer and it is this pathway which must be open to record the CVP. Pressure in the vena cava displaces or equilibrates with the pressure exerted by the column of fluid in the manometer, and the point at which the fluid level settles is recorded as the CVP.

To obtain an accurate measurement, the patient should be flat, with the zero point of the manometer at the same level as the right atrium. This level corresponds to the midaxillary line of the patient or can be determined by measuring approximately 5 cm below the sternum. However, consistency is the important detail, and all readings should be taken with the patient in the same position and the zero point calculated in the same manner. If deviations from the routine procedure must be made, as when the patient cannot tolerate being flat and the reading must be taken with the patient in a semi-Fowler's position, it is valuable to note this on the patient's chart or care plan to provide for consistency in future readings.

A patent system is assured when the fluid column falls freely and slight fluctuation of the fluid column is apparent. This fluctuation follows the patient's respiratory pattern and will fall on inspiration and rise on expiration due to changes in interpulmonic pressure. If the patient is being ventilated on a respirator, a falsely high reading will result. If possible, the respirator should be discontinued momentarily for maximum accuracy. If the patient cannot tolerate being off the respirator for even this short period, significant trends in the CVP can still be determined if consistency in taking the readings is followed.

Variations in CVP. As noted earlier, changes in CVP must be interpreted in terms of the clinical picture of the patient. There are, however, some situations which commonly produce an *elevated CVP.* These include congestive heart failure when the heart can no longer effectively handle the venous return, cardiac tamponade, a vasoconstrictive state, or states of increased blood volume such as overtransfusion or overhydration.

A *low CVP* usually accompanies a hypovolemic state due to blood or fluid loss or drug-induced vasodilation. Increasing the rate of fluid administration or replacing blood loss is indicated in this situation.

Joan Mersch

HEMODYNAMIC PRESSURE MONITORING

The concept of pressure is a key parameter in patient assessment. Mathematically, pressure is defined as the product of flow and resistance:

$$pressure = flow \times resistance$$

Blood pressure is one of the "vital signs" routinely obtained, reported, and recorded.

For the critical care nurse to make important clinical decisions, the knowledge of pressure concepts must be incorporated into patient evaluation. The purpose of this section is to describe a current method of measuring heart and blood pressures; to discuss normal and abnormal hemodynamic pressures; and to assist the nurse in determining the physiological importance of these pressures.

METHOD OF MEASURING HEART AND BLOOD PRESSURES

Advances in medical technology have made it possible to measure pressures directly within the

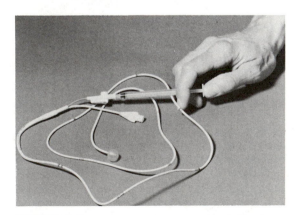

FIGURE 10-41.
Flow-directed catheter.

chambers of the heart and great vessels. Essential to direct measurement of hemodynamic pressures are catheters, a transducer, and a pressure module.

Essentials

CATHETERS

Flow-Directed (Swan-Ganz). The development of the flow-directed catheter has made possible the measurement of pulmonary artery wedge (PAW) pressure at the bedside. This pressure is an index of left ventricular function.

The catheter has two lumens, one for intravenous fluid to assure catheter patency and the second for the balloon (see Fig. 10-41). At the tip of the radiopaque catheter is a balloon, which when inflated causes the tip of the catheter to become buoyant. If then advanced, the catheter will float in the direction of blood flow. Introduced into either a brachial or a femoral vein, it can be passed into the superior or inferior vena cava respectively. It then can be passed to the right atrium, through the tricuspid valve into the right ventricle, through the pulmonary valve into the pulmonary artery. And, if advanced further, the catheter will obstruct forward blood flow, which allows *left* heart pressures to be reflected through the catheter tip. Because of the catheter size, it obstructs forward flow in a small pulmonary artery.

Right atrial (RA), right ventricular (RV), and pulmonary artery (PA) pressures give precise information on heart valve function and circulatory volume. The value of the flow-directed catheter lies in the fact that left ventricular function can be determined by inserting a catheter into the right side of the heart. This procedure has fewer risks and is simpler to perform than measuring left ventricular pressures directly.

Arterial. The ability to measure arterial pressures directly has been available for a longer time. A simple catheter inserted into an artery suffices. Directly measuring arterial pressure affords the nurse precise blood pressure readings and easy access to arterial blood samples. In addition, it saves the patient from numerous arterial punctures.

TRANSDUCER

The transducer is the second essential component for measuring pressure. It is an electrical device which converts one form of energy into another. Specifically, it senses mechanical energy—pressure—and converts it into electrical energy—the waveform. The pressures generated by myocardial contraction and relaxation are reflected through the lumen of the catheter to the transducer, where the pressure is converted to an electrical waveform. For the waveform to have meaning, two conditions must be met, a zeroing condition and a calibrating condition.

For accurate pressure measurement, the transducer must be placed at a standard level in relation to patient position—mid-chest suffices as a reference level.

1. To meet the *zeroing condition,* the transducer must be set at an arbitrarily assigned zero value pressure. This can be done by opening the transducer to room air or atmospheric pressure (760 mm Hg at sea level) and assigning that pressure zero value in millimeters Hg (0 mm Hg).
2. The second necessary condition for the transducer is the *calibrating condition.* That is, the amplitude of the electrical signal (height of the waveform) must be assigned a value in millimeters of mercury pressure. The trans-

ducer is calibrated when a numerical value in millimeters Hg pressure is assigned to each centimeter of waveform amplitude. For instance, 1 cm = 4 mm Hg or 1 cm = 20 mm Hg.

PRESSURE MODULE

The pressure module allows the transducer to be zeroed and calibrated and allows the pressure waveform to be displayed on an oscilloscope or paper tracing. Different pressure modules and transducers require varying techniques for zeroing and calibrating. Though the technical procedure changes according to specific equipment, the principles for zeroing and calibrating are the same.

Preparation for Pressure Measurement

Prepare for pressure measurement by (A) gathering supplies and (B) assembling supplies.

A. Gather supplies
1. Intravenous (IV) fluid in a plastic bag
2. Heparin (1 ml/1,000 units) and syringe

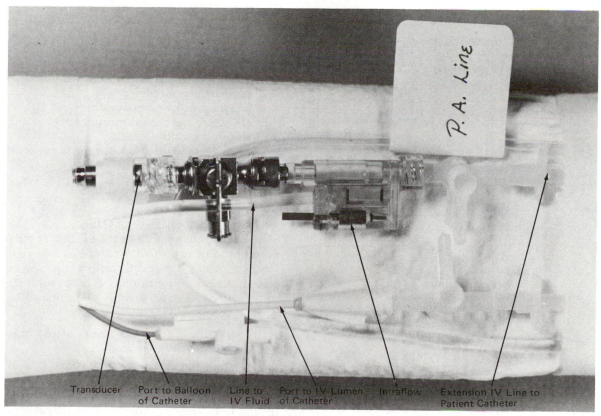

Transducer | Port to Balloon of Catheter | Line to IV Fluid | Port to IV Lumen of Catheter | Intraflow | Extension IV Line to Patient Catheter

FIGURE 10-42.
Arterial line set-up.

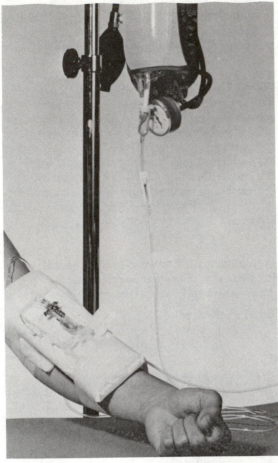

FIGURE 10-43.
Assembled set-up for monitoring hemodynamic pressures.

3. Pressure bag
4. IV tubing (15 gtt/ml)
5. Pressure valve (C.S.F. ®Intraflo, Continuous Flush System)*
6. Three 3-way stopcocks (2 plain, 1 with Luer-Lok)
7. IV extension tubing
8. Transducer
9. Pressure module

B. Assemble supplies
1. Heparinize the IV solution in the plastic bag by adding 1 unit of heparin per ml IV fluid. Label solution.
2. Connect the IV tubing to the IV solution in the plastic bag (Fig. 10–42).
3. Place the IV solution bag in the pressure bag and inflate to 300 mm Hg pressure.

*Sorenson Research Company, Salt Lake City, Utah.

4. Connect the IV tubing to the IV port of the pressure valve.
5. Connect the 3-way stopcock with Luer-Lok to the pressure valve port which is at the same end as the IV port.
6. Attach transducer to stopcock, Step 5.
7. Fill dome of transducer with IV fluid (fluid without air bubbles must fill dome for accurate pressure measurement).
8. Attach a 3-way stopcock to the distal port of the pressure valve.
9. Connect IV extension tubing to the stopcock, Step 8.
10. Attach a 3-way stopcock to the other end of the IV extension tubing.
11. Flush the line with IV fluid and connect it to the patient's flow-directed or arterial catheter. The assembled setup is shown in Figure 10–43.

Pressure Measurement
Following are the steps for pressure measurement:
1. Flush line with IV fluid.
2. Open stopcock attached to transducer to room air.
   a. Zero transducer.
   b. Calibrate transducer.
3. Open stopcock attached to transducer to patient pressure.
4. Assess quality of waveform.
5. Measure and record pressures.
6. Flush line with IV fluid.
7. Adjust treatment according to pressure values.

NORMAL PRESSURE VALUES
An understanding of the physiological mechanisms producing normal pressure is necessary to knowledgeably care for the patient requiring invasive pressure monitoring. A systematic approach to waveform analysis is essential. One such approach is to

1. Review the mechanical events of the heart and the normal pressures.
2. Learn the normal waveform characteristics.
3. Correlate the electrical and mechanical events of the heart.

In the following section this approach will be employed to analyze normal pressure tracings. Under the subheading Waveform Interpretation, the mechanical events, waveform characteristics, and normal pressure values will be discussed. The correlation between electrical and mechanical events will be discussed under the subheading Comparison of ECG with Waveform. The following abbreviations will be used throughout when referring to pressures:

- right atrial — RA
- right ventricular — RV
- right ventricular end-diastolic pressure — RVEDP
- pulmonary artery — PA
- pulmonary artery diastolic — PAd
- pulmonary artery wedge — PAW
- left atrial — LA
- left ventricular — LV
- left ventricular end-diastolic pressure — LVEDP
- aortic — Ao
- mean arterial pressure — MAP

Although the most frequently monitored pressures in the critical care setting are pulmonary artery, pulmonary artery wedge, and arterial, this section will discuss normal pressure values within all chambers of the heart and great vessels, emphasizing the process of waveform analysis.

Right Atrial Pressure

Visualize the catheter tip in the right atrium. The pressure created during RA systole, contraction, is greater than during RA diastole, relaxation. During RA systole, the tricuspid valve will open when RA pressure exceeds RV pressure. When the RV contracts, the tricuspid valve will be closed. The pulmonary artery cusps will open when the RV pressure exceeds the pressure in the pulmonary artery.

An RA pressure tracing appears as shown in Figure 10-44.

WAVEFORM INTERPRETATION

The right atrial waveform has three positive waves: *a, c,* and *v*. The *a* wave represents RA systole. The *v* wave represents RA diastole. Following RA systole, the tricuspid valve closes, the RA is filling with blood, and the RV is beginning to contract. At this point, the pressure within the RA briefly increases because the force of RV contraction causes the tricuspid valve to balloon into the RA, producing the *c* wave. Thus the *c* wave is caused by the closed tricuspid valve's pushing into the RA during RA diastole.

Sometimes the *c* wave is superimposed on the *a* wave and is not distinguishable, or it appears as a notch in the *a* wave.

The RA pressure tracing has three negative waves or descents: x, x^1 and y. The descents are of less significance and will be briefly mentioned here. The x descent follows the *a* wave and represents right atrial relaxation. The x^1 descent follows the *c* wave and represents atrioventricular movement during ventricular contraction. The y descent follows the *v* wave and represents passive right atrial emptying immediately after opening of the tricuspid valve just before right atrial systole.

The right atrium is a low-pressure chamber; the significant RA pressure is the mean or midpoint between the systolic and diastolic pressures. Normal right atrial mean $(\overline{RA})$ pressure is < 6 torr.

COMPARISON OF ECG WITH WAVEFORM

The electrical energy of the heart is demonstrated by the ECG; the mechanical energy is demonstrated by the pressure waveform. The electrical events precede and cause the mechanical events. On the ECG, the P wave represents the discharge of electrical current from the SA node (see Fig. 10-44). Following electrical activation, the atria contract. In comparing the ECG with the pressure waveform, it can be seen that the P wave on the ECG precedes the *a* wave, atrial systole, on the pressure tracing. The QRS complex represents ventricular depolarization, and it precedes ventricular systole. While the right ventricle is contracting, the right atrium is relaxing. Thus, on the ECG, the QRS complex will precede the *v* wave on the RA pressure tracing.

The *v* wave frequently extends beyond the T wave, which demonstrates ventricular repolarization on the ECG.

If the *c* wave is visible, it will occur between the *a* and *v* waves, and it will occur immediately after the QRS complex. Early in ventricular systole, the pressure within the ventricle pushes the closed tricuspid valve into the right atrium, causing a slight increase in RA pressure, demonstrated by the *c* wave on the RA pressure tracing.

Right Ventricular Pressure

Again, visualize the flow-directed catheter in the right atrium. When the balloon at the tip of the catheter is inflated, the catheter tip will become

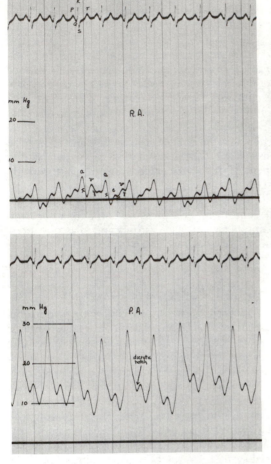

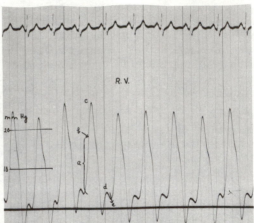

FIGURE 10-44.
(Top left) Right atrial pressure recording.

FIGURE 10-45.
(Top right) Right ventricular pressure recording.

FIGURE 10-46.
(Left) Pulmonary artery pressure recording.

buoyant. The catheter will tend to float in the direction of blood flow. If it is advanced, the slack in the line will allow the catheter to float through the open tricuspid valve into the ventricle. At this point, Figure 10-45 shows how the right ventricular waveform would be seen on the oscilloscope.

WAVEFORM INTERPRETATION

In order to identify the specific mechanical events causing the right ventricular waveform configuration, arbitrary letters *a* through *e* have been assigned to simplify the discussion. The initial rapid rise in the right ventricular waveform represents isovolumetric contraction, *a*. That is, the tricuspid and pulmonary valves are closed, and the volume of blood within the right ventricle remains constant while the pressure increases. When RV pressure exceeds PA pressure, the pulmonary valve opens, *b*. Blood is then ejected from the right ventricle into the pulmonary artery. Maximum RV systolic pressure is presented by point *c* on the waveform.

The pulmonary valve closes, and the RV pressure rapidly decreases. The tricuspid valve opens, and the right ventricle passively fills with blood from the right atrium. Point *d* represents right atrial contraction, with *e* representing right ventricular end diastole.

Note that the RV pressure waveform goes below baseline. It is generally characteristic of both right ventricular and left ventricular waveforms to return to or to go below baseline. Significant RV pressures are systolic and end-diastolic. RV systolic pressure is < 30 torr and RVEDP is < 5 torr.

COMPARISON OF ECG WITH WAVEFORM

The P wave on the ECG generally precedes two positive deflections on the right ventricular waveform. Following electrical activation of the atrium (P wave), the tricuspid valve opens, and the right ventricle passively fills with blood, causing an increase in RV diastolic pressure. The second positive deflection is caused when the atrium contracts, *d,* emptying the right atrium more completely, which increases RV diastolic pressure. Ventricular depolarization demonstrated by the QRS complex on the ECG precedes ventricular contraction, causing a rapid increase in the RV pressure wave. Following the electrical event of ventricular depolarization, the mechanical event of isovolumetric contraction occurs. During ventricular repolarization (T wave on the ECG), maximum ejection, reduced ejection, pulmonic valve closure, and rapid decrease in pressure occur.

Sometimes a slight increase in pressure can be seen following reduced ejection on the downward slope of the right ventricular tracing. Immediately after closure of the pulmonic valve, the pressure in the right ventricle increases slightly as the column of blood behind the closed valve pushes toward the ventricular chamber.

Pulmonary Artery Pressure

To float the catheter from the right ventricle into the pulmonary artery, the balloon is inflated and the catheter is advanced. The PA pressure tracing is shown in Figure 10-46.

WAVEFORM INTERPRETATION

The rapid rise in the pulmonary artery waveform represents right ventricular ejection. The dicrotic notch in the downward slope corresponds with pulmonary valve closure. Note that the pulmonary artery waveform always has a positive pressure; at no time does the pressure wave fall to zero or reach baseline. Normal PA pressures are systolic < 30 torr, diastolic < 10 torr, and mean < 20 torr.

Under normal conditions, the mean pulmonary artery ($\overline{PA}$) pressure will be closer to diastolic pressure than to systolic pressure. This pressure is not a true mathematic mean because systolic pressure is sustained approximately one-third of the cardiac cycle, whereas diastole lasts about two-thirds of the cycle. The diastolic pressure, therefore, contributes more in determining the $\overline{PA}$. As heart rate increases, systole changes little, but diastole is shortened; likewise, as heart rate slows, systole changes minimally, but diastole is prolonged. Thus, as heart rate increases, diastole contributes less to the mean value, while, as heart rate decreases, diastolic pressure contributes more to the mean pressure value.

COMPARISON OF ECG WITH WAVEFORM

Immediately after ventricular depolarization (QRS complex) ventricular ejection occurs. As the ventricle contracts, blood is ejected into the pulmonary artery causing the rapid rise in PA pressure. Maximum PA pressure is reached during ventricular repolarization (T wave). Closure of the pulmonary valve, dicrotic notch, corresponds with the end of ventricular repolarization.

Pulmonary Artery Wedge Pressure

A flow-directed catheter in the pulmonary artery can be wedged in the pulmonary capillary bed by advancing the catheter or by inflating the balloon (see Fig. 10-47). When forward blood flow is prevented, the catheter is wedged. The PAW pressure reflects left heart pressures. That is, it reflects LA mean and LVEDP. When the catheter is advanced from the pulmonary artery to the pulmonary artery wedge position, the waveform configuration will change as shown in Figure 10-48.

WAVEFORM INTERPRETATION

The pulmonary artery wedge tracing has an *a* wave and a *v* wave. The *a* wave reflects left atrial contraction and, in addition, left ventricular relaxation. The *v* wave reflects left atrial relaxation and left ventricular contraction. Mean PAW pressure is < 12 torr.

COMPARISON OF ECG WITH WAVEFORM

The P wave on the ECG will precede the *a* wave on the pulmonary artery wedge tracing. On the ECG, the QRS complex will precede the *v* wave of the pressure recording. Note that the QRS precedes both the *a* wave and the *v* wave because of delay in PAW pressure transmission (see Fig. 10-48).

Left Atrial Pressure

The LA pressure is rarely measured in the critical care setting. It is, however, measured in the cardiac catheterization laboratory. A special catheter, one which can be passed transseptally from the right atrium to the left atrium, is used. The LA pressure is shown in Figure 10-49.

WAVEFORM INTERPRETATION

The LA pressure tracing has the same characteristics as the PAW pressure tracing. It has an *a* wave and a *v* wave. The *a* wave corresponds with left atrial contraction, whereas the *v* wave corresponds with left atrial relaxation. A *c* wave is not generally seen on an LA pressure tracing; however, it may be seen as the *c* wave on the RA

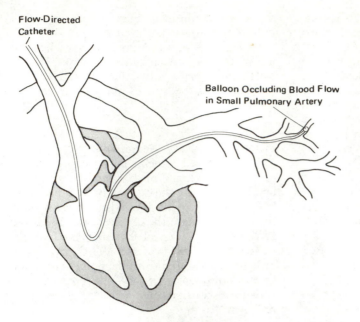

Flow-Directed Catheter

Balloon Occluding Blood Flow in Small Pulmonary Artery

FIGURE 10-47.
(Left) Diagram of catheter wedged in pulmonary capillary bed.

FIGURE 10-48.
(Bottom left) Pulmonary artery wedge pressure recording.

FIGURE 10-49.
(Bottom right) Left atrial pressure recording.

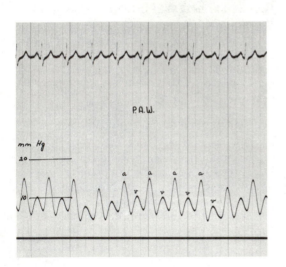

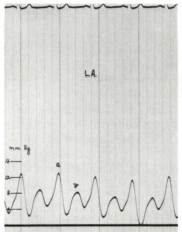

pressure tracing. Left atrial mean ($\overline{LA}$) pressure is < 12 torr.

COMPARISON OF ECG WITH WAVEFORM
The P wave precedes the *a* wave since the electrical events precede and cause the mechanical events; likewise, the QRS complex precedes the *v* wave.

Left Ventricular Pressure
The configuration of the LV pressure waveform is comparable to that of the right ventricular waveform. The significant difference is the pressure that each ventricle can generate. An LV pressure tracing appears in Figure 10-50.

WAVEFORM INTERPRETATION
Again, arbitrary letters have been assigned to various points in the waveform for ease of discussion. Interval *a* represents left ventricular isovolumetric contraction. As the pressure within the left ventricle exceeds the pressure in the aorta, the aortic valve is forced open, point *b*. Maximum ejection pressure is shown by *c*. The point at which the aortic valve closes, *d*, is followed by a rapid decrease in LV pressure. Open-

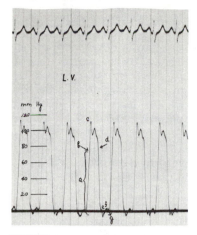

FIGURE 10-50.
Left ventricular pressure recording.

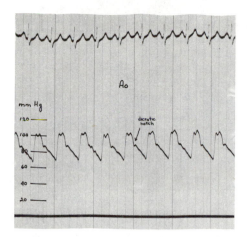

FIGURE 10-51.
Aortic pressure recording.

ing of the mitral valve, *e,* allows passive left ventricular filling; and *f* demonstrates the increases in LV pressure because of left atrial contraction. Point *g* represents LVEDP.

LVEDP is an indication of function. It is not customary to measure LV pressures directly; therefore, the flow–directed catheter is used. The value of this catheter lies in the following relationships (≈ means "is approximately equal to"):

$$PAd \approx \overline{PAW}$$
$$\overline{PAW} \approx \overline{LA}$$
$$\overline{LA} \approx LVEDP$$

The normal, significant LV pressures are systolic < 140 torr and end–diastolic < 12 torr.

COMPARISON OF ECG WITH WAVEFORM

Following atrial depolarization, P wave, the mitral valve opens, causing a slight increase in pressure, *e* on the pressure recording. Left atrial contraction, *f,* causes a second positive wave during ventricular diastole. The QRS complex precedes the systolic component of the left atrial waveform. As the ventricles repolarize, maximum LV pressure, *c,* is attained. The dicrotic notch represents aortic valve closure, *d,* and occurs at the end of repolarization.

Arterial Wave Pressure

Radial or femoral arteries are common sites for arterial lines. The arterial pressure waveform has the same configuration as that of the pulmonary artery. The primary difference is that the sys-

temic arteries support greater pressures than the pulmonary artery.

WAVEFORM INTERPRETATION

When LV systolic pressure exceeds Ao pressure, the aortic valve opens. On the arterial pressure tracing, this is the point at which the pressure rapidly rises. On the LV pressure tracing, it is point *b,* the end of isovolumetric contraction. The rapid rise in arterial pressure occurs after left ventricular ejection. An arterial line measuring pressure within the aorta will have a systolic pressure rise at the time of ventricular contraction; however, a line measuring radial artery pressure will have a delayed pressure rise because the artery is more distal to the left ventricle. Even though the line is in a distal artery, the dicrotic notch, which indicates aortic valve closure, can generally be seen (see Fig. 10-51). Arterial pressures are systolic < 140 torr, diastolic < 90 torr, and mean 70 to 90 torr.

COMPARISON OF ECG WITH WAVEFORM

The rapid rise in arterial pressure follows electrical depolarization of the ventricles, QRS complex. The more distal the artery is to the left ventricle, the greater the delay in systolic pressure rise. For instance, the time interval between the QRS complex and a radial artery pressure waveform will be greater than between the QRS complex and an Ao pressure tracing. The dicrotic notch occurs at the end of ventricular repolarization, T wave.

ABNORMAL PRESSURE VALUES

Before proceeding, the importance of understanding the normal mechanisms of hemodynamic pressures will be emphasized. In the previous discussion of normal pressures, the following components and pressures were identified as important:

Table 10-2
Significant Hemodynamic Pressures and Waveform Components

Chamber or Vessel	Significant Components of Waveform	Significant Pressure
RA	a wave	$\overline{RA}$ (< 6 torr)
	c wave	
	v wave	
RV	systole	RV systole (< 30 torr)
	end diastole	RVEDP (< 5 torr)
PA	systole	PA systole (< 30 torr)
	diastole	PA diastole (< 10 torr)
		$\overline{PA}$ (< 20 torr)
PAW	a wave	$\overline{PAW}$ (< 12 torr)
	v wave	
LA	a wave	$\overline{LA}$ (< 12 torr)
	v wave	
LV	systole	LV systole (< 140 torr)
	end diastole	LVEDP (< 12 torr)
Ao	systole	systole (< 140 torr)
	diastole	diastole (< 90 torr)
		$\overline{Ao}$ or MAP (70-90 torr)

A working knowledge of the normal hemodynamic pressures serves as the basis for identifying and interpreting abnormal pressures. A nurse with this knowledge will feel at ease with the systematic approach to waveform analysis and will automatically consider the following:

1. The mechanical events of the heart and the normal pressures
2. The characteristics of each waveform
3. The correlation between the electrical and mechanical events of the heart

From this the nurse will be able to

1. Identify the abnormal component(s).
2. Identify the mechanical events that cause and that affect the abnormal portion of the waveform.
3. Enumerate the possible physiological reasons.
4. Review the goals of treatment.
5. Evaluate the effectiveness of treatment.

It is not within the realm of this section to address steps 4 and 5, but they are mentioned here because they, too, are necessary steps for the nurse to take in order to assure sound clinical decisions. Steps 1 through 3 outline the approach used in this section to analyze abnormal hemodynamic pressures. Under the subheadings, the components of each waveform will be discussed. The process for determining abnormal pressures will be emphasized.

Right Atrial Waveform Abnormalities

Normal $\overline{RA}$ pressure is < 6 torr. $\overline{RA}$ pressure is equivalent to central venous pressure. A catheter in the right atrium reflects systemic venous pressure; in addition, it reflects pressures beyond the right atrial chamber. Problems that affect systemic venous resistance, pulmonary vascular resistance, tricuspid or pulmonary valves, or myocardial contraction or relaxation will be reflected by changes in $\overline{RA}$ pressure. Both increased vascular tone and hypervolemia elevate systemic venous pressure and, likewise, increase $\overline{RA}$ pressure, whereas loss of systemic venous tone and hypovolemia would decrease $\overline{RA}$ pressure. Pulmonary vascular resistance is increased in pulmonary hypertension, and as the right ventricle fails, the $\overline{RA}$ pressure would increase. Valvular problems, notably tricuspid stenosis and tricuspid insufficiency, elevate $\overline{RA}$ pressure. Problems that affect the ability of the myocardium to contract and relax include right heart failure, constrictive pericarditis, and pericardial tamponade, all of which elevate $\overline{RA}$ pressure.

a-WAVE CHANGES

On an RA pressure tracing, the *a* wave represents right atrial contraction and follows the P wave when compared with the ECG. The electrical impulse that causes atrial depolarization, the P wave on the ECG, initiates atrial contraction. In cardiac arrhythmias such as atrial fibrillation and junctional rhythms, there are no P waves, no organized atrial contraction, and therefore no *a* wave on a right atrial tracing.

When the right atrium must generate increased systolic pressure in order to eject blood into the right ventricle, the *a* wave would be elevated. In tricuspid stenosis, the right atrioventricular valve is narrowed, and the right atrium must contract with greater force to squeeze blood through the stenotic opening. Conditions beyond the right atrial chamber that cause increased pressure will be reflected in an elevated *a* wave. For instance, right ventricular hypertrophy causes the right ventricle to contract with greater force, which, in turn, causes the right atrial *a* wave to have a higher pressure than normal. Such conditions include pulmonary stenosis and pulmonary hypertension.

Pathologic conditions that cause changes in myocardial tissue itself or prevent the heart muscle from relaxing completely would elevate the ventricular filling pressure, and thus cause the *a* wave to be elevated. When fibrotic changes occur in the myocardium, as in constrictive pericarditis, the elevated RV diastolic pressure would be reflected in the RA pressure tracing by an elevated *a* wave.

Cardiac tamponade occurs when fluid collects under pressure in the cardiac sac between the visceral and parietal pericardium. With fluid filling this space, the heart muscle is restricted and prevented from filling normally. Fluid compressing the myocardium during ventricular diastole causes an elevated *a* wave on the RA pressure tracing. Severe cases of both constrictive pericarditis and pericardial tamponade cause pressure changes in all chambers of the heart. These two conditions elevate RA, LA, RVED, and LVED pressures.

v-WAVE CHANGES

The *v* wave on an RA pressure tracing corresponds with right atrial filling and right ventricular systole. It occurs after the T wave and precedes the P wave when compared with the ECG. On an RA tracing, the *v* wave will be elevated in conditions that cause an increase in RA filling pressure. For example, in tricuspid insufficiency, the tricuspid valve is incompetent. The valve remains open, when, under normal conditions, it should be closed. With the tricuspid valve open during right ventricular contraction, blood regurgitates from the right ventricle into the right atrium, causing an increased *v* wave.

c-WAVE CHANGES

A normal variant of the RA pressure tracing can demonstrate the absence of a *c* wave or a *c* wave superimposed on the *a* wave. Since the *c* wave occurs because of the ballooning of the closed tricuspid valve into the right atrium during right ventricle contraction, it is not seen in the pressure tracing of a patient with tricuspid insufficiency. No *c* wave is seen because the valve leaflets do not close and cannot bulge into the right atrium, causing a slight pressure increase.

Right Ventricular Waveform Abnormalities

Normal significant RV pressures are systolic < 30 torr and end-diastolic < 5 torr. Abnormal RV pressures are seen in right ventricular failure, pulmonary stenosis, pulmonary insufficiency, and pulmonary hypertension. Eventually, untreated left ventricular failure would cause RV pressures to be elevated; however, other signs and symptoms would be obvious to the nurse before the RV pressures become elevated.

RIGHT VENTRICULAR SYSTOLIC CHANGES

RV systolic pressures would be elevated in conditions that require greater force to eject the blood. For example, in pulmonary stenosis the right ventricle must generate enough pressure to overcome the resistance caused by the narrowed pulmonary valve. Pulmonary hypertension is a common cause of elevated RV systolic pressure and usually occurs because of left ventricular failure.

RIGHT VENTRICULAR END DIASTOLIC CHANGES

Under normal conditions the pulmonary valve is closed during right ventricular diastole. The right ventricle fills with blood only from the right atrial, and the RVEDP is < 5 torr. When the pulmonary valve is incompetent, blood regurgitates through the opened pulmonary cusps from the pulmonary artery into the right ventricle. In severe cases of pulmonary insufficiency, the additional blood volume because of regurgitant flow causes an elevated RVEDP.

RIGHT VENTRICULAR SYSTOLIC AND END-DIASTOLIC CHANGES

Initially, in right ventricular failure the right ventricular tracing would show a decreased systolic and an increased end-diastolic pressure. As the failure increases, systolic pressure would decrease, the body's compensatory mechanisms would fail, and cardiac output would decline. Thus, the RV systolic pressure may be low or within normal limits, but the end-diastolic pressure would remain elevated, indicating decreased right ventricular output because of reduced ventricular contractile force. In this situation, a larger volume of blood remains in the ventricle at the end of diastole.

Pulmonary hypertension elevates the RV systolic and end-diastolic pressures. The more severe the pulmonary hypertension, the greater the RV pressures. Eventually the right ventricle fails, at which point the pressures vary according to the pressure changes seen in right ventricular failure.

Pulmonary Artery Waveform Abnormalities

Normal PA pressure values are systolic < 30 torr, diastolic < 10 torr and mean < 20 torr. The pulmonary artery diastolic (PAd) pressure is an approximation of the mean pulmonary artery wedge ($\overline{PAW}$) pressure, which reflects mean left atrial ($\overline{LA}$) pressure, which indicates left ventricular function. For this reason, the PAd is the most significant PA pressure. The exception occurs in pulmonary hypertension, which causes elevated PA systolic, diastolic, and mean pressures but a normal PAW pressure. PA pressures are elevated in pulmonary vascular disease, mitral stenosis, and left ventricular failure.

PULMONARY ARTERY DIASTOLIC CHANGES

In the absence of pulmonary vascular disease, PAd pressures accurately reflect pressures in the left chambers of the heart. Conditions which require increased LA systolic pressures increase PA pressure values. For example, the LA systolic *a*-wave pressure would be elevated if the mitral valve were narrowed. This increase in LA *a*-wave pressure would be reflected in the pulmonary system. The PAd pressure would be abnormally high because the left atrium must contract with greater force to eject the blood through the stenotic mitral valve. Thus, in mitral stenosis, the PAd pressure would be elevated. In the presence of mitral stenosis, a simultaneous PA and LV pressure tracing would demonstrate a pressure difference between the PAd and the LVEDP. Recall the following:

$$PAd \approx \overline{PAW}$$
$$\overline{PAW} \approx \overline{LA}$$
$$\overline{LA} \approx LVEDP$$

Normally, none of these pressures vary more than 1 to 3 torr. When the difference among these pressures is > 1 to 3 torr, pathology exists.

PULMONARY ARTERY SYSTOLIC AND DIASTOLIC CHANGES

Left ventricular failure is reflected in the pulmonary artery tracing by an elevation of all pressures. Early in left ventricular failure, the loss of left ventricular compliance causes the LVEDP to be elevated. The heart rate increases in an attempt to compensate for the decreased force of left ventricular contraction. With the increase in heart rate, diastole is shortened and there is less time for ventricular filling. With decreased ventricular filling time and loss of compliance, the blood volume ejected from the left ventricle is less, and cardiac output falls. LV systolic pressure decreases as the left ventricular compliance decreases. Concurrently, the LVEDP increases because of the increased blood volume remaining in the ventricle. This cycle is reflected in the pulmonary artery, and eventually causes the PA pressures to be elevated.

Pulmonary Artery Wedge Abnormalities

PAW pressure is < 12 torr. It reflects left ventricular function. The catheter is wedged in the pulmonary capillary bed, pressures from the right heart are blocked, and only pressures forward to the catheter are sensed. PAW pressures are elevated in mitral stenosis, mitral insufficiency, and left ventricular failure. When aortic stenosis and aortic insufficiency are severe, the elevated LV pressures are also reflected in the pulmonary artery wedge tracing.

a-WAVE CHANGES

The *a* wave of the pulmonary artery wedge tracing corresponds with left atrial systole and will therefore be elevated in conditions that elevate LA systolic pressure. LA systolic pressure is elevated in mitral stenosis. This increase in LA systolic pressure will cause the *a* wave of the PAW pressure to be elevated.

v-WAVE CHANGES

The *v* wave on the PAW pressure tracing reflects left atrial filling and left ventricular contraction. Conditions that cause the LA diastolic pressure to be elevated will cause the PAW *v* wave to be elevated. In mitral regurgitation, the LA diastolic pressure is increased because of blood regurgitation from the left ventricle, through the incompetent mitral leaflets. This additional volume of blood in the left atrium during left atrial relaxation elevates the *v* wave on the pulmonary artery wedge tracing.

a-WAVE AND *v*-WAVE CHANGES

Both *a* waves and *v* waves will be elevated on the pulmonary artery wedge tracing in left ventricular failure. The myocardium loses elasticity, compliance, and its ability to contract. In early left ventricular failure, the LVEDP is elevated. The heart rate increases to compensate for the decreased force of contraction. Diastole is shortened, less blood is ejected, more blood remains in the ventricle, and the LVEDP increases. An elevated *a* wave on the PAW tracing reflects this increase in pressure. The *v* wave pressure would likewise increase, reflecting the increase in LV pressure. The $\overline{PAW}$ pressure is elevated since it is an approximation of the LVEDP.

The abnormal pressures discussed heretofore are pressures with which the critical care nurse will become familiar. These pressure abnormalities were discussed in detail so that the nurse will have the understanding necessary to make sound clinical judgments in caring for the patients who require invasive monitoring. The following abnormal pressure tracings are ones commonly seen in the cardiac catheterization laboratory rather than the critical care setting.

Left Atrial Waveform Abnormalities

Mean LA pressure is < 12 torr. The *a* waves and *v* waves of the LA pressure tracing are elevated in the same pathologic conditions that cause the pulmonary artery wedge waveforms to be elevated. Since they are elevated for the same reasons that were previously discussed, the rationale will not be reiterated.

Left Ventricular and Aortic Waveform Abnormalities

The LV and Ao pressures will be discussed together because most frequently the pressures are measured simultaneously. Normal LV pressures are systolic < 140 torr and end-diastolic < 12 torr. Normal Ao pressures are systolic < 140 torr, diastolic < 90 torr, and mean 70 to 90 torr. LV and Ao systolic pressures are equal. Differences between these pressures indicate a gradient across the aortic valve and demonstrate pathology. The diagnosis of aortic valvular problems is made by a composite patient examination that includes palpation, auscultation, phonocardiogram, and catheterization.

Left Ventricular and Aortic Systolic Pressure Differences

In the presence of aortic stenosis, the left ventricle must contract with greater force to overcome resistance caused by the narrowed orifice. LV systolic pressure would be elevated; however, Ao systolic pressure would be within normal limits. The millimeters of mercury pressure difference between these two systolic values demonstrates the pressure gradient across the aortic valve. As the degree of stenosis increases, the left ventricle would require increasing pressure in order to eject blood out the aortic valve and maintain cardiac output. A simultaneous LV and Ao pressure tracing would demonstrate (1) systolic pressure differences between the left ventricle and aorta, and (2) a slowly rising initial aortic systolic upstroke. The obstructed aortic valve prevents the normal rapid ejection of blood from the left ventricle into the aorta causing the delayed pressure rise. Study the pressure tracing shown in Figure 10-52.

Left Ventricular and Aortic Diastolic Pressure Changes

In aortic insufficiency, blood regurgitates from the aorta into the left ventricle during diastole, which elevates the LVEDP. As the aortic valve deteriorates, the Ao diastolic pressure decreases, which increases the pulse pressure. The characteristics of aortic insufficiency on a simultaneous LV and Ao pressure tracing are the following: (1) an elevated LVEDP, (2) a pulse pressure < 100 torr and (3) no dicrotic notch on the Ao pressure waveform. Since the dicrotic notch is caused by aortic valve closure, which does not occur in aortic regurgitation, no dicrotic notch is seen. Study the pressure tracing shown in Figure 10-53.

Nonphysiological Waveform Changes

When changes occur in waveform configurations, one way to identify the problem is to consider possible causes. Begin by checking with the patient to ascertain if the problem is with the hardware. Once you have confirmed no patient change in status, start the equipment check: Are the electrical plugs secure in the outlet? Is the power on? If you find no problem, proceed to the transducer. The transducer needs to be covered with fluid; air cannot be in the dome of the transducer. All connections must be secure. Stopcocks connecting lines must be turned correctly to (1) zero and calibrate the transducer, (2) measure patient pressures, and (3) aspirate blood samples. Continue the problem identification search until the cause is found. Then proceed with the problem-solving process.

A waveform which becomes flattened is said to be damped. Figure 10-54 shows a damped waveform.

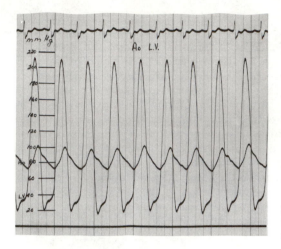

FIGURE 10-52.
Simultaneous aortic and left ventricular pressure recordings from patient with aortic stenosis.

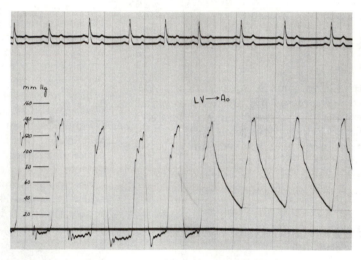

FIGURE 10-53.
Left ventricular pressure recording with catheter pull-back to aorta in patient with aortic insufficiency. Note that the LVEDP is not elevated in this patient at rest.

Damped waveforms occur when there is air in the fluid line, when intravenous flow rate decreases and blood stasis occurs, when a fibrin clot is at the catheter tip, or when the catheter adheres to the vessel wall. A damped waveform indicates that air needs to be evacuated from the line, that the line needs to be flushed with heparinized saline, or that the line tip needs to be rotated or moved slightly. To flush the line, use the pressure valve or a bolus of 10 ml heparinized saline.

The flow-directed catheter can become wedged in the pulmonary capillary bed by (1) inflating the balloon or (2) advancing the catheter into the pulmonary artery. When the catheter goes from the pulmonary artery into the pulmonary artery wedge position, the waveform on the oscilloscope will change and appear as shown in Figure 10-55.

Noting a tracing such as in Figure 10-55 or seeing a pulmonary artery wedge waveform on the oscilloscope, the nurse would first consider that the catheter balloon may be inflated and second, that the catheter tip may have floated into the wedge position. Pulmonary infarction has occurred when the flow-directed catheter was unintentionally in the wedge position. Because of this danger, the catheter balloon must be deflated or the catheter must be withdrawn into the pulmonary artery immediately.

Occasionally, the Swan-Ganz catheter floats from the pulmonary artery to the right ventricle. The pattern on the oscilloscope would change from the pulmonary artery to the right ventricular waveform as shown in Figure 10-56.

To correct this situation, inflate the balloon with air and allow the catheter to float from the right ventricle into the pulmonary artery.

The pressure tracing shown in Figure 10-57 demonstrates catheter fling.

Catheter fling is caused when the catheter can move laterally in the vessel. It produces spiked

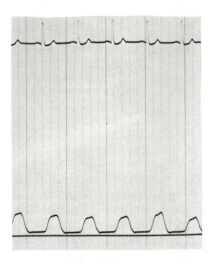

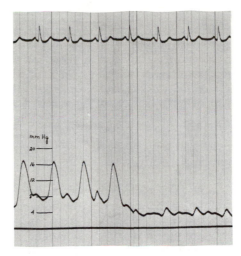

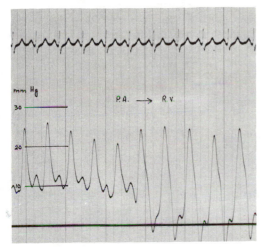

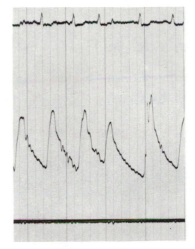

FIGURE 10-54.
(Top left) Damped pressure waveform.

FIGURE 10-55.
(Top right) Pulmonary artery and pulmonary artery wedge pressure recording.

FIGURE 10-56.
(Bottom left) Pulmonary artery pressure recording with catheter pull-back to right ventricle.

FIGURE 10-57.
(Bottom right) Aortic pressure recording demonstrating catheter fling.

waves, distorting the waveform configuration and pressure values. To remedy the problem, add IV extension tubing between the patient line and the pressure valve.

NURSING CONSIDERATIONS

The Nurse-Patient Relationship

The nurse who desires to care for the patient requiring hemodynamic pressure monitoring must know normal physiology, normal pressure values, the reasons for abnormal pressures, and problem-solving procedures. It is essential to be at ease with the technical and theoretic components of invasive monitoring in order to work with each patient as an individual and to establish a therapeutic nurse-patient relationship.

Nurses have the responsibility to create an environment in which the patient is free to ask questions, express concerns, participate in patient care and decision making, and relate to family and friends. Some patients requiring invasive monitoring are severely weakened by their cardiac problem, whereas others are stronger and more troubled by the activity restriction imposed because of the lines. These patients have individual concerns, but they also have common concerns and potential problems that the nurse can alleviate, prevent, or correct.

Patient fear and anxiety are allayed by the nurse who is confident in knowledge, skill, and problem-solving abilities. This nurse is free to listen to the patient's fears and concerns and to watch for nonverbal cues which need to be clarified. A caring attitude includes an explanation of the routines and reasons for them. Family members should be included in this education process. Both patient and family members need to realize that the nurse cares for the patient as a whole individual and that the technical equipment assists the nurse in monitoring parameters necessary for optimal care.

Prevention of Problems

Circulation and Exercise. Patients need instruction to exercise the extremities where the lines are inserted. Exercising the fingers and toes

and contracting and relaxing arm and leg muscles will promote circulation in the extremity. Most patients requiring invasive monitoring have compromised circulation. Inactivity further adds to this problem. Patients unable to exercise extremities need to have routine passive exercises done for them.

Catheter Care. The presence of a catheter in a vessel increases the likelihood of inflammation, leading to the development of *phlebitis*. The catheter site should be looked at several times daily for early signs of inflammation, such as tenderness, changes in local temperature, redness, and swelling. The dressing should be changed every 8 hours; the insertion site is cleansed with soap and water, and antiseptic ointment, sponges, and tape are applied in a secure but comfortable manner. The previously pictured method for securing the lines and transducers on a short armboard recommended for patient safety and nurse convenience is shown again in Figure 10-58.

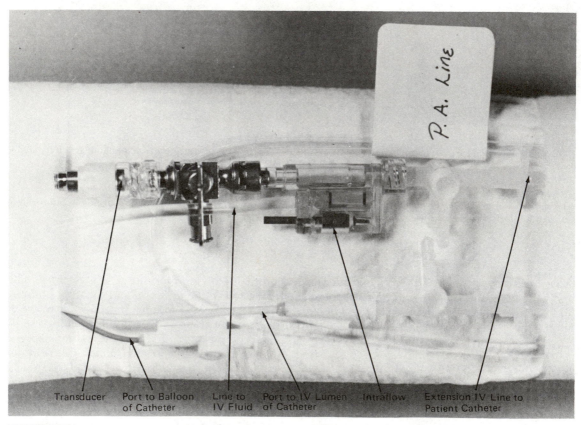

FIGURE 10-58.
Pressure lines mounted on armboard.

Deep Breathing. Individuals confined to bed rest for several days need to consciously take slow, deep breaths, using their abdominal muscles. Reminding the patient to breathe in this manner ten times an hour while awake will expand the alveoli and prevent atelectasis. Although pressures are generally recorded with the patient in the supine position, he should be encouraged to rest on either side between pressure readings.

Pressure is an essential concept for the critical care nurse to understand because it affects all body systems. Along with basic knowledge of the body systems, the critical care nurse must possess a questioning mind and a caring spirit. An inquisitive nurse will formulate questions in a methodic, scientific manner, seek answers, and find new questions. The analytic approach to patient care fosters improved patient care. The critical care nurse is well named because a caring spirit makes the nurse's efforts complete by combining the science and art of nursing intervention.

Shirley J. Hoffman

DIRECT CARDIAC OUTPUT MEASUREMENT

Cardiac output refers to the amount of blood that is pumped out of the heart and is expressed in liters per minute. It is a function of stroke volume and heart rate. Flow is determined by the ratio of pressure to resistance; thus, cardiac output is determined by the ratio of mean arterial pressure to total peripheral resistance.

Any condition that causes uncompensated changes in arterial pressure or peripheral resistance will cause a change in cardiac output. Since many disease states, as well as their modes of therapy, affect arterial pressure, peripheral resistance, and cardiac output, it is often important that the critically ill patient's cardiac output be measured in order to provide optimal medical and nursing care.

Normal Cardiac Output and Cardiac Index

Normal cardiac output at rest is considered 4 to 7 liters per minute; however, actual cardiac output is related to body size. The cardiac index is a more realistic guide for evaluating the cardiac output of any one individual. The cardiac index is obtained by dividing cardiac output by the body surface area. Body surface area can be determined by using the Dubois body surface chart (see Fig. 10-59). A straight line drawn between the patient's height in the left-hand column and his weight in the right-hand column will cross the number in the middle column that represents his body surface area in square meters. Normal cardiac index is 2.5 to 4 liters per minute per square meter.

Low Cardiac Output

Many disease states may decrease the pumping effectiveness of the left ventricle, resulting in a decrease in the pressure generated within the ventricle. This in turn will cause the cardiac output to fall. Myocardial infarction is the most common cause of compromised pumping ability of the left ventricle. Other causes include valvular heart disease, congestive heart failure, myocarditis, cardiac tamponade, and some congenital anomalies. In monitoring therapy in patients who are critically ill because of these disease states, cardiac output determinations, in conjunction with various intracardiac and pulmonary pressure measurements, can be very helpful.

Venous return to the right side of the heart is a major factor in determining cardiac output. The heart can pump out only the volume presented to it. If inadequate blood volume is present, the cardiac output must, of necessity, fall. In the critical care unit, low cardiac output because of decreased venous return is commonly caused by severe hemorrhage and dehydration.

It must be remembered that any patient who receives mechanical ventilation with positive pressure breathing may have a decreased cardiac output because of increased intrathoracic pressure and decreased venous return. In the patient with acute respiratory distress syndrome who is being treated with positive end-expiratory pressure (PEEP), cardiac output monitoring may help determine the level of PEEP that will pro-

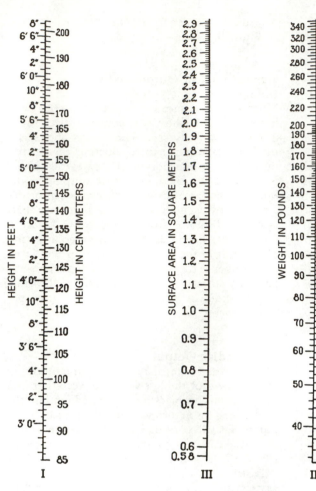

FIGURE 10-59.
Dubois body surface chart (as prepared by Boothby and Sandiford of the Mayo Clinic). To find body surface of a patient, locate the height in inches (or centimeters) on scale I and the weight in pounds (or kilograms) on scale II and place a straight edge (ruler) between these two points which will intersect scale III at the patient's surface area.

duce the optimum pO_2 with minimal decrease in cardiac output.

High Cardiac Output

Normally the cardiac output increases with exercise as a result of increased oxygen consumption at the cellular level. The trained athlete may raise his cardiac output to several times normal during strenuous exercise. Stimulation of the sympathetic nervous system will also increase cardiac output by increasing heart rate and the contractile force of the left ventricle.

In the critical care unit, septic shock is one of the causes of abnormally high cardiac output. This occurs because of massive vasodilation, probably from the toxic substances produced by sepsis, thus decreasing peripheral resistance. The cardiac output in septic shock may increase to three or four times normal.

The thiamine deficiency associated with beriberi may also cause vasodilation and high cardiac output.

Because of their effects on peripheral resistance, many of the potent antihypertensive drugs used in the critical care unit should be titrated by monitoring the pressures obtained from a Swan-Ganz catheter and cardiac output determinations.

A high rate of metabolism, such as is found in thyrotoxicosis, fever, and in certain tumors, may also cause an increase in cardiac output because of increased oxygen consumption.

Measurement of Cardiac Output

METHODS

The Fick method of measuring cardiac output involves determining the difference in oxygen concentration of mixed venous blood and arterial blood and measuring oxygen consumption in the lungs. The cardiac output is then calculated from a formula. The indicator dilution method is accomplished by injecting dye into a large vein or into the right side of the heart, obtaining a time-concentration curve from peripheral artery sampling, and calculating cardiac output. Neither of these methods is feasible in the clinical setting.

With the advent of the four-lumen Swan-Ganz thermodilution catheter and cardiac output computers, it is now a relatively simple procedure for the critical care nurse to measure cardiac output at the patient's bedside. The thermodilution method is similar to the indicator dilution method. When thermodilution is used, the indicator is cold solution injected into the right atrium, and the sampling device is a thermistor near the end of the catheter in the pulmonary artery (see Fig. 10-60). The thermistor continuously measures the temperature of the blood flowing past it. The catheter is connected to a cardiac output computer that computes the cardiac output from the time-temperature curve resulting from the rate of change in temperature of the blood that flows past the thermistor. Because of the number of variables inherent in the procedure, an average of several consecutive cardiac output determinations will assure greater accuracy.

INITIAL CONSIDERATIONS

It is important for the critical care nurse to eliminate as many potential sources of error as possible in order to obtain an accurate cardiac output. The procedure should be done at a time when the patient is in a quiet, steady state. Agitation increases the cardiac output, and the measurement will not be meaningful relative to the resting output or those obtained during various degrees of agitation. It is felt by some that respiratory variations may cause changes in the temperature of the blood in the pulmonary circulation and thus render the cardiac output measurement something less than accurate. This possible source of error may be avoided if the determination is done when the patient is breathing quietly.

The *Swan-Ganz thermodilution catheter* should be checked for proper functioning before beginning the procedure (see Fig. 10-61). If the proximal lumen of the catheter is not fully patent, the cardiac output measurement will be inaccurate. The proximal lumen should be flushed before injecting the cold solution. If the proximal lumen is being used for the administration of intravenous medications, slow flushing before injection will also preclude the administration of a bolus of the infusing medication.

The *thermistry circuit* in the catheter and the

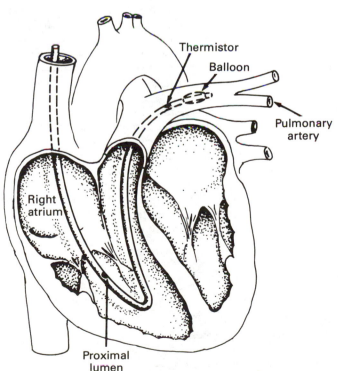

FIGURE 10-60.
Swan-Ganz thermodilution catheter in place.

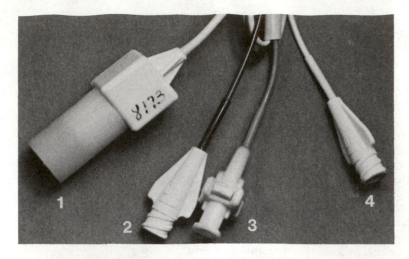

FIGURE 10-61.
Entry sites for the four lumens of the Swan-Ganz thermodilution catheter. *1.* Thermistor. *2.* Proximal (right atrium). *3.* Balloon inflation. *4.* Distal (pulmonary artery).

cardiac output computer should be checked for proper functioning before each set of cardiac outputs is determined. This requires connection of the catheter thermistry circuit to the computer cable. Care must be taken to avoid damaging or breaking the relatively fragile connector mechanism. Follow the directions in the cardiac output computer operator's manual for checking the catheter and computer. This should also be done at any time a cardiac output determination that does not correlate with the patient's clinical condition is obtained.

The *computation constant* should be checked and set on the cardiac output computer to reflect the volume and temperature of the injectate being used. This number also takes into account catheter size and the rise in temperature of the injectate as it is being injected through the catheter. A table of computation constants will be found in the cardiac output computer operator's manual.

INJECTATE

The injectate solution used for the procedure is usually sterile 5% dextrose in water, although sterile normal saline may be used. Either 5 or 10 ml may be used, although 10 ml allows for more accuracy in the cardiac output determination.

Either glass or plastic Luer-Lok syringes may be used; "control" syringes, which have two finger rings attached to the barrel and a thumb ring at the end of the plunger, facilitate the speed of injection and also allow for holding the syringe without handling the barrel (see Fig. 10-62).

The injectate can be used at room temperature, but optimum accuracy is attained at 0° to 4°C. The injectate can be cooled by a variety of methods. Electrical coolers manufactured for this purpose are available. An ice bath may also be used, and alcohol may be added to the ice bath for faster cooling. (One should take care when using an electric cooling plate or when adding alcohol to the ice bath that the solution in the syringes does not freeze.) Refrigeration of the injectate solution will also allow for faster cooling.

Each syringe should be filled with sterile injectate and the sterile cap replaced over the tip of the syringe. The syringes can be placed in a container that is then immersed in the ice bath, or placed directly into the cooler.

An extra syringe must be filled with the same amount of injectate, the sterile cap replaced, and the plunger removed from the barrel. This syringe is placed in the container with the other

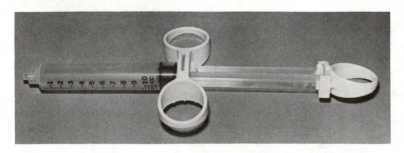

FIGURE 10-62.
"Control" syringe.

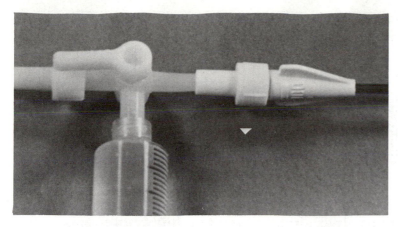

FIGURE 10-63.
Attachment of injectate syringe to three-way stopcock between proximal lumen of Swan-Ganz thermodilution catheter on right and intravenous tubing on left. Handle on stopcock points to "off."

syringes, and the injectate temperature probe is placed into the solution in this syringe. The probe is connected to the computer, which measures the temperature of the injectate. All the syringes, including the one containing the temperature probe, should be filled from the same container of solution to ensure that the initial temperature of the injectate in each is the same. Since the temperature of the solution actually being injected is not measured, the solution in which the temperature *is* being measured should simulate the injectate as closely as possible. The assumption is that the temperature of the solution in all the syringes is the same.

After the cardiac output determinations have been made, it is helpful to fill a new set of syringes to cool in preparation for the next set of determinations. Be certain to replace the temperature probe syringe along with the injectate syringes, since they must all have the same initial temperature.

INJECTION

When the injectate solution has cooled to 0° to 4°C as indicated by the cardiac output computer, injection can be accomplished with optimum accuracy. Because significant warming of the injectate can result from holding the syringe in the hand, the syringe should be handled using the finger and thumb rings, avoiding contact of the hands with the syringe barrel. Make certain that the syringe has been filled to the *exact* volume indicated by the computation constant used, usually 10 ml. Use of inaccurately measured injectate volume will result in inaccurate cardiac output measurements. Follow the cardiac output computer manufacturer's directions in operating the computer.

Attach the injectate syringe to the proximal lumen of the Swan-Ganz catheter. A three-way stopcock between the proximal lumen and intra-

venous tubing allows maintenance of a closed system and facilitates rapid attachment of the syringe (see Fig. 10-63). Inject the solution into the proximal line at the time the computer indicates readiness. Injection should be accomplished during the end-expiratory phase of the respiratory cycle to minimize the effects of blood temperature variations from respirations. Injection time for 10 ml of solution should be 4 seconds or less. The elapsed time from removal of syringe from the cooling mechanism until injection should be as short as possible to avoid environmental warming of the injectate.

The cardiac rhythm should be observed immediately after injection because the sudden bolus of cold solution into the right atrium may precipitate atrial or ventricular arrhythmias. The pulmonary artery pressure waveform should also be observed after injection for migration of the catheter into the wedge position or retrograde into the right ventricle. Remove and discard the empty syringe after injection.

Measurements may be repeated when the computer signifies readiness. Disconnect the catheter thermistry circuit from the computer cable after the entire procedure is completed. Replace the protective cap over the end of the thermistry circuit "tail" of the Swan-Ganz catheter.

Some cardiac output computers are equipped with strip chart recorders, so that the thermodilution curve can be observed and recorded. The curve should have a smooth upstroke, peak, and smooth downstroke. If the curve is distorted because of poor injection technique or improper catheter positioning, that cardiac output measurement should be rejected (see Fig. 10-64).

AVERAGING CARDIAC OUTPUTS

The average of several cardiac outputs is more accurate than using one isolated determination

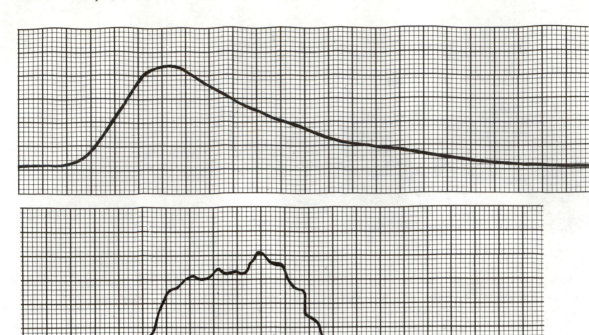

FIGURE 10-64.
Examples of accurate and distorted thermodilution curves as produced on strip chart recorder. *(A)* Smooth recording is accurate. *(B)* Irregular recording is distorted.

because of the number of possible variables in the patient and procedure performance. Four consecutive determinations should be obtained if possible. If one measurement is unduly high or low relative to the others in the series, it should be discarded as inaccurate. To assure optimum accuracy, the measurements should be within 0.5 liter per minute of each other. The remaining determinations are then averaged for the measurement to be recorded in the patient's chart. Calculate the cardiac index as described earlier and also record this in the chart.

Electrical Safety

An electrically safe environment must be maintained at all times for the critical care patient. This is especially important when cardiac output determinations are being made by the Swan-Ganz catheter, which traverses the heart.

The following guidelines should be used to maintain electrical safety for the patient with a Swan-Ganz thermodilution catheter:

- The patient should be in a nonelectric bed. If an electric bed must be used, it should be unplugged from the wall outlet.
- Bed linens should be changed immediately when wet.
- The amount of electrical equipment in the immediate environment should be minimal and, when required for patient care, properly grounded.
- Cardiac output computer cable should be inspected for continuity before use.
- Protective cap should be in place over thermistry tail on catheter when not in use.
- Catheter should not be connected to computer cable during insertion procedure.
- Computer should be on battery power, not AC power, when connected to catheter.
- Electrical cooler should be disconnected from wall outlet or temperature probe removed from cooler while catheter is connected to computer cable.
- Personnel handling catheter should not be in simultaneous contact with any other electrical equipment.

- Computer and cable should be kept dry and clean.
- Computer should not be operated in the presence of explosive anesthetic agents.

Evaluation of Cardiac Output and Cardiac Index

The cardiac output and index should always be evaluated in conjunction with other assessed parameters and the clinical status of the patient. For example, one would expect the patient in cardiogenic shock to have a low cardiac output and cardiac index and high pulmonary capillary wedge (PCW) and pulmonary artery diastolic (PAd) pressures. With improvement in the patient's clinical status, the cardiac output and index should rise, and the PCW and PAd pressures should decrease. If one of the above measurements does not reflect the trend of the others and the patient's clinical status, then the nurse should suspect an error in technique or equipment malfunction and begin troubleshooting or repeating measurements. One of the reasons for determining multiple hemodynamic measurements is to use each determination to verify the others.

The gamut of measured hemodynamic parameters can be used to calculate other parameters that cannot be measured directly. Calculators that can be programmed to calculate such information as stroke volume, right and left ventricular stroke work, and systemic and pulmonary vascular resistance from measured parameters are now available. Systemic vascular resistance can be hand-calculated as follows:

$$\frac{(\text{mean arterial pressure} - \text{PCW}) \times 80}{\text{cardiac output}}$$

The patient who has a low mean arterial pressure (MAP), high cardiac index, and low systemic vascular resistance (such as seen in septic shock) may best be treated with additional circulatory volume and vasoconstrictor therapy. The patient who has cardiogenic shock may demonstrate a low MAP, low cardiac index, and high systemic vascular resistance because of maximal vasoconstriction and may best be treated with circulating volume, vasodilator therapy, and inotropic agents.

In the patient with acute myocardial infarction, cardiac outputs can be evaluated in conjunction with changes in PCW pressures. By relating these two measurements, it may be possible to modify therapy to obtain a PCW pressure that will result in optimal cardiac output and arterial pressure for that patient.

It is obvious that these hemodynamic parameters can be very useful in assessing the efficacy of vasodilators, vasoconstrictors, additional volume, diuretics, and inotropic agents.

It is important that the critical care nurse be adept at setting up, maintaining, and troubleshooting all types of hemodynamic and cardiac monitoring equipment in the critical care unit. Measurements of the various parameters must be made with accuracy and evaluated in conjunction with one another and with the patient's clinical status. Appropriate use of these determinations will aid in medical diagnosis, choice of therapy, monitoring of therapy, and anticipation of prognosis. The ultimate goal in the use of these hemodynamic parameters is the reduction of morbidity and mortality in critically ill patients.

BIBLIOGRAPHY

Buchbinder N, Ganz W: Hemodynamic monitoring: Invasive techniques. Anesthesiology 45, No. 2:146–155, 1976

Davies H, Nelson WP: Understanding Cardiology. Boston, Butterworths, 1978

Editorial: Swan-Ganz catheters, Lancet 2, No. 8085: 357–358, 1978

Forrester JS et al: Medical therapy of acute myocardial infarction. Reprint from N Engl J Med 295:1356–1362, 1404–1413, 1976

Guyton AC: Basic Human Physiology: Normal Function and Mechanisms of Disease. Philadelphia, W. B. Saunders, 1977

Hathaway R: The Swan-Ganz catheter: A review. Nurs Clin North Am 13, No. 3:389–407, 1978

Kaplan JA: Hemodynamic Monitoring and Ischemic Heart Disease. Edwards Laboratories, Div. of American Hospital Supply Corp, October 1979

Levett, JM, Replogle RL: Current research review: Thermodilution cardiac output: A critical analysis and review of the literature. J Surg Res 27:392–404, 1979

O'Connor L: Hemodynamic Monitoring and Cardiovascular Medicine. Edwards Laboratories, Div. of American Hospital Supply Corp, November 1979

Schroeder J, Daily E: Techniques in Bedside Hemodynamic Monitoring. St. Louis, C. V. Mosby, 1976

Shapiro B, Harrison R, Trout C: Clinical Application of Respiratory Care. Chicago, Year Book Medical Publishers, 1975

Understanding Hemodynamic Measurements Made with the Swan-Ganz Catheter. Edwards Laboratories, Div. of American Hospital Supply Corp, May 1978

Section B   Respiratory System

Barbara Fuller

Normal Structure and Function of the Respiratory System 11

Oxygen is required for the complete catabolism of chemicals that occurs in the production of cellular energy. Although some energy can be stored, cells differ in the amount of energy they can store. Neurons, for example, are thought to have less capacity to store energy than skeletal muscle cells. Also, the amount of energy stored can fuel cell activities for only a short time. Neuronal energy storage and the duration of cell life it will support is reflected by the limited time available in which cardiopulmonary resuscitation can be started.

Catabolic energy-producing reactions produce carbon dioxide. High levels of this waste product can seriously impair cell function. Thus, there is a critical need for providing oxygen to body cells and at the same time removing carbon dioxide from the body. Strictly defined, *resuscitation* is the exchange and transport of oxygen and carbon dioxide between cells (of the body) and the external environment (atmosphere).

Accomplishing this in vertebrates (including humans) involves both the respiratory and the cardiovascular systems: the former to provide exchange of these gases between atmosphere and blood, the latter to transport these gases to and from the cells of the body. At times it is difficult to establish priorities between these two systems; it is better to consider them as being equally critical to the dynamic stability of the human body.

In this chapter, we shall examine four general phases or areas of respiration in the following order:

1. Pulmonary ventilation—actual flow of air in and out between the atmosphere and the alveoli of the lung
2. Exchange of oxygen and carbon dioxide between the alveoli and the blood
3. Transport of oxygen and carbon dioxide in the blood and body fluids to and from the cells
4. Regulation of ventilation by control mechanisms of the body with regard to rate, rhythm, and depth

VENTILATION

Mechanics of Respiration

The downward and upward movement of the diaphragm, which lengthens and shortens the chest cavity, combined with the elevation and depression of the ribs, which increases and decreases the anteroposterior diameter of the cavity, causes the expansion and contraction of the lungs. It is estimated that about 70% of the expansion and contraction of the lungs is accomplished by the change in anteroposterior measurement and about 30% by the change in length due to movement of the diaphragm.

Respiratory Pressures

The lungs—two air-filled spongy structures—are attached to the body only at their hila. Thus the outer surfaces have no attachment. However, the membrane lining the interpleural space constantly absorbs fluid or gas that enters this area, thereby creating a partial vacuum. This phenomenon holds the visceral pleura of the lungs tightly against the parietal pleura of the chest wall.

As the volume of the chest cavity is increased by the muscles of inspiration, the lungs also enlarge; as it is decreased during expiration, the lungs in turn become smaller. The two pleurae slide over each other with each inspiration and expiration, lubricated by the few millimeters of tissue fluid-containing proteins in the intrapleural space.

With each normal inspiration, the pressure within the alveolar sacs, the intra-alveolar pressure, becomes slightly negative (−3 torr) with regard to the atmosphere. This slightly negative pressure sucks air into the alveolar sacs through the respiratory passage.

During normal expiration and resultant compression of the lungs, the intra-alveolar pressure builds to about +3 torr and forces air out of the respiratory passages. During maximum respiratory efforts, the intra-alveolar pressure can vary from −80 torr during inspiration to +100 torr during expiration.

The lungs continually tend to collapse. Two factors are responsible for this phenomenon. First, there are many elastic fibers contained within the lung tissue itself that are constantly attempting to shorten. The second and more important factor contributing to this tendency to collapse is the high surface tension of the fluid lining the alveoli. A lipoprotein substance called *surfactant,* which is constantly secreted by the epithelial alveolar lining, decreases the surface tension of the fluids of the respiratory passages 7- to 14-fold. The lack of the ability to secrete surfactant in the newborn is called *hyaline membrane disease* or *respiratory distress syndrome.*

No single factor or phenomenon is responsible for the body's ability to maintain inflated functional lungs; rather, it is the combination of all of these factors.

Compliance and Respiratory "Work"

As can be seen from the preceding discussion, both the lungs and the thorax itself have elastic characteristics and thus exhibit expansibility. This expansibility is called *compliance* and is expressed as the volume increase in the lung for each unit increase in intra-alveolar pressure. Normal total pulmonary compliance, that is, both lungs and thorax, is 0.13 liter per centimeter of water pressure. Or, in other words, every time alveolar pressure is increased by an amount necessary to raise a column of water 1 cm in height, the lungs expand 130 ml in volume.

Conditions or situations that destroy lung tissue, cause it to become fibrotic, produce pulmonary edema, block alveoli, or in any way impede lung expansion and expansibility of the thoracic cage reduce pulmonary compliance and decrease the efficiency of meeting the need for oxygen to carry on the necessary functional activities of the total organism.

It is extremely important to emphasize that when the lungs are expanded and contracted through the action of the respiratory muscles, energy is required for the muscular activity involved.

In addition to this work, energy is also required to overcome two other factors that tend to prevent expansion of the lungs: (1) nonelastic tissue resistance, and (2) airway resistance, meaning that energy is required to rearrange the large molecules of viscous tissues of the lung itself so that they slip past one another during respiratory movements. In the presence of tissue edema, the lungs lose many of their elastic qualities, and increased viscosity of the tissues and fluids increases the nonelastic resistance. Thus the work of breathing is increased, and the energy expended to accomplish the task is also greatly increased.

Under normal conditions, the airway resistance is low, and the amount of energy required to move air along the passages is only slight. When the airway becomes obstructed, such as in obstructive emphysema, asthma, or diphtheria, then airway resistance is greatly increased, and the energy required simply to move air in and out is greatly increased.

Ventilatory Function Tests

Ventilatory function tests can be subdivided into tests to measure static values and capacities and tests to measure dynamic values and capacities. These measurements will be influenced by exercise and disease. Age, sex, body size, and posture, when measured, are other variables that are taken into consideration when the test results are interpreted. Static values for females are usually 25% less than those for males.

STATIC MEASUREMENTS

There are eight static measurements: four volumes and four capacities.

- *Tidal volume* (V_T) is the volume of air moved in and out with each normal respiration and measures about 500 ml in normal young males.
- *Inspiratory reserve volume (IRV)* represents forced inspiration over and beyond V_T, amounting to about 3000 ml.
- *Expiratory reserve volume (ERV)* is the volume of a forced expiration following the normal tidal expiration and amounts to about 1100 ml.
- *Residual volume (RV)* is the volume of air remaining following forced expiration. This volume can be measured only by indirect spirometry while the others can be measured directly.

When one studies the actual moment-to-moment events of the pulmonary cycle, it is sometimes more convenient to consider some volumes in combination with others. These various combinations are known as the four pulmonary capacities:

- *Inspiratory capacity (IC)* is equal to the V_T plus the IRV. This is about 3500 ml and is that amount of air which, when starting from normal expiratory level, can be forcibly inspired.
- *Functional residual capacity (FRC)* is the sum of the ERV and the RV. It is the amount of air remaining in the lungs at the end of normal expiration, about 2300 ml.
- *Vital capacity (VC)* is the sum of the IRV, V_T, and ERV. Stated another way, it is the maximum amount of air that can be forcibly expired following a forced maximal inspiration. This volume is about 4500 ml in a normal male.
- *Total lung capacity (TLC)* is equal to the volume to which the lungs can be expanded with greatest inspiratory effort. The volume of the capacity is about 5800 ml.

These static volumes and capacities provide information about compliance. In persons with reduced compliance (restrictive) disorders, these measurements will be reduced. Increases in TLC, FRC, and RV may occur in persons with obstructive disorders that have resulted in chronic hyperinflation of the lungs. In contrast, the dynamic measurements provide data about airway resistance and the energy expended in breathing (respiratory work).

DYNAMIC MEASUREMENTS

There are eight such dynamic measures.

- *Respiratory rate or frequency (f)* is the number of breaths per minute. At rest, f equals about 15.
- *Minute volume,* sometimes called minute ventilation (V_E) is the volume of air inhaled and exhaled per minute. As such, it is calculated by multiplying V_T by f. At rest V_E equals approximately 7500 ml/minute.
- *Dead space* (V_D) is that part of the V_T which does not participate in alveolar gas exchange. V_D (measured in ml) comprises the air contained in the airways (anatomical dead space) plus the volume of alveolar air that is not involved in gas exchange (*e.g.,* air in an unperfused alveolus due to pulmonary embolism or, more commonly, air in underperfused alveoli). V_D is obtained by subtracting the partial pressure of arterial carbon dioxide ($PaCO_2$) from the partial pressure of the carbon dioxide of alveolar air ($PACO_2$). The normal value of V_D in healthy adults is typically less than 40% of the V_T. This value of the V_D/V_T ratio is used to follow the effectiveness of mechanical ventilation.
- *Alveolar ventilation* is the complement of V_D expressed as the *volume of tidal air that is involved in alveolar gas exchange.* This volume is repre-

sented as volume per minute by the symbol V_A. As such, V_A indicates effective ventilation. It is more relevant to the blood gas values than is either V_D or V_T because these latter two measures include physiological dead space. V_A is calculated by subtracting V_D from V_T and multiplying the result by the respiratory rate/minute:

$$V_A = (V_T - V_D) \times f$$

About 2300 ml of air (FRC) remains in the lung at the end of expiration. Each new breath introduces about 350 ml of air into the alveoli. The ratio of new alveoli air to total volume of air remaining in the lungs is $\frac{350 \text{ ml}}{2300 \text{ ml}}$. Thus, new air is only about one-seventh of the total volume contained within the lungs. The normal V_A is 5250 ml/minute (350 ml/breath $\times$ 15 breaths/min = 5250 ml/min).

A normal breath (V_T) can replace 7500 ml of air per minute (500 ml/breath $\times$ 15 breaths/min = 7500 ml/min), requiring a time of .008 second per ml ($\frac{1 \text{ min}}{7500 \text{ ml}} \times \frac{60 \text{ sec}}{1 \text{ min}}$ = .008 sec/ml). Thus, the FRC of the lungs can be completely replaced in 18.4 seconds (2300 ml $\times$ .008 sec/ml = 18.4 sec), assuming uniform air diffusion. This slow turnover rate prevents rapid fluctuations of gas concentrations in the alveoli with each breath.

Lung Resistance. In order for these volumes to be moved into and out of the lungs, work must occur to overcome the resistance of the abdomen, thorax, and lung tissue. This work is the amount of energy expended to operate the chest bellows. The energy required for ventilation is proportional to the nature of lung resistance encountered. There are two kinds of such resistance: (1) elastic, which is measured by compliance indices, and (2) nonelastic, which is best reflected by measures of airway diameters — patency.

Compliance may refer to distensibility of lung or thorax. This data is collected by simultaneous measurement of intraesophageal balloon pressure (as a reflection of intrapleural pressure) and of lung volume (using a manometer attached to an oval or nasal breathing tube). The subject then inflates the lungs to varying degrees and the two measurements attained at each point are plotted on a graph. The slope of this pressure-volume curve reflects compliance. The equation is as follows:

$$\text{compliance} = \frac{\text{change in lung volume (liters)}}{\text{change in balloonic measure (cm/H}_2\text{O)}}$$

Elasticity in the alveolar walls and the presence of normal amounts of surfactant contribute to normal compliance. Fibrosis, atelectasis, or fluid in (pneumonia) or around (edema) the alveoli will decrease compliance. With decreased compliance, a greater pressure is associated with a given volume than would be normally seen. With increased compliance, the reverse would occur.

Common measures of airway diameters are the forced expiratory volume (FEV), the forced vital capacity (FVC), and the maximal mid-expiratory flow (MMEF).

- *FVC* measures the amount of air in a forceful maximal expiration. Normally it is approximately the same as the VC.
- *FEV* is the volume of air exhaled in a given time period — usually during the first second of the FVC (FEV_1).
- *MMEF* is the volume of air that is exhaled during the midpoint record of the FVC.

The FEV is expressed in terms of the FVC or the VC. Normally, the FEV_1 is about 80% of a VC. In obstructive disorders such as chronic bronchitis or emphysema, this FEV_1 is a smaller percentage of the VC (or FVC).

As stated before, the work of breathing is proportional to the compliance and airway resistance (diameters). A normal person at rest expends less than 6% of his total bodily oxygen consumption upon the work of breathing. This percentage increases as the airway diameters (FEV, MMEF) or compliance decreases.

VENTILATION–PERFUSION

Maximal efficiency in the exchange of gases between blood and alveolus results when ventilation and perfusion correspond equally. In other words, if an acinus (group of alveoli — the basic unit of respiration) is less ventilated, it needs less perfusion; if it is more ventilated, then perfusion must be increased. Ventilation would be, in effect, wasted on an unperfused unit. Similarly, perfusion would be wasted on an unventilated unit. Two reflexes operate normally to facilitate such matching of ventilation and perfusion.

One reflex adjusts perfusion to ventilation. Here, a low concentration of alveolar oxygen (PAO_2) causes a lowered PaO_2, which, in turn, triggers vasoconstriction of nearby pulmonary arterioles. This effectively shunts blood away from an un(der)ventilated area. The other reflex adjusts ventilation to perfusion. If perfusion through an area is impeded (*e.g.,* an embolus plugging the vessel), it will result in a local decrease in $PaCO_2$. This will cause a decrease in $PACO_2$ which, in turn, will cause a constriction of the bronchioles and smaller bronchi in the underperfused area. Thus, the underperfused area is not ventilated as much as before. These reflexes serve to keep the ventilation (V = 4 liters/min) to perfusion (Q = 5 liters/min) ratio at 4:5. Thus, the V/Q ratio is 0.8 under normal circumstances. V/Q mismatch occurs in many respiratory disorders. If ventilation is in excess of perfusion, the disorder is termed a *dead space-producing* one (with a V/Q > 0.8). When perfusion exceeds ventilation, the disorder is a *shunt-producing* one (with a V/Q < 0.8).

Exchange of Gases Through the Pulmonary Membrane

The pulmonary membrane in humans is made up of all the surfaces in the respiratory wall that are thin enough to permit the exchange of gases between the lungs and the blood. The total area of this membrane in the average normal adult male is about 60 sq m, or about the size of a moderate-sized classroom. It is 0.2μ to 0.4μ thick, or less than the thickness of the average red blood cell. These two outstanding features combine to allow large quantities of gases to diffuse across the pulmonary membrane in a very short period of time.

PARTIAL PRESSURE

The air that is taken into the respiratory passages is a mixture of primarily nitrogen and oxygen (99.5%) and a small amount of carbon dioxide and water vapor (0.5%). The molecules of the various gases behave as in solution and exhibit Brownian movement. Thus, a mixture of gases such as air has all molecular species evenly distributed throughout the given volume. Because of this constant molecular bombardment, the volume of gases exerts pressure against the walls of the container. This pressure can be defined as the force with which a gas or mixture of gases attempts to move from the confines of the present environment. Therefore, each of the components of a mixture such as air will account for part of the total pressure of the entire mixture. Consequently, if we take 100 volumes of air and place them in a container under 1 atmosphere of

pressure (760 torr), by analysis we would find that nitrogen makes up 79 of the 100 volumes and oxygen makes up 21 volumes, or 79% and 21% concentration, respectively.

Both these gases are contained at 760 torr pressure in this container. If we now take the same volume of nitrogen and move it to a container of the same volume and allow to expand until it completely fills all of the volume (100%), we will observe that the pressure in the second container drops from 760 to 600 torr. If we do the same thing with the 21 volumes of oxygen and allow them to expand to 100% of the volume, we observe that the pressure in the third container drops from 760 to 160 torr. We conclude then that in the original container the *part* of the total pressure due to nitrogen was 600 torr and the *part* due to oxygen was 160 torr. This pressure of nitrogen is called the *partial pressure* of nitrogen (PN_2) and that of oxygen the *partial pressure* of oxygen (PO_2).

The partial pressure of a gas in a given volume is the force it exerts against the walls of the container. If the walls of the container are permeable, like the pulmonary membrane, then the penetrating or diffusing power of a gas is directly proportional to its partial pressure.

It is extremely important to point out that atmospheric air differs from alveolar air in partial pressures of the components. The comparative concentrations of each are shown in Table 11-1.

The difference between atmospheric air and alveolar air is in the increased concentration of carbon dioxide and water in alveolar air. The reasons for these differences are twofold. First, the air is humidified as it is inspired by the moisture of the epithelial lining of the respiratory tract. At normal body temperature, water vapor has a partial pressure of 47 torr and mixes with and dilutes the other gases, decreasing their partial pressures.

Table 11-1
Comparison of Gases in Atmospheric and Alveolar Air

Gas	Atmospheric air, %	Alveolar air, %
N_2	78.62	74.90
O_2	20.84	13.60
CO_2	0.04	5.30
H_2	0.50	6.20
	100.00	100.00

Second, molecules in a given volume of gas behave like molecules in a solution and diffuse from an area of high concentration to one of lower concentration.

FACTORS AFFECTING DIFFUSION

The factors that govern the rate of diffusion of the gases through the pulmonary membrane are as follows.

- First, the greater the pressure difference across the membrane, the faster the rate of diffusion.
- Second, the larger the area of the pulmonary membrane, the larger the quantity of gas that can diffuse across the membrane in a given period of time. The thinner the membrane, the more rapidly do gases diffuse through it to the compartment on the opposite side.
- Finally, the diffusion coefficient is directly proportional to the solubility of the gas in the fluid of the pulmonary membrane and inversely proportional to molecular size. Therefore, small molecules that are highly soluble diffuse more rapidly than do large molecular gases that are less soluble.

The diffusion coefficients are as follows:

- Oxygen   1
- Carbon dioxide   20.3
- Nitrogen   0.53

These three gases are very similar to one another with regard to molecular size but have quite different solubilities in the fluids of the pulmonary membrane. It is these differences that account for the difference in the rate of diffusion of the gases through the pulmonary membrane.

Transport of Oxygen and Carbon Dioxide Through the Tissues

As oxygen diffuses from the lungs to the blood, a small portion of it becomes dissolved in the plasma and cell fluids, but more than 60 times as much combines immediately with hemoglobin and is carried to the tissues. Here the oxygen is used by the cells, and carbon dioxide is formed.

As the carbon dioxide diffuses into the interstitial fluids, about 5% is dissolved in the blood, and the remainder diffuses into the red blood cells where one of two things occurs:

- Carbon dioxide combines with water to form carbonic acid and then reacts with the acid base buffer and is transported as the bicarbonate ion.

- A small portion of the carbon dioxide combines with hemoglobin at a different bonding site than oxygen and is transported as carbaminohemoglobin.

Nitrogen diffuses from the alveolus into the blood. Since there is no carrier mechanism and under standard conditions nitrogen has only slight solubility in tissue fluid, it quickly establishes an equilibrium state on either side of the membrane and thus is essentially inert.

The relative partial pressure (torr) in the various compartments is summarized in Table 11-2.

It can readily be seen that concentration gradients are established that then foster the diffusion of these gases in the direction that is physiologically advantageous.

Figure 11-1 summarizes the events of gaseous diffusion through pulmonary membrane and transport to and from the tissues.

OXYHEMOGLOBIN DISSOCIATION CURVE

The influence of PaO_2 (the arterial level of oxygen) upon the attachment of oxygen to hemoglobin is not a straight-line function. In other words, the relationship is not directly proportioned on a 1:1 basis. The relationships involved are shown in Figure 11-2.

The upper right hand corner illustrates conditions in arterial blood when the normal PaO_2 is at about 100 torr. Then, as the blood circulates through the capillaries, losing oxygen to the interstitial fluid, the curve falls until the PO_2 of venous fluid (40 torr) is reached. At a PO_2 of 40, hemoglobin molecules are still about 70% to 75% saturated (combined) with oxygen. This provides a reserve supply of oxygen that can be provided to the tissues in cases of emergency or strenuous exercise. Thus, only about 25% to 30% of the arterial oxygen supply is used to meet tissue needs.

Due to the relationships represented by this curve, oxygen can be applied to the tissues even

Table 11–2
Relative Partial Pressures

Gas	Atmospheric Air	Alveolar Air	Venous Blood	Arterial Blood
PO_2	159	104	40	100
PCO_2	0.15	40	45	40
PN_2	597	569	569	569

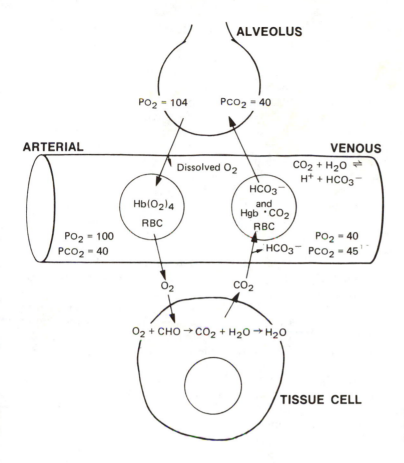

FIGURE 11-1.
Gaseous diffusion through pulmonary
membrane in respiration.

if the PaO_2 is under 100 (hypoxemia or high altitude living). Indeed, oxygen administration with a PaO_2 of 80 will raise the hemoglobin saturation only slightly.

Several factors influence the affinity of hemoglobin for oxygen. Clinically important are the pH, PCO_2, and temperature. These factors exert a Bohr effect upon the oxyhemoglobin dissociation curve: that is, they shift it to the right or left. A shift to the right is caused by acidity, hypercarbia, and elevation in temperature and means a decrease in the affinity of hemoglobin for oxygen. This means that less oxygen can be picked up in the lungs but that oxygen is more readily given up to the tissues in the capillaries. A shift to the left, as produced by alkalinity and a fall in PCO_2 and temperature, will increase the affinity of hemoglobin for oxygen. Thus, more oxygen can be picked up in the lungs, but oxygen is less readily released in the capillaries. This could cause tissue hypoxia even in the face of adequate PaO_2. Respiratory alkalosis (*e.g.*, as caused by mechanical hyperventilation) has the greatest clinical potential for producing such a condition.

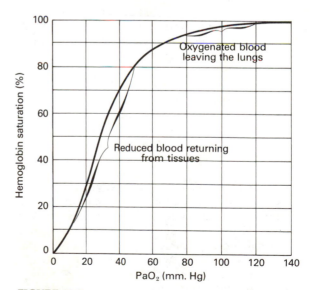

FIGURE 11-2.
Oxyhemoglobin dissociation curve. (From Guyton AC: Textbook of Medical Physiology. Philadelphia, WB Saunders, 1976)

REGULATION OF RESPIRATION

Brain Stem Centers

Unlike the heart, the lungs have no spontaneous rhythm. Ventilations depend upon rhythmic operation of brain stem centers and intact pathways from there to the respiratory muscles. There are two centers in the medulla: (1) a center that stimulates inspiration by diaphragmatic contraction (by way of phrenic nerves) and (2) another center that innervates both inspiratory and expiratory intercostal and accessory muscles.

The pons also contains two centers included in respiration. One is called the *pneumotaxic* center. The other, the *apneustic* center, produces sustained inspiration when stimulated. Voluntary and involuntary control is further established by descending fibers from other brain centers. (These facilitate the alterations in respiration seen, for example, during swallowing, coughing, yawning, and willed action.)

In breathing at rest, the following sequence is thought to occur. The neurons innervating the inspiratory muscles fire bursts of impulses to these muscles. These neurons also stimulate the pneumotaxic center. This center, in turn, fires inhibitory impulses back to these inspiratory neurons. This causes a halt in inspiration. Expiration is thought to passively follow. After this the inspiratory neurons are again stimulated to automatically fire. During exercise or other occasions when more vigorous ventilation occurs, the expiratory neurons of the medulla are postulated to actually participate in this sequence. A more comprehensive picture of the breathing process awaits further data.

External Regulations

The rate and depth of ventilations are potentially influenced by four factors: concentrations of (1) hydrogen ions, (2) carbon dioxide, (3) oxygen, and (4) exercise.

Carbon Dioxide. The most powerful stimulus for the respiratory center is the carbon dioxide content of the blood and tissue fluids of the body. When the carbon dioxide level rises above normal, both inspiratory and expiratory neurons are stimulated, and thus both rate and depth of respiration are increased. Approximately one-half of the effect of carbon dioxide on respiration is due to its direct effect on the respiratory neurons themselves. The other half is due to the indirect effect of carbon dioxide in the cerebrospinal fluid. As carbon dioxide diffuses into the cerebrospinal fluid, it combines with water to form carbonic acid, which then dissociates to hydrogen and bicarbonate ions. The increased hydrogen-ion concentration directly stimulates the neurons of the respiratory center as the fluid bathes the sides of the brain stem.

The respiratory system's response to carbon dioxide concentrations is extremely important because it is the main pathway for regulating carbon dioxide levels in body fluids. Should carbon dioxide accumulate in the tissues and fluids of the body, all chemical reactions of the body are essentially inhibited. If the carbon dioxide level drops too low, alkalosis develops, which is also incompatible with life.

Hydrogen-Ion Concentration. As implied in the previous section, hydrogen-ion concentration is the second most powerful influence on alveolar ventilation. In the equation showing carbon dioxide combining with water in body fluids, it is noted that the reactions are reversible. Therefore, if there is an accumulation of hydrogen-ion concentration (a low pH tending toward acidemia), the center neurons respond, increasing the rate of respiration, which drives the reaction to the left and lowers the hydrogen-ion concentration. If the hydrogen-ion concentration is low (high pH tending toward alkalemia), alveolar ventilation is depressed, and the reaction is driven to the right. This response of the respiratory system in conjunction with the kidneys to a large extent controls the acid–base balance of the body.

Oxygen. Although normally hemoglobin is almost completely saturated with oxygen, the body does have chemoreceptors located in the carotid bodies in the neck and in the aortic arch that monitor blood oxygen levels. These receptors are sensitive to oxygen diffusion, and the respiratory center is stimulated by the vagus and glossopharyngeal nerves.

The chemoreceptor mechanism is not as powerful a respiratory stimulus as either carbon dioxide or hydrogen-ion concentration, but it is important in persons with chronic obstructive pulmonary disease (COPD). These persons eventually become physiologically acclimated to their chronically high $PaCO_2$. Their hydrogen-ion mechanisms no longer operate to stimulate ventilation. Instead, they rely on the PaO_2 mechanism. Thus, giving oxygen to a COPD patient can actually depress ventilation and even cause respiratory arrest if it raises PaO_2 levels high enough.

There is also a mechanism for preventing lung overinflation. It is called the *Hering-Breuer reflex*. Scattered throughout the lung tissue (between acini) are stretch receptors. When they are stimulated by lung inflation, they cause sensory impulses to travel up fibers in the vagus. These impulses reflexively cause inhibition of the inspiratory center, which halts further inhalation and consequent stretch.

Exercise. The rate and depth of respiration are directly proportional to the amount of work done during exercise. It is not the chemical factors that appear to cause increased rate and depth of respiration during exercise, except secondarily. The primary cause of increased respiration during exercise is the simultaneous stimulation (by the cerebral cortex) of the muscle exercised and of the sensory pathway from the cord that stimulates the respiratory center.

The Respiratory System and *p*H Homeostasis

Erythrocytes contain the enzyme carbonic anhydrase, which catalyzes the formation of carbonic acid from carbon dioxide and water ($CO_2 + H_2O \rightarrow H_2CO_3$). Carbonic acid readily dissociates to form a hydrogen ion (H^+) and a bicarbonate radical (HCO_3^-). It may be remembered that acidity represents the concentration of unattached or free hydrogen ions. Thus, the more carbon dioxide in the blood, the more free hydrogen ions or acidity that may be produced. The less carbon dioxide, the less acid (or more boric) the blood.

The hydrogen ions produced in this way are normally buffered, thereby maintaining homeostasis of extracellular fluid (ECF) *p*H. However, if there is more carbon dioxide-produced acid than the buffers can handle, acidosis will result. This is called *respiratory acidosis*. It occurs whenever there is a situation that produces alveolar hypoventilation and consequent decrease in the elimination of carbon dioxide from the bloodstream (*e.g.,* depression of the respiratory centers in the brain by certain drugs). Conversely, hyperventilation reduces the amount of carbon dioxide in the bloodstream. Less carbon dioxide means fewer hydrogen ions. This results in respiratory alkalosis.

In addition to its potential for causing *p*H imbalances, the respiratory system also plays a role in compensating for metabolically caused acidosis or alkalosis. Respiratory compensation for metabolically caused acidosis is hyperventilation. This maneuver decreases the plasma carbon dioxde, thereby decreasing the plasma hydrogen-ion concentration. Fewer hydrogen ions mean less acidosis. For metabolic alkalosis, respiratory compensation involves decreased ventilation. This increases plasma carbon dioxide (or free hydrogen ions), thereby reducing the alkalosis. Such compensation can occur immediatcly when blood and time buffers are inadequate to handle the *p*H imbalance. In 48 to 72 hours the renal compensatory mechanism also comes into play in order to restore *p*H homeostasis.

BIBLIOGRAPHY

Ganong WF: Review of Medical Physiology. Los Altos, Lang, 1977

Price SA, Wilson LM: Pathophysiology: Clinical Concepts of Disease Processes. New York, McGraw-Hill, 1978

Stephens G: Pathophysiology for Health Practitioners. New York, Macmillan, 1980

Joseph O. Broughton

Pathophysiology of the Respiratory System
12

A broad definition of the function of the respiratory system is (1) to provide adequate oxygenation to all body tissues and (2) to eliminate excess carbon dioxide gas produced by the tissues. Performance of these functions requires not only normally functioning lungs and thorax, but also a normally functioning medullary respiratory center and cardiovascular system, normally functioning aortic and carotid chemoreceptors, and a normal amount of functioning hemoglobin. Malfunction of any of these components can cause respiratory failure—inadequate oxygenation of the tissues, inadequate elimination of carbon monoxide gas, or both. Since hypoxemia and hypercapnia are the essence of respiratory failure, they deserve special attention.

PULMONARY DISORDERS

Normal function of the lungs and thorax may be impaired by various disease processes. These pulmonary diseases are often placed into two main categories: (1) airway obstructions and (2) restrictive defects.

Airway Obstruction

The obstructive diseases seen most commonly are

- Chronic bronchitis
- Asthma
- Emphysema

Frequent subjection to irritants, allergens, and infections can cause gradual but definite tissue changes. In chronic bronchitis and asthma, the airways may be obstructed by mucosal edema, increased mucus in the lumen, and presumably by spasms of the muscle encircling the bronchi and bronchioles. In chronic bronchitis there may also be an increased number of mucous glands, and in emphysema there may be loss of support for the walls of the airways so that they collapse rapidly on expiration, like a wet straw.

Rarer causes of airway obstructions are aspirated foreign bodies (most often in children); bronchial or tracheal stenosis from scarring (often from a previous tracheostomy); intrabronchial tumors; occasionally silicosis, tuberculosis, and other granulomatous diseases; and sometimes the frothy, bubbly secretions of severe pulmonary edema. Upper-airway obstruction from large tonsils and adenoids has on occasion been the cause of respiratory failure in children.

On pulmonary function tests, obstructive diseases are manifested by slowing of expiratory flow ratio; that is, reduced FEV_1 (forced expiratory volume in 1 second), FEV/VC (forced expiratory volume/vital capacity) ratio of less than 75% and reduced FEF 25% to 75% (MMEF). If severe, obstructive diseases usually cause hypoxemia and hypercapnia.

Restrictive Defects

Although many conditions can cause restrictive pulmonary problems, obstructive problems are more common. *Restrictive* refers to any situation which makes it difficult to expand the lungs. Diffuse interstitial pulmonary fibrosis, either idiopathic or associated with sarcoid, causes fibrosis inside the lung. The stiffness or noncompliance of the tissue restricts lung expansion. Fibrosis outside the lung, as in pleural thickening or fibrosis, can also make it difficult to expand the lungs and is therefore a restrictive process.

Abdominal distention and/or abdominal pain can limit movement of the diaphragm, thereby restricting lung expansion. Failure of the left ventricle results in pulmonary vascular congestion, another restrictive process. Skeletal abnormalities such as kyphoscoliosis and ankylosing spondylitis, as well as neuromuscular disorders such as Guillain-Barré syndrome, also restrict chest expansion.

On pulmonary function tests, restrictive problems are reflected by low vital capacity and reductions in all other lung volumes. They do not often cause blood gas abnormalities unless they are associated with another abnormality, that is, diffusion (gas transport) problems.

DIFFUSION PROBLEMS

When restriction to lung expansion is caused by *interstitial fibrosis,* there is usually interference with transport of oxygen from the alveoli into the bloodstream, and this is reflected by a low PO_2. If the diffusion problem is severe, there may be hypoxemia at rest, but if the condition is mild or moderate, the PO_2 at rest is usually normal and exercise is required to demonstrate the hypoxemia. With exercise, blood flows through the lung faster than at rest, so blood may not remain in the pulmonary capillaries long enough to pick up oxygen if the oxygen is delayed in getting into the capillaries because of a diffusion problem.

Pulmonary edema is another cause of diffusion problems. It may take longer for oxygen to diffuse from the alveoli through alveolar edema, through the interstitial edema, and into the capillary. In other conditions such as emphysema there may be a diffusion abnormality because of a lack of alveoli and/or pulmonary capillaries, thus less opportunity for gas transport.

If the PO_2 is normal, 97% of the oxygen-carrying capacity of hemoglobin is used. Even though the PO_2 may rise as high as five times normal when a person breathes 100% oxygen, the hemoglobin can carry only 3% more oxygen.

HEMOGLOBIN SATURATION

There are certain disease states in which the hemoglobin is abnormal and carries either more or less oxygen for a given PO_2 than does normal hemoglobin. When a certain type of hemoglobin carries less oxygen than normal at a given PO_2, it is the same as having the oxyhemoglobin dissociation curve shifted to the right.

When hemoglobin does not carry its full amount of oxygen, it assumes a blue or dark color. Generally *cyanosis* is recognized when there are 5 g or more of hemoglobin that are not saturated with oxygen. (Occasionally because of hypoxemia the body may make too many red blood cells [RBC] and too much hemoglobin.) When there is more than the usual amount of hemoglobin and when the circulation moves the RBC slowly, more unsaturated hemoglobin is present, so that cyanosis is more apparent. Sometimes, then, cyanosis may be present — particularly in the extremities — when the arterial oxygen concentration is normal, if there is an excess of hemoglobin or reduction in blood flow. Much more common is the opposite situation in which arterial oxygen concentration is low but no cyanosis is recognizable. If one relies on cyanosis to diagnose significant hypoxemia, many instances of hypoxemia will be missed completely and others will be discovered late. Cyanosis is especially hard to diagnose in anemic patients.

In spite of the unreliability of cyanosis as an early indicator of hypoxia, many nurses nevertheless continue to rely on the absence of cyanosis to indicate adequate oxygenation, to the detriment of the patient.

Hypoxemia

Hypoxia may be caused by hypoventilation, diffusion problems, living at high altitudes, right-to-left shunts, and ventilation/perfusion (V/Q)mismatching.

Conditions that cause just hypoxemia may be even less obvious than those associated with hypoxemia and hypercapnia. A pulmonary embolus may cause or intensify hypoxemia. Other causes of chest pain, such as fractured ribs, may cause decreased expansion of part of the lung and lead to hypoxemia.

V/Q Problems. V/Q inequality, or more simply stated, mismatching of ventilation and perfusion, is probably the most common cause of hypoxemia. If any area of the lung is underventilated, for instance, because its bronchus is partially obstructed by a mucus plug with that part of the lung still receiving its normal blood supply, then there is relatively too little ventilation for the amount of perfusion (blood flow); this situation might be represented as v/Q as compared to the normal V/Q. The blood going to this part of the lung does not have the opportunity to pick up its full quota of oxygen because of the reduction in ventilation. If the bronchus to an area of the lung were completely obstructed while the perfusion remained normal, it would represent a right-to-left shunt; that is, unsaturated venous blood would flow from the right ventricle through the lungs without picking up any oxygen, mix with blood from other parts of the lungs, and then be pumped by the left ventricle into the systemic circulation.

Incidentally, just the opposite type of V/Q problem may occur yet may not cause hypoxemia. For instance, the pulmonary artery to part of the lung might be occluded, but the ventilation to that part of the lung might be maintained, and there would therefore be excessive ventilation in respect to perfusion, which could be represented as V/q. This is called *wasted ventilation*. This condition does not necessarily cause serious problems but is often associated with excessive work of breathing.

Usually the lung reflexively reduces ventilation to match reduced perfusion, and vice versa. However, in some disease states these reflex changes do not occur. For instance, in patients who have severe pathology in the upper abdomen such as pancreatitis, or who have just undergone gastric surgery or cholecystectomy, pain or tight bandages may prevent the diaphragm from descending normally with inspiration, thereby reducing ventilation in the lung bases. Sometimes the chest roentgenogram shows atelectasis or sometimes just a high diaphragm, but underventilation may occur without noticeable radiographic changes. If perfusion remains normal, some blood flows through underventilated bases without becoming oxygenated, so that the systemic arterial blood shows hypoxemia.

As mentioned above, this type of reduced ventilation in relation to perfusion in some lung areas can occur in many different diseases and is probably the most common cause of hypoxemia. It occurs in many ill patients who would not be expected to have respiratory failure — patients with shock, gastrointestinal bleeding, heart failure — in fact, in almost any patient sick enough to be in the intensive care or coronary care unit.

Diffusion Problems usually occur with interstitial lung disease such as diffuse interstitial pulmonary fibrosis and metastatic carcinoma spreading through the lymphatics of the lung in the interstitial spaces (between alveoli). Diffusion problems also may occur in pulmonary edema, in which edema fluid is found in the interstitial space and often in the alveoli as well.

With diffusion problems the PO_2 may be normal at rest, but with exercise the PO_2 falls; in more severe diffusion problems the PO_2 may be low even at rest.

Generally the patient with a diffusion problem hyperventilates in an effort to move adequate amounts of oxygen from the alveoli through the widened interstitial space into the capillary blood. As a result of this hyperventilation, the PCO_2 is lowered.

Usually in diffusion problems there is no difficulty in getting air through the airways. In severe pulmonary edema, however, because of the frothy, bubbly secretions occluding the airways, there may be enough obstruction to airflow to cause a rise in PCO_2.

In summary, diffusion problems show hypoxemia first only with exercise and later even at rest. The hyperventilation necessary to keep PO_2 up causes a low PCO_2. Only in severe problems such as severe pulmonary edema is the PCO_2 elevated.

Living at high altitudes, even with normal ventilation, is associated with hypoxemia because the inspired oxygen concentration is low. The hypoxemia usually leads to hyperventilation in an effort by the body to raise the PO_2, and the hyperventilation causes a low PCO_2. For instance, the normal PCO_2 in Denver is 36 torr (mm Hg) as compared with the normal at sea level of 40 torr.

Right-to-left shunts, which may occur with ventricular septal defects, for example, are associated with hypoxemia because part of the blood from the right heart that is destined to be oxygenated in the lungs bypasses the lungs and is shunted directly into the systemic arterial circulation. The resulting systemic arterial hypoxemia may lead to hyperventilation and therefore to low PCO_2. Occasionally right-to-left shunting occurs through abnormal vascular channels in the lung.

Hypoventilation from any cause leads to hypoxemia and hypercapnia. The hypoventilation is most frequently associated with airway obstruction such as emphysema or chronic bronchitis, or even the obstruction due to the frothy secretions that occur in severe pulmonary edema. Hypoventilation also may occur with a variety of neurologic problems such as myasthenia gravis, Guillain-Barré syndrome, and polio. Hypoventilation may occur with some head injuries or with oversedation. Rarely hypoventilation may be caused by restrictive pulmonary problems such as large pleural effusion, immobile chest with ankylosing spondylitis, and so forth.

The hypoventilation that occurs with airway obstruction may be due to retained secretions, airway narrowing due to edema or swelling of the mucosal lining, bronchospasm, or airway collapse. Increase in secretions is due to increase in output of the goblet cells and submucosal glands. The submucosal glands are stimulated to produce mucus by the vagus nerve and local irritants in the tracheobronchial tree; the goblet cells are stimulated to produce mucus mainly by local irritants.

In many diseases of the respiratory tract such as asthma and bronchitis, there is edema of the mucosal lining. Treating bronchospasm without treating the associated mucosal edema is treating only half of the problem, so we should usually combine an inhaled vasoconstrictor with an inhaled bronchodilator. In conditions such as emphysema there is often a rapid collapse of the trachea and bronchi during expiration, which causes airway obstruction during expiration.

Assessment Factors. Hypoxemia caused by hypoventilation is accompanied by hypercapnia, but hypoxemia due to any of the other causes is usually associated with hyperventilation and therefore low PCO_2.

Therefore, when hypoxemia is associated with a high PCO_2, it generally means that hypoxemia is due to hypoventilation. When hypoxemia is associated with a low or normal PCO_2, it may be caused by diffusion problems, V/Q mismatching, right-to-left shunting, or living at high altitude. The latter is obvious. Diffusion problems usually respond by a return of arterial oxygen concentrations to normal with low-to-moderate amounts of supplemental oxygen, while V/Q mismatching and shunts usually require high levels of oxygen to bring the arterial oxygen concentrations to normal, and even then the arterial oxygen sometimes does not return to normal.

Hypercapnia

Hypercapnia (also called *hypercarbia*) is easier to explain than hypoxemia. It always means alveolar hypoventilation. The most common causes of hypoventilation are mentioned above. Hypoventilation (and therefore hypercapnia) of limited degree may also be due to compensation of nonrespiratory alkalosis. With more significant hypoventilation, however, there is hypoxemia, which is a strong stimulus to ventilation. This hypoxemia, then, increases ventilation and therefore prevents severe hypoventilation from occurring in compensation for nonrespiratory alkalosis.

There is only one cause of hypercapnia—hypoventilation. There are several causes of hypoxemia, one of which is hypoventilation. Therefore hypercapnia is a better reflector of hypoventilation than is hypoxemia.

Compliance

The work of breathing is often increased in diseases in which the lungs fail, and this increased work of breathing may be due to reduced compliance, increased airway resistance, or both. Reduced compliance occurs in restrictive conditions such as diffuse interstitial pulmonary fibrosis or conditions in which there is reduced surfactant—adult and newborn respiratory distress syndromes. Increased airway resistance occurs with anything that causes airway obstruction, as listed above. In both increased airway resistance and reduced compliance, increased pressure is required to deliver a normal tidal volume. This is easily recognized in patients on ventilators. Increased airway resistance is noted by an initial high pressure that then falls to a lower level, and increase in compliance is noted by a sustained high pressure.

RESPIRATORY FAILURE

Assessment Factors

Arbitrary values for defining when respiratory failure is present have been proposed. Respiratory failure is said to be present when the PO_2 falls below 50 torr (oxygen saturation below 85%) or when PCO_2 rises above 50 torr. However, numbers are not the perfect way to diagnose a complicated situation such as respiratory failure. Some persons are in mild respiratory failure even before the PO_2 falls below 50 torr or before the PCO_2 rises above 50 torr. Others who have increased PCO_2 and/or decreased PO_2 are in a stable state, often still working, because they have adapted to the abnormal blood gases. In spite of these exceptions, *blood gases* are by far the best means of detecting respiratory failure.

It is easy to understand how respiratory failure occurs in one of the airway obstructive diseases—that is, emphysema, chronic bronchitis, or asthma. A very important fact is that these diseases account for fewer than half of the cases of respiratory failure that occur in a general hospital.

It is most important to be able to diagnose respiratory failure at an early stage when treatment is most likely to be successful. Even more desirable is the recognition of *impending* respiratory failure. This can be accomplished by

- Knowing the setting in which respiratory failure is most likely to occur
- Being aware that there are many nonspecific signs and symptoms that are indicators of early or impending respiratory failure
- Being inquisitive enough to obtain *arterial blood gases* when the question of respiratory failure enters your mind (see the discussion of blood gases in Chapter 14).

Settings

Drugs such as sedatives, tranquilizers, sleeping pills, or analgesics—and rarely, alcohol—may cause depression of respiratory drive and may allow the PCO_2 to rise significantly while the patient is under the influence of the drug. Once the effect of the drug is gone, the remaining elevation of PCO_2 is often enough to cause continuing respiratory depression. It is important to remember that a small rise in PCO_2 is a large stimulus to breathing, but that larger rises in PCO_2 can cause depression of the respiratory center, resulting in hypoventilation. Other brain functions may also be depressed. If the PCO_2 is already elevated enough to cause respiratory depression, the carotid chemoreceptors may sense hypoxemia and respond to this last remaining stimulus to breathing. If oxygen is administered because the patient is cyanotic or appears to have labored breathing, the final stimulus to respiration, hypoxemia, may be removed, causing the patient to have even less ventilation. Such a patient who has respiratory center depression due to drugs, a significantly elevated PCO_2 or both, when given enough oxygen to reduce his respiratory drive may no longer appear cyanotic, and as he ventilates less, he may no longer appear to be laboring to breathe. In fact, he may become quieter and go to sleep. It is extremely important to recognize the set of circumstances mentioned above, for it happens daily in chronic airway obstruction (CAO) patients in hospitals across the country. Usually if low flows (2 to 3 liters/min) of oxygen or low percentages (24% to 28%) of oxygen are given—just enough oxygen to raise PO_2 to 60 torr—the hypoxic ventilatory drive will not be significantly reduced.

Misdiagnoses. Often respirtory failure is misdiagnosed as congestive heart failure, as a stroke, or as "pneumonia occurring in a patient with a lousy personality." Usually the personality improves as the pneumonia clears, yet the diagnosis of respiratory failure was never made.

The patient who is semiconscious and flaccid in all extremities may be said to have suffered a stroke, when in reality there is no localizing finding of a cerebral thrombosis or hemorrhage, and instead hypoxia and hypercapnia cause the impaired consciousness and impaired motor function. Unless someone has a high degree of suspicion, the patient may die of respiratory failure masquerading as a stroke. On the other hand, it is certainly possible for a patient with a typical stroke to retain enough secretions in his respiratory tract to develop respiratory failure.

Most common are the patients with obvious

right-sided congestive heart failure. The cause of right-sided congestive heart failure—lung failure—often goes unrecognized. Fortunately, many of these patients improve just with treatment of the heart failure, but they would improve more if respiratory failure and its cause were recognized and treated.

Asthma.   It is easy to recognize the respiratory distress present in a patient with asthma, but it is often difficult to tell when the patient is in real danger. The physical exam can be misleading. Occasionally, in asthma, little or no wheezing is heard because there is virtually no air exchange. The patient may appear to be making normal, though labored, respiratory movements, while in fact exchanging very little air. The earliest blood gas abnormality in an asthmatic is hypoxemia. The hypoxemia may be worsened by treatment with the usual bronchodilators, even though the wheezing is decreasing. The worsening hypoxemia is probably due to changing V/Q relationships. The hypoxemia causes hyperventilation, which in turn causes hypocapnia. In spite of attempts at hyperventilation, if the asthma becomes more severe with increasing airway obstruction, the PCO_2 rises to normal. As the situation worsens, even mild elevations of PCO_2 combined with the hypoxemia (if the patient has not been treated with oxygen) signify severe asthma. In asthma, slight elevation of PCO_2 signifies impending crisis, while similar elevations of PCO_2 in chronic bronchitis or emphysema have much less significance. As in other respiratory problems, the best indicators are arterial blood gases, but the interpretation of blood gases must be related to the clinical situation.

Chronic Airway Obstruction.   Usually some additional insult occurs in patients with CAO that either (1) increases airway obstruction or (2) reduces respiratory drive. Both of these cause hypoventilation and result in an increase in PCO_2 and a decrease in PO_2. The additional insult that causes the patient with CAO to develop respiratory failure may be (1) infection such as pneumonia or acute bronchitis (*Hemophilus influenzae* and *Diplococcus pneumoniae* are the most common organisms in outpatients), (2) pulmonary embolus, (3) congestive heart failure or fluid overload, and (4) increasing bronchospasm.

Often the patient with CAO is getting by with only marginal lung function, and even minor insults tip him over into frank respiratory failure. Such an insult may be an infectious process leading to bronchial mucosal edema, increased mucus production, bronchospasm, increased airway obstruction, and worsening hypercapnia and hypoxemia.

Nonspecific Signs and Symptoms

There are also a number of situations in which anyone can recognize respiratory failure; for example, patients with cardiac arrest, those with drug overdose or head injury who stop breathing, and those with cyanosis and labored breathing. However, in many patients the presence of respiratory failure may not be so obvious. The signs and symptoms may be nonspecific and manifested as lethargy, irritability, headaches, confusion (sometimes intermittent), vagueness, facetiousness, jerky motions, and asterixis (flapping tremor of hand). Other less specific manifestations may be sweating, mydriasis, tachycardia, hypotension, anorexia, impaired motor function, impaired judgment, and coma.

Respiratory failure occurs in a variety of clinical settings and is associated with a variety of signs and symptoms. One must be exceedingly astute to recognize respiratory failure every time it occurs, and perhaps all that can be expected is that one should learn to develop a high index of suspicion regarding the existence of respiratory failure and be eager to obtain arterial blood gases when a suspicion of respiratory failure exists.

Treatment

The treatment of respiratory failure is designed to raise the PO_2 to normal or reduce the PCO_2 to normal. Usually this can be accomplished by initially supplying supplemental oxygen and treating the factors which are causing the altered physiology; for example, bronchospasm, infection, mucosal edema, and retained secretions. This treatment, if instituted early enough, usually allows the patient to increase his own ventilation so that in most cases of respiratory failure, ventilators are not required. It is most important for the patient to receive adequate oxygen—just enough to raise his PO_2 to about 60 torr while the other treatment is being instituted. Raising the PO_2 to 60 will help to prevent secondary problems such as the development of heart failure or worsening coma. Hypoxemia can cause death in minutes, but it takes hours or days for hypercapnia to become marked enough to cause death.

Management Modalities: Respiratory System* 13

Patricia K. Brannin

RESPIRATORY DISEASES AND MANAGEMENT

The continuing growth of critical care nursing challenges nurses to expand their scope to meet the needs of this rapidly advancing specialty. Increased accountability for nursing practice demands continual development of the knowledge base from which the critical care nurse operates. The purpose of this chapter is to enable nurses to enhance their knowledge of the respiratory system and its acute disorders and to recall knowledge of normal pulmonary functions and apply it to abnormal situations when assessing, applying, and evaluating therapeutic modalities. Patient observation and recognition of the signs of pulmonary insufficiency—tachypnea, tachycardia, diaphoresis, and anxiety—are the keys to recognizing abnormal pulmonary function. The ability of the clinician to anticipate, recognize,

*We wish to acknowledge the contribution of Susan Kudla, R.N., M.S., to this chapter in the previous edition.

Anatomical Shunt ($\dot{Q}$S anat.)

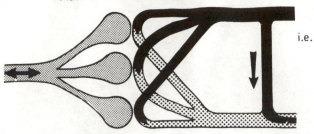

i.e. portion of cardiac output bypassing pulmonary capillaries

Capillary Shunt ($\dot{Q}$S cap.)

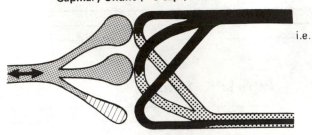

i.e. portion of cardiac output perfusing nonventilating alveoli (Atelectasis)

Physiological Shunt ($\dot{Q}$S phys.)

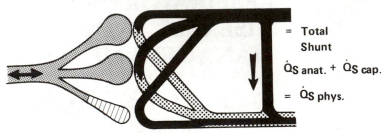

= **Total Shunt**

$\dot{Q}$S anat. $^{+}$ $\dot{Q}$S cap.

= $\dot{Q}$S phys.

FIGURE 13-1.
Subdivisions of the physiological shunt. (Bendixen HH et al: Respiratory Care, p 13. St. Louis, C.V. Mosby, 1965)

and intervene to treat pulmonary disorders may modify and/or prevent common lung disorders.

ATELECTASIS

Atelectasis can be defined as a diminution of volume or collapse of lung units.[1] Several etiologic factors may precipitate atelectasis.

Reabsorption atelectasis occurs when communications between the alveoli and trachea are obstructed, for example, by plugging of a bronchus with mucus. The alveolar gas is rapidly absorbed into the circulation and due to the obstruction cannot be replenished; hence, alveolar collapse ensues.

Passive atelectasis occurs when air and/or fluid in the pleural space prevents normal alveolar filling.

Compression atelectasis occurs in the presence of a space-occupying lesion such as a pulmonary mass.[2] Atelectasis may also occur in patches, which may be caused by mucus plugging or altered compliance in the atelectatic area.[3]

Atelectasis results in a pathologic shunting of blood from the right side of the heart to the left, resulting in desaturation of blood entering the systemic circulation. The degree of shunt present depends upon the severity of the atelectasis. In the normal lung there is a small amount of unoxygenated blood entering the systemic circulation. Contributing to the normal shunt are those vessels whose venous outflow bypasses pulmonary capillaries. Shunting is increased by atelectasis because blood flow passes through the pulmonary capillaries that are in contact with nonventilated alveoli (see Fig. 13-1).

Signs and symptoms vary with the severity of atelectasis and degree of shunt present. With severe shunts (*i.e.,* large areas of atelectasis) cyanosis may become evident. Arterial blood gases will reflect the degree of hypoxemia as well as the adequacy of alveolar ventilation. There is frequently roentgenographic evidence of atelectasis. In compression atelectasis there is roentgenographic evidence of air or fluid collection in the pleural space, resulting in atelectasis. All the roentgen signs are based on diminished volume of the affected lobe or segment.[4] Cyanosis may become evident as atelectasis increases. Large areas of atelectasis may cause a shift of the mediastinal structures toward the affected side, which may be demonstrated roentgenographically. Auscultatory examination reveals decreased breath sounds over the atelectatic lung. There may be diminished chest expansion of the affected side. The patient may complain of shortness of breath (s.o.b.), dyspnea on exertion (d.o.e.), and weakness. He may have tachypnea, tachycardia, fever, anxiety, restlessness, and confusion.

Treatment is based upon the etiology of the atelectasis. Meticulous bronchial hygiene (see discussion later in this chapter), mobilization of the patient when appropriate, and administration of oxygen in pharmacologic doses comprise the basic framework of therapy.

PNEUMONIA

Pneumonia is an inflammatory process in which alveolar gas is replaced by cellular material. The etiology may be due to viral, bacterial, fungal, protozoan, or rickettsial causes or to hypersensitivity, resulting in the primary presenting illness. Pneumonia may also result from aspiration.

The signs and symptoms will depend on the location and extent of involvement (*i.e.,* segmental or lobar) and etiology of the pneumonia. Subjective findings include dyspnea, tachypnea, pleuritic chest pain, fever, chills, hemoptysis, and cough productive of rusty or purulent sputum. Objective findings include fever, splinting of involved hemithorax, hypoxemia, percussion dullness, coarse inspiratory rales, and diminished breath sounds over the involved area.

Treatment of pneumonia is dependent upon etiology, as shown in Table 13-1. Observation of the patient for tachycardia, tachypnea, diaphoresis, restlessness and confusion (signs of hypoxemia), increased sputum production and increased splinting is essential in determination of progression or regression of the process. Careful attention must be directed to improving ventilation through adequate pain medication followed by bronchial hygiene.

Complications of pneumonia include abscess formation, pleural effusion, empyema, bacteremia, and septicemia. Superinfection may occur as a complication of pharmacologic treatment.

PLEURAL EFFUSION

The pleural space is a potential space between the visceral and parietal pleura that line the lungs and interior chest wall. This space normally contains a small amount of fluid. Excess fluid may accumulate in neoplastic, thromboembolic, cardiovascular, and infectious disease processes. This is due to at least one of four basic mechanisms:[5]

- Increased pressure in subpleural capillaries or lymphatics
- Decreased colloid osmotic pressure of the blood
- Increased intrapleural negative pressure
- Inflammatory or neoplastic involvement of the pleura

Subjective findings include shortness of breath and pleuritic chest pain, depending on the amount of fluid accumulation. Objective findings include tachypnea and hypoxemia if ventilation is impaired, dullness to percussion, and decreased breath sounds over the involved area.

Removal of the pleural effusion by thoracentesis or chest tubes is palliative treatment. Major treatment is that directed toward the underlying cause.

Empyema

Empyema is a collection of purulent material in the pleural space secondary to an inflammatory

Table 13-1
Antibiotic Therapy in Pulmonary Disease

Pulmonary Complication	Antibiotic	Dosage
Pneumococcal pneumonia with or without COPD	Penicillin	600,000 U procaine penicillin IM q12hr (a blood level of 0.02 mg/ml 12 hours after start of drug is adequate to kill organism) or IV prep: aqueous penicillin 400,000–600,000 U IV q3–4 hr
Staphylococcal pnemonia (production of enzymes that destroy lung tissue)	Antistaphylo-coccal agents: Nafcillin Methicillin Cloxacillin Penicillin	1–2 g IV q4hr
Klebsiella pneumonia (gram-negative): a very severe pneumonia with high mortality; seen more commonly in chronic/debilitated states	Gentamicin	Dosage will be related to renal function (*i.e.,* creatinine clearance); commonly, 3–5 mg/kg/24 hr. Aim to achieve a trough blood level not less than 1.5 mg/ml and a peak level not over 10 mg/ml
Pseudomonas pneumonia (gram-negative)	Tobramycin	3–5 mg/kg/24 hr, producing blood levels of 2.5 mg/ml in presence of normal renal function
	Gentamicin	3–5 mg/kg/24 hr (see Klebsiella pneumonia, above)
Hemophilus influenza	Ampicillin	2.0–6.0 g/24 hr, increasing to 8–12 g/24 hr for serious infections
	Chloramphenicol	3.0–4.0 g/24 hr PO (50–100 mg/kg/24 hr)

A complete discussion of antibiotic therapy related to pulmonary disease and/or complications is beyond the scope of this chapter.

process of the mediastinum, lung, esophagus, or subdiaphragmatic space. The symptom complex may include shortness of breath and pleuritic chest pain. A major objective finding is continued fever during antibiotic administration. Other findings include those of pleural effusion. Treatment consists of rigorous antibiotic therapy and chest tube drainage (see discussion of chest tubes, later in this chapter). A serious complication of empyema is irreversible fibrotic changes that compromise pulmonary ventilation, due to trapping of the lung on the involved side.

BRONCHOSPASM

Bronchospasm implies a narrowing of the airways resulting in increased airway resistance, which can be caused by a variety of mechanisms: (1) inhalation of toxic or irritating substances such as smoke, pollens, dust, or noxious gases;

(2) bronchitis; (3) severe coughing episodes; (4) extreme cold; and (5) exercise. Although bronchospasm is usually associated with asthma, these mechanisms may precipitate bronchospasm in anyone.

Signs and symptoms vary with the degree of bronchospasm. The patient may complain of shortness of breath associated with wheezing respirations. Further findings include tachycardia, tachypnea, retractions, restlessness, anxiety, inspiratory/expiratory wheezing, hypoxemia, hypercapnia, cyanosis, and coughing. One must be aware that a decrease in wheezing does not necessarily mean decreased bronchospasm, but rather progression of airway narrowing and markedly decreased ventilation.

Treatment is directed at removing the cause of bronchospasm and initiating bronchodilator therapy (see Table 13-2). The patient must be observed for increasing bronchospasm and deteriorating pulmonary function manifested by a rising PCO_2.

Table 13–2
Pulmonary Drugs and Their Sites of Action

Sites of Drug Actions

1. Receptors of Smooth Muscle – Airways

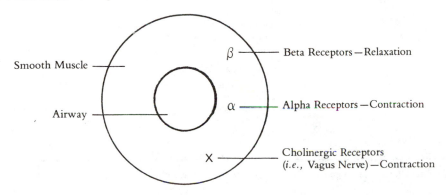

β ——— Beta Receptors — Relaxation

α ——— Alpha Receptors — Contraction

X ——— Cholinergic Receptors
(*i.e.,* Vagus Nerve) — Contraction

Smooth Muscle

Airway

2. Cellular Metabolism

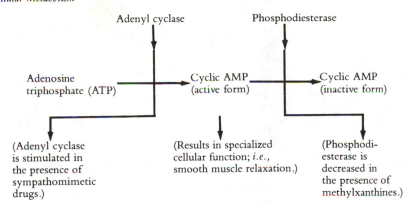

Adenyl cyclase

Phosphodiesterase

Adenosine
triphosphate (ATP)

Cyclic AMP
(active form)

Cyclic AMP
(inactive form)

(Adenyl cyclase
is stimulated in
the presence of
sympathomimetic
drugs.)

(Results in specialized
cellular function; *i.e.,*
smooth muscle relaxation.)

(Phosphodi-
esterase is
decreased in
the presence of
methylxanthines.)

Cyclic AMP is one of the intermediaries of cellular metabolism in the sequence
of energy production. It is present in almost all cell membranes and is influenced
by a variety of agents, such as hormones and drugs.

3. Mast cells

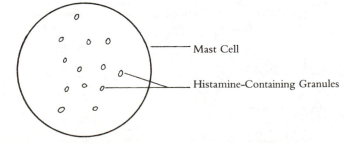

Mast Cell

Histamine-Containing Granules

Mast cells with histamine-containing granules are abundant in allergic asthmatics.

Table 13–2 *(Continued)*

Pulmonary Drugs	Action	Dosage	Side-Effects
1. *Bronchodilators* Methylxan- thines	↓ phosphodiester- ase with ↑ cyclic AMP (active form)	IV: loading — 5 mg/kg; maintenance — 0.9 mg/kg PO: aminophyl- line — 1200 mg/ 24 hr; oxtriphyl- line (Choledyl) — 1600 mg/24 hr NB: Dosages adjusted to maintain serum theophylline levels 10 μg–20 μg/ ml	Nausea Vomiting Nervousness Arrhythmias Seizures

> Theophylline — dosage increased by 50% for smokers who can tolerate the drug if effect is less than optimum
> dosage decreased by 50% for patients with liver failure, heart failure, hypox- emia and in shock

Pulmonary Drugs	Action	Dosage	Side-Effects
Sympathomi- metics	Beta (β) stimu- lants		Relatively few side- effects with recom- mended dosages
Isoetharine (Bronkosol)	Stimulates adenyl cyclase with ↑ cyclic AMP (active form)	Delivered via nebulizer — either hand- powered or IPPB 0.5 ml with sterile water or normal saline (1:3 conc.) q4hr	Tachycardia Palpitations Nausea Headache Changes in blood pressure Nervousness
Terbutaline (Brethine)	Stimulates adenyl cyclase with ↑ cyclic AMP (active form)	5 mg PO q8hr; 0.25 mg SC not to exceed 0.5 mg q4hr	↑ Heart rate Nervousness Tremor Palpitations Dizziness Usually transient and do not require treatment
Metaproter- enol (Alupent, Metaprel)	Stimulates adenyl cyclase with ↑ cyclic AMP (active form)	Metered dose device: 0.65 mg/metered dose; 20 mg PO t.i.d.	Tachycardia Hypertension Palpitations Nervousness Tremor Nausea and vomiting
2. *Steroids*	Stimulate adenyl- ate cyclase with ↑ cyclic 3′, 5′ — AMP; may facili- tate use of β- stimulants; anti-inflammatory agents		

Table 13–2 *(Continued)*

Pulmonary Drugs	Action	Dosage	Side-Effects
Prednisone		Variable; *e.g.*, 40–60 mg PO initially and decreasing according to PFT and eosinophil counts (in patients with ↑ Eos 2° to allergin mediated responses)	Formation of glucose from body protein→ ↑ blood sugar Depletion of bone calcium — osteoporosis Increase in fat production Impairment of immunologic response Reduction of inflammatory response Increase in gastric acidity Elevation of blood pressure Acne
Methyl-prednisolone (Solu-Medrol)		Variable; *e.g.*, 100 mg IV and repeat with one-fourth original dose q6hr	Same as for prednisone
Beclomethasone (Vanceril)	Virtually same as above except it is an inhaled preparation with high topical effect on the airways and low systemic activity	Inhalation device; 2 inhalations (100 μg) q.i.d.	Oral candidiasis Mild oropharyngeal symptoms — discomfort and dryness of throat
3. *Cromolyn sodium* (Aarane, Intal)	Prophylactic bronchospasmolytic in allergic asthma; *not* useful in acute bronchospasm; probably strengthens mast cell membrane, preventing release of histamine and therefore decreases bronchospasm in the allergic asthmatic	1 capsule via inhaler device q.i.d.	Maculopapular rash Urticaria Cough and/or bronchospasm

CHRONIC OBSTRUCTIVE PULMONARY DISEASE (COPD)

The common pulmonary complications discussed above are potentially reversible causes of respiratory insufficiency, but several disease entities result in COPD. These include chronic bronchitis, emphysema, and asthma. COPD is a national health problem second only to heart disease, and it is the most common cause of respiratory insufficiency.

Chronic Bronchitis

Chronic infection or irritation of the bronchi may result in bronchitis. The mucus-secreting glands of the tracheobronchial tree become

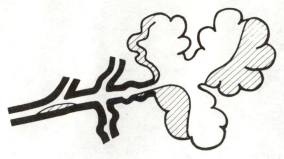

FIGURE 13-2.
Bronchitis. Inflammation, thickening produce narrowing of airways. Lined areas indicate secretions.

thickened and encroach on the diameter of the airway lumen (see Fig. 13-2). In addition there is increased mucus production in peripheral airways. By far the most common cause is tobacco smoking.

The two most common bacterial organisms isolated from the secretions of the chronic bronchitic are *Hemophilus influenzae* and pneumococcus. Exacerbation of chronic bronchitis with resultant respiratory insufficiency most often results from an acute bacterial inflammation of the bronchial tree. An essential prophylactic measure in preventing an acute inflammatory process is rigorous bronchial hygiene to promote clearance of secretions that provide an ideal medium for bacterial growth in the peripheral airways. In contrast to emphysema, chronic bronchitis may have a reversible component if the source of chronic infection or irritation is treated.

Emphysema
Emphysema is an anatomic alteration of the terminal air spaces, the acini, where exchange of oxygen and carbon dioxide takes place. Emphysema is an irreversible abnormal dilatation of the acinus accompanied by destructive changes of acinar walls, with resultant loss of lung elastic recoil.[6] The destructive process resulting in airway obstruction develops insidiously. In contrast to the chronic bronchitic, patients with emphysema usually have mild chronic hypoxemia because destruction of acinar walls is accompanied by destruction of corresponding vasculature. The ratio of ventilated to perfused lung tissue remains stable (see Fig. 13-3).

The majority of patients with COPD will have a mixture of chronic bronchitis and emphysema rather than "pure" bronchitis or emphysema (see Table 13-3).

Asthma
In comparison with emphysema and, to a lesser extent, chronic bronchitis, asthma is a reversible

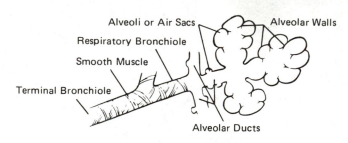

Alveoli or Air Sacs

Alveolar Walls

Respiratory Bronchiole

Smooth Muscle

Terminal Bronchiole

Alveolar Ducts

With Breakdown of Alveolar Walls

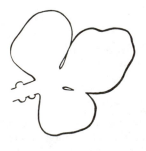

Emphysematous Bulla at Surface of Lung

Pleura

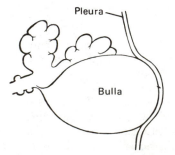

Bulla

FIGURE 13-3.
Emphysema. Airway showing normal primary lobule *(top)* and emphysematous lobule *(bottom)*. (Introduction to Lung Diseases, 6th ed, p 71. New York, American Lung Association, 1975)

Table 13-3
COPD: Features that Distinguish Bronchitis and Emphysema

Features	Bronchitis	Emphysema
Clinical Exam		
History	Often recurrent chest infections	Frequently only insidious dyspnea
Chest exam	Noisy chest, slight over-distention	Quiet chest, marked over-distention
Sputum	Frequently copious and purulent	Usually scanty and mucoid
Chronic cor pulmonale	Common	Infrequent
Physiological Tests		
Chronic hypoxemia	Often severe	Usually mild
Chronic hypercapnia	Common	Unusual
Pulmonary hypertension	Often severe	Usually mild
Cardiac output	Normal	Often low
Therapeutic Modalities		
Bronchial hygiene	Very important for clearance of secretions	Less important unless patient has respiratory infection

Adapted from Burrows B et al: Respiratory Insufficiency. Chicago, Year Book Medical Publishers, 1975

obstructive pulmonary disease in which hyper-reactive bronchial airways respond to a variety of irritating stimuli (*e.g.,* allergens, infections, exercise, and emotional factors) by widespread narrowing and subsequent bronchospasm (see Fig. 13-4).[7] Figure 13-5 illustrates a series of events that may become a vicious cycle resulting in life-threatening status asthmaticus unless bronchospasm is controlled.

Spontaneous remission of bronchospasm may occur; however, use of bronchodilating agents (see Table 13-2) in addition to rigorous bronchial hygiene is the usual mode of treatment. The potential severity of an asthma attack is frequently minimized by these means.

According to Petty (1975), status asthmaticus is defined as "unrelenting acute wheezing dyspnea not responsive to oral, inhaled or subcuta-

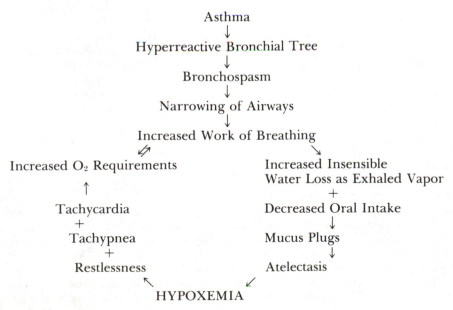

FIGURE 13-4.
Sequence of events leading from asthma to hypoxemia.

Bronchiole Obstructed on Expiration by:

1. Muscle Spasm

2. Swelling of Mucosa

3. Thick Secretions

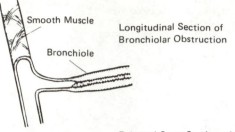

Smooth Muscle

Longitudinal Section of
Bronchiolar Obstruction

Bronchiole

Enlarged Cross-Section of Same

Muscle in Spasm

Swollen Mucous Membrane

Thick Secretions

FIGURE 13-5.
Pathophysiological changes in bronchial asthma. (Introduction to Lung Disease, 6th ed, p 63. New York, American Lung Association, 1975)

neous sympathomimetic amines or connectional doses of oral or rectal methylxanthines."[8] The patient manifests a dramatic picture of acute anxiety, marked labored breathing, tachycardia, or diaphoresis. Deterioration of pulmonary function results in alveolar hypoventilation with subsequent hypoxemia, hypercapnia, and acidemia. A rising PCO_2 in a patient with an acute asthmatic attack is often the first objective indication of status asthmaticus.

Multiple therapeutic modalities must be instituted. All patients in status asthmaticus demonstrate hypoxemia and require oxygen therapy. Dehydration usually exists and requires correction. Pharmacologic agents consist of methylxanthines, sympathomimetic amines, and corticosteroids. If pulmonary function cannot be improved and respiratory failure ensues, the patient may require intubation and assisted ventilation.

BRONCHIAL HYGIENE

Bronchial hygiene consists of any one or a combination of the following measures: aerosol therapy, deep breathing, coughing, and postural drainage. The therapeutic goals of bronchial hygiene are removal of secretions, improved ventilation, and oxygenation. Specific bronchial hygiene is dependent upon existing pulmonary dysfunction.

The need for an effectiveness of various modalities of bronchial hygiene must be evaluated frequently.

The following discussion is not intended as a specific instructional guide for bronchial hygiene. Techniques in delivery of bronchial hygiene are paramount in the prevention and treatment of pulmonary complications. The reader is referred to the bibliography for further references.

Intermittent Positive Pressure Breathing (IPPB)

IPPB treatments are used for improved administration and deposition of aerosols. Successful IPPB treatments will be determined by the patient's position, ventilatory pattern, and ability to cooperate and follow instructions.

An adequate ventilatory pattern during an IPPB treatment consists of a deep inspiration aimed at increasing normal tidal volume two to three times. The patient is then instructed to hold his breath briefly to provide greater depth and deposition of aerosolized medication, water, or saline. Exhalation should take twice as long as inspiration, resulting in complete exhalation.

Contraindications of IPPB therapy may include pneumothorax, active pulmonary tuberculosis in which infection or hemoptysis is hazardous, and hemoptysis. Caution should be taken in the use of IPPB treatment immediately following lung resection because of potential bronchial leakage.

The use and value of IPPB therapy have become controversial issues.

Inhaled Moisture

The primary purposes of inhaled moisture are hydration of normal mucociliary clearance mechanisms and liquefaction of secretions. Adequate systemic hydration is essential for optimum results of inhaled moisture.

The most important aspect of inhaled moisture therapy is active deep breathing by the patient followed by brief breath holding to allow deposition of aerosolized particles and slow, complete exhalation.

Potential hazards that may exist include bronchospasm in patients with hyperreactive airways and infection from contaminated equipment. The ultimate success of inhaled moisture therapy will depend upon clearance of secretions with forceful rigorous coughing.

Effective Cough

An effective cough is an essential prerequisite for clearance of secretions. Various techniques are available to assist the patient in achieving an effective cough, such as a maximal exhalation followed by a maximal inspiration followed by a forceful cough. Gentle pressure to the trachea above the manubrial notch may be used to stimulate cough production in the comatose or uncooperative patient.

Chest Physiotherapy

Inadequate clearance of secretions dictates the need for chest physiotherapy. Chest physiotherapy includes use of gravity to aid flow of secretions to a point where they can be expectorated with forceful coughing maneuvers or suctioned with a catheter. The effectiveness of positioning may be augmented by chest percussion.[9] (Figure 13-6 demonstrates the positions for postural drainage.)

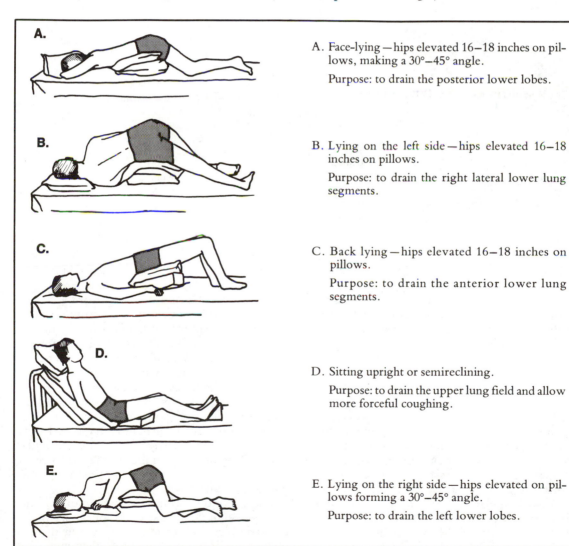

A. Face-lying—hips elevated 16–18 inches on pillows, making a 30°–45° angle.

Purpose: to drain the posterior lower lobes.

B. Lying on the left side—hips elevated 16–18 inches on pillows.

Purpose: to drain the right lateral lower lung segments.

C. Back lying—hips elevated 16–18 inches on pillows.

Purpose: to drain the anterior lower lung segments.

D. Sitting upright or semireclining.

Purpose: to drain the upper lung field and allow more forceful coughing.

E. Lying on the right side—hips elevated on pillows forming a 30°–45° angle.

Purpose: to drain the left lower lobes.

FIGURE 13-6.
Positions used in lung drainage.

Anatomical Deadspace (V_D anat.)

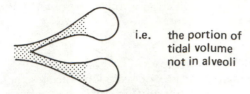

i.e. the portion of tidal volume not in alveoli

Alveolar Deadspace (V_D alv.)

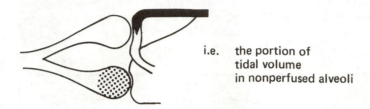

i.e. the portion of tidal volume in nonperfused alveoli

Physiological Deadspace (V_D phys.)

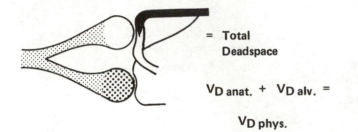

= Total Deadspace

$$V_D \text{ anat.} + V_D \text{ alv.} = V_D \text{ phys.}$$

FIGURE 13-7.
Subdivisions of physiological dead space. Only that part of the volume of ventilation which enters perfused alveoli is effective in blood-gas exchange and is labelled as alveolar ventilation. The remainder is wasted or dead space ventilation. Total ventilation may be subdivided accordingly.

Total
ventilation
(V)
−
Alveolar
ventilation
(V_A)
=
Dead space
ventilation
(V_D)

This division applies equally to minute ventilation and to the individual tidal volumes. Dividing by the respiratory frequency we get

Tidal
volume
(V_T)
−
Alveolar
tidal
volume
=
Physiological
dead space
($V_{D\text{phys.}}$)

(Berdixen HH et al: Respiratory Care, p 17. St. Louis, C.V. Mosby, 1965)

Modification or contraindication of chest physiotherapy may be necessary in the following: increased intracranial pressure, intravascular bleeds, cervical cord trauma, unstable vertebral fractures, chest and abdominal trauma, hiatal hernia, obesity, osteoporosis, and orthopaedic appliances.

PULMONARY EMBOLI

Pulmonary emboli may occur as a complication of many medical conditions that predispose to venous thrombosis, including postoperative states, prolonged bed rest, and trauma. Deep venous thrombosis, particularly in the lower extremities, is the main predisposing factor for pulmonary emboli.

Both pulmonary and hemodynamic changes occur as a result of occlusion of a pulmonary artery by an embolus. Alveoli are ventilated but not perfused, thereby producing areas of ineffective ventilation, that is, increased respiratory dead space (see Fig. 13-7).

Pneumoconstriction resulting from a lack of carbon dioxide normally present in pulmonary arterial blood shifts ventilation from the underperfused alveoli. The decrease in pulmonary blood flow due to an embolus results in deficient nutrients for surfactant production, ultimately resulting in atelectasis. The severity of hemodynamic changes depends upon the size of the embolus. Increased pulmonary vascular resistance occurs, which, if pulmonary blood flow remains constant, may result in right ventricular failure.[10] Pulmonary embolus may resolve or infrequently may lead to death of tissue, that is, pulmonary infarction.

The symptom complex of a pulmonary embolus depends upon its size. Dyspnea, one of the most frequent complaints, is often out of proportion to the physical findings. Tachypnea and tachycardia may be present in varying degrees. Mild fever may exist although leukocytosis is rare.[11] It should be noted that pleuritic chest pain and hemoptysis are associated with pulmonary infarction rather than with pulmonary embolus.

Massive pulmonary embolization results in a more dramatic clinical manifestation of acute illness. The patient develops pronounced tachypnea, usually with cyanosis, tachycardia, restlessness, confusion, and hypotension. The resulting shock state produces concomitant changes of decreased urinary output and cold clammy skin.

A suspected pulmonary embolus may be confirmed by radioactive lung scanning and pulmonary angiography. Treatment is anticoagulation and correction of predisposing causes of venous thrombosis. Anticoagulant therapy is administered by various ways in different institutions. The nurse must be aware that multiple drug interactions may occur with use of anticoagulant therapy.

HEMOTHORAX/PNEUMOTHORAX

A pneumothorax occurs when air enters the pleural space between the visceral and parietal pleurae. Blood in this location is called a *hemothorax.*

There are two types of pneumothorax, spontaneous and tension pneumothorax.

A *spontaneous pneumothorax* may result from the rupture of a subpleural alveolar cyst or an emphysematous bleb. The signs and symptoms will vary with the size of the pneumothorax and may range from mild shortness of breath to chest pain and signs of increasing respiratory distress. Physical examination reveals decreased breath sounds and decreased respiratory movement on the affected side. The diagnosis is confirmed by roentgenography.

Chest trauma, IPPB, positive end expiratory pressure (PEEP), cardiopulmonary resuscitation, thoracic and high abdominal surgery, and thoracentesis may precipitate an iatrogenic pneumothorax or hemothorax.[12] A pneumothorax, regardless of etiology, becomes life-threatening as tension in the pleural space occurs.

When a *tension pneumothorax* develops, the tear in lung bronchus or chest wall acts as a one-way valve that allows air to enter the pleural space on inspiration, but not escape on expiration. If it is not immediately recognized and treated, massive atelectasis will result. In addition, the mediastinal structures are displaced toward the unaffected side, and tracheal deviation may be especially prominent. This mediastinal shift will result in a decreased venous return, decreased cardiac output, and ultimately death.

Clinically, the patient manifests severe respiratory distress. Agitation, cyanosis, and tachypnea are severe. Tachycardia and the initial increase in blood pressure are followed by hypotension as cardiac output decreases. The diagnosis is based on the clinical manifestations as well as the clinical setting. Any patient who is being ventilated and suddenly develops acute respiratory distress during ventilation evidenced by markedly increased inspiratory pressures is a prime candidate for a tension pneumothorax. Treatment must be immediate.

A 16- to 18-gauge needle inserted into the second, third, or fourth intercostal space at the midclavicular line on the affected side will relieve the pressure. Once this has been accomplished, a chest tube should be inserted and underwater seal drainage instituted to prevent any further development of tension.

FLAIL CHEST

Trauma to the thorax resulting in a flail chest is caused by the disruption of the normally semirigid structure of the chest cage from (1) fracture of three or more adjoining ribs in one or more places, (2) rib fracture(s) with costochondral separation, or (3) sternal fractures. Wherever fractures occur, that segment loses continuity with the remaining intact chest wall and subsequent paradoxical movement occurs.

During paradoxical ventilation, as the intact chest expands, the injured "flail" segment is depressed, thereby limiting the amount of negative intrathoracic pressure needed to move air into the lungs. During expiration the flail segment bulges outward, thus interfering with exhalation. The degree of ventilatory impairment that results from a flail chest is proportional to the extent of injury. The occurrence of concomitant hemothorax/pneumothorax further impairs ventilation.

During inspiration, the intrapleural pressures on the unaffected side are greater, thus displacing the mediastinum toward it. Conversely, during expiration the negative pressure on the unaffected side is less than on the affected side, and the mediastinum shifts toward the affected side. This phenomenon, known as *mediastinal flutter,* further impairs ventilation as well as cardiac output. Normally venous return to the right heart is enhanced during inspiration. Reduced intrapleural negative pressure during inspiration impairs circulating dynamics, thus decreasing venous return to the heart, right atrial filling, and ultimately cardiac output.

Frequent patient assessment, including anterior and posterior visual inspection of chest movement, is essential for evaluation and intervention in the treatment of a patient with a flail chest.

Treatment is directed toward improvement of ventilation and oxygenation as well as stabilization of the chest wall. The increased ventilatory effort that is needed for adequate ventilation is difficult for the patient to maintain because of the pain caused by injury. A mechanically controlled volume ventilator, which will enhance chest wall stability and improve alveolar ventilation, is the treatment of choice. Ventilatory support is needed for approximately 14 to 21 days or until the chest is adequately stabilized.

A hemothorax or pneumothorax is treated by chest tubes, underwater seal drainage, and surgical intervention when repair of structural damage is necessary. Chest tubes with underwater seal drainage systems are usually maintained during the entire time the patient needs ventilatory assistance to manage not only the initial hemothorax/pneumothorax, but any which occur as a complication during positive pressure mechanical ventilation.

UNDERWATER SEAL DRAINAGE

It is important to recall several principles to understand underwater seal drainage. There is normally negative (less than atmospheric) pressure in the pleural space, which ranges from minus 5 to 3 cm of water during expiration.[13] The development of negative pressure during inspiration allows air to enter the lungs. As the extrapulmonary and atmospheric pressures equalize, active inspiration ceases, and passive exhalation occurs. When the integrity of the pleural space is disrupted, the air or fluid that accumulates prevents the development of negative pressure necessary for normal ventilation.

Chest drains and underwater seal drainage are used to restore the physiological integrity of the pleural space. A chest tube (drain) inserted into the pleural space will remove air or fluid. The underwater seal drainage to which the chest tube is connected prevents backflow into the pleural space (see Fig. 13-8).

A glass rod under water in a bottle establishes negative pressure in the water seal system. The depth of the rod in the water determines the degree of negative pressure. A basic law of physics states that gases and fluids move from areas of greater pressure to areas of lesser pressure. Therefore, the air or fluid disrupting the normal pressures in the pleural space will drain into the chest bottle in an attempt to equalize the more negative pressure of the underwater seal drainage system. The air vent in the chest bottle allows the drained air to escape, preventing pressure buildup in the bottle.

Larger amounts of blood or fluid draining from the pleural space necessitate modification of the underwater seal system. A second bottle may be added to accommodate large amounts of fluid (see Fig. 13-9).

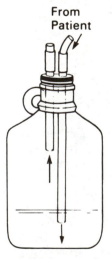

FIGURE 13-8.
One-bottle system underwater seal drainage.

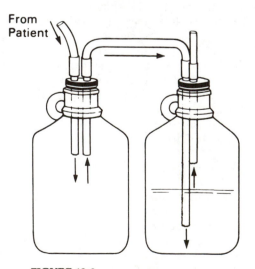

FIGURE 13-9.
Two-bottle system underwater seal drainage.

Suction may be added to the system if the air leak into the pleural space accumulates faster than the system can remove it (see Fig. 13-10). A single self-contained underwater seal drainage unit which has the capacity to function as a two- or three-bottle system with suction has been developed.

The system must remain patent. Malfunction of the chest tube or underwater seal drainage system may result in inadequate removal of air or fluid from the pleural space. Occlusion of the system at any point may result in the development of a tension pneumothorax. The life-threatening seriousness of a tension pneumothorax has led to the consensus that clamping of chest tubes for more than a few seconds is a dangerous practice.[14]

NONPULMONARY RESPIRATORY COMPLICATIONS

Patients who have surgery, notably high abdominal thoracic and low abdominal resection, are especially susceptible to respiratory embarrassment. The mechanism of pulmonary compromise is a restrictive entity in which there is a reduction of vital capacity, thus resulting in a limited ventilatory reserve. The major restrictive insult occurs sometime in the first 24 hours postoperatively.[15] Patients without complications gradually resume their preoperative ventilatory status.

Postoperative pulmonary complications may be avoided or minimized by adequate preoperative cardiopulmonary evaluation by the critical care nurse. The nurse may thereby institute those measures that are directed toward monitoring pulmonary status and providing modalities aimed toward improving vital capacity.

Pharmacotherapy. Appropriate administration of narcotics and sedatives is a necessary adjunct to pulmonary care. The use of these drugs must be guided by the patient's clinical status. The aim of pharmacologic therapy is to minimize pain so that the patient will tolerate respiratory therapy and other therapeutic modalities. On the other hand, overzealous use of sedatives and narcotics may result in respiratory depression and acute respiratory failure.

The patient with a sedative or narcotic overdosage presents with respiratory insufficiency. The severity of the respiratory insufficiency is dependent upon the specific drug(s), amount ingested, time of ingestion, and rate of metabolism of the drug(s).

Factors that may alter drug effects include multiple drug ingestion, hepatic or renal function abnormalities, and preexisting pulmonary disease such as COPD.

Care of patients with drug overdose is guided by this information as well as by the knowledge that patients with certain types of drug ingestion (*e.g.,* glutethimide) may show a fluctuation in level of consciousness. This presents a problem in the maintenance of an adequate airway. It must not be assumed that a patient who at one time appears alert and able to maintain his airway will continue to do so.

There are also drugs that in normal phar-

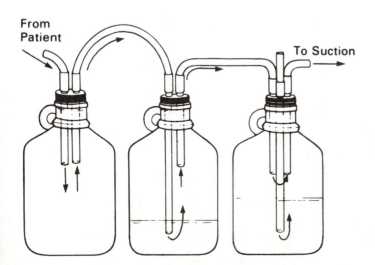

FIGURE 13-10.
Underwater seal drainage with suctioning.

macologic doses can cause neuromuscular blockade with resultant respiratory paralysis. These include kanamycin, gentamicin, streptomycin, neomycin, and polymyxin B.

Neuromuscular Involvement.   Disease states or trauma involving the neuromuscular system may affect pulmonary function. The degree of dysfunction will depend upon the extent of respiratory muscle involvement.

In certain neurologic diseases the gag and cough reflexes may be diminished, resulting in aspiration of food, fluid, or secretions. The aspirated contents can cause atelectasis and pneumonia which, if not recognized, will lead to progressive respiratory failure. As impairment of respiratory muscles progresses, there is a resultant decrease in vital capacity.

Taking serial measurements of the vital capacity is an important method of assessing adequacy of pulmonary function. This assessment can be done quite readily by the nurse. Cardinal signs of respiratory embarrassment, pulmonary function measurements, and arterial blood gas analysis must be correlated with the clinical status of the patient.

Long-term management of a patient with a neuromuscular disorder includes maintenance of a patent airway, rigorous clearance of secretions, treatment of infections, maximum mobilization of the patient, and ventilatory assistance when indicated.

Restrictive Disorders.   Several entities restrict chest wall expansion with resultant compromised pulmonary function. These include kyphoscoliosis, rheumatoid spondylitis, scleroderma, pectus excavatum, and use of orthopaedic appliances such as spica casts. These patients may, in a stable environment, have normal pulmonary function. A crisis such as trauma or a major medical illness such as drug overdose may precipitate severe respiratory impairment. In the management of these patients the nurse must use those measures that maximize ventilation and minimize pulmonary complications.

ACUTE RESPIRATORY FAILURE (ARF)

ARF may be defined as respiratory dysfunction of such a degree that gas exchange is no longer

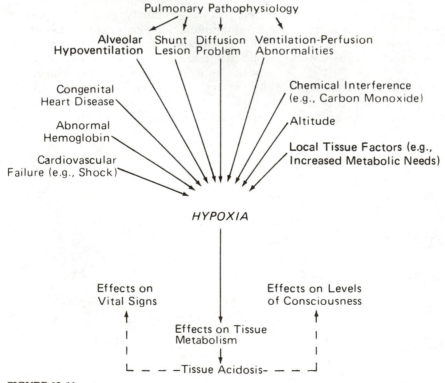

FIGURE 13-11.
Hypoxia: mechanisms and effects. (Brannin P: Oxygen therapy and measures of bronchial hygiene. Nurs Clin North Am 9, No. 1:111, 1974)

adequate to maintain normal arterial blood gases.[16] Quantitatively, ARF may be defined as a $PO_2 < 50$ torr with or without a $PCO_2 > 50$ torr[17] (see Fig. 13-11).

ARF may result from a variety of insults including pneumonia, atelectasis, and pneumothorax. Neuromuscular disease, drugs, toxins, and trauma may also lead to ARF.

The key to treatment of ARF is anticipation of its subsequent development in the face of a precipitating event. Management of the patient in the presence of ARF is twofold:

1. Establishment of adequate arterial oxygenation, thereby providing adequate tissue perfusion
2. Amelioration of the underlying cause(s) of ARF

Patient Management

Rigorous bronchial hygiene and carefully monitored oxygen therapy may eliminate the need for an artificial airway or ventilatory support. When these measures fail to provide adequate oxygenation and removal of carbon dioxide, an artificial airway or ventilatory support becomes mandatory.

Artificial Airway

Artificial airways have a threefold purpose:

1. Establishment of an airway
2. Protection of the airway, with the cuff inflated
3. Provision of continuous ventilatory assistance

Artificial airways require knowledgeable and aggressive nursing care to maintain the patency of the airway and maximize therapeutic effects while minimizing damage to the patient's natural airway.

The selection of the appropriate artificial airway is most important. Any artificial airway will increase airway resistance; therefore it is essential that the largest tube possible be used for intubation. The cuff on the endotracheal or tracheostomy tube must be low compliance (soft), thereby minimizing barotrauma to the trachea, vocal cords, and subglottic area. The competency of the cuff must be established prior to intubation. Approximately 10 ml of air is injected into the cuff prior to use.

Placing the Tube. Once an artificial airway is placed, it must be in the proper location and remain there. In order to properly ascertain tube placement, the cuff must be inflated. Anterior and lateral auscultation of the chest bilaterally aids in evaluation of tube position. It must be remembered that breath sounds can be transmitted to the nonventilated or inadequately ventilated lung field. The final analysis of tube placement must depend on roentgenography. Because of normal airway anatomy, endotracheal tubes have a tendency to enter the right main stem bronchus. Chest radiographs should be ordered immediately after tube placement. Evaluation of tube placement should be ongoing, since endotracheal and tracheostomy tubes may become dislodged during routing care.

Proper securement of an endotracheal or tracheostomy tube must ensure airway patency, proper alignment, and stability of the tube, and should minimize pressure at the insertion site. The tube should be immobilized so that it will not ride, slip, and twist unnecessarily and injure tissue with which it comes in contact (see Fig. 13-12).

It should be noted that an endotracheal tube is a round tube that is inserted through an elliptic opening, the vocal cords. Therefore a pathway is established for continual flow of oropharyngeal secretions and flora, which become potential pathogens to the lower respiratory tract. Use of minimal air leak technique reduces the flow of secretions and flora.

Inflating the Cuff. Appropriate inflation of a cuff on an artificial airway is based on the following rationale:

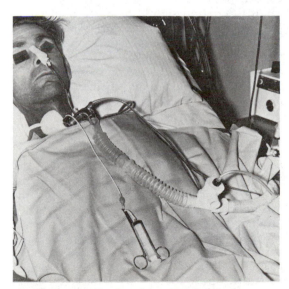

FIGURE 13-12.
Proper alignment for securing endotracheal tubing.

- It protects the airway in the presence of copious secretions
- It establishes a seal necessary for ventilatory support

An inflated cuff requires only that amount of air necessary to achieve a minimal air leak. A minimal air leak may be achieved and ascertained by the application of positive pressure (ventilator or self-inflating bag) to the patient's airway, during which time air is injected into the cuff until no leak is heard over the trachea or felt over the mouth or nose. Once this is achieved, ½ to 1 ml of air is removed and a minimal air leak is therefore achieved. This method of cuff inflation minimizes airway trauma due to excessive cuff pressures.

Deflating the Cuff. *It has been proved that periodic deflation of a cuff of an endotracheal or tracheostomy tube is of no value in minimizing tracheal damage.*[18]

Intelligent rationale for cuff deflation is based on

- The presence and amount of upper airway secretions
- Continuous ventilatory support
- The patient's ability to protect his airway

The purpose of cuff deflation is to remove pooled secretions that have accumulated above the cuff, which may seed the upper airway with potentially pathogenic bacterial growth. The frequency of cuff deflation is dictated by individual patient needs.

Cuff deflation should be performed while positive pressure is applied during inspiration. This establishes retrograde flow of secretions into the oropharynx, where rapid removal of these secretions is achieved by suctioning. The minimal air leak is then quickly reestablished to provide adequate ventilation and protection of the airway.

Suctioning

The presence of an artificial tube prevents the patient from coughing, which functions as the normal clearing mechanism. It also increases production of secretions due to the presence of a foreign object.[19] Suctioning therefore becomes paramount to remove secretions and maintain patency. The need for suctioning is determined by visual observation of secretions and, more importantly, by chest auscultation to determine the presence of secretions or mucus plugs in major airways. The authors recommend the following suctioning procedure:

1. Hyperoxygenate the patient with 100% oxygen using a bag or the ventilator (this can be done while the nurse is preparing for suctioning).
2. Assemble the following equipment:
   a. Atraumatic sterile catheter
   b. Glove
   c. Sterile irrigation container
   d. Sterile normal saline
   e. Syringe containing sterile normal saline for tracheal irrigation when indicated
3. Once the above two steps have been completed, a sterile catheter is quickly but gently inserted as far as possible into the artificial airway without application of suction. It is then withdrawn 1 to 2 cm and intermittent suction is applied as the catheter is simultaneously rotated and removed. The aspiration should not exceed 8 to 10 seconds. Prolonged aspiration can lead to severe hypoxemia, changes in pulmonary pressure and volume, and ultimately cardiac arrest.[20]
4. Reestablish ventilatory assistance, allowing the patient to receive 3 to 5 breaths before the procedure is repeated.

It should be noted that patients not on ventilators also need to be hyperoxygenated. The patient should be instructed to take deep breaths while connected to a 100% oxygen source. Patients incapable of taking a deep breath should be assisted by a positive pressure device.

If secretions are tenacious, 3 to 5 ml of sterile normal saline may be injected into the artificial airway. Secretions should be monitored for amount, consistency, odor, and color, and the observations recorded. Changes in any of these characteristics may necessitate changes in therapy. Laboratory analysis of secretions must be performed, based on patient assessment and response to existing therapy.

Humidification

An artificial airway excludes normal physiological airway humidification. Therefore, artificial humidification is essential for maintenance of airway patency and clearance of secretions. Determination of adequate airway humidification is based upon the consistency and amount of secretions as well as condensation visible in the oxygen tubing leading to the patient. The humidification devices attached to oxygen therapy equipment often become media for bacterial growth. Appropriate care should therefore be taken in the maintenance of all oxygen therapy equipment. Policies should be established to monitor, by culture, the presence of organisms.

Ventilators

When ventilatory support is required, the nurse must be aware of the degree of hypoxemia present, the percentage of oxygen required, and the underlying cause and subsequent management of ARF.

Ventilatory assistance does not negate the need for continued monitoring of the patient for signs of ARF but actually increases the need for rigorous assessment and aggressive pulmonary care. Ventilatory assistance in a sense buys time for the patient, and the amount we buy for a given patient is a direct reflection of the adequacy of management. Detailed information of ventilatory support is found in the next section of this chapter and in Chapter 14.

ADULT RESPIRATORY DISTRESS SYNDROME (ARDS)

ARDS is a sudden and severe form of respiratory failure that usually occurs in previously healthy individuals who have been exposed to a variety of pulmonary or systemic insults. Some precipitating factors include near drowning, fat emboli, sepsis, pancreatitis, pulmonary emboli, aspiration, and hemorrhage and trauma of any kind that occur 1 to 96 hours prior to onset of ARDS. Table 13-4 provides an extensive list of disorders associated with ARDS. This distinct clinical syndrome of diverse etiology appears to manifest common pathogenesis regardless of causative factors.

Pathogenesis

The common pathogenesis is damage to the alveolar capillary membrane. The exact mechanisms are unclear; however, in 1977, Hopewell and coworkers postulated a series of events in this pathogenesis. The events occur sequentially after the alveolar-capillary membrane has been damaged. The cells that produce surfactant, type II pneumocytes, may be damaged with a resultant decrease or inactivation of surfactant. The latter may lead to interstitial and alveolar edema which, in turn, also decreases surfactant. Alveolar or airway filling or closure may be affected by either the decrease of surfactant or the development of interstitial and alveolar edema. In-

Table 13-4
Disorders Associated With ARDS

Shock of any etiology	Inhaled toxins:
	Oxygen
Infectious causes:	Smoke
Gram-negative sepsis	Corrosive chemicals
Viral pneumonia	
Bacterial pneumonia	Hematologic disorders:
Fungal pneumonia	Intravascular coagulation
Pneumocystic carinii	Massive blood transfusion
	? Postcardiopulmonary bypass
Trauma:	
Fat emboli	Metabolic disorders:
Lung contusion	Pancreatitis
Nonthoracic trauma	Uremia
Head injury	Paraquat ingestion
Liquid aspiration:	Miscellaneous:
Gastric juice	Lymphangitic carcinomatosis
Fresh and salt water	Increased intracranial pressure
Hydrocarbon fluids	Eclampsia
	Postcardioversion
Drug overdose:	Radiation pneumonitis
Heroin	
Methadone	
Barbiturates	

Hopewell PC: ARADS. Basics of RD 17(4), 1979

creased permeability of endothelium and epithelium following alveolar-capillary membrane injury may also lead to interstitial and alveolar edema and thus, decreased alveolar or airway filling or closure.[21] The net effect of the above postulated events is threefold: (1) reduced functional residual capacity (FRC), (2) intrapulmonary shunting, and (3) reduced lung compliance.

Certain iatrogenic maneuvers may also effect various events in the aforementioned sequence thereby producing the same result.[22] Some of these maneuvers are

- High fraction of inspired oxygen (FIO_2) — above 0.5 torr O_2 may cause increased permeability of endothelium and epithelium
- Overhydration — may cause interstitial and alveolar edema
- Overexpansion of alveoli secondary to ventilatory assistance — may result in decreased surfactant

An increase in alveolar-capillary permeability leads to subsequent interstitial and alveolar edema and microatelectasis. Therefore, the amount of air remaining in the lungs at the end of a normal expiration, functional residual capacity (FRC), is decreased.

Mechanical properties of the lungs change. Lung distensibility (compliance) is decreased.

The lungs become stiff. Therefore, greater than normal ventilator pressures will be needed to maintain minute ventilation.

The pathogenesis of ARDS also includes markedly abnormal gas exchange. Hypoxemia is a cardinal feature of ARDS. This may be secondary to extensive interstitial and alveolar edema, decreased surfactant, atelectasis, shunting, or ventilation/perfusion (V/Q) imbalance.

Assessment

The clinical presentation of ARDS consists primarily of extreme tachypnea, tachycardia, refractory hypoxemia, and decreased lung compliance. Chest roentgenograms reveal bilateral alveolar infiltrate secondary to increased alveolar-capillary permeability and flux of fluid and protein into interstitium and alveoli.

Prevention

Prevention *must include anticipation.* Which patients have pulmonary or nonpulmonary trauma or disease entities known to be potential causes of ARDS? Train yourself to be an astute observer. Monitor the patients for early clues indicative of abnormal lung function — arterial blood gases, vital signs, and sensorium.

Treatment

Treatment consists of fluid management, ventilatory support, oxygen therapy, prevention of atelectasis, corticosteroids, treatment of infections, adequate nutritional support, and extracorporeal oxygenation.

Fluid management is *crucial.*   Recall the pathogenesis of increased alveolar-capillary permeability which results in interstitial and alveolar edema. Excessive administration of fluid in normal individuals can produce pulmonary edema and cause respiratory failure. As a rule of thumb, intravenous fluids should be administered in an amount appropriate to maintain adequate tissue perfusion with as little effect as possible on pulmonary wedge pressure.[23] (See Chapter 10, Hemodynamic Pressure Monitoring.)

An important aspect of treatment of true ARDS is mechanical ventilation and prevention. (For a detailed discussion of general and specific principles of ventilatory management the reader is referred to the ventilatory sections of Chapters 13 and 14.) A therapeutic goal of this treatment modality is to provide ventilatory support until the integrity of the alveolar-capillary membrane is reestablished.[24] Two additional goals are

- Maintenance of adequate ventilation and oxygenation during the critical period of severe hypoxemia
- Reversal of the etiologic factors that initially caused the respiratory distress to occur[25]

To facilitate reversal or prevention of atelectasis, tidal volumes of 10 to 15 ml/kg of body weight are recommended.

Positive End Expiratory Pressure (PEEP). Adequate ventilation and oxygenation are provided by a mechanical ventilator to which PEEP may be added. PEEP is maintained in the alveoli throughout the entire respiratory cycle, thereby preventing or minimizing alveolar collapse at the end of expiration (see Fig. 13-13). The goal of continuous PEEP is improved oxygenation with subsequent decrease in inspired oxygen concentration needed to correct life-threatening hypoxemia.

PEEP may alter intrathoracic pressures so that venous return and ultimately cardiac output are decreased. Careful monitoring of the patient's blood pressure, pulse, urine output, and sensorium is necessary. PEEP may also increase the patient's susceptibility to developing a pneumothorax and, more significantly, a tension pneumothorax. Anticipation of such an occurrence and immediate intervention will minimize the deleterious effects of pneumothorax.

Continuous clinical observation of the patient's response to ventilatory therapy is essential. Arterial blood gas determinations and measurement of vital signs guide oxygen therapy and application of PEEP. The altered alveolar-capillary permeability renders the patient with ARDS susceptible to dangerous fluid overload. Transudation of fluid into the alveoli impairs adequate ventilation. Fluid therapy must be carefully monitored with respect to the patient's ventilatory and hemodynamic status.

The patient's response to therapy and ultimate recovery are dependent upon the rapidity and adequacy of treatment of the ARDS and its precipitating and etiologic factor(s).

Oxygen Therapy.   Oxygen is a drug with essential therapeutic properties and potentially toxic side-effects. A cardinal manifestation of ARDS is refractory cyanosis — profound hypoxemia. However, the injudicious prescribing of oxygen in these patients may result in oxygen

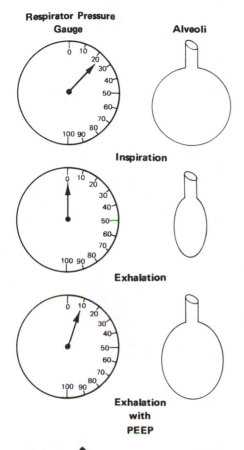

Respirator Pressure Gauge

Alveoli

Inspiration

Exhalation

Exhalation with PEEP

PEEP: Desired effect is: ↑ FRC (Functional Residual Capacity) ↓ F_IO_2 (Fraction of Inspired Oxygen)

FIGURE 13-13.
With PEEP, the alveoli have more gas remaining after exhalation for O_2/CO_2 exchange to take place.

toxicity. The toxic events of the latter include endothelial proliferation and perivascular edema. Recall that pathogenesis of ARDS includes increased permeability of alveolar-capillary membrane and both alveolar and interstitial edema.[26] Therefore, the least amount of oxygen should be administered to achieve adequate oxygenation. According to Bone, inspired oxygen concentrations of less than 50% do not appear to result in clinical manifestations of oxygen toxicity in the adult.[27]

Corticosteroids. The use of corticosteroids is controversial. Possible therapeutic effects include (1) reduction of the severity of lung injury, if given in large doses to stabilize lysosomal membranes and (2) reduction of pulmonary fibrosis.[28]

Monitoring for Infection. A questionable infection warrants thorough evaluation. A sample of pulmonary secretions is aspirated for a Gram

stain and culture. Invasive procedures such as fiberoptic bronchoscopy may be performed with relative ease on the intubated or ventilated patient—making certain adequate oxygenation and ventilation are maintained throughout the procedure. Other invasive procedures include thoracentesis and open-lung biopsy. Specific therapy needs to be initiated once an organism is identified. Pulmonary secretions must be monitored constantly for signs indicative of infection.

Nutritional management of ARDS is commonly overlooked during the early, as well as the late, stages. Optimal nutrition may be difficult to achieve, but the establishment and maintenance of an adequate feeding program will be imperative for the successful management of every patient with this syndrome.

In order for the body to adapt to the additional energy demands produced by trauma, sepsis, major surgery, and so forth, it must depend on body fuel reserve, ability to mobilize these reserves, and lastly, the ability to tolerate and use exogenous sources of essential fuels to prevent depletion of limited reserves.

A discussion of individual nutrients and minerals is beyond the scope of this chapter. However, it would be advantageous to briefly discuss proteins and the mineral phosphorus—both essential for adequate nutritional balance.

Protein is stored as a nitrogen reservoir. In addition, each molecule of protein is either part of the contractile force in muscle, part of cellular content or membrane, or an enzyme. Protein depletion is loss of essential function. Skeletal muscle provides the largest part of protein loss in starvation, with a resultant poor energy supply of less than 1 calorie per gram of muscle.[29]

The mineral element, phosphorus, probably has more functions than any other. It is essential for building bones and teeth, nucleic acids of all cells, phospholipids that regulate absorption and transportation of fats, enzymes involved in energy metabolism, buffer salts in the regulation of acid-base balance, and compounds involved in the sequential phases of muscle contraction. In other words, this mineral is involved in many metabolic pathways. The normal serum phosphate level is 2 to 5 mg/dl. Hypophosphatemia is said to occur with a serum level less than 1 mg/dl. A patient with ARDS who has hypophosphatemia may be very difficult to wean off the ventilatory support system.

In conclusion, to maintain an essential, adequate, nutritional balance during this acute syndrome, intravenous hyperalimentation should be considered as a primary therapeutic modality (see Chapter 27).

SUMMARY

Three phases of lung function—ventilation, diffusion, and perfusion—exist simultaneously to provide oxygenation and removal of carbon dioxide from tissues. Pulmonary and nonpulmonary pathophysiological states may exist and interfere with normal function at any one of these three levels. The critical care nurse must have a thorough understanding of normal lung function to be able to assess the patient's respiratory status, anticipate compromised lung function, and intervene appropriately.

REFERENCES

1. Burrows B et al: Respiratory Insufficiency, p 118. Chicago, Year Book Medical Publishers, 1975
2. Fraser R et al: Diagnosis of Disease of the Chest, Vol 1, pp 196–239. Philadelphia, W. B. Saunders, 1970
3. Burrows: Respiratory Insufficiency, p 119
4. Felson B et al: Principles of Chest Roentgenology, p 127. Philadelphia, W. B. Saunders, 1965
5. Burrows: Respiratory Insufficiency, p 116
6. Thurlbeck W: Chronic bronchitis and emphysema. Basics of RD, p 3. New York, American Thoracic Society, 1974
7. Thurlbeck W: Chronic Airflow Obstruction in Lung Disease, p 386. Philadelphia, W. B. Saunders, 1976
8. Petty T: Status asthmaticus, lecture given at a pulmonary medicine course, March 11–14, 1975, Continuing Medical Education, University of Colorado School of Medicine
9. Brannin P: Oxygen therapy and measures of bronchial hygiene. Nurs Clin North Am 9, No. 1:116–121, 1974
10. Moser K: Diagnostic measures in pulmonary embolism. Basics of RD, p 1. New York, American Thoracic Society, 1975
11. Fitzmaurice J et al: Current concepts of pulmonary embolism: Implications for nursing practice. Heart Lung 3, No. 2:210–211, 1974
12. Bendixen H: Pneumothorax. In Weil M, Shubin H (eds): Critical Care Medicine, p 28. John W. Kolen, 1974
13. Kersten L: Chest tube drainage system: Indications and principles of operation. Heart Lung 3, No. 1:97, 1974
14. Morgan C et al: The care and feeding of chest tubes. Am J Nurs 72, No. 2:307, 1972
15. Shapiro B et al: Clinical Application of Respiratory Care, pp 362–363. Chicago, Year Book Medical Publishers, 1975
16. Burrows: Respiratory Insufficiency, p 91
17. Brannin: Oxygen therapy, p 111
18. Bryant L et al: Reappraisal of the chest injury from cuffed tracheostomy tubes. JAMA 215, No. 4:624–628, 1971
19. Kudla M: The care of the patient with respiratory insufficiency. Nurs Clin North Am 8, No. 1:184, 1973
20. *Ibid.,* p 184
21. Hopewell PC et al: Chapter 5. In Shibel EM et al: Respiratory Emergencies, pp 101–128. St. Louis, C. V. Mosby, 1977
22. *Ibid.*
23. *Ibid,* p 115
24. Bone RC: Treatment of severe hypoxemia due to the adult respiratory distress syndrome. Arch Intern Med 140:85–89, 1980
25. Petty: lecture
26. Hopewell: Respiratory Emergencies, pp 101–128
27. Bone: Treatment of hypoxemia, pp 85–89
28. Hopewell: Respiratory Emergencies, pp 101–128
29. Henry RH: Surgical nutrition: Parenteral and oral. In Kinney JM et al (eds): Manual of Preoperative and Postoperative Care, pp 75–108. Philadelphia, W. B. Saunders, 1971

BIBLIOGRAPHY

Demos RR et al: Criteria for optimum PEEP. Respir Care, 22, No. 6:596–601, 1977
Harper HA: Review of Physiological Chemistry, pp 392–412. Los Altos, Land Medical Publications, 1971
Koda-Kimble MA et al (eds): Applied Therapeutics for Clinical Pharmacists, 2nd ed. San Francisco, Applied Therapeutics, 1978
Springer RR et al: The influence of PEEP on survival of patients in respiratory failure. Am J Med 66:196–200, 1979

Eileen Brent

VENTILATORY SUPPORT

Once a patient has been intubated and resuscitated successfully, the commitment to mechanical ventilation has been made. This commitment poses a high financial and psychological burden on the patient and family. Since mortality is reduced very little, every effort and consideration must be given to prevent mechanical ventilation.

Two approaches that may eliminate the need for mechanical ventilation are:

- Identification of high-risk patients
- Institution of appropriate measures to forestall or prevent respiratory failure

Patients are predisposed to developing respiratory failure when any of the systems involved in respiration are compromised or overwhelmed (see Table 13-5). The degree of risk for developing respiratory failure depends on the patient's ability to move air, secretions, and blood. Inability to do the latter is reflected clinically as pulmonary edema due to poor cardiac output.

ASSESSMENT

Respiratory failure is defined as an inability to maintain an adequate pH, $PaCO_2$, and PaO_2. *Adequate* means a pH greater than 7.25, a $PaCO_2$ less than 50 torr, and a PaO_2 greater than 50 torr with the patient on oxygen. As the arterial blood gases deteriorate and the patient fatigues, mechanical ventilatory support is indicated.

Many times, it is the nurse who initially recognizes the onset of respiratory failure. Simple bedside monitoring can alert the nurse to signs of patient decompensation. Two simple, noninvasive and inexpensive indicators that can be used are respiratory rate and vital capacity.

Normal *respiratory rate* is 16 to 20 breaths per minute. If the rate increases to 25 breaths per minute, the patient's status must be evaluated

Table 13-5
Body Systems and Possible Events Leading to Respiratory Failure

Systems	Events
1. Nervous system:	Head trauma
Brain stem	Polio
Spinal cord and nerves	Cervical (C1–C6) fractures
	Overdose
2. Muscular system:	Myasthenia gravis
Primary —diaphragm	Guillain-Barré
Secondary —respiratory	
3. Skeletal system:	Flail chest
Thorax	Kyphoscoliosis
4. Respiratory system:	Obstruction
Airways	Laryngeal edema
	Bronchitis
	Asthma
Alveoli	Emphysema
	Pneumonia
	Fibrosis
5. Cardiovascular system	Congestive heart failure
	Fluid overload
	Cardiac surgery
	Myocardial infarction

and appropriate measures instituted: that is, suctioning, postural drainage, and cupping. (See previous section on management modalities.) Once the rate reaches 40 or more per minute, the "work of breathing" to maintain less than acceptable blood gas values is high. Eventually, exhaustion occurs, and ventilatory assistance is required. This process may occur over hours or minutes, depending upon the patient's respiratory reserve (see Table 13-6).

Vital capacity, the second parameter, is a measure of ventilation. Using a simple bedside spirometer, the patient is asked to take a deep breath and exhale through the spirometer until he has completely emptied his lungs. If the vital capacity is less than 10 to 20 ml/kg, respiratory reserve is minimal. Serial monitoring of this parameter is more meaningful than a one-spot check. A good clinical example is a patient with a cervical spine injury. Serial monitoring of vital capacity may show the progression of ascending edema and dictate elective rather than crisis intubation and resuscitation.

In summary, identification of high-risk patients, serial monitoring and evaluation of progressive respiratory status, and institution of appropriate measures may forestall or negate the need for mechanical ventilation.

Table 13–6
Indications for Mechanical Ventilation

Parameters	Values	Action
Respiratory rate	< 10 breaths/min (diminished drive to breathe)	Evaluate patient and eliminate cause
	16–20 breaths/min	Normal
	28–40 breaths/min	Evaluate patient and institute appropriate measures
	> 40 breaths/min	Consider elective intubation/ventilation
Vital capacity	< 10–20 ml/kg (poor ventilatory reserve)	Watch for signs of respiratory failure; Prepare to initiate ventilatory support
Arterial Blood Gases		
pH	< 7.25	Evaluate in combination with $PaCO_2$, if it is rising
$PaCO_2$	> 50 torr	Evaluate in combination with pH, if it is decreasing
PaO_2	< 50 torr while on oxygen	Evaluate in combination with the pH and $PaCO_2$
Chest auscultation	Diminished or no breath sounds	Deliver 100% oxygen; Prepare ventilatory support
Heart rate and rhythm	Pulse over 120, arrhythmias	Monitor for arrhythmias
Activity	Extreme fatigue	Evaluate with above and take appropriate measures
Mental status	Confusion, delirium, somnolence	Monitor for hypoxic seizure activity

MECHANICAL VENTILATORS

Generally, today's ventilators can be divided into two categories—*volume* cycled and *pressure* cycled. Realistically, the type selected will depend upon the models present in the hospital and the familiarity of the physicians with one type over the other. Regardless of which type or model is used, the ventilator's function and limitations must be intimately known. A mechanical device used to sustain life is only as good as its design and the patient team using it.

Ambu Bag

Before discussing the two above-mentioned types, a brief note about a simple, man-powered ventilator is necessary. Frequently overlooked is the nurse's first important line of defense for acute respiratory failure (ARF)—the ambu bag. This respiratory bag provides a satisfactory method of artificial resuscitation. Connected to an oxygen source with a reservoir bag or cuff, it can deliver close to 100% oxygen. Knowledge of the bag, along with skill in using it, is vital. The function of this simple ventilator can be compared to the more sophisticated models. With the ambu bag,

- The *force* of squeezing the bag determines *tidal volume* (V_T) delivered to the patient
- The *number* of hand squeezes per minute determines the *rate*
- Both the *force* and *rate* at which the nurse squeezes the bag determine the *peak flow*

When the bag is used, careful observation of the patient's chest is vital to determine if the bag is performing properly and if any gastric distension is developing. In addition, the ease or resistance encountered can roughly indicate lung compliance. If a patient becomes progressively harder to "bag," an increase in secretions, hemothorax, pneumothorax, or worsening bronchospasms must be considered.

The following criteria are suggested for selection of an ambu bag:

- The ability of the ambu bag to deliver 100% oxygen in acute situations. (In nonacute maintenance situations, less oxygen concentration is acceptable.)
- If used with a face mask, the need for the mask to be transparent to enable visualization of vomitus or blood, which is a potential for aspiration
- A valve system that functions without jamming in acute situations
- The cleaning and recycling endurance of the bag

Volume Ventilators

The volume ventilator is the most frequently used type in critical care settings. The basic principle of this ventilator is that once a *designated volume* of air is delivered to the patient, inspiration is terminated. A piston or bellows pushes a predetermined volume (V_T) into the patient's lungs at a set rate. Oxygen concentrations can be varied from 21% to 100%. The advantage of a volume ventilator is that despite changing patient lung compliance, a consistent V_T will be delivered.

Some examples of volume ventilators are the MA-1, MA-2, Ohio, Monaghan, Emerson, Bourns-Bear-1, Searle, and the Engstrom.

Pressure Ventilators

In contrast to the volume ventilator, the pressure-cycled ventilator works under the basic principle that once a *preset pressure* is reached, inspiration is terminated. At this pressure point, the inspiratory valve closes and exhalation occurs passively. Ultimately this means that if a patient's lung compliance or resistance to flow changes, the *volume* of air delivered will *vary*.

Clinically, as a patient's lungs become stiffer (less compliant), the volume of air delivered to the patient will drop—sometimes drastically. Consequently, to ensure adequate minute ventilation and to detect any changes in lung compliance and resistance, inspiratory pressure, rate, and *exhaled* V_T must be monitored frequently. In a patient whose pulmonary status is unstable, the use of a pressure ventilator is not recommended. However, in a very stable patient with compliant lungs, pressure ventilators are adequate and can also be used as a weaning tool in selected patients.

Examples of pressure ventilators are the Bird, Mark-1, the Bennett PR-1 and PR-11.

Ventilator Controls

Most ventilators have dials that are similar in function regardless of terminology. Understanding each dial's function will enable the nurse to manipulate the function of the ventilator to meet the changing needs of the patient.

Fraction of Inspired Oxygen (FIO$_2$) Most recent models enable direct dial-in oxygen percentage, FIO$_2$. However, do not assume that because 100% is dialed-in, the patient is receiving 100%. When a patient requires 50% or more of FIO$_2$ concentrations, the ventilator needs to be checked daily for accuracy with an oxygen analyzer. The newer models of volume ventilators, such as the MA-II or Bear, have oxygen analyzers in circuit with constant digital readouts of oxygen concentrations. However, the older models, such as the MA-I or Monaghan, have no oxygen analyzers in circuit. Indeed, as long as 50 psi (pounds per square inch) of compressed air is connected, the ventilator will function.

Respiratory Rate. The number of breaths per minute delivered to the patient can be directly dialed-in. In some models, the numbers are marked, whereas in models such as the Monaghan, the rate is timed for a full minute with a watch, and the dial set accordingly. Again, do not assume just because the ventilator is set at a specified number of breaths per minute that this is what is being delivered. Double check the functioning of the ventilator with a watch having a second hand. The possibility of mechanical failure is ever present.

In the pressure ventilator, the inspiratory time flow-rate control determines the duration of inspiration by regulating the velocity of gas flow. The higher the flow rate, the faster peak airway pressure is reached and the shorter the inspiration. The lower the flow rate, the longer the inspiration. A high flow rate produces turbulence, shallow inspirations, and uneven distribution of volume.

Tidal Volume. In the volume ventilator, a dial or crank is turned to the number of milliliters of air to be delivered with each breath. Again, in the pressure ventilator, manipulaton of the in-

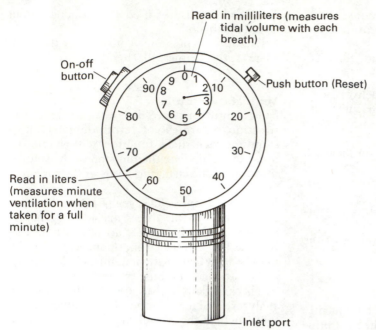

Read in milliliters (measures tidal volume with each breath)

On-off button

Push button (Reset)

Read in liters (measures minute ventilation when taken for a full minute)

Inlet port

FIGURE 13-14.
Wright respirometer—newer model.

spiratory time flow-rate control determines the magnitude of inspiration. A low flow rate increases V_T and produces better alveolar ventilation than a high flow rate. Use of a Wright Respirometer to measure exhaled air checks that the V_T dialed-in is being delivered (see Figs. 13-14 and 13-15).

Peak Flow. This is the velocity of air flow per unit of time and is expressed as liters per minute. In the volume ventilator, this is a separate knob. In the pressure ventilator, this is manipulated,

again, with the inspiratory time flow-rate control.

Installation of a demand valve in the newer volume ventilators enables a patient to receive the flow of air as he demands. The older models dump the air at the set rate (peak flow) dialed-in. The demand valve, in addition to decreasing airway turbulence, also enhances patient comfort.

Pressure Limit. On the volume-cycled ventilators, this knob limits the highest pressure

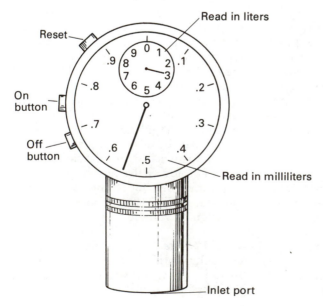

Reset

Read in liters

On button

Off button

Read in milliliters

Inlet port

FIGURE 13-15.
Wright respirometer—older model.

allowed in the ventilator circuit. Once the high pressure limit is reached, inspiration is terminated. Thus, if the pressure limit is being constantly reached, the designated V_T is not being delivered to the patient. Causes of this can include coughing, accumulation of secretions, kinked ventilator tubing, pneumothorax, decreasing compliance, or simply a pressure limit set too low.

Positive End Expiratory Pressure (PEEP).
The PEEP knob adjusts the pressure that is maintained in the lungs at the end of expiration. If an intermittent mandatory ventilation (IMV) model is used, this knob may be labeled continuous positive airway pressure (CPAP). CPAP indicates that spontaneous breathing through the ventilator circuit is occurring (non-IMV breaths) and that at the end of these breaths, positive airway pressure is being maintained. PEEP can be visualized on the respiratory pressure gauge. Instead of dropping to zero at the end of expiration, the pressure needle drops to PEEP level (see Figure 13-13).

In the newer ventilators, PEEP is built-in. The process by which PEEP is obtained on these ventilators is by keeping the exhalation valve inflated throughout the expiratory phase with a pressure equal to the amount of desired PEEP.

Several other devices can be used to apply PEEP externally on a ventilator or t-piece. They range from spring-loaded diaphragms and plastic cylinder ball valves to a container of water. These devices are applied on the exhalation port of the ventilator circuit. If water is used, for each 1 cm of exhalation tubing extending into the water, 1 cm of PEEP will be generated.

Sensitivity.
This controls the amount of patient effort as expressed by negative inspiratory pull needed to initiate an inspiration. Increasing the sensitivity decreases the amount of work the patient must do to initiate a ventilatory breath. Likewise, decreasing sensitivity increases the amount of negative pressure that the patient needs to initiate inspiration and increases the work of breathing. In some models, sensitivity may be totally dialed-out so that the ventilator is controlling the patient.

Sigh.
To understand the function of this knob, a little history of initial attempts at mechanical ventilation must be reviewed. Since normal breathing consists of V_Ts at 5 ml/kg of body weight, patients were initially ventilated at these volumes. However, subsequent studies on dogs showed that atelectasis developed. In an attempt to mimic normal breathing, rather than V_T, a sigh mode was incorporated. A sigh mode delivers a bigger breath to patients at a designated volume and rate per hour. Presently, mechanical ventilation is performed at twice normal V_T; hence, with this practice, the need for sighs has been negated except in special cases such as refractive atelectasis.

Ventilatory Modes
Several different modes of ventilatory control can be found on ventilators. These modes can be separate dials, or they can be incorporated in the function of another knob such as sensitivity. Some of these modes are *assist, control, assist-control,* and *IMV.*

In the *assist mode,* only the breaths triggered by the patient at the designed V_T are delivered to the patient. In this mode, the patient *must* have a drive to breathe. If the patient is unable to trigger a breath, air will not be delivered.

In the *control mode,* the ventilator controls the patient. Breaths delivered to the patient will be at the rate and volume dialed-in on the ventilator, regardless of the patient's attempts to initiate an inspiration. If the patient is not unconscious or paralyzed, this mode can provoke high anxiety and discomfort.

The *assist-control mode* incorporates the above two. A basic rate can be set. If the patient wishes to breathe faster, he can trigger the ventilator (providing the sensitivity allows). If the patient's drive to breathe is negated, the ventilator will "kick-in" at the preset rate. This ensures that the patient will never stop breathing while on the ventilator.

The *IMV mode* allows intermittent mandatory ventilation. As in the control mode, the rate and V_T are preset. If the patient wishes to breathe above this rate, he may. However, unlike the assist-control mode, any breaths he takes above the set rate are spontaneous breaths taken through the ventilator circuit. The V_T of these breaths may vary drastically from the V_T set on the ventilator because it is determined by the patient's ability to generate negative pressure in his chest. V_Ts may vary from zero to one liter.

To understand IMV, the basic functioning of the ventilator must be reviewed. Instantaneously, as the ventilator delivers a preset volume to the patient, a burst of air inflates a balloon in the exhalation port, forcing the air in only one direction — into the patient. When inspiration is terminated, the balloon deflates and

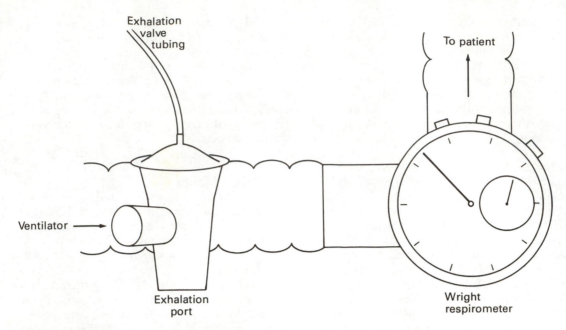

FIGURE 13-16.
Wright respirometer in-line circuit.

air rushes into the area of least resistance — out the exhalation port. This occurs with every ventilator cycle in assist, control, and assist-control modes.

However, when the IMV mode is used, the balloon is inflated *only* during the *mandatory cycles.* The rate and V_T are dialed-in for only the IMV breaths. As the patient triggers above this rate, the balloon is not inflated. These are non-IMV breaths. Because the balloon is not inflated during these breaths, the ventilator bellows "dump" and air is delivered to the area of least resistance. If the patient generates negative pressure in his chest, some or all of the V_T dumped may be delivered to the patient. If the patient is unable to generate adequate negative pressure, all of the V_T dumped rushes out the exhalation port with none reaching the patient.

Because of this, accurate monitoring of *inspired* V_T must be done. On the newer ventilators, this is accomplished by a continuous digital readout of inspired V_T with alarms set accordingly. On the older models, such as the Monaghan, there are no such monitoring systems. The nurse or respiratory therapist *is* the *alarm system.* In these ventilators, Wright Respirometers must be placed in line of the ventilator circuit between the patient and the exhalation port (see Fig. 13-16). A total minute ventilation (MV) is calculated. From this, the IMV MV is subtracted to obtain the patient's MV.

$$\begin{array}{r} \text{Total MV} \\ \underline{- \text{ IMV}} \\ = \text{Patient's MV} \end{array}$$

For example: the total MV, as measured in-line on the Wright Respirometer, is 20 liters, and the ventilator is set for an IMV rate of 10 and V_T of 800. The following calculations produce the amount of patient's contribution to ventilation.

Total MV	20 liters	
−IMV MV	8 liters	$(V_T \times \text{rate})$
Patient's MV	12 liters	

If the patient fatigues and drops his contribution to 5 liters, an arterial blood gas must be obtained to evaluate the $PaCO_2$. When the IMV rate is set very low and the patient fatigues, MV is reduced drastically. Because of this, the $PaCO_2$ elevates rapidly and the patient may have an arrest — on a mechanical ventilator. Use of IMV as a weaning tool will be discussed in Chapter 14.

When selecting a patient for IMV, compliance and respiratory reserve must be evaluated. When compliance and reserve are both low and IMV is instituted, the work of breathing increases dramatically.

In the IMV mode, the mandatory breaths are delivered at a set rate regardless of whether the patient is in inspiration or expiration. Some ventilators have the IMV mode synchronized

(SIMV) so that the mandatory breaths are delivered in synchrony with patient triggering.

PHYSIOLOGICAL EFFECTS OF MECHANICAL VENTILATION

To understand the effects of mechanical ventilation, a review of normal respirations and their physiological effects is necessary.

With a normal respiration, *inspiration* is an *active* process. The intercostal muscles contract, pulling the rib cage upward and outward, and the diaphragm contracts downward, creating a *negative* pressure in the pleural cavity. When this subatmospheric pressure is generated, air moves into the lungs and ventilation occurs. In *expiration,* the thoracic cavity and lung tissue recoil, pushing air out of the lung and creating a *positive* pressure. This process is usually *passive.*

Hemodynamically, during inspiration, the fall in extrathoracic pressure decreases pressure in the great veins and atrium and acts as a suction pump. Venous return to the atrium is increased, resulting in increased ventricular output. During expiration, because of the positive pressures generated in the chest, venous return and cardiac output decrease.

In mechanical ventilation, the relationship between pressures in inspiration and expiration is *reversed.* The ventilator delivers air by virtually pumping it into the patient; thus, pressures during inspiration are positive. When a patient is placed on mechanical ventilation, hypotension may develop due to the hemodynamic effects of the positive intrathoracic pressure. As PEEP is instituted, cardiac output may be affected even more because PEEP continues to keep positive pressure in the chest at all times. In addition, large V_Ts, greater than 10 to 12 ml/kg, which generate pressures greater than 40 cm H_2O, may not only influence the cardiac output but also increase the risk of pneumothorax.

The movement of air through the airways creates friction and turbulence. The more the flow, the more friction. If the airway is narrowed, the friction increases even more. Thus, when inspiration is spontaneously generated, more negative pressure must be generated for a given flow of air to occur. During mechanical ventilation, more positive pressure is needed to deliver air through the narrowed airway.

Compliance.   The lungs hold a volume of air. As more air is added, the lungs expand. Compare this with stretch or degree of elasticity. The

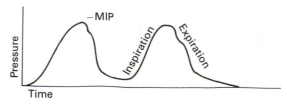

FIGURE 13-17.
Graph depicting maximum inspiratory pressure. *(MIP)* maximum inspiratory pressure.

resistance to stretch or lack of elasticity is compliance. Since volume determines stretch, compliance is equal to changes in volume divided by changes in pressure.

$$compliance = \frac{volume \ (ml)}{pressure \ (cm \ H_2O)} = ml/cm$$

Normal lung compliance is 200 ml/cm H_2O. Once the rib cage is added, this compliance drops to 100 ml/cm H_2O. As a lung becomes stiffer, as in adult respiratory distress syndrome (ARDS), increasing pressures are required to deliver the same volume. Therefore, compliance decreases. In contrast, where there is destruction of lung tissue, as in emphysema, elasticity is lost and the lung is more compliant. Compliance is frequently compared to a balloon. Initially it is hard to inflate, until it is stretched. After repeated inflations the elasticity is lost, and the balloon becomes very easy to blow up.

As the volume of gas is delivered to a patient on a mechanical ventilator, the respirator pressure gauge will slowly rise from zero to maximum inspiratory pressure (MIP). The rise in pressure is caused by resistance to flow or resistance to lung and chest wall inflation. A graph of pressure over time, depicting inspiration, would look like that shown in Figure 13-17.

Dynamic pressures and MIP can give an indication of flow properties of the airways (see Table 13-7).

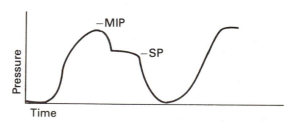

FIGURE 13-18.
Graph depicting static pressure. *(MIP)* maximum inspiratory pressure; *(SP)* static pressure.

Table 13–7
Factors Influencing MIP
(Maximum Inspiratory Pressure)

Flow resistance	Peak flow
	Size of airways
	Airway obstructions
	External obstructions
	(*i.e.,* kinked ventilator
	tubing or water in the
	tubing)
Lung resistance	Chest size
	Volume of air
	Elasticity of lung
Chest wall resistance	Chest wall deformities
	Position of patient
	External compression of
	chest wall or diaphragm
	(*i.e.,* distended
	abdomen)

Static Pressure. Another measurement used to obtain compliance is static pressure (SP). SP is obtained by kinking the exhalation valve line when the patient is in maximum inspiration. This holds the volume of delivered air in the patient's chest by preventing exhalation. The pressure recorded at this moment is SP and reflects the force necessary to deliver the preset volume of air to the patient and hold the airways open. Graphically, it would appear as in Figure 13–18. Thus, dividing the V_T by the SP yields compliance.

Application. Clinically, compliance and airway dynamics can be applied in various situations. For example, an asthmatic patient being mechanically ventilated has a basic disease process affecting airway resistance with normal lung elasticity. In this situation, dynamic pressure would be high in contrast to SP, which would be near normal. When nebulized bronchodilators are administered, airway resistance decreases, and the respirator pressure gauge will reflect this by showing a lower dynamic pressure. In this way, the effectiveness of bronchodilators can objectively be evaluated.

In contrast, a patient with ARDS may have airway resistance near normal while compliance is very low, indicating a stiffness of the lung tissue. As the patient improves, compliance improves.

BIBLIOGRAPHY
Bone RC: Compliance and dynamic characteristic curves in acute respiratory failure. Crit Care Med 4, No. 4:173–179, 1976
Egan DF: Fundamentals of Respiratory Therapy, 3rd ed. St. Louis, C. V. Mosby, 1977
Guenter CA (ed): Pulmonary Medicine. Philadelphia, J. B. Lippincott, 1977
Martin, R, Rogers RM: Treatment of acute respiratory failure without mechanical ventilation. Resident Staff Physician, May 1979, pp 41–48
Mitchell RS (ed): Synopsis of Clinical Pulmonary Disease. St. Louis, C. V. Mosby, 1978
Moses RM, Steinberg S: Does the MA-1 respirator make you nervous? RN, April 1979, pp 34–44
Respiratory function: 4-Monitoring artificial ventilation. Nursing Times, April 1978 (Suppl)
Suter P et al: Optimum end-expiratory airway pressure in patients with acute pulmonary failure. N Engl J Med 292:284–288, 1975

Eileen Brent

GUIDELINES FOR VENTILATORY MANAGEMENT

In most hospitals, the philosophy of respiratory care and ventilatory management is dependent upon the philosophy of the pulmonary or anesthesia physicians who direct respiratory care. It is important that each team member be well acquainted with the basic guidelines of their philosophy.

ASPECTS OF THE MECHANICAL VENTILATOR

Humidification and Temperature

Mechanical ventilation bypasses the upper airway, thus negating the body's protective mechanism for humidification and warming. These two processes must be added—a humidifier with a temperature control. All air delivered by the ventilator passes through the water in the humidifier, being warmed and saturated. Because of this, no insensible water loss occurs. In most instances, the temperature of the air will be near body temperature. In some rare instances (severe hypothermia), the air temperature may be increased. Caution is advised because prolonged, high, inhaled temperatures can cause tracheal burns. Contrary to a dangerous myth, a dry humidifier does *not* decrease pulmonary edema! It only contributes to drying the airway, with resultant mucus plugging and an inability to suction-out secretions.

As the air is passed through the ventilator to the patient, large droplets are rained-out in the corrugated hose. This moisture is considered contaminated and must be drained into a receptacle and not back into the sterile humidifier. If the water is allowed to build up, resistance is developed in circuit and positive end expiratory pressure (PEEP) is generated. In addition, if left unchecked, the water may be aspirated by the patient. Attention to this is a primary nursing responsibility.

Initial Setting

Before placing a patient on a ventilator, attach it to a test lung to adjust the settings to the standard guidelines.

Standard setting

- Fraction of inspired oxygen (FIO_2) — 100%
- Tidal volume (V_T) — 10–15 ml/kg body weight
- Respiratory rate (RR) — 10–15 breaths/min
- Inspiratory flow — 40–60 liters/sec
- Sensitivity — −2 cm H_2O
- Sigh rate (optional) — 1–2/min, V_T 20 ml/kg
- Positive end expiratory pressure (PEEP) — zero

Settings for the patient will be determined by the goals of the therapy, and changes of the settings will be determined by the patient's response as reflected in arterial blood gases.

Fraction of Inspired Oxygen (FIO_2)

Initially the patient without a previous blood gas analysis is usually placed on 100% oxygen. When the PaO_2 on 100% has been established, calculation by the alveolar air equation can be used to determine an FIO_2 concentration for a *target* PaO_2 (See accompanying chart).

CALCULATING ALVEOLAR AIR

PAO_2 = partial pressure of O_2 in alveolus
PaO_2 = partial pressure of O_2 in arteries
PIO_2 = partial pressure of inspired O_2
$PACO_2$ = partial pressure of CO_2 in alveolus
$PaCO_2$ = partial pressure of CO_2 in arteries
($PACO_2$ = the patient's $PaCO_2$)
R = respiratory quotient = 1 on O_2 = .8 on room air and reflects $\dfrac{CO_2 \text{ production}}{O_2 \text{ consumption}}$
P_B = barometric pressure
P_{H_2O} = water pressure

Alveolar Air Equation: $PAO_2 = PIO_2 - \dfrac{PACO_2}{R}$

STEP 1: $PIO_2 = FIO_2 (P_B - P_{H_2O})$

STEP 2: Substituting the following given values,
a P_B of 647 torr
P_{H_2O} of 47 torr
and a patient on 100% O_2 with a $PaCO_2$ of 40 torr, the equation would read:
$$PAO_2 = 1.00 (647 - 47) - \frac{40}{1}$$
$$= 1.00 (600) - 40$$
$$= 600 - 40$$
$$= 560 \text{ torr}$$

STEP 3: Blood gases are drawn on 100% FIO_2 with the following results:
$$pH = 7.40$$
$$PaO_2 = 300 \text{ torr}$$
$$PaCO_2 = 40 \text{ torr}$$

STEP 4: To calculate *target* PaO_2, set PaO_2 and PAO_2 in ratio form.
Since normal PaO_2 in Denver is 65–75 torr, target PaO_2 would be 75 torr.
(Equation) $\dfrac{PAO_2}{PaO_2}$ (Blood gas) $= \dfrac{560}{300} = \dfrac{x}{75}$
x = the PAO_2 to give a target PaO_2 of 75 torr
$$(560) 75 = 300x$$
$$\frac{(560) 75}{300} = x$$
$$140 = x$$
From these calculations, to have a PaO_2 of 75 torr, a PAO_2 of 140 is needed.

STEP 5: Now to find the FIO_2 that gives a PAO_2 of 140, substitute the values into the alveolar air equation. (Assume everything else stays constant.)
$$140 = x (647 - 47) - \frac{40}{1}$$
x = target FIO_2
$$140 = x (600) - 40$$
$$180 = 600x$$
$$.30 = x$$

STEP 6: Therefore, for a target PaO_2 of 75 torr, the FIO_2 on the ventilator can be reduced to 30%.

Respiratory Rate and Tidal Volume

RR times the V_T determines minute ventilation (MV). In turn, MV determines alveolar ventilation. These two parameters are adjusted according to the $PaCO_2$. Increasing MV decreases $PaCO_2$, and conversely, decreasing MV increases $PaCO_2$. There are special cases, however, in which hypoventilation or hyperventilation may be desired. For example, in a head injury, the neurosurgeon may wish a respiratory alkalosis to occur to promote cerebral vasoconstriction. In this case, the V_T and RR are increased to achieve the desired alkalotic pH by $PaCO_2$ manipulation. In contrast, chronic obstructive pulmonary disease (COPD) patients whose baseline arterial blood gases consist of elevated carbon dioxide need to be mechanically hypoventilated at their baseline, $PaCO_2$. These patients usually have a large acid load, and lowering their carbon dioxide levels rapidly may result in seizures. Patients with restrictive diseases need careful monitoring of their blood gases because they may need lower V_T and higher RR.

Peak Flow

If MV is high, peak flow may need to be increased to provide time for exhalation before a new inhalation is triggered. However, remember that increasing peak flow increases turbulence, which is reflected in increasing airway pressures.

Positive End Expiratory Pressure

Institution of PEEP or CPAP is primarily indicated for refractive hypoxemia. However, if a patient requires FIO_2 greater than 50% for prolonged periods of time, the risk of oxygen toxicity increases. Oxygen is time-dose related, and PEEP may decrease the need for high FIO_2 concentrations. It is important to weigh the risks of PEEP against the effects of long-term oxygen administration. The physiological effects on cardiac output and tissue oxygenation must be monitored. Mixed venous blood drawn from the distal end of a Swan-Ganz catheter reflects tissue oxygenation and helps evaluate the effects of PEEP.

PEEP is usually begun in increments of 5 cm of water pressure. Mixed venous and arterial blood gases should be drawn beforehand for baseline values and repeated 20 minutes after settings are adjusted.

PEEP holds the alveoli open by maintaining a pressure greater than atmospheric pressure in the alveoli at the end of expiration. This end expiratory pressure increases fractional residual capacity (FRC) by reinflating collapsed alveoli, keeping the alveoli open, and decreasing the pressure needed to ventilate them. In addition, there is some evidence that suggests that keeping the alveoli open may enhance surfactant regeneration. If a patient requires high levels of PEEP for a prolonged period of time, decreasing PEEP must be done slowly over a period of time. Within 4 hours, after PEEP is decreased, airways may start to collapse again due to hypoxia.

Sensitivity

Sensitivity in some machines is set by turning the knob (increasing sensitivity) to the point that the ventilator "chatters." Chatter comes from the sound of the ventilator constantly dumping. The dial is then slowly decreased to the point where the chattering stops. At this point, the ventilator can be triggered when a -2 cm is generated.

Some physicians prefer to have the patient trigger the ventilator. Keeping the patient in control of the ventilator enables him to adjust his own MV as needed. This will also be of benefit to the patient when he is weaned from the ventilator. In contrast, some physicians prefer to paralyze, anesthetize, dial-out the sensitivity, or increase MV so the patient does not initiate respiration on the ventilator. They prefer to rest the patient while the ventilator does the work of breathing. In the latter case, psychological support must be provided if the patient is alert and awake.

Addition of PEEP may change the sensitivity on a ventilator. For example, if the machine is set so that generation of -2 cm initiates respiration, the patient triggers the ventilator by "sucking" the dial from zero to -2. If 10 cm of PEEP are added, the ventilator is still triggered at a -2 cm. However, now the patient must suck the needle from 10 to -2 (-12 cm pressure) to initiate a breath. This increases the patient's work of breathing. Because of this increased work, the patient may stop triggering the machine, decreasing his MV. To correct this, the sensitivity is increased so that inspiration is initiated at 8 cm of pressure. Thus, when the patient sucks the needle from 10 cm to 8 (-2 cm), the work of breathing is decreased to the initial level. If PEEP is decreased to levels less than 8 cm, sensitivity must also be decreased or oversensitivity occurs,

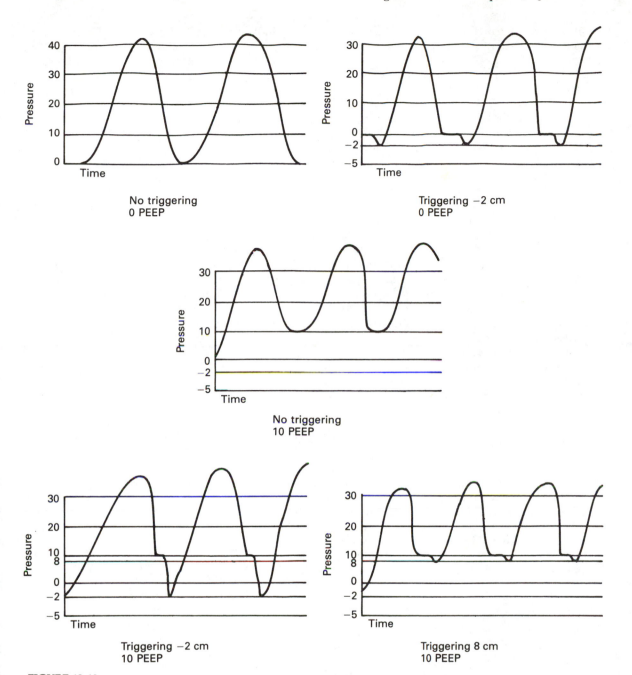

FIGURE 13-19.
Respiratory wave forms with different settings of PEEP and triggering.

resulting in a severe respiratory alkalosis from mechanical hyperventilation. (See Fig. 13-19.)

Dead Space

Dead space is a term designating the addition of tubing between the patient and the exhalation valve. In essence the patient is rebreathing his exhaled CO_2. Indication for additional dead space is a respiratory alkalosis not mechanically correctable through manipulation of RR and V_T. Clinically, for some physiological reason, the patient is hyperventilating. This type of high ventilatory output failure is often times seen in adult respiratory distress syndrome (ARDS). Since it is desirable to correct this alkalosis by correcting the primary arterial blood gas abnormality (increased $PaCO_2$), dead space is sometimes added.

When adding dead space, an MV must be calculated before and after application. Some patients appear very sensitive to $PaCO_2$ levels. Indeed, if 5 inches of dead space are added, they may increase their MV so that the effect on the $PaCO_2$ values is negligible, and continued addition of vast inches of dead space may force the patient into agonal breathing.

There is no set formula for calculating inches of dead space for rises in $PaCO_2$. This is a trial and error process. Since 5 inches is a negligible amount, 10 inches is usually applied initially.

It must be stressed that *mechanical manipulation of $PaCO_2$ must be based on pH values.* In other words, if a patient is in metabolic acidosis and his $PaCO_2$ is low because of this, dead space is not indicated. Additional dead space at this time would force the patient into a more severe acidosis.

Lastly, since the partial pressures of CO_2 and O_2 largely determine the total pressure of inhaled gas on a ventilator, increasing the $PaCO_2$ may slightly lower the oxygen values.

Alarm Systems

Mechanical ventilators are used to support life. Alarm systems are necessary to warn the nurse of developing problems. Alarm systems can be categorized according to volume versus pressure and high versus low. Low pressure alarms warn of disconnection from the patient. High pressure alarms warn of rising pressures. Low volume alarms warn of leaks. Electrical failure alarms are a *must* for all ventilators.

NURSING CARE

The patient who needs ventilatory support also needs primary nursing care. Intensive care units, mechanical ventilators, and intubation naturally evoke psychological stress. Communications are frustrating and anxiety-producing because the intubated patient will not be able to speak. Each patient must be told that the tube prevents him from talking and that there is nothing wrong with his voice. Perhaps he can write or use sign language to indicate his messages, and the nurse can be more aware of nonverbal communications and body language.

Airway care must consist of adequate humidification, suctioning, and monitoring.

Humidification and warming (discussed earlier) are accomplished by mechanical additions to the ventilator to prevent airway obstruction from dry secretions and mucus plugs.

Suctioning is done hourly *and* whenever necessary. Aseptic technique is used to reduce airway contamination, and the patient must be oxygenated with 100% oxygen both before and after suctioning.

Routine auscultation of the chest enables monitoring of results from therapy and alerts the nurse to any problems such as increasing fluid overload, secretions, bronchospasms, or slippage of the tube into the right main stem bronchus. If bronchospasms are present, administration of bronchodilators needs to be considered. When secretions become a problem, vigorous suctioning and "bagging" after postural drainage, percussion, and vibration must be instituted. The reader is referred to previous sections in Chapter 13 for details.

Tube Care. All endotracheal tubes must be anchored securely to prevent tube movement (see Fig. 13-12). If taping obscures skin areas, septum or lip necrosis may occur. Since oral hygiene is given everyday, it is an opportune time to inspect the skin, nose, and mouth for tissue breakdown. Placement of an oral bite block will prevent the patient from biting on the tube or displacing the tube with his tongue. The use of a swivel connector (connecting the tube to the ventilator circuit), along with anchoring a large loop of tubing to the bed, will facilitate patient movement without tube movement.

Tube cuff pressures are monitored every shift to prevent overdistension and excess pressure on the tracheal wall. When a patient is on the ventilator, the best pressure is the lowest possible pressure without having a leak of V_T. Physiologically, arterial circulation to the tracheal wall is obliterated by pressures around 30 torr. If a cuff leak is suspected by a discrepancy in actual versus measured V_T, auscultation at the neck for air turbulence can determine if the seal is adequate. If the patient is not on a ventilator, the pressure is arbitrarily set at 20 torr. Figure 13-20, cuff monitoring, shows the procedure:

1. The pilot balloon tubing is attached to a syringe and mercury manometer by a four-way stopcock.
2. The stopcock is turned off to the patient.
3. Air pressure is added to the system by compressing the syringe until the mercury manometer reads 20 torr.

4. The stopcock is then turned on to the patient, manometer, and syringe. Pressure can be increased or decreased by manipulation of the syringe.
5. After the pressure is set, preferably at 20 or less, the stopcock is closed to the pilot balloon and the manometer.
6. The pressures are then recorded on the ventilator flowsheet.

Gastrointestinal (GI) Care. Due to the increased physical and psychological stress, GI bleeds are a potential occurrence. Hourly antacids instilled by way of a nasogastric tube help neutralize gastric acidity. Also, Cimetidine can be given prophylactically.

Other measures, such as skin care by frequent turning, maintenance of muscle strength by ROM and ambulation, and good nutrition, are not included here. They are still vital to the patient and his plan of care. They cannot be negated; hence, sometimes it may require two staff people to provide all the care needed. Psychologically and physically, care of the ventilated patient takes a toll on the nursing team because it demands vigilance to details and repetition of basic nursing procedures.

COMPLICATIONS OF MECHANICAL VENTILATION

The patient on a mechanical ventilator requires observant, skillful, and *repetitive* nursing care. Complications that may occur with this therapy can be minimized—*prevention* is the key.

Airway Complications

Aspiration can occur before, during, or after intubation. The risk of aspiration after intubation can be minimized by securing the tube,

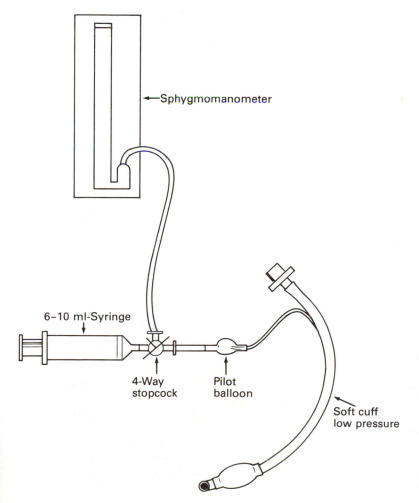

Sphygmomanometer

6–10 ml-Syringe

4-Way stopcock

Pilot balloon

Soft cuff low pressure

FIGURE 13-20.
Monitoring cuff pressures.

maintaining an inflated cuff, and continuing adequate tube or oral suctioning. If resuscitation was prolonged and gastric distention occurred, the airway must be secured before passing a nasogastric tube for stomach decompression. Once aspiration does occur, the potential for the development of ARDS increases.

Most ventilator patients need to be restrained on both hands because self-extubation with aspiration is an ever present complication. In addition, self-extubation with an inflated cuff can result in vocal cord damage.

The procedure of intubation itself is a high risk. Examples of situations that increase the risk are

- Prolonged and complicated intubation⟶increased hypoxia and tracheal trauma
- Mainstem intubation (usually right)⟶unequal ventilation, increasing the mortality rate
- Intubation of pyriform sinus (rare)⟶pharnygeal abscess

Mechanical Complications

Ventilator malfunctioning is a potentially serious problem at all times. Hourly checks of the ventilator by the nurse can minimize or spot potentials for existing problems. At this time, alarms must be checked for proper functioning and be noted.

If the tube is placed nasotracheally, a severe sinus infection can develop. Or, because of the position of the tube in the pharynx, the orifice to the inner ear may become occluded, resulting in a severe otitis media. Whenever a patient complains of ear or sinus pain, or develops a fever of unknown etiology, the sinuses and ears must be checked for possible sources of infection.

Some degree of tracheal damage results from prolonged intubation. Tracheal stenosis and malacia can be minimized if cuff pressures are minimized. Arterial circulation is occluded around cuff pressures of 30 torr. A decreased incidence of both stenosis and malacia has been reported when cuff pressures are kept around 20 torr. If laryngeal edema is present, life-threatening postextubation stridor can occur.

Pseudomonas pneumonia frequently develops in cases of prolonged intubation and is always a potential possibility from contaminated equipment.

The last frequently encountered problem involves alveolar ventilation. Alveolar hypoven-

tilation is significantly associated with COPD and hypotension, while alveolar hyperventilation is associated with prolonged time on the ventilator. Hypoventilation increases the mortality of ventilation. Hyperventilation may or may not increase mortality, but it does produce a high alkalotic pH that can result in seizures and a significant drop in cardiac output. With a right mainstem intubation, the right lung is overventilated and develops significant atelectasis. The incidence of pneumothorax increases.

WEANING FROM MECHANICAL VENTILATION

From the time the patient is placed on mechanical ventilation, the goal of weaning is present. The process to achieve this goal includes

- Correction of the cause of respiratory failure
- Maintenance of muscle strength
- Proper nutrition

Each of these phases is as important as the other for a successful discontinuance of ventilatory support.

Each patient is evaluated daily for the possibility of weaning. Generally, patients are categorized as

- Short-term ventilation with uncomplicated extubation
- Long-term ventilation with prolonged weaning time

The former usually requires only a short trial of 20 minutes before extubation; the latter requires a tedious 3 to 4 weeks of weaning associated with numerous problems.

The criteria listed in Table 13-8 are suggested for assessing the patient's potential to be weaned. All criteria must be evaluated within the context of the patient's disease process and his capabilities.

Minute Ventilation. If MV is higher than 20 liters, the work of breathing is high. The patient may well wean, but after a couple of hours may fatigue and need to be reintubated. When MV is less than 6 liters, hypoventilation will occur. The etiology for hypoventilation needs to be investigated because often the cause will be sedation.

Maximum Voluntary Ventilation (MVV) is obtained by having the patient breathe as hard and as fast as he can for 15 seconds. Multiply this by 4 and the answer is total MVV for one minute.

MVV is an objective measurement of the patient's ventilatory reserve. If the patient's work of breathing postextubation is increased and ventilatory reserve is low, reintubation may be needed.

Inspiratory Pressure. Inspiratory pressure gives an indication of inspiratory muscle strength. A pressure less than -20 ml/cm H_2O pressure indicates muscle weakness. The work of breathing will be very costly and fatigue will result.

Vital Signs and Blood Gases. When the decision has been made to have the patient try spontaneous breathing, baseline vital signs and arterial blood gases are obtained. It is preferable that the patient be well rested and that he receive an inhaled bronchodilator prior to weaning. Blood pressure, pulse, and respiratory rates are monitored frequently during the weaning, and at the end of 20 to 30 minutes arterial blood gases are drawn along with measurements of V_T, MV, and RR. These results will indicate the appropriateness of extubation.

Nutrition and Muscle Strength. For the long-term patient, the weaning process *must* proceed slowly. All energy areas, such as nutrition, muscle strength, and lung status, must be maximized. Nutrition and muscle strength need emphasis because many intensive care unit patients exist in a semistarved state. Starvation decreases not only the energy available to breathe but also the drive to breathe. To improve the patient's nutritional status, frequent small feedings with high-protein supplements may be sufficient. If not, a nasogastric or gastrostomy tube may be inserted, or hyperalimentation may be considered. Although good nutrition will improve muscle strength, appropriate muscle building exercises, active and passive, will also increase respiratory muscle strength. It is not uncommon that the first time off the ventilator, the patient will "forget" how to breathe and will need reminding.

The decision to wean a patient from ventilatory support needs to be realistically evaluated, based on the prognosis of the patient. Once a patient is considered a candidate for weaning, a consistent team approach determines the success or failure of this goal.

Table 13-8
Criteria for Potential Weaning From Ventilator

RR	—15–20 breaths/min
MV	— 6–12 liters
V_T	— 5 ml/kg of body weight
VC	—10 ml/kg of body weight
MVV*	—12–20 liters
Inspiratory pressure	—20 cm H_2O
Compliance	—> 20 ml/cm H_2O pressure
FIO_2 requirements	—< 50%
No PEEP	
Adequate ABG values†	
Physiologically stable	

*MVV, total maximum voluntary ventilation.
†ABG, arterial blood gas.

BIBLIOGRAPHY

Adams NR: The nurse's role in systematic weaning from a ventilator. Nursing, 34–41, August 1979

Arora N, Rochester DF: Effects of nutrition on respiratory muscle strength and endurance (abstr). Mimeographed. University of Colorado Health Sciences Center, 1980

Burton G et al (eds): Respiratory Care: A Guide to Clinical Practice. Philadelphia, J. B. Lippincott, 1977

Feldtman RW, Andrassy R: Meeting exceptional nutritional needs. Post Grad Med, 65–71, September 1978

Martz KV et al: Management of the Patient-Ventilator System: A Team Approach. St. Louis, C. V. Mosby, 1979

Moir J: Nursing care of patients on ventilators. Nursing Times, 492–500, March 1978

Petty TL: Complications occurring during mechanical ventilation. Heart Lung, 112–118, January-February 1976

Sahebjami H et al: Lung mechanics and ultrastructure in prolonged starvation. Am Rev Respir Dis, 117:77–83, 1978

Sahn SA et al: Weaning from mechanical ventilation. JAMA, May 1976, 2208–2212

Sahn S, Lakshminarayan S: Bedside criteria for discontinuation of mechanical ventilation. Chest, 1002–1005, June 1973

Stauffer J et al: Complications of endotracheal and tracheotomy: A prospective study of 150 critically ill patients (abstr). Mimeographed. University of Colorado Health Sciences Center, 1980

Zwillich CW et al: Effects of hypermetabolism on ventilation and chemosensitivity. J Clin Invest, 900–906, October 1977

Joseph O. Broughton

Assessment Skills for the Nurse: Respiratory System 14

UNDERSTANDING BLOOD GASES

Blood gases are obtained in a variety of clinical situations, but they are obtained for two major reasons:

- To determine if the patient is well oxygenated
- To determine the acid–base status of the patient, concentrating on either the respiratory component, the metabolic (nonrespiratory) component, or most often, both respiratory and metabolic components.

In the following discussion, the term *nonrespiratory* will be used interchangeably with the term *metabolic*.

ARTERIAL VS VENOUS BLOOD MEASUREMENTS

Most often blood gases are measured on arterial blood rather than on venous blood for two reasons.

- Studying arterial blood is a good way to sample a mixture of blood that has come from various parts of the body.
- Arterial blood gives the added information on how well the lungs are oxygenating the blood.

Blood obtained from a vein in an extremity gives information mostly about that extremity and can be quite misleading if the metabolism in the extremity differs from the metabolism of the body as a whole, as it often does. This difference is accentuated if the extremity is cold or underperfused as in a patient in shock, if the patient has done local exercise with the extremity such as opening and closing his fist, if there is local infection in the extremity, and so forth.

Sometimes blood is sampled through a central venous catheter (CVP catheter) in hopes of getting mixed venous blood, but even in the superior vena cava or right atrium, where a CVP catheter ends, there is usually incomplete mixing of venous blood from various parts of the body. For complete mixing of the blood, one would have to obtain a blood sample from the pulmonary artery through a Swan-Ganz catheter, for example; even then one would not get information about how well the lungs are oxygenating the blood.

The second reason for selecting arterial blood is that it gives the added information of how well the lungs are oxygenating the blood. Oxygen measurements of mixed venous blood can tell if the tissues are getting oxygenated but cannot separate the contribution of the heart from that of the lungs. In other words, if the mixed venous blood oxygen is low, it means that either heart or lungs or both are at fault, and this may indicate either (1) that the lungs have not oxygenated the arterial blood well and that when the tissues extract their usual amount of oxygen from arterial blood, the resulting venous blood has a low oxygen concentration, or (2) that the heart is not circulating the blood well so that it is taking blood a long time to circulate through the tissues. The tissues, therefore, must extract more than the usual amount of oxygen from each cardiac cycle because the blood is flowing slowly. This produces a low venous oxygen concentration.

If it is known that the arterial oxygen concentration is normal (indicating that the lungs are doing their job), but the mixed venous oxygen concentration is low, then one can infer that the heart and circulation are failing.

One advantage of using mixed venous blood instead of arterial blood is that if the oxygen concentration in mixed venous blood is normal, one can infer that the tissues are receiving enough oxygen—usually this means that both ventilation and circulation are adequate.

OXYGEN

There are three ways to measure oxygen in blood:

- Oxygen content, which is the number of milliliters of oxygen carried by 100 ml of blood
- The PO_2, or pressure exerted by oxygen dissolved in the plasma
- The oxygen saturation of hemoglobin, which is a measure of the percentage of oxygen that hemoglobin is carrying related to the total amount the hemoglobin could carry, or

$$O_2 \text{ sat} = \frac{\text{amount of oxygen that hemoglobin is carrying}}{\text{maximum amount of oxygen that hemoglobin can carry}} \times 100$$

PROCEDURE FOR DRAWING BLOOD FOR ARTERIAL BLOOD GAS ANALYSIS

A. Equipment
1. 5-ml or 10-ml glass syringe
2. 10-ml bottle of heparin, 1000 units/ml (reusable)
3. No. 21, No. 22 needle or even No. 25 disposable needle (short level)
4. Cork
5. Alcohol swab
6. Container of ice (emesis basin or cardboard milkshake cup or plastic bag)
7. Request slip on which to write patient's clinical status, etc., including
   a. Name, date, time
   b. Whether receiving O_2, and if so how much and by what route
   c. Whether in shock
   d. Recent bicarbonate Rx, etc.
   e. If on continuous ventilation: tidal volume, respiratory frequency, and inspired oxygen concentration (FIO_2), amount of PEEP or CPAP

B. Technique
1. Call the lab to notify them you plan to draw a blood gas sample so that they can be calibrating equipment for 15 to 30 minutes.
2. Patients should be in steady state for at least 15 minutes (no recent change in inspired O_2, etc.).
3. Brachial artery is generally preferred, though radial may be used. Femoral artery sometimes must be used in hypotensive patients but should be avoided if possible.
4. Elbow is hyperextended and arm is externally rotated.
   a. Very important to have elbow *completely straight*—usually a folded towel or pillow under the elbow accomplishes this.
   b. For radial artery puncture, wrist is hyperextended after supporting lower arm on towels.

(continued)

5. 1 ml of heparin is aspirated into the syringe, barrel of the syringe is wet with heparin, and then the excess heparin is discarded through the needle, being careful that the hub of the needle is left full of heparin and there are no bubbles.
6. Brachial or radial artery is located by palpation with index and long fingers, and point of maximum impulse is found.
7. Needle is inserted into the area of maximum pulsation. This is easiest with the syringe and needle approximately perpendicular to the skin; however, if the needle is inserted at a more acute angle (such as used for venipunctures), there may be better hemostasis after the needle is removed.
8. Often the needle goes completely through both sides of the artery and only when the needle is slowly withdrawn does the blood gush up into the syringe.
9. The only way to be certain that arterial blood is obtained is the fact that the blood pumps up into the syringe under its own power.
   a. If one has to aspirate blood by pulling on the plunger of syringe — as is sometimes required with a tighter fitting plastic syringe — it is impossible to be positive that blood is arterial.
   b. *The blood gas results do not allow one to determine whether blood is arterial or venous.*
   c. If one suspects that blood may be venous, then draw another sample of obviously venous blood and compare the two samples. If the two samples are similar, then the first sample also was venous, but if the PO_2 and O_2 saturation on the second (obviously venous) sample are significantly lower than the first sample, then the first sample is probably arterial.
10. After 5 to 10 ml of blood are obtained, the needle is withdrawn and the assistant puts constant pressure on site of arterial puncture for at least 5 minutes.
    a. If the patient is anticoagulated, hypertensive, or has a bleeding disorder, a longer period of pressure — 10 minutes — is required.
    b. Even if attempt is unsuccessful, pressure must be applied.
11. Any air bubbles should be squirted out of the syringe and needle immediately, for these can change the blood gas values. The needle is then stuck into a cork, and the syringe is shaken to ensure that the blood mixes with the heparin.

12. Corked syringe and needle are labeled and immediately placed into ice or ice water, then taken to the lab.
13. Minimal analyses required are
    a. pH
    b. PCO_2 (by direct electrode or Astrup tonometer technique)
    c. PO_2
    d. Hgb.
    Base excess and actual bicarbonate should be calculated (standard bicarbonate may be substituted for actual bicarbonate). Other calculated values such as buffer base should not be reported, because they just tend to be confusing.
14. *Other*
    a. If O_2 saturation is also measured, this provides a cross-check for accuracy of the PO_2 (use PO_2 and pH to calculate O_2 saturation on blood gas slide rule and see if this calculated O_2 saturation agrees with the measured O_2 saturation.
    b. If CO_2 content is also measured, this provides a cross-check for accuracy of PCO_2. (Use PCO_2 and pH to calculate CO_2 content on blood gas slide rule and see if this calculated CO_2 content agrees with the measured CO_2 content.)
15. Another way to insure accuracy is to run the tests in duplicate on two different blood gas analyses. If there is a discrepancy in the two determinations, it must be run a third time.
16. Results should be reported back to the unit on the same request slip that includes the patient's status, as listed in A-7 above, so that results of blood gases can be related to clinical condition. (If all information is not on the same slip, it becomes impossible to interpret data hours, days, or weeks later. For instance, PO_2 has little meaning unless FIO_2 is known.
17. The technician performing analysis should report any suspicion that results are not reliable. For instance
    a. If syringe comes to her with air bubbles in it
    b. If she introduces air into the sample inadvertently
    c. If calculated O_2 saturation and measured O_2 saturation do not agree
    d. If calculated CO_2 content and measured CO_2 content do not agree
    e. If equipment does not appear to be functioning correctly

Table 14–1
How Oxygen is Carried in Blood

Dissolved in plasma	0.3 ml/100 ml blood	Reflected by PO_2 90 torr
Combined with Hgb.	19.4 ml/100 ml blood	Reflected by O_2 sat Hgb. 97%
Total in whole blood	19.7 ml/100 ml blood	

The first of these three methods is the easiest to understand but the most difficult to measure, so it is not used routinely. The latter two methods, which are used routinely, are more understandable when compared with the first method in Table 14–1.

The table reminds us that the majority of oxygen carried by the blood is carried by hemoglobin, and that a very small amount is dissolved in plasma. The percent saturation of hemoglobin with oxygen, then, gives a close estimate of the total amount of oxygen carried in blood.

The PO_2 measurement, however, tells only of the pressure exerted by the small amount of oxygen that is dissolved in plasma.

PO_2 is widely used and is valuable because PO_2 (pressure of oxygen dissolved in plasma) and oxygen saturation of hemoglobin (which is closely related to the total oxygen content of whole blood) are related to each other in a definite fashion, and the relationship has been charted—the *oxyhemoglobin dissociation curve* (see Fig. 14–1).

When the PO_2 in plasma is high, hemoglobin carries much oxygen. When the PO_2 is low, hemoglobin carries less oxygen. Once this relationship is known, PO_2 is just as valuable as a measurement of total O_2 content or the percentage of oxygen that hemoglobin is carrying.

Oxygen Content

Oxygen content refers to the total amount of oxygen that is present in blood in any form. Oxygen is carried in blood just two ways: (1) dissolved in the plasma and (2) combined with hemoglobin. By far the larger amount of oxygen is carried in combination with hemoglobin, and a very small amount is dissolved in plasma (see Table 14–1). Oxygen is not very soluble in plasma or water, so only a very small amount can dissolve in plasma. Oxygen content and oxygen saturation of hemoglobin are indicators of the *amount* of oxygen in blood or in the red blood cells respectively.

PO_2 Measurement

The oxygen that is combined with hemoglobin exerts no pressure, but the oxygen that is dissolved in plasma exerts a pressure or tension.

The pressure or tension of oxygen dissolved in plasma can be readily measured and is known as PO_2. The hemoglobin oxygen dissociation curve (Fig. 14–1) defines the relationship between the pressure exerted by dissolved oxygen and the amount of oxygen carried by hemoglobin. It should be made quite clear, though, *that PO_2 is a measure of the pressure or tension exerted by dissolved oxygen, and PO_2 is not a measure of the* amount *of oxygen in blood.*

Partial Pressure and Barometric Pressure. An explanation of PO_2 must start with an explanation of barometric pressure. Barometric pressure may be thought of as the weight of the atmosphere or the pressure exerted by the atmosphere. At sea level barometric pressure is 760 torr. We are not conscious of the weight or pressure exerted on us by the atmosphere, partly because the atmosphere is made up of gases. If we dive into water, we are much more aware of the weight or pressure exerted on us by the water, and this pressure increases as we dive deeper because there is progressively more water above us. Just as in water, the deeper we are in the atmosphere, the higher the barometric pressure. So, at the top of Pike's Peak (elevation 14,110 feet above sea level) we are near the top of the atmosphere and the barometric pressure is lower—425 torr. Denver and the cities of Colorado and Wyoming are between these two extremes. The average barometric pressure in Denver is 625 torr. (Of course, as weather fronts approach, the barometric pressure may fluctuate slightly even though the elevation is constant.) With high-pressure weather fronts, the barometric pressure may increase by 5 to 10 torr, and with low-pressure fronts the barometric pressure may fall by 5 to 10 torr. In blood gas laboratories a barometer is necessary for determining the barometric pressure each day.

If one takes a bottle in which a vacuum has been created and inverts this bottle in a pan of water, when the cork is removed from the bottle the water in the pan will rise in the bottle (see Fig. 14–2). The force that makes the water rise in the bottle is the difference between the barometric pressure exerted on the pan and the absence of barometric pressure in the vacuum bottle.

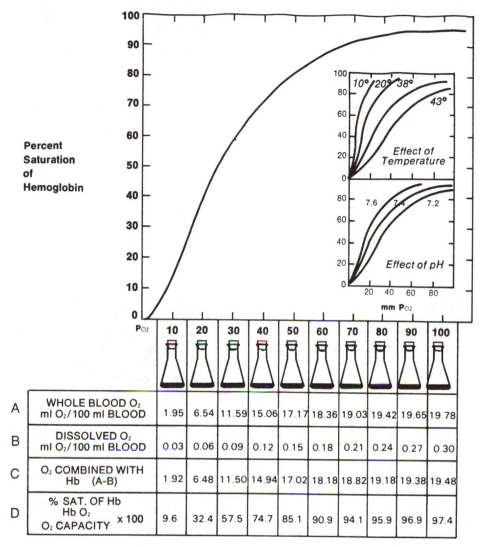

		P_{O_2}	10	20	30	40	50	60	70	80	90	100
A	WHOLE BLOOD O_2 ml O_2/100 ml BLOOD		1.95	6.54	11.59	15.06	17.17	18.36	19.03	19.42	19.65	19.78
B	DISSOLVED O_2 ml O_2/100 ml BLOOD		0.03	0.06	0.09	0.12	0.15	0.18	0.21	0.24	0.27	0.30
C	O_2 COMBINED WITH Hb (A-B)		1.92	6.48	11.50	14.94	17.02	18.18	18.82	19.18	19.38	19.48
D	% SAT. OF Hb $\dfrac{\text{Hb } O_2}{O_2 \text{ CAPACITY}}$ x 100		9.6	32.4	57.5	74.7	85.1	90.9	94.1	95.9	96.9	97.4

FIGURE 14-1.

HbO_2 dissociation curves. The large graph shows a single dissociation curve, applicable when the pH of the blood is 7.40 and temperature 38°C. The blood O_2 tension and saturation of patients with CO_2 retention, acidosis, alkalosis, fever, or hypothermia will not fit this curve because the curve shifts to the right when temperature, pH, or P_{CO_2} is changed. Effects on the HbO_2 dissociation curve of change in temperature and in pH are shown in the smaller graphs. (Comroe JH: Physiology of Respiration, 2nd ed. Copyright © 1974 by Year Book Medical Publishers, Inc., Chicago. Used by permission.)

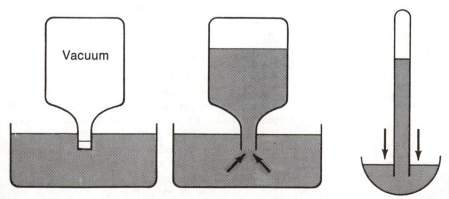

FIGURE 14-2.
Effects of barometric pressure.

Table 14-2
Comparison of PO_2 at Sea Level with PO_2 at Denver

At Sea Level		At Denver		Remarks
760		630	torr	Average barometric pressure
−47		−47	torr	Water vapor pressure at body temperature (subtracted because in the body this pressure is exerted by water vapor)
713		583	torr	Corrected barometric pressure (in body or completely humidified air at body temperature)
×21%		×21%		Percent of oxygen in the atmosphere
150	torr	123	torr	PO_2 in air that is completely humidified
−40		−36		PCO_2—pressure exerted by CO_2 in alveolus
110	torr	87	torr	PO_2 in alveolus
−5	torr	−5	torr	Gradient for diffusion of O_2 from alveolus into capillary
105	torr	82	torr	PO_2 in capillary blood in lungs
−10	torr	−10	torr	Due to venous shunting
95	torr	72	torr	PO_2 in arterial blood

If we substitute a long tube for the bottle, create a vacuum in the tube, and invert the tube in a container of mercury instead of a pan of water, we have a barometer. Since the vacuum in the tube remains constant, the only factor influencing how high mercury rises in the tube is the barometric pressure (or weight of the atmosphere) pressing down on the mercury in the container.

Table 14-2 is a simplified explanation of why the arterial PO_2 in Denver is about 72 torr and at sea level about 95 torr.

It should be pointed out that the percentage of oxygen in the atmosphere is 21% (actually 20.93%) everywhere in the atmosphere and that changes in PO_2 with altitude are due to changes in barometric pressure with altitude and not due to changes in percentage of oxygen present.

Hemoglobin Saturation

Each gram of hemoglobin in 100 ml of blood can carry a maximum of 1.34 ml of oxygen. As stated earlier in this chapter, the percent saturation of hemoglobin is defined as the amount of oxygen that hemoglobin *is* carrying compared with the amount of oxygen that hemoglobin *can* carry, expressed as a percentage:

Percent O_2 saturation of Hgb. =

$$\frac{\text{Amount } O_2 \text{ Hgb. is carrying}}{\text{Amount } O_2 \text{ Hgb. can carry}} \times 100$$

Since the amount of oxygen that hemoglobin can carry is a constant 1.34 ml/g hemoglobin, then,

1.34 ml × g Hgb. × % saturation Hgb. =
No. of ml O_2 that Hgb. is carrying

(It should be noted that there are rare abnormal types of hemoglobin that cannot carry 1.34 ml oxygen/g. There are also rare situations in which normal hemoglobin has been poisoned so that it cannot carry 1.34 ml oxygen/g—sulfhemoglobin or methemoglobin, for example.)

In 100 ml of blood

$$\begin{cases} 1 \text{ g Hgb. can carry } 1.34 \text{ ml } O_2 \\ 15 \text{ g Hgb. can carry } 15 \times 1.34 \text{ ml } O_2 \end{cases}$$

In Denver, the normal oxygen saturation of hemoglobin in arterial blood is 93% (*i.e.,* hemoglobin *is* carrying 93% of the total amount of oxygen it *can* carry), then 93% of 20.1 ml equals 18.7 ml of oxygen carried by hemoglobin in Denver. At sea level, arterial oxygen saturation of hemoglobin is 97%, so hemoglobin is carrying 97% of 20.1 ml or 19.4 ml of oxygen.

The major factor that determines how much oxygen hemoglobin *is* carrying is the PO_2 that the hemoglobin is exposed to. At high PO_2 hemoglobin carries more oxygen; at low PO_2 hemoglobin carries less oxygen. The exact relationship between the amount of oxygen that hemoglobin is carrying and the PO_2 is shown by the oxyhemoglobin dissociation curve in Figure 14-1.

OXYHEMOGLOBIN DISSOCIATION CURVE

The relationship between PO_2 and oxygen saturation of hemoglobin is not a linear one, so that for a given rise or fall in PO_2 there is not always the same amount of rise or fall in oxygen saturation of hemoglobin. Instead, for very low PO_2, a rise in PO_2 is associated with a more rapid rise in oxygen saturation; and for PO_2 in the normal range or higher, a rise in PO_2 is associated with a very small rise in oxygen saturation.

This relationship is much easier to understand if one looks at the oxygen dissociation curve for hemoglobin (see Fig. 14-1). In simple terms, the dissociation curve indicates that in environments in which the PO_2 is high, such as the capillaries of the lungs, hemoglobin combines with and carries a high percentage of the total oxygen it could carry; in environments in which the PO_2 is low, such as the capillaries in the tissues, hemoglobin carries a lower percentage of the total oxygen it could carry, having given up the difference in oxygen for use by the tissues.

Shifts in the Curve. The dissociation curve presented applies only to normal conditions. In the presence of *acidosis* or fever, the entire dissociation curve is shifted to the right, so that for a given oxygen saturation the PO_2 is greater than usual, and more oxygen is available for the tissues. In the presence of *alkalosis,* hemoglobin is more stingy, and for a given oxygen saturation, the PO_2 is lower than usual.

Certain abnormal types of hemoglobin may shift the dissociation curve to the right or the left, and the presence of certain compounds such as 2,3 diphosphoglycerate (2,3 DPG) may also shift the dissociation curve. Normal or high amounts of 2,3 DPG shift the curve to the right, thereby making more oxygen available to the tissues for a given oxygen saturation of hemoglobin because 2,3 DPG decreases the affinity of hemoglobin for oxygen. Conversely, blood with low amounts of 2,3 DPG, such as transfused blood from a blood bank, has a left-shifted oxyhemoglobin dissociation curve, which makes less oxygen available to the tissues because this hemoglobin has a greater than normal affinity for oxygen. The measurement of P_{50} (partial pressure of oxygen when hemoglobin is exactly 50% saturated) allows one to detect the shifted oxyhemoglobin dissociation curve, so that P_{50} is greater than 27 when the curve is shifted to the right and less than 27 when it is shifted to the left.

Fraction of Inspired Oxygen (FIO$_2$). One should always relate the oxygen content of blood to the FIO_2. For instance, an oxygen saturation of hemoglobin of 96% is normal if the patient is breathing room air, which has an FIO_2 of 21, but is quite abnormal if the FIO_2 is −40. Some hospitals formally measure the A-a oxygen gradient (the difference between PO_2 in alveolar air and PO_2 in arterial blood), but much the same information can be obtained if one compares the PaO_2 or oxygen saturation of hemoglobin with the FIO_2. The normal range for A-a oxygen gradient increases with age. In young people the A-a oxygen gradient may normally be as high as 15 torr, while in elderly people it may be as high as 27 torr.

As previously mentioned, the normal values for oxygen in arterial blood in Denver or any other place above sea level are lower than those at sea level because there is progressively lower PO_2 in the ambient air as one ascends (see Table 14-3).

In mixed venous blood the normal values for oxygen may be slightly lower in Denver than at sea level, but not enough lower to warrant remembering a second set of values.

Oxygen Transport

The amount of oxygen that is transported to the tissues is more important than the PO_2. The PO_2 is a measure of intensity or pressure due to oxygen, and oxygen content is a measure of amount of oxygen.

$$O_2 \text{ transport to the tissues} = \text{arterial } O_2 \text{ content} \times \text{cardiac output}$$

Table 14-3
Oxygen Values in Denver vs Sea Level

	Denver	Sea Level
Arterial Blood O$_2$		
Oxygen content	18.9 ml O_2/100 ml of blood	19.7
PO_2	70 torr (range 65–75)	> 80 torr
O_2 saturation of Hgb.	93% (range 92%–94%)	> 95%
Mixed Venous Blood O$_2$		
Oxygen content	14–16 ml O_2/100 ml of blood	
PO_2	35–40 torr	
O_2 saturation of Hgb.	70%–75%	

The oxygen transported to the tissues depends on: (1) the amount of oxygen in arterial blood (arterial oxygen content) and (2) the ability of the heart to pump this blood containing oxygen around to the tissues.

The arterial oxygen content depends in turn on: (1) how well the lungs are able to get oxygen from air into the blood and (2) a normal amount of functioning hemoglobin to carry the oxygen.

In summary, oxygenation of the tissue depends on:

1. Arterial O_2 content, which depends on
   a. Lungs' ability to get O_2 into blood
   b. Ability of hemoglobin to hold enough O_2
2. Cardiac output (circulation)

Tissue Hypoxia

There are varied pulmonary and nonpulmonary causes for tissue hypoxia, which results from insufficient oxygenation. Four pulmonary reasons can be listed to explain why arterial blood may not be carrying the normal amount of oxygen.

- Alveolar hypoventilation.
   Associated with high PCO_2
- Diffusion defect (at alveolar–capillary level).
   Associated with low or normal PCO_2
- Right-to-left shunt (in lung or heart).
   Associated with low or normal PCO_2
- Mismatching of ventilation and blood flow in the lungs. (Blood goes by alveoli that are poorly ventilated. This blood, as it passes through the lungs, picks up little oxygen. This poorly oxygenated blood then returns to the heart and is pumped out into the arteries to the body, therefore causing arterial blood to have less than the normal amount of oxygen.)
   Associated with low or normal PCO_2

The nonpulmonary causes of tissue hypoxia are (1) reduced blood flow to the tissues (reduced cardiac output); (2) anemia — not enough hemoglobin to carry oxygen; (3) nonfunctioning hemoglobin — enough hemoglobin but hemoglobin that exists cannot carry oxygen because it has been "poisoned"; and (4) right-to-left cardiac shunts — most frequently seen in cyanotic congenital heart disease.

- *Reduced blood flow* to the tissues (reduced cardiac output) might be caused by
   Myocardial infarction
   Abnormal cardiac rhythm
   Reduced cardiac function (other causes): congestive heart failure, valvular heart lesion, etc.
   Hypovolemia (intimately related to anemia)

- *Anemia:* 1 g Hgb. carries 1.34 ml O_2 and normally there are 15 g Hgb. to carry 15×1.34 ml O_2 or 20.1 ml O_2. If there is anemia so that only 7.5 g Hgb. are present, then 7.5×1.34 ml $O_2 = 10$ ml O_2 are all that can be carried; if anemia is milder (between 7.5 and 15 g Hgb.), more O_2 can be carried; if anemia is more severe (less than 7.5 g Hgb.), even less O_2 can be carried. Usually the body compensates for anemia by having the heart circulate faster the lesser amount of hemoglobin that is present.
- *Nonfunctioning hemoglobin:* A few rare conditions exist in which there might be a normal amount of hemoglobin, but even this normal amount cannot function because it has been poisoned. Some examples of this are
   Carbon monoxide poisoning
   Methemoglobinemia
   Sulfhemoglobinemia
   In each of these situations something (carbon monoxide, for example) has combined with hemoglobin, making it hard for oxygen to combine with and be carried by this hemoglobin.
- In *right-to-left cardiac shunts,* oxygen gets through the lungs normally into the bloodstream, there is enough functioning hemoglobin to carry the oxygen, and the heart is strong enough to circulate the oxygenated blood. However, some venous blood that never passes through the lungs to get oxygenated is *shunted* into the systemic arterial system, and the combination of oxygenated blood plus venous unoxygenated blood is carried through the arteries to the tissues, supplying them with less oxygen than they need.

COMPENSATORY MECHANISMS

The patient who is hypoxemic compensates for hypoxia in the following ways:

- Tachypnea (rapid breathing)
- Tachycardia (rapid heartbeat)
- Erythrocytosis (high hemoglobin and hematocrit)

The tachypnea and tachycardia represent extra energy expenditure by the patient. Erythrocytosis simply means increased production of red blood cells by the hypoxic patient's bone marrow in an attempt to get more oxygen to the tissues. If the fault is lack of enough red blood cells, this can be remedied. But if the fault is in getting enough oxygen through the lungs, increasing the number of red blood cells helps little or not at all. The hypoxemic patient tries all these means of compensating for hypoxemia, and often all of them together are inadequate.

Hypoxia often leads to pulmonary hyperten-

Table 14-4
Normal Blood Gas Values

	Arterial Blood	Mixed Venous Blood
pH	7.40 (7.35–7.45)	7.38 (7.33–7.43)
PO_2	80–100 torr	35–40 torr
O_2 sat	95% or greater	70%–75%
PCO_2	35–45 torr	41–51 torr
HCO_3	22–26 mEq/liter	24–28 mEq/liter
Base excess (B.E.)	−2–+2	0–+4

sion (high blood pressure in the arteries of the lungs), and this can lead to strain or failure of the right side of the heart.

OXYGEN THERAPY

If oxygen is administered to the patient to treat his hypoxemia, tachypnea and tachycardia do not occur, no erythrocytosis occurs, and pulmonary hypertension may go away. Complete compensation is possible with oxygen treatment, but sometimes patient compensation is not complete.

It can be seen that supplemental oxygen is rational treatment for the patient with hypoxemia, but long-term continuous oxygen is usually reserved for the patient who, when completely stable, has a PO_2 below 50 torr (oxygen saturation below 85%) and who also has one or more of the following:

- Right heart failure that is difficult to manage with digitalis and diuretics
- Significant secondary erythrocytosis
- A progressive downhill course with weight loss, progressive muscle wasting, or decreased mental function

Often such a patient responds to nocturnal oxygen (oxygen for 8 hours at night), or if the patient is living at a high altitude, a move to a lower altitude may make supplemental oxygen unnecessary.

Possible CO_2 Retention.
Oxygen treatment may lead to CO_2 retention if the oxygen is not carefully controlled.

There are two major reflex stimuli to breathing:

- CO_2 retention (hypercapnic stimulus to breathe)
- Low PO_2 (hypoxic stimulus to breathe)

Small elevations of PCO_2 are a major stimulus to breathing. Increasing the PCO_2 by 4 torr can cause a 100% increase in ventilation. Large elevations in PCO_2 reduce the amount of ventilation by reducing all brain functions including function of the respiratory center.

In patients with large elevation of PCO_2, hypoxemia may be the most important stimulus to breathe. If a patient who no longer has a hypercapnic stimulus to breathing is treated with oxygen, thereby eliminating the hypoxic stimulus to breathe, he may breathe even less, significantly worsening his condition. It has become apparent that giving a controlled amount of oxygen (just enough to raise the PaO_2 to approximately 60 torr) allows the patient to benefit from the oxygen and usually does not reduce ventilation.

It should be clear that oxygen therapy, though often given in a haphazard fashion, requires just as much understanding and precision in dosage as any other form of drug therapy.

BLOOD GAS ANALYSIS

Normal Values
Normal values for blood gases are given in Table 14-4. Following this the main emphasis will concern acid-base interpretation (see Table 14-5).

Note that in Table 14-4 only two measurements—PO_2, and PCO_2—are actually measurements of gases. However, all should be determined in blood gas analyses. It is imperative that a measure of the nonrespiratory (meta-

Table 14-5
Definitions

Acid: A substance that can donate hydrogen ions, H^+.
Example:
$$H_2CO_3 \longrightarrow H^+ + HCO_3^-$$
(acid)

Base: A substance that can accept hydrogen ions, H^+.
All bases are alkaline substances. Example:
$$HCO_3^- + H^+ \longrightarrow H_2CO_3$$
(base)

Table 14–6
Acid-Base Terms

---

pH measurement = Only way to tell if body is too acid or too alkaline

Acidemia = Acid condition of the blood —pH < 7.35

Alkalemia = Alkaline condition of the blood —
pH > 7.45

Acidosis = Process causing acidemia

Alkalosis = Process causing alkalemia

---

bolic) component be included, and actual HCO_3^- and base excess are the most useful. Many other terms may be given on a blood gas report, but one need be concerned only with those listed in Table 14-4.

Older persons have values for PO_2 and oxygen saturation near the lower part of the normal range, and younger people tend to have high normal values.

Normal values for mixed venous blood are more variable than for arterial blood, but representative normals are given in Table 14-4. Because there is not much difference in normal values of HCO_3^- and base excess between arterial and mixed venous blood and because venous blood is not often used, one does not need to remember a different set of values for venous blood.

An acid is any substance that can donate a hydrogen ion, H^+. H^+ can be thought of as the most important part of an acid.

Many substances may include H in their chemical structure, but some cannot donate the H because it is too tightly bound. Only those substances that can give up their H^+ are acids.

Bases are substances that can accept or combine with H^+. The terms *base* and *alkali* are used interchangeably. (See Table 14-6.)

Each of the acid–base terms in Table 14-6 will now be discussed in more detail.

The pH measurement is the only way to tell if

Table 14–7
PCO₂, the Respiratory Parameter

PCO_2 = pressure (tension) of dissolved CO_2 gas in blood; influenced only by respiratory causes

Food $\xrightarrow[\text{by body}]{\text{converted}}$ $H_2O + CO_2$ + energy

$CO_2 + H_2O \rightleftharpoons H_2CO_3 \rightleftharpoons HCO_3^- + H^+$

Normal PCO_2 = normal ventilation

High PCO_2 = hypoventilation

Low PCO_2 = hyperventilation

---

the body is too acid or too alkaline. Low pH numbers (below 7.35) indicate an acid state, and high pH numbers (above 7.45) indicate an alkaline state.

If the numbers are lower than 7.35, there is acidemia, and if higher than 7.45, alkalemia. Aci*demia* refers to a condition in which the *blood* is too acid. Aci*dosis* refers to the *process* in the patient that causes the acidemia, and the adjective for the process is acid*otic*. Alkal*osis* refers to the *process* in the patient that causes the alkalemia, and the adjective for this process is alkal*otic*.

This much time has been spent in defining the terms because later it will be seen that in a patient there may be more than one process occurring at a time. For instance, if both an acidosis and an alkalosis are occurring at once, then the pH will tell us which is the stronger of the two processes. The pH will be below 7.35 if the acidosis is the stronger, above 7.45 if the alkalosis is the stronger, and between 7.35 and 7.45 if the acidosis and alkalosis are of nearly equal strength. The pH value of blood represents an average of the acidoses and alkaloses that may be occurring.

Respiratory Parameter: PCO₂

The PCO_2 refers to the pressure or tension exerted by dissolved CO_2 gas in the blood (see Table 14-7). The PCO_2 is influenced *only* by respiratory causes. Although this is an oversimplification, remember that PCO_2 *is influenced only by the lungs.*

Where does the CO_2 come from? It is present only in very tiny amounts in the air we breathe. It comes directly from foods we eat. As a result of metabolism for the production of energy, foods are converted by the body tissues to water and CO_2 gas. When the pressure of CO_2 in the cells exceeds 40 torr (the normal arterial value), the CO_2 spills over from the cells into the plasma. In plasma, CO_2 may combine with H_2O to form H_2CO_3 (carbonic acid), but there is actually 800 times as much CO_2 in the form of dissolved gas in plasma as is converted to H_2CO_3.

You should consider CO_2 gas an acid substance because when it combines with water, an acid is formed — carbonic acid, H_2CO_3.

H_2CO_3 dissociates into hydrogen ion, H^+, and bicarbonate, HCO_3^-. Much of the H^+ forms a loose association with the plasma proteins (is buffered), thus reducing the free H^+.

The body has to get rid of the waste product, CO_2, and can do so in two ways:

Table 14–8
Respiratory Abnormalities

Parameter	Condition	Mechanism
↑ PCO_2	Respiratory acidosis	Decreased elimination by lungs of CO_2 gas (Hypoventilation)
↓ PCO_2	Respiratory alkalosis	Increased elimination by lungs of CO_2 gas (Hyperventilation)

- The less important way is by converting the CO_2 gas to carbonic acid, H_2CO_3, which dissociates to H^+ and HCO_3^-. The H^+ can be excreted by the kidneys, mainly in the form of NH_4^+.
- A much more important way is to have the lungs get rid of the CO_2.

Getting rid of CO_2 gas, then, is one of the main functions of the lungs, and a very important relationship exists between the amount of ventilation and the amount of PCO_2 in blood. If the PCO_2 in blood (*i.e.,* the dissolved CO_2 gas in blood) is too high, it means that the lungs are not providing enough ventilation. This is called *hypoventilation*. Hypoventilation can thus be detected by finding high levels of PCO_2 in the blood. If the PCO_2 is too low, there is excessive ventilation by the lungs, or *hyperventilation,* and if the PCO_2 is normal, there is exactly the right amount of ventilation.

PCO_2 is much more important than PO_2 in judging whether there is normal ventilation, hyperventilation, or hypoventilation, because there are other factors (such as shunting, diffusion abnormalities, etc.) which lower the PO_2 without reducing ventilation.

As seen in Table 14–8 there are only two abnormal conditions associated with abnormalities in PCO_2: respiratory acidosis (high PCO_2) and respiratory alkalosis (low PCO_2).

RESPIRATORY ACIDOSIS

The term *respiratory acidosis* means elevated PCO_2 due to hypoventilation. The causes of respiratory acidosis (high PCO_2) are:

- Obstructive pulmonary disease (mainly chronic bronchitis, emphysema, and occasionally asthma)
- Oversedation, head trauma, anesthesia, and other causes of reduced function of the respiratory center
- Neuromuscular disorders such as myasthenia gravis or the Guillain-Barré syndrome

- Hypoventilation with a mechanical ventilator
- Other rarer causes of hypoventilation (such as the Pickwickian syndrome) (see Table 14–9)

It should be noted that *respiratory* acidosis may occur even with normal lungs if the respiratory center is depressed.

RESPIRATORY ALKALOSIS

The term *respiratory alkalosis* means low PCO_2 due to hyperventilation. The causes are hypoxia, congestive heart failure, anxiety, pulmonary emboli, pulmonary fibrosis, pregnancy, hyperventilation with mechanical ventilator, gram-negative septicemia, hepatic insufficiency, brain injury, salicylates, fever, asthma, and severe anemia (see Table 14–10). In gram-negative sep-

Table 14–9
Causes of Respiratory Acidosis (↑ PCO_2)

1. Obstructive lung disease
2. Oversedation and other causes of reduced function of the respiratory center (even with normal lungs)
3. Neuromuscular disorders
4. Hypoventilation with mechanical ventilator
5. Other causes of hypoventilation

Table 14–10
Causes of Respiratory Alkalosis (↓ PCO_2)

1. Hypoxia
2. Nervousness and anxiety
3. Pulmonary embolus, fibrosis, etc.
4. Pregnancy
5. Hyperventilation with mechanical ventilator
6. Brain injury
7. Salicylates
8. Fever
9. Gram-negative septicemia
10. Hepatic insufficiency
11. Congestive heart failure
12. Asthma
13. Severe anemia

ticemia, the hyperventilation may precede other evidence of septicemia. In patients with congestive heart failure, pneumonia, asthma, pulmonary emboli, and pulmonary fibrosis, the hyperventilation (respiratory alkalosis) continues even if the hypoxia is corrected; hence, hypoxia is not the only cause in these conditions.

Nonrespiratory (Metabolic) Parameters: HCO_3^- and Base Excess

The term *base excess* refers principally to bicarbonate but also to the other bases in blood (mainly plasma proteins and hemoglobin). Bicarbonate and base excess are influenced *only* by nonrespiratory causes, not by respiratory causes. Again, this is a simplification, but a very important fact to remember—*bicarbonate and base excess are influenced only by nonrespiratory processes.*

For our purposes we can define a *metabolic process* as anything other than respiratory causes that affects the patient's acid-base status. Examples of common metabolic (nonrespiratory) processes would be diabetic acidosis and uremia.

When a nonrespiratory process leads to the accumulation of acids in the body or losses of bicarbonate, bicarbonate values drop below the normal range, and base excess values become negative. On the other hand, when a nonrespiratory process causes loss of acid or accumulation of excess bicarbonate, bicarbonate values rise above normal, and base excess values become positive. Base excess may be thought of as representing an excess of bicarbonate or other base. Bicarbonate, then, is base—or in other words, an alkaline substance.

As seen in Table 14–11, there are only two abnormal conditions associated with abnormalities in HCO_3^- or base excess: metabolic alkalosis and metabolic acidosis. (Nonvolatile acid is any acid other than $PCO_2 - H_2CO_3$.)

METABOLIC ALKALOSIS

The *causes* of metabolic alkalosis (increased HCO_3^- and base excess) are (1) loss of acid-containing fluid from the upper gastrointestinal tract as by nasogastric suction or vomiting (this loss of acid from the stomach leaves the body with a relative excess of alkali); (2) rapid correction of chronic hypercapnia (it will take the body several days to correct its compensation for hypercapnia—accumulation of excess HCO_3^-—after the hypercapnia is suddenly relieved); (3) diuretic therapy with mercurial diuretics, ethacrynic acid, furosemide, and thiazide diuretics; (4) Cushing's disease; (5) treatment with corticosteroids (*i.e.*, prednisone or cortisone); (6) hyperaldosteronism; (7) severe potassium depletion; (8) excessive ingestion of licorice; (9) Bartter's syndrome; (10) alkali administration; and (11) nonparathyroid hypercalcemia.

A rare cause of nonrespiratory alkalosis, which unfortunately is not reflected by an elevated bicarbonate in the blood, is the intravenous infusion of phenytoin (Dilantin), which has a very alkaline *p*H. Infusion of this alkaline substance causes a short-lived alkalemia not associated with elevated HCO_3^-.

Hypokalemia and Hypochloremia. The first three causes of alkalosis listed above—fluid losses from the stomach, rapid correction of chronic hypercapnia, and diuretic therapy—will all show correction of the alkalosis in response to administration of sodium chloride. Treatment with potassium chloride may be more reasonable if the potassium is low or if one is trying to prevent accumulation of salt and water. Treatment with two other diuretics, spironolactone (Aldactone) and triamterene (Dyrenium), does not cause metabolic alkalosis. With causes 4 through 9 in Table 14–12, the metabolic alkalosis cannot be corrected by administration of sodium chloride. With the last two causes listed, the response of sodium chloride is variable.

Table 14–11
Metabolic Abnormalities

Parameter	Condition	Mechanism
↑ HCO_3^- or ↑ B.E.	Nonrespiratory (metabolic) alkalosis	1. Nonvolatile acid is lost, or 2. HCO_3^- is gained
↓ HCO_3^- or ↓ B.E.	Nonrespiratory (metabolic) acidosis	1. Nonvolatile acid is added (using up HCO_3^-) or 2. HCO_3^- is lost

Table 14–12
Causes of Metabolic (Nonrespiratory) Alkalosis (↑ HCO₃⁻)

1. Fluid losses from upper GI tract — vomiting or nasogastric tube causing loss of acid
2. Rapid correction of chronic hypercapnia
3. Diuretic therapy — mercurial, ethacrynic acid (Edecrin), furosemide (Lasix), thiazides
4. Cushing's disease
5. Therapy with corticosteroids (prednisone, cortisone, etc.)
6. Hyperaldosteronism
7. Severe potassium depletion
8. Excessive ingestion of licorice
9. Bartter's syndrome
10. Alkali administration
11. Nonparathyroid hypercalcemia

The following is an explanation of the relationship between hypokalemia (low K^+), hypochloremia (low Cl^-), and metabolic alkalosis. Normally in the kidney sodium (Na^+) and chloride (Cl^-) pass from the blood into the urine at the glomerulus. Further along in the tubules of the kidney this Na^+, which is in the urine, must be reabsorbed from the urine into the kidney tubule cells and then into the blood.

Because Na^+ has a positive charge (+), when it is reabsorbed into the cells, the Na^+ must either

• Be reabsorbed with something that has a negative charge (−) like Cl^- or

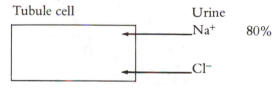

• Enter the tubule cell in exchange for something else that has a positive charge, like K^+ or H^+ (which passes from the tubule cell to the urine)

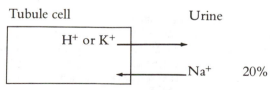

Normally, 80% of the Na^+ is reabsorbed while accompanied by Cl^-, and 20% is exchanged for K^+ or H^+. (See Fig. 14–3.)

When there is hypochloremia (↓ Cl^-), the amount of Na^+ that is reabsorbed in the company of Cl^- is reduced, and more Na^+ must be exchanged for K^+ or H^+. When Na^+ is exchanged for K^+ and H^+, the loss of H^+ represents a loss of acid, leaving the patient alkalotic — therefore a hypochloremic alkalosis.

When Na^+ is exchanged for K^+ or H^+, only a small amount of K^+ is available, and when this is used up the patient becomes hypokalemic, and H^+ is lost. The loss of H^+ is a loss of acid, leaving the patient with an alkalosis — hypokalemic alkalosis.

METABOLIC ACIDOSIS

Substances that have a negative charge are attracted to an anode and are called *anions*. The anions that are normally measured (specified) are HCO_3^- and CL^-. The anions that are not regularly measured but are normally present in blood are called *unspecified* or *unmeasured* anions. They are phosphates, sulfates, creatinates, and proteinates.

The causes of nonrespiratory (metabolic) acidosis (low HCO_3^- and low base excess) can be divided into those causes in which there is an increase in the unspecified anions and those

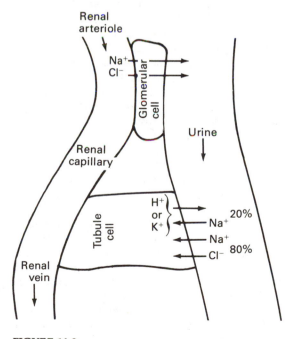

FIGURE 14-3.
Process by which low Cl^- and low K^+ can cause metabolic alkalosis.

Table 14–13
Causes of Metabolic (Nonrespiratory) Acidosis
(↓ HCO_3^- and ↓ B.E.)

With Increase in Unspecified Anions	*Without Increase in Unspecified Anions*
Diabetic ketoacidosis	Diarrhea
Starvation ketoacidosis	Drainage of pancreatic juice
Alcoholic ketoacidosis	Ureterosigmoidostomy
Poisonings	Obstructed ileal loop
Salicylate	Therapy with acetazolamide (Diamox)
Ethylene glycol	Therapy with ammonium chloride (NH_4Cl)
Methyl alcohol	Renal tubular acidosis
Paraldehyde (rarely)	Intravenous hyperalimentation (rarely)
Lactic acidosis	Dilutional acidosis
Renal failure	

causes in which bicarbonate has been lost and there is no such increase in unspecified anions (see Table 14-13).

The normal value for unspecified anions is 12 ± 3.

An increase in unspecified anions may be due to accumulation of phosphates, sulfates, and creatinates, as seen in renal failure or the accumulation of an unusual negatively charged substance such as lactic acid, ketoacids, or the like. Often the unspecified anions are referred to as the *anion gap.* If one subtracts the sum of HCO_3^- and Cl^- concentration from Na^+ concentration and finds a difference greater than 15, there is said to be an increase in unspecified anions (increased anion gap). Conditions causing this are diabetic ketoacidosis, alcoholic ketoacidosis, poisonings (salicylate, ethylene glycol, methyl alcohol, paraldehyde), lactic acidosis, and renal failure. In these cases there is accumulation of or ingestion of an unusual acid.

Conditions that cause a metabolic acidosis *without an increase in unmeasured anions* are associated with a high serum chloride. These conditions are diarrhea, drainage of pancreatic juice, ureterosigmoidostomy, obstructed ileal loop, treatment with acetazolamide (Diamox), renal tubular acidosis, treatment with ammonium chloride or arginine monohydrochloride, and intravenous hyperalimentation. In most of these latter conditions, there is a deficit of bicarbonate, leaving relatively too much acid.

In all of the conditions in the left-hand column in Table 14-13, there is an accumulation of an abnormal acid substance in blood, which then reacts with and uses up some of the usual amount of bicarbonate, leaving the patient with reduced levels of bicarbonate and base excess.

One of the most important causes of metabolic acidosis is *lactic acidosis.* Whenever body tissues do not have enough oxygen, they lose their ability to metabolize lactic acid, which then accumulates in the blood. This lactic acid then combines with some of the normal amount of bicarbonate, using up the bicarbonate.

In a cardiac arrest, we customarily administer bicarbonate, about 1 ampul (44.6 mEq) every 5 minutes, to resupply the bicarbonate which is used up by combining with lactic acid. Other conditions besides cardiac arrest that may be associated with lactic acidosis are shock, severe heart failure, and severe hypoxemia. Tissue hypoxia, seen in all of these conditions, leads to the lactate production.

If a patient has a metabolic acidosis with an anion gap of greater than 15, the nurse can consult Table 14-13, left column, and ask the lab to measure whichever unspecified anion she guesses might be elevated; for example, if the patient is an uncontrolled diabetic, measure ketoacids; if the patient is in shock, measure lactic acid.

CO_2 Content

PCO_2 is the respiratory parameter, is a gas, is an acid, and is regulated by the lungs. HCO_3^- and base excess are nonrespiratory parameters occurring in solution, are bases (alkaline substances), and are regulated mainly by the kidneys (not by the lungs). To summarize

- PCO_2 — respiratory parameter
  Gas
  Acid
  Regulated by the lungs

Table 14–14

HCO_3^-	24 mEq/liter
Dissolved CO_2 gas	1.2 mEq/liter = 40 torr PCO_2
CO_2 content	25.2 mEq/liter

- HCO_3^- or base excess — nonrespiratory parameter
  Solution
  Base
  Regulated mainly by the kidneys

Where does the CO_2 content fit in this scheme? Determination of electrolytes consists of Na^+, K^+, Cl^-, and CO_2. In this case CO_2 is an abbreviation for CO_2 content, which is composed mainly of bicarbonate; if the term *CO_2 content* were used, it would improve understanding. Note that in conversation CO_2 is sometimes used to mean CO_2 content (mainly bicarbonate) and sometimes to mean CO_2 gas. This double use of the term CO_2 is one of the main difficulties in understanding acid-base problems. Use the terms *CO_2 content* and *CO_2 gas* to avoid confusion. Better yet, some hospitals are reporting HCO_3^- in place of CO_2 content when electrolytes are ordered.

Table 14–14 shows that CO_2 content is made up mainly of bicarbonate (HCO_3^-) and to a lesser extent, dissolved CO_2 gas. The normal value of CO_2 content, 25.2 mEq/liter, consists of 24 mEq/liter of HCO_3^- and 1.2 mEq/liter of dissolved CO_2 gas. The 1.2 mEq/liter of dissolved CO_2 gas i expressed in different terminology: PCO_2 of 40 torr equals 1.2 mEq/liter. To convert from torr to mEq/liter, the conversion factor is 0.03, so 40 torr $\times$ 0.03 = 1.2 mEq/liter.

HCO_3^-/CO_2 Ratio. In Table 14–14 you will note that the ratio of HCO_3^- to PCO_2 is 24:1.2 or 20:1. The body always tries to keep this ratio of HCO_3^- to PCO_2 stable at 20:1. That is, the ratio of alkali (HCO_3^-) to acid (PCO_2) is normally 20:1. As long as the ratio remains 20:1, the *p*H remains normal. If bicarbonate (HCO_3^-) or base excess increases, there is alkalosis, causing the *p*H to rise. If HCO_3^- or *base excess falls, there is acidosis, and the pH falls. If the pH change is due mainly to change in bicarbonate (or base excess), it is said to be due to nonrespiratory (metabolic) causes.*

Just the opposite happens with PCO_2 which, remember, is an acid substance. If the PCO_2 rises, there is an acidosis, causing the *p*H to fall. If the PCO_2 falls, there is an alkalosis, and the *p*H rises. *If the pH change is due mainly to changes in PCO_2, it is said to be due to respiratory causes.*

As seen in Table 14–15, acid-base abnormalities can be separated into just four categories to make understanding them easier. First they are divided by *p*H into either alkalemia or acidemia. Next they are subdivided into either nonrespiratory (metabolic) or respiratory causes. This is the procedure one uses in interpreting acid base abnormalities.

*p*H Factor

***p*H and Alkalemia.** If *p*H is high, there is an alkalemia. There may be two types of alkalemia:

- Nonrespiratory, in which the primary abnormality is due to an increase in bicarbonate. An example of this is a person who has taken too much bicarbonate or baking soda.
- Respiratory, in which the primary abnormality is hyperventilation with loss of CO_2 gas. CO_2 gas is an acid substance; when CO_2 gas is lost (due to hyperventilation), an alkalosis occurs. An example would be a nervous person having a hyperventilation attack.

Table 14–15
Causes of Alkalemia and Acidemia

Types		Primary Abnormality
Alkalemia (high *p*H)	Nonrespiratory (metabolic)	$\uparrow HCO_3^-$
	Respiratory	$\downarrow PCO_2$
Acidemia (low *p*H)	Nonrespiratory (metabolic)	$\downarrow HCO_3^-$
	Respiratory	$\uparrow PCO_2$

pH and Acidemia.   If the *p*H is low, there is an acidemia, of which there are just two types:

- Nonrespiratory, in which the primary abnormality is loss of HCO_3^-, usually due to reaction with excessive metabolic acids. An example is diabetic acidosis in which ketoacids accumulate; these acids then react with the normal amount of HCO_3^-, using up HCO_3^- and leaving HCO_3^- and base excess levels low.
- Respiratory, in which there is an accumulation of CO_2 gas (high PCO_2) which, you remember, is an acid substance. An example is a patient with acute respiratory failure who *hypo*ventilates because his airways are obstructed by mucus. In respiratory acidosis there is an accumulation of volatile acid—CO_2 gas, but in nonrespiratory acidosis the acids with accumulate are not gases.

pH and Combined Acidosis – Alkalosis. There may be more than one primary acid-base disturbance occurring at the same time. Occasionally two disturbances will be of equal magnitude, and if one is an acidosis and the other an alkalosis, they will balance each other and the *p*H will remain normal. On another occasion there may be several acidoses, for instance, occurring at the same time, all adding their effects to make the *p*H more acidemic than one alone would.

pH Compensation and Correction.   There are two ways in which an abnormal *p*H may be returned toward normal: (1) compensation and (2) correction (see Table 14–16).

In *compensation,* the system not primarily affected is responsible for returning the *p*H toward normal. For example, if there is respiratory acidosis (high PCO_2) the kidneys *compensate* by retaining bicarbonate to return the ratio of HCO_3^- to PCO_2 to 20:1, when the ratio is 20:1, the *p*H is normal.

Table 14–16
Compensation vs. Correction of Acid-Base Abnormalities

In both:	Abnormal *p*H is returned toward normal.
Compensation:	Abnormal *p*H is returned toward normal *by altering the component not primarily affected, i.e.,* if PCO_2 is high, HCO_3^- is retained to compensate.
Correction:	Abnormal *p*H is returned toward normal *by altering the component primarily affected, i.e.,* if PCO_2 is high, PCO_2 is lowered, correcting the abnormality.

Compensation is complete only in chronic respiratory alkalosis. In the other acid-base disorders the *p*H is returned nearly but not completely to normal because the compensation is not complete.

In *correction,* the system primarily affected is repaired, returning the *p*H toward normal. For example, if there is respiratory acidosis (high PCO_2) vigorous bronchial hygiene and bronchodilators may improve ventilation and lower PCO_2, returning the *p*H toward normal.

In most cases, physicians, nurses, and paramedical persons are more interested in correcting the abnormality than in helping the body to compensate. In both compensation and correction the *p*H is returned toward normal. The body tries hard to maintain a normal *p*H because the various enzyme systems in all organs function correctly only when the *p*H is normal. Using newer terminology, the term *acute* respiratory acidosis means *uncompensated; chronic* respiratory acidosis means *compensated.*

Compensatory Mechanisms

Next we will discuss how the body compensates for the various acid-base abnormalities. Remember, the body compensates for abnormalities by trying to return the ratio of HCO_3^- to PCO_2 to 20:1, for if this ratio is 20:1, the *p*H is normal. If the primary process is respiratory, then the compensating system is metabolic, and vice versa. When the lungs compensate for a nonrespiratory abnormality, compensation occurs in hours, but the kidneys take 2 to 4 days to compensate for a respiratory abnormality.

Remember, the PCO_2 in torr must be converted to mEq/liter by multiplying it by 0.03 before trying it in the 20:1 ratio mentioned above; for example, PCO_2 of 40 torr × 0.03 = 1.2 mEq/liter.

In four examples in Table 14–17, the first column lists normal values for the parameters listed in the second column. The uncompensated state is listed in the third column, and the last column demonstrates how compensation takes place. The primary abnormality is enclosed in a box.

In *primary respiratory acidosis,* characterized by elevated levels of PCO_2 (an acid), the system at fault is the respiratory system, and compensation occurs through metabolic process. To compensate, the kidneys excrete more acid and less HCO_3^-, thus allowing levels of HCO_3^- to rise, returning the ratio of HCO_3^- to PCO_2 toward 20:1, and therefore returning *p*H toward normal.

Table 14–17
Compensation for Acidosis and Alkalosis

Normal		Abnormal	Compensated
Respiratory Acidosis			
24	HCO_3^- mEq/liter	24	36
1.2	PCO_2 mEq/liter	1.8	1.8
40	PCO_2 torr	60	60
20:1	ratio	13:1	20:1
7.40	*p*H	7.23	7.40
Respiratory Alkalosis			
0	B.E.	+2.5	−5
24	HCO_3^- mEq/liter	24	18
1.2	PCO_2 mEq/liter	0.9	0.9
40	PCO_2 torr	30	30
20:1	ratio	27:1	20:1
7.40	*p*H	7.52	7.40
Metabolic Acidosis			
0	B.E.	−17	−10
24	HCO_3^- mEq/liter	12	12
1.2	PCO_2 mEq/liter	1.2	0.6
40	PCO_2 torr	40	20
20:1	ratio	10:1	20:1
7.40	*p*H	7.11	7.40
Metabolic Alkalosis			
0	B.E.	+13	+9
24	HOC_3^- mEq/liter	36	36
1.2	PCO_2 mEq/liter	1.2	1.8
40	PCO_2 torr	40	60
20:1	ratio	30:1	20:1
7.40	*p*H	7.57	7.40

If the PCO_2 is high (respiratory acidosis) but the *p*H is normal, it means that the kidneys have had time to retain HCO_3^- to compensate for the elevated PCO_2 and that the process is not acute (has been present at least a few days to give the kidneys time to compensate). Usually the body does not fully compensate for respiratory acidosis.

In *primary respiratory alkalosis,* characterized by low PCO_2, compensation occurs through metabolic means. The kidneys compensate by excreting HCO_3^-, thus returning the ratio of HCO_3^- to PCO_2 back toward 20:1; this compensation by the kidneys takes 2 to 3 days.

Of the four acid-base abnormalities, it is only in compensation for respiratory alkalosis that the body is able to fully return the ratio to 20:1 and return *p*H entirely to normal.

In *primary metabolic acidosis,* the major abnormality is low HCO_3^- or base excess. In most cases excess acids, such as ketoacids in diabetic ketoacidosis, have reacted with the normal amounts of HCO_3^-, using up some of the HCO_3^- and leaving a low level of HCO_3^-. The body compensates by hyperventilating, thus lowering the PCO_2 so that the ratio of HCO_3^- to PCO_2 returns toward 20:1. Because the compensating system is the lungs, compensation can occur in hours. However, if the metabolic acidosis is severe, the lungs may not be able to blow off enough CO_2 gas to compensate fully. Actually, in metabolic acidosis the body never compensates fully (never gets the ratio back to 20:1 or the *p*H back to 7.40).

In *metabolic alkalosis* (i.e., presence of excess HCO_3^-), the body compensates with the respiratory system by hypoventilating so that PCO_2 rises and the ratio of HCO_3^- to PCO_2 is returned toward the normal of 20:1, therefore returning the *p*H to normal. The body is usually unable to completely compensate for metabolic alkalosis. In this instance respiratory compensation is by hypoventilation, and this occurs over one or several hours. Hypoventilation allows PCO_2 to rise only to a maximum of 50 to 60 torr before other stimuli of ventilation such as hypoxia take over to prevent further hypoventilation.

In compensating for one abnormality, high HCO_3^-, the body creates another abnormality, high PCO_2, but in doing so brings the ratio of HCO_3^- to PCO_2 to 20:1, allowing the pH to return to normal in spite of two abnormalities. These two abnormalities balance each other.

Treatment

It is important to realize that in each of these situations the body's compensation is only an effort to return the pH toward normal, and the primary abnormality is not corrected. The physician's definitive treatment is aimed at correcting the primary abnormality.

Metabolic (nonrespiratory) alkalosis (excess HCO_3^-) is treated by getting rid of excess HCO_3^- rather than just allowing PCO_2 to rise and normalize the ratio. Excess HCO_3^- can be corrected by giving the patient acetazolamide (Diamox) to make his kidneys excrete more HCO_3^-, or more commonly by giving KCl to allow the kidneys to excrete K^+ and Cl^- rather than acids. Sometimes ammonium chloride (NH_4Cl), arginine monohydrochloride, or even hydrochloric acid (HCl) is given to react with the excessive HCO_3^-, thereby correcting the metabolic alkalosis.

Respiratory alkalosis (low PCO_2) is treated by getting the patient to stop hyperventilating.

Metabolic (nonrespiratory) acidosis, in which excess acids have used up HCO_3^- or HCO_3^- has been lost, is treated by supplying HCO_3^- in the form of sodium bicarbonate ($NaHCO_3$) orally or intravenously while also treating the cause of acid accumulation or HCO_3^- loss. Multiplying the body weight (in kg) by the deficiency of HCO_3^- (in mEq/liter) by 0.3 gives a rough guide to the amount of $NaHCO_3^-$ (in mEq) that should be administered. Thus a 60 kg patient with an HCO_3^- of 4 would be given 360 mEq $NaHCO_3^-$, or

$$24 - 4 = 20 \times .3 \times 60 = 360$$

Giving large doses of $NaHCO_3^-$ can give the patient a large osmotic load, which may be more detrimental than the acidemia; hence, metabolic acidosis is not usually treated with $NaHCO_3^-$ unless the pH is below 7.25.

Respiratory acidosis (high PCO_2) is treated by increasing ventilation, enabling the lungs to get rid of the CO_2. Although *overtreatment* may occur, *overcompensation* by the body usually does not occur. In fact, complete compensation seldom occurs, so that instead of the ratio returning to 20:1, it returns to nearly 20:1, and pH, instead of returning to 7.40, returns almost to this point. (See Fig. 14-3 and the explanation that goes with it.)

pH AS A DETERMINANT

It is the fact that the pH usually does not return completely to 7.40 that allows us in some cases to decide just from blood gas values which is the primary process and which is the compensating process. We first look at the pH to see which side of 7.40 it is on. Even though it is in normal range, pH is usually either above or below 7.40. If the pH is above 7.40, the primary process is probably alkalosis, and if below 7.40, the primary process is probably acidosis. For example

pH 7.42
PCO_2 52 torr .... Respiratory acidosis
HCO_3^- 33 mEq/liter ... Metabolic alkalosis

Which is the primary process, respiratory acidosis or metabolic alkalosis? If one consults Figure 14-4, he finds that these numbers can be interpreted in either of two ways, for they fit into two 95% confidence bands: that is, those for chronic (fully compensated) metabolic alkalosis and chronic (fully compensated) respiratory acidosis. However, following our rule, we see that the pH, though normal, is tending toward alkalemia. Therefore, the primary process is probably alkalemia. So this is a metabolic alkalosis with nearly complete compensation. Often it is clinically obvious which is the primary abnormality, but sometimes this is not clinically apparent.

It must be pointed out that there may be more than one *primary* acid-base abnormality; so, if there is both a respiratory and a nonrespiratory acid-base abnormality, instead of one compensating for the other, both may be acidoses or both alkaloses, in which case the pH deviates more from normal than if either of the abnormalities was present alone.

Examples
1. Here is an example of blood gases to interpret:

pH 7.24
PCO_2 38 torr
HCO_3^- 15.5 mEq/liter
B.E.   −11

Coronary care nurses deciphering an arrhythmia are taught to first find the P wave; in

pH ISOBARS

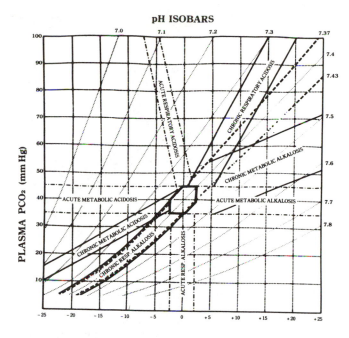

FIGURE 14-4.
Ninety-five percent confidence limits of respiratory or metabolic compensation.

trying to interpret an acid-base abnormality, one must look first at the pH to see if there is an alkalemia or an acidemia. Here we have an acidemia because the pH is low.

Next look at the PCO_2 to see if there is a respiratory abnormality. Here there is no abnormality; the PCO_2 is normal.

Next, look at either HCO_3^- or base excess to see if there is a metabolic abnormality. The HCO_3^- and the base excess are low, indicating a metabolic acidosis. We have an acidemia caused by a metabolic acidosis.

Consulting Figure 14-4, one sees that the example falls in the area labeled acute (uncompensated) metabolic acidosis.

2. Next is a tougher example:

pH	7.20
PCO_2	55 torr
HCO_3^-	20.5 mEq/liter
B.E.	−8

First, look at the pH to see if there is an alkalemia or an acidemia. Here the pH is low, indicating an acidemia.

Does the PCO_2 indicate a respiratory abnormality? Yes, PCO_2 is high, indicating respiratory acidosis.

Does the HCO_3^- or B.E. indicate a nonrespiratory abnormality? Yes, HCO_3^- and base excess are low, indicating nonrespiratory (metabolic) acidosis.

Therefore, this is an acidemia caused by combined respiratory and metabolic acidoses.

Consulting Figure 14-4, one sees that this example falls in the area between acute metabolic acidosis and acute respiratory acidosis, indicating that both are occurring.

THE NOMOGRAM

The foregoing is all that is necessary to solve most acid-base problems. Some experts feel that the use of "confidence limits" is a big help or even a necessity in solving acid-base problems. This concept will be briefly discussed below and may help to explain some of the intricacies of acid-base problems. The use of a nomogram will also be presented.

Some of the statements made in the preceding sections are true most of the time but not all of the time. For instance, because of the equation $CO_2 + H_2O \rightleftarrows HCO_3^- + H^+$ it can be seen that elevations of PCO_2 will raise the HCO_3^- just because of the chemical reaction. Later—several days later—the HCO_3^- is elevated further because the kidneys excrete less HCO_3^- in an effort to compensate.

Ninety-five percent confidence limits have been compiled so that if, for example, the primary problem is chronic respiratory acidosis (fully compensated respiratory acidosis), one can look up the level of HCO_3^- that would be expected in 95% of the cases of chronic respiratory acidosis.

In Figure 14-4, base excess values are plotted

DEFINITIONS FOR ACID-BASE DISTURBANCES

1. H^+: Hydrogen ion
2. $[H^+]$: Hydrogen ion concentration
3. pH: The negative log of the hydrogen ion concentration, or simply, a way of representing the free H^+ in a solution. The pH of a solution is inversely proportional to the concentration of H^+ in the solution.
4. Acid: A substance that can donate hydrogen ions, H^+.

   Example: $\underset{\text{(acid)}}{H_2CO_3} \rightarrow H^+ + HCO_3^-$

5. Base: A substance that can accept hydrogen ions, H^+.

   All bases are alkaline substances.

   Examples: $OH^- + H^+ \rightarrow H_2O$

   $\underset{\text{(bases)}}{HCO_3^-} + H^+ \rightarrow H_2CO_3$

6. Acidemia: Arterial pH below 7.35
7. Alkalemia: Arterial pH greater than 7.45
8. PCO_2: The tension exerted by carbon dioxide gas. The P in PCO_2 stands for pressure or tension exerted by CO_2 gas. CO_2 written without the preceding P does not refer to CO_2 gas, but usually refers to total CO_2 content. (Usually CO_2 gas is dissolved in a solution.) Any deviation from the normal carbon dioxide tension (PCO_2) reflects a respiratory acid-base disturbance, either primary or compensatory. CO_2 combines reversibly with water to form carbonic acid, H_2CO_3.

   $$CO_2 + H_2O \leftrightarrows H_2CO_3$$

   In blood, there is 800 times as much CO_2 in the form of a gas, dissolved CO_2, as there is in the form of an acid, H_2CO_3. PCO_2 should be thought of as an acid. PCO_2 is inversely related to ventilation; hence, it tells a great deal about the lungs' function.

9. Base excess: Expresses directly, in mEq/liter, the amount of strong base (or acid) added per liter of blood with normal arbitrarily fixed at 0 (range of normal -2 to $+2$). Positive values express excess of base (or deficit of acid) and negative values express deficit of base (or excess of acid). Base excess reflects mainly the concentration of bicarbonate and is affected only by metabolic processes. Positive values reflect metabolic alkalosis, and negative values reflect metabolic acidosis.

10. Standard bicarbonate: The actual bicarbonate concentration measured at 37°C on blood that has been equilibrated to a high oxygen tension to completely saturate the hemoglobin and to a PCO_2 of 40 torr, thereby correcting any respiratory abnormalities that might have existed in the patient when the blood was drawn. Any abnormality remaining in standard bicarbonate, then, is due to metabolic causes.

11. Actual bicarbonate: The actual amount of bicarbonate, HCO_3^-, expressed in mEq/liter of plasma as it existed in the patient. (If the patient had a PCO_2 of 40 torr, completely saturated hemoglobin, and a temperature of 37°C, then actual bicarbonate and standard bicarbonate are identical.)

12. Total CO_2 content (sometimes abbreviated as just CO_2): The amount of CO_2 gas extractable from plasma in the presence of a strong acid. Total CO_2 content consists of bicarbonate (HCO_3^-), carbonic acid (H_2CO_3), and dissolved carbon dioxide gas (PCO_2).

$$HCO_3^- + \text{dissolved } CO_2 \text{ gas and } H_2CO_3 = \text{total } CO_2 \text{ content}$$

Since there is 800 times as much dissolved CO_2 gas at equilibrium as H_2CO_3, and since CO_2 gas and H_2CO_3 are interchangeable anyway, dissolved CO_2 gas is used instead of H_2CO_3.

$$HCO_3^- + \text{dissolved } CO_2 \text{ gas} = \text{total } CO_2 \text{ content}$$

$$HCO_3^- + PCO_2 = \text{total } CO_2 \text{ content}$$

(Capital P stands for the pressure or tension exerted by the dissolved gas.)

To convert PCO_2 from torr to mEq/liter, it is multiplied by 0.03

$$HCO_3^- + (0.03 \times PCO_2) = \text{total } CO_2 \text{ content}$$

Example: 24 mEq/liter + (0.03 × 40 torr)
$$= \text{total } CO_2 \text{ content}$$
24 mEq/liter + 1.2 mEq/liter
$$= 25.2 \text{ mEq/liter}$$

In normal plasma, more than 95% of the total

CO_2 content is contributed by HCO_3^-, the other 5% being contributed by dissolved CO_2 gas and H_2CO_3. Dissolved CO_2 gas (which is regulated by the lungs), therefore, contributes little to the total CO_2 content. Total CO_2 content gives little information about the lungs.

13. Buffer: A substance which minimizes any change in pH when either acid or base is added to a solution containing the buffer.

Approximate Contribution of Individual Buffers to Total Buffering in Whole Blood

Individual Buffers	% Buffering in Whole Blood	
Hemoglobin & oxyhemoglobin	35	
Organic phosphate	3	Total nonbicarbonate — 47%
Inorganic phosphate	2	
Plasma proteins	7	
Plasma bicarbonate	35	Total bicarbonate — 53%
RBC bicarbonate	18	

14. Metabolic acidosis: An abnormal physiological process characterized by the primary gain of strong acid or primary loss of bicarbonate from the extracellular fluid.

15. Metabolic alkalosis: An abnormal physiological process characterized by primary gain of strong base (or loss of strong acid) or the primary gain of bicarbonate by the extracellular fluid.

16. Respiratory acidosis: An abnormal physiological process in which there is a primary reduction in the rate of alveolar ventilation relative to the rate of CO_2 production.

17. Respiratory alkalosis: An abnormal physiological process in which there is a primary increase in the rate of alveolar ventilation relative to the rate of CO_2 production.

18. Henderson-Hasselbalch equation: (small "p" stands for negative logarithm of a number)

$$pH = pK + \log \frac{HCO_3^-}{\left[\begin{array}{c}\text{dissolved } CO_2 \text{ gas} \\ \text{and } H_2CO_3\end{array}\right]}$$

Although the equation is usually written simply:

$$pH = pK + \log \frac{[HCO_3^-]}{[H_2CO_3]}$$

It is understood that most of the H_2CO_3 is in the form of dissolved CO_2 gas. In clinical practice we measure the pressure exerted by the dissolved CO_2 gas, so the equation could be rewritten:

(Capital "P" stands for pressure or tension exerted by dissolved gas.)

$$pH = pK + \log \frac{[HCO_3^-]}{[PCO_2 \text{ in torr}]}$$

To convert PCO_2 from torr to mEq/liter, multiply by 0.03.

$$pH = pK + \log \frac{[HCO_3^-]}{[0.03 \times PCO_2]}$$

(pK is a constant 6.10)

Example: $7.40 = 6.10 + \log \dfrac{[24 \text{ mEq/liter}]}{[0.03 \times 40]}$

$$7.40 = 6.10 + \log \frac{24 \text{ mEq/liter}}{1.2 \text{ mEq/liter}}$$

$$7.40 = 6.10 + \log 20$$

(log of 20 is 1.30)

$$7.40 = 6.10 + 1.30$$

$$7.40 = 7.40$$

19. P_{50}: The partial pressure of oxygen (PO_2) when hemoglobin is exactly 50% saturated. This measurement is used to detect a shift in the oxyhemoglobin dissociation curve; *i.e.,* if the P_{50} is greater than 27, the curve is shifted to the right, and if the P_{50} is less than 27, the curve is shifted to the left.

20. Acute respiratory acidosis: Uncompensated respiratory acidosis

21. Chronic respiratory acidosis: Compensated respiratory acidosis

22. Acute metabolic acidosis: Uncompensated respiratory acidosis

23. Chronic metabolic acidosis: Compensated metabolic acidosis

24. Fully compensated: Compensated to the greatest extent that the body can in 95% of the cases

25. Completely compensated: Compensated to the extent that the pH is within the normal range

on the horizontal axis and PCO_2 values are plotted on the vertical axis; pH isobars are the sweeping lines of small dots. Cohen, the author who produced this figure, prefers the narrow range of 7.37 to 7.43 for the normal pH range instead of 7.35 to 7.45. Cohen plotted 95% confidence bands for the acute and chronic (uncompensated and compensated) forms of each of the four basic acid-base disturbances. If one knows any two of the three parameters (pH, PCO_2, B.E.), one can calculate the third and also name the process and determine whether it is acute or chronic (fully compensated) or somewhere in between. Without using the 95% confidence limits or consulting the nomogram, one may occasionally miss the less obvious part of a combined acid-base problem.

Based on Figure 14-4, a computer program for acid-base interpretation has been developed.

BIBLIOGRAPHY

Cohen ML: A computer program for the interpretation of blood gas analysis. Computers in Biomed Res 2:549–557, 1969

Comroe JH Jr: Physiology of Respiration, 2nd ed. Chicago, Year Book Medical Publishers, 1974

Masoro EJ, Siegel PD: Acid-Base Regulation: Its Physiology, Pathophysiology and the Interpretation of Blood Gas Analysis, 2nd ed. Philadelphia, W. B. Saunders, 1977

Murray JF: The Normal Lung. Philadelphia, W. B. Saunders, 1976

Schrier RW (ed): Renal and Electrolyte Disorders. Boston, Little, Brown & Co., 1976

Schwartz AB, Lyons H (eds): Acid-Base and Electrolyte Balance. New York, Grune & Stratton, 1977

Schwartz WB: Disturbances of acid-base equilibrium. In Beeson PB, McDermott W (eds): Textbook of Medicine, 14th ed., pp 1589–1955. Philadelphia, W. B. Saunders, 1975

Snider GL: Interpretation of the arterial oxygen and carbon dioxide partial pressures. Chest 63:801–806, 1973

Thomas HM et al: The oxyhemoglobin dissociation curve in health and disease. Am J Med 57:331–348, 1974

Winters RW, Engel K, Dell RB: Acid-Base Physiology in Medicine, 2nd ed. Cleveland, The London Company of Cleveland and the Radiometer A/S of Copenhagen, 1969

CHEST PHYSICAL ASSESSMENT

Nurses contribute significantly to the care of patients with respiratory problems by performing chest physical examinations on these patients. This examination allows the nurse an opportunity to establish a "baseline" of information and provides a framework to detect some of the rapid changes in the patient's condition. Since the nurse is with the patient more frequently than the physician is, it makes sense that it will often be the nurse who detects the patient's changing condition rather than the physician, who visits the patient only once or twice a day, and who, even with the information provided by daily chest roentgenograms, is less likely to be alert to changes in the status of the patient.

Sometimes a chest examination by the nurse is the quickest and most reliable assessment of the situation.

Example:
A 69-year-old hypertensive man fainted in the shower and fell, breaking five ribs on the left side. When he recovered consciousness, it was clear that he had had a cerebrovascular accident (CVA), with left-side hemiparesis. He did well until the third day of hospitalization, when he developed respiratory distress. The working diagnosis was congestive heart failure, but the nurse was able to convince those in attendance that the breath sounds and thoracic movement on the left side—which everyone agreed were depressed due to rib fractures—were more depressed than they had been previously. A chest roentgenogram showing atelectasis of the entire left lung, confirmed her observations. The roentgenogram showed the lung returned to normal the next day after tracheostomy, vigorous bronchial hygiene, and tracheal suction.

This is just one of many examples in which the nurse's ability to do a competent chest physical examination led to improved patient care.

Physical diagnosis of the chest includes four examinations:
- Inspection, or looking at the patient (see Fig. 14-5)
- Palpation, or feeling the patient
- Percussion, or thumping on the patient
- Auscultation, or listening to the patient's chest with a stethoscope

INSPECTION

Inspecting the patient involves checking for the presence or absence of several factors.

Cyanosis is one of the factors in which we are most interested. Cyanosis is notoriously hard to detect when the patient is anemic, and the patient who is polycythemic may have cyanosis in his extremities even when he has a normal oxygen tension.

We generally differentiate between *peripheral* and *central* cyanosis: peripheral cyanosis occurs in the extremities or on the tip of the nose or ears, even with normal oxygen tensions, when there is diminished blood flow to these areas, particularly if they are cold or dependent (see Fig. 14-6). Central cyanosis, as noted on the tongue or lips (see Fig. 14-7), has a much greater significance; it means the patient actually has a low oxygen tension.

Labored breathing is an obvious sign to check; we are particularly interested in knowing if the patient is using the accessory muscles of respiration. Sometimes the number of words a patient can say before having to gasp for another breath is a good measure of the amount of labored breathing. *An increase in the anteroposterior (AP) diameter of the chest* — that is, an increase in the size of the chest from front to back is also checked.

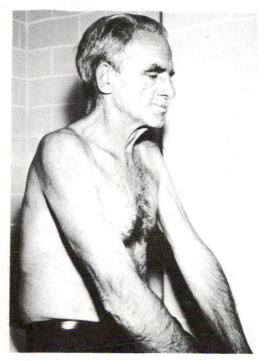

FIGURE 14-5.
Frequently observe the patient's overall aspect.

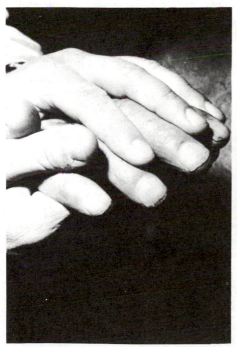

FIGURE 14-6.
Feel the patient's extremities and assess their temperature.

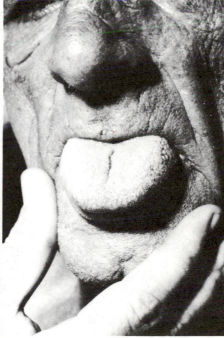

FIGURE 14-7.
Examine the tongue and lips for cyanosis.

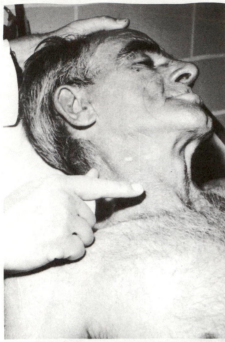

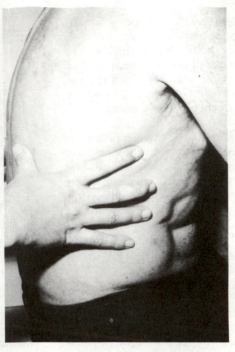

FIGURE 14-8.
Note the position of the trachea.

FIGURE 14-9.
Note the general chest expansion.

This is often due to overexpansion of the lungs from obstructive pulmonary disease, but an increase in AP diameter may also be present in a patient who has kyphosis (forward curvature of the spine).

Chest deformities and scars are important in helping us to determine the reason for respiratory distress. For instance, a scar may be our first indication that the patient has had part of his lung removed. A chest deformity such as kyphoscoliosis may indicate why the patient has respiratory distress.

The patient's posture must also be noted, for patients with obstructive pulmonary disease often sit and prop themselves up on outstretched arms, or lean forward with their elbows on a desk in an effort to elevate their clavicles, thereby giving them a slightly greater ability to expand their chests.

The position of the trachea is also an important factor to observe (see Fig. 14-8). Is the trachea in the midline as it should be, or deviated to one side or the other? A pleural effusion or a tension pneumothorax usually deviates the trachea away from the diseased side. On the other hand, atelectasis often pulls the trachea toward the diseased side.

The respiratory rate is an important parameter to follow; it should be counted over at least a 15-second period, rather than just estimated.

Often the respiratory rate is recorded as 20 breaths/minute, which frequently means the rate was estimated rather than counted.

The depth of respiration is often as meaningful as the respiratory rate. For instance, if a patient were breathing 40 times/minute, one might think he had severe respiratory problems, but if he were breathing quite deeply 40 times/minute, it might mean that he had Kussmaul respirations due to diabetic acidosis or other acidosis. However, if the respirations were shallow at a rate of 40 times/minute, it might mean he had severe respiratory distress from obstructive lung disease, restrictive lung disease, or other pulmonary problems.

The duration of inspiration versus the duration of expiration is important in determining whether or not there is airway obstruction. In patients with any of the obstructive lung diseases, expiration is prolonged, requiring more than one and one-half times as long for expiration as for inspiration.

General chest expansion is an integral part of examining a patient. Normally we expect about a 3-inch expansion from maximum expiration to maximum inspiration (see Fig. 14-9). Ankylosing spondylitis, or Marie-Strümpell arthritis, is one condition in which general chest expansion is limited. We compare the expansion of the upper chest with that of the lower chest and use of the diaphragm to see if the patient with obstructive pulmonary disease is concentrating on expanding his lower chest and using his diaphragm properly. We look at the expansion of one side of the chest versus the other side, realizing that atelectasis, especially atelectasis caused by a mucus plug, may cause unilateral diminished chest expansion.

A pulmonary embolus, pneumonia, pleural effusion, pneumothorax, or any other cause of chest pain, such as fractured ribs, may lead to diminished chest expansion. An endotracheal or nasotracheal tube inserted too far, so that it extends beyond the trachea into one of the main stem bronchi (usually the right), is a serious and frequent cause of diminished expansion of one side of the chest. When the tube slips into the right main stem bronchus, the left lung is not expanded, and the patient usually develops hypoxemia and atelectasis on the left side. Fortunately the nurse who is aware of this potential problem usually recognizes it.

If present, *intercostal retractions,* that is, sucking in of the muscles and skin between the ribs during inspiration, usually mean that the patient is making a larger effort at inspiration than normal. Usually this signifies that the lungs are less compliant (stiffer) than usual.

A patient's cough, its effectiveness and frequency, are important to note, as are sputum characteristics such as amount, color, and consistency.

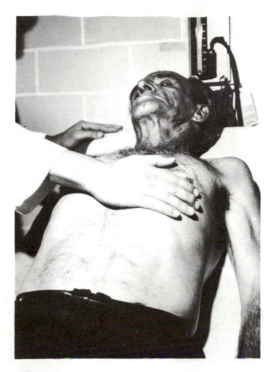

FIGURE 14-10.
In palpation, place the heel of your hand flat against the patient's chest.

PALPATION

Palpation of the chest is done with the heel of the hand flat against the patient's chest (see Fig. 14-10). Often we are determining whether tactile fremitus is present. We do this by having the patient speak, particularly asking him to say "ninety-nine." Normally, when a patient speaks, or says a word such as "ninety-nine," a vibration is felt by the hand on the outside of the chest. This is similar to the vibration one feels when putting one's hand on the chest of a cat when the cat is purring. In normal patients tactile fremitus is present. It may be diminished or absent when there is something that comes between the patient's lung and the hand on the chest wall. For instance, when there is a pleural effusion, thickened pleura, or pneumothorax, either it is impossible to feel this vibration or the vibration is diminished. When the patient has atelectasis due to an occluded airway, the vibration also cannot be felt. Tactile fremitus is slightly increased in conditions of consolidation, but detection of this

slight increase may be difficult. Just by palpating over the patient's chest with quiet breathing, one may sometimes feel palpable rhonchi that are due to mucus moving in large airways.

PERCUSSION

In percussing a patient's chest (see Fig. 14-11), one must use a finger that is pressed flat against the patient's chest; this finger is struck over the knuckle by the end of a finger from the opposite hand. Normally the chest has a resonant or hollow percussion note. In diseases in which there is increased air in the chest or lungs, such as pneumothorax or emphysema, there may be hyperresonant (even more drumlike) percussion notes. Hyperresonant percussion notes, however, are sometimes hard to detect. More important is a dull or flat percussion note such as is heard when one percusses over a part of the body that contains no air. A dull or flat percussion note is heard when the lung underneath the examining hand has atelectasis, pneumonia, pleural effusion, thickened pleura, or a mass lesion. A dull or flat percussion note is also heard when one is percussing over the heart.

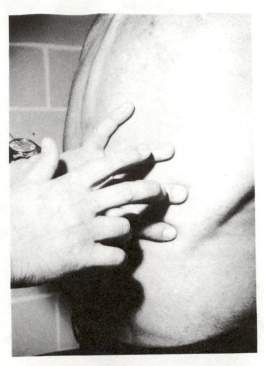

FIGURE 14-11.
In percussion, press a finger flat against the patient's chest or back and strike this finger over the knuckle with the end of a finger from the opposite hand.

AUSCULTATION

In auscultation, one generally uses the diaphragm of the stethoscope and presses this firmly against the chest wall (see Fig. 14-12). It is important to listen to the intensity or loudness of breath sounds, and to realize that normally there is a fourfold increase in loudness of breath sounds when a patient takes a maximum deep breath as opposed to quiet breathing. The intensity of the breath sounds may be diminished due to decreased airflow through the airways or due to increased insulation between the lungs and the stethoscope. In airway obstruction, such as chronic obstructive pulmonary disease or atelectasis, the breath sound intensity is diminished. With shallow breathing there is diminished air movement through the airways, and the breath sounds are also not as loud. With restricted movement of the thorax or diaphragm, there may be diminished breath sounds in the area of restricted movement. In pleural thickening, pleural effusion, pneumothorax, and obesity there is an abnormal substance (fibrous tissue, fluid, air, or fat) between the stethoscope and the underlying lung; this substance insulates the breath sounds from the stethoscope, making the breath sounds seem less loud.

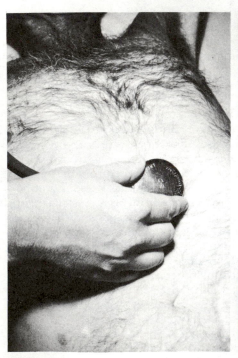
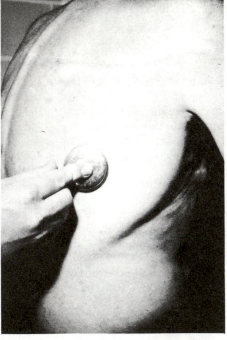

FIGURE 14-12.
In auscultation press the stethoscope firmly against the chest wall *(left)* or the back *(right)*.

CHECKLIST OF ABNORMAL RESPIRATORY FINDINGS

Bronchitis
Occasional increased respiratory rate
Occasional use of accessory muscles
Occasional intercostal retraction
Prolonged expiratory phase (often)
Increased AP diameter of the chest (often)
Decreased motion of the diaphragm (often)
Decreased intensity of breath sounds
Fine, medium, and coarse rales (rhonchi)
Wheezes (often)
Often coarse rales (rhonchi) and wheezes clear after cough

Pneumothorax
Increased respiratory rate
Trachea deviated to side of pneumothorax
Occasional cyanosis
Decreased movement of chest on side of pneumothorax (splinting)
Hyperresonance (unreliable sign)
Decreased breath sounds
Decreased tactile fremitus and decreased vocal fremitus (the most reliable signs)

Emphysema
Increased respiratory rate (often)
Use of accessory muscles (neck)
Intercoastal retractions
Propped up on outstretched arms
Prolonged expiratory phase
Increased AP diameter
Decreased chest expansion
Decreased motion of diaphragm
Hyperresonance to percussion
Decreased intensity (loudness) of breath sounds
Little or no increase in loudness of breath sounds with deep breath
Fine rales at bases (often)
Occasional wheeze

Pneumonia
Increased respiratory rate
Occasional cyanosis
Decreased expansion (splinting) (often)
Increased fremitus (tactile and vocal)
Occasional palpable rhonchi—usually are removed by coughing or suctioning
Dullness to percussion
Bronchial breathing, whispered pectoriloquy, and E to A changes (usual if consolidation is extensive)
Fine or medium rales
Occasional coarse rales (rhonchi)—clear with cough or suctioning, usually
Occasional pleural friction rub

Atelectasis
Increased respiratory rate
Increased pulse
Cyanosis (often)
Trachea deviated to side of atelectasis
Decreased chest expansion on side of atelectasis (splinting)
Decreased fremitus (tactile and vocal)
Dull or flat percussion note
Decreased breath sounds
Occasional rales

Pleural effusion
Occasional increase in respiratory rate
Trachea deviated away from side of effusion
Decreased fremitus (tactile and vocal)
Decreased breath sounds
Above effusion
    Bronchial breathing ⎫ due to compressed
    E to A changes ⎬ lungs with open
    Whispered pectoriloquy ⎭ airway
Friction rub—after fluid is removed and visceral pleura rubs against parietal pleura

Large mass lesion (tumor)
Dullness over tumor
Fine rales (often)
Decreased breath sounds if airway is occluded
Bronchial breathing, E to A changes, and whispered pectoriloquy if airway is open
Occasional pleural friction rub

Subcutaneous emphysema
Crackling sounds similar to rales that come from air outside the chest in the soft tissue

Pulmonary edema (congestive heart failure)
Increased respiratory rate
Cyanosis (often)
Use of accessory muscles (usually)
Apprehension
Sitting upright (often)
Increased fremitus (due to interstitial edema)
Dull percussion note (due to interstitial edema)
Bronchovesicular sounds (due to interstitial edema often obscured later by rales)
Fine rales → medium rales later
Occasional coarse rales (rhonchi)
Occasional wheezing

Pulmonary interstitial fibrosis
Increased respiratory rate (often)
Intercostal retractions
Cyanosis (late)
High-pitched, fine, and medium rales
Occasional bronchovesicular breathing

Generally, there are three types of sounds that are heard in the normal chest:

- Vesicular breath sounds, which are heard in the periphery of the normal lung
- Bronchial breath sounds, which are heard over the trachea
- Bronchovesicular breath sounds, which are heard in most areas of the lung near the major airways

Bronchial breath sounds are high-pitched, seem to be close to the ear, are loud, and there is a pause between inspiration and expiration. *Vesicular breath sounds* are of lower pitch, having a rustling quality, and there is no noticeable pause between inspiration and expiration. *Bronchovesicular breath sounds* represent a sound halfway between the other two types of breath sounds.

Bronchial breathing, in addition to being heard over the trachea of the normal person, is also heard in any situation in which there is consolidation—for instance, pneumonia. *Bronchial breathing* is also heard above a pleural effusion in which the normal lung is compressed. Wherever there is bronchial breathing, there may also be two other associated changes: (1) "E to A" changes and (2) whispered pectoriloquy.

An *E to A change* merely means that when one listens with a stethoscope and the patient says "E," what one hears is actually an A sound rather than an E sound. This occurs where there is consolidation.

Whispered pectoriloquy is the presence of a loud volume as heard through the stethoscope when the patient whispers. For bronchial breathing and these two associated changes to be present there must be either (1) an open airway and compressed alveoli, or (2) alveoli in which the air has been replaced by fluid.

Extra sounds that are heard with auscultation include rales, rhonchi, wheezes, and rubs.

Rales are divided into three categories: fine, medium, and coarse. Fine rales are also called *crepitant rales,* and are produced in the small airways in patients with diseases such as pneumonia and heart failure. Medium rales are sounds produced in the medium airways and occur later in pneumonia, heart failure, and pulmonary edema. Coarse rales, also called *rhonchi,* are continuous, bubbling, gurgling, or rattling sounds, often musical and usually coming from the large airways.

Extra sounds such as wheezing mean there is airway narrowing. This may be caused by asthma, foreign bodies, mucus in the airways, stenosis, and so forth. If the wheeze is heard only in expiration, it is called a *wheeze;* if the wheezing sound occurs in both inspiration and expiration, it is usually due to retained secretions and is best called a *rhonchus.*

A *friction rub* is heard when there is pleural disease such as a pulmonary embolus, peripheral pneumonia, or pleurisy and is often difficult to distinguish from a rhonchus. If the abnormal noise clears when the patient coughs, it usually means that it was a rhonchus rather than a friction rub.

Certainly, critical care nurses and respiratory nurse therapists and, hopefully, unit nurses and inhalation therapy technicians should learn to participate in chest physical diagnosis so that they can detect changes in the patient's condition as soon as they occur, rather than waiting for the physician's visit once or twice a day or depending on a daily chest x-ray.

Section C Renal System

Barbara Fuller

Normal Structure and Function of the Renal System
15

NORMAL STRUCTURE OF THE KIDNEY

The regulation and concentration of solutes in the extracellular fluid of the body is the primary function of the kidney. This is accomplished by removing waste products of metabolism and excess concentrations of constituents and by conserving those substances that are present in normal or low quantities. Figure 15-1 is a schematic representation of the general macroscopic and microscopic structure of the kidney.

Urine, the end product of kidney function, is formed from the blood by the *nephron* and flows from the nephrons through *collecting tubules* to the *pelvis* of the kidney. From here it leaves the kidney itself by way of the *ureters* and flows into the *urinary bladder*. Each human kidney contains about one million nephrons, all of which function identically, and thus kidney function can be explained by describing the function of one nephron.

Figure 15-2 is a composite drawing of a functional nephron. Each nephron is made up of two major components: the *glomerulus*, in which water and solutes are filtered from the blood; and the *tubules*, which reabsorb essential materials from the filtrate and permit waste substances and unneeded materials to remain in the filtrate and flow into the renal pelvis as urine.

For purposes of further describing these two major divisions of the nephron, a more schematic diagram appears in Figure 15-3.

The *glomerulus* consists of a tuft of capillaries fed by the *afferent arteriole*, drained by the *efferent arteriole*, and surrounded by *Bowman's capsule*.

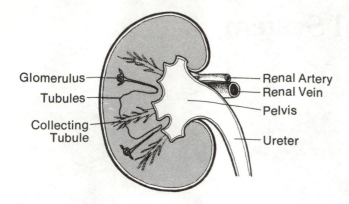

Figure 15-1.
General characteristics of kidney structure. Note that the glomerulus is in the cortex of the kidney while the proximal, distal, and collecting tubules are in the medulla.

Fluid that is filtered from the capillaries into this capsule then flows into the tubular system. The first section is called the *proximal tubule;* the second, the *loop of Henle;* the third, the *distal tubule;* and last, the *collecting tubule.*

Most of the water and electrolytes are reabsorbed into the blood in the *peritubular capillaries* and the *vasa recta,* while the end products of metabolism pass into the urine.

NORMAL RENAL PHYSIOLOGY

The Glomerulus and Filtration

The glomerular capillaries, nestled in Bowman's capsule, are composed of three layers: (1) an inner endothelium, (2) a glycoprotein-constituted basement membrane, and (3) an outer epithelial layer continuous from that lining Bowman's capsule.

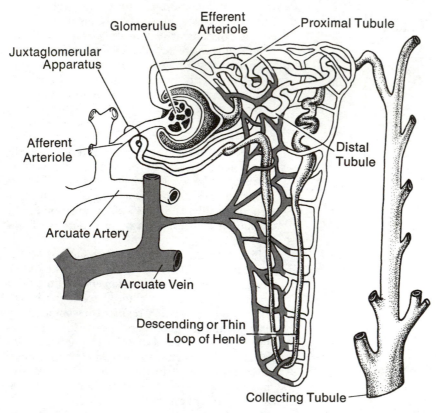

Figure 15-2.
The nephron. (Guyton AC [ed]: Textbook of Medical Physiology, p. 439. Philadelphia, WB Saunders, 1976)

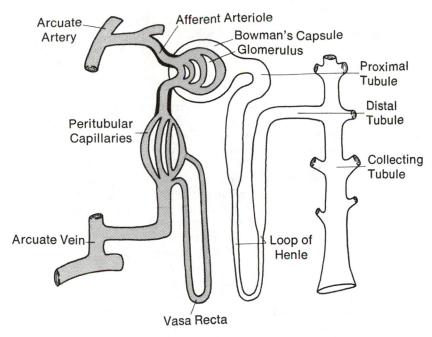

Figure 15-3.
Schematic representation of the nephron. (Guyton AC: Function of the Human Body. Philadelphia, WB Saunders, 1969)

Pore size determines permeability. Like other body capillaries, the glomerular capillaries are relatively impermeable to large plasma proteins and are quite permeable to water and smaller solutes such as electrolytes, amino acids, glucose, and nitrogenous waste. Unlike other capillaries in the body, the glomerular capillaries have an elevated hydrostatic (blood) pressure (70 torr versus 10–30 torr). This increased hydrostatic pressure in part forces (or squeezes) water and permeable solutes from the bloodstream into Bowman's capsule. This process is termed *glomerular filtration.* The material entering Bowman's capsule is called the *filtrate.*

The *hydrostatic pressure* of the glomerulus does not operate alone. Three other factors participate: the hydrostatic pressure (HP) of the filtrate fluid (in Bowman's capsule); the osmotic pressure (OP) of the blood; and the osmotic pressure (OP) of the filtrate (in Bowman's capsule). Figure 15-4 illustrates the interaction of these factors. HP can be thought of as a "pushing" force while OP can be viewed as a "pulling or attracting" force. Thus, the plasma HP (70 torr) cooperates with filtrate OP (close to zero) to move water and permeable solutes from plasma to Bowman's capsule, while the filtrate HP (20 torr) cooperates with the plasma OP to move

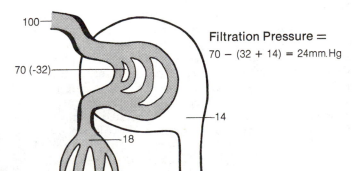

Filtration Pressure =

70 − (32 + 14) = 24mm.Hg

Figure 15-4.
Normal fluid pressures at various points in the nephron. (Guyton AC: Function of the Human Body, p. 197. Philadelphia, WB Saunders, 1969)

water in the opposite direction (*i.e.,* from the capsule to bloodstream). Net effective forces can be equated as

from blood to capsule   versus   from capsule to blood
70 + 0   20 + 30

As can be noted, the left side of this equation has a greater force (70 torr) than the right side (50 torr). Hence, there is a pressure gradient of about 20 torr (70 − 50 = 20) that causes water and permeable solutes to filter out of the glomerulus into Bowman's capsule.

The *rate* at which the filtrate is formed is termed the *glomerular filtration rate (GRF)*. In the typical healthy person, this amounts to the formation of 125 ml of filtrate per minute. Major factors that influence the GFR are the glomerular plasma HP and OP. Subnormal plasma OP, such as in hypoproteinemia, will increase the GRF. A fall in glomerular HP such as from systemic hypotension or hypovolemia would decrease the GFR. Other factors that will decrease the HP and, hence, the GFR, are afferent arteriole constriction and renal artery stenosis.

Because of the influence of HP upon the GFR, the kidneys were long thought to function in the normal homeostasis of systemic blood pressure. But we now know that the GFR is relatively stable over fluctuations of 20 to 30 torr in arterial blood pressure. The reason for this stability is that the afferent arterioles adjust their diameter in response to the pressure of blood coming to them. If the blood pressure decreases (*e.g.,* 10 torr), the smooth muscles of the afferent arterioles relax. This causes dilation of these arterioles which, in turn, increases the perfusion of the glomeruli and maintains the GFR at its normal rate; conversely, with an increase in blood pressure, these vessels constrict. There is a limit, however, to this autoregulatory mechanism. If the systemic blood pressure falls greatly, such as in shock, the GFR will fall to near zero, thereby producing near anuria.

The Glomerular Filtrate
The glomerular filtrate is an ultrafiltrate of plasma containing only a small (.03%) amount of protein. Approximately 125 ml of filtrate are produced each minute. This totals 180 liters/day, about 4½ times the total amount of fluid in the body. As this filtrate passes through the remainder of the nephrons, all but about 1.5 liters/day will be returned to the bloodstream by way of the peritubular capillaries (see Fig.

15–3). The volume and content of the urine are the result of tubular reabsorption (accomplished by active transport, osmosis and diffusion, and tubular secretion). Reabsorption occurs in all parts of the nephron, whereas only tubule cells perform secretion.

Active transport involves the binding of a molecule to a carrier, which then moves the molecule from one side of the membrane to the other. The carrier acts somewhat like a pump. This process moves the transported molecule either into or out of a cell. In tubular cells, the carrier is located in the cell membrane nearest the peritubular capillaries, and it transports material out of the tubular cell into the peritubular fluid. This lowers the intracellular concentration of the type of molecule being transported. The decreased concentration enables more of those molecules to diffuse into the tubule cell. These molecules, in turn, exit the cell and enter the peritubular fluid by active transport. The movement of molecules increases the peritubular fluid concentration of the molecule, and this increase, in turn, stimulates the diffusion of the molecule into the peritubular capillaries. Thus, in the nephrons, active transport removes molecules from the filtrate (urine) back to the bloodstream.

Tubular secretion, thought also to be used as a carrier system, moves molecules from the bloodstream into the filtrate by a process similar to, but the reverse of, active transport. The carrier mechanism of both processes (active transport and secretion) requires energy (in the form of high energy adenosine triphosphate [ATP] bonds), the provision of which requires a healthy tubule cell. Hence, tests of secretion, for example, provide valuable data regarding tubular cell health. Similarly, a sign of diminished reabsorption of sodium (supernormal urinary sodium) provides evidence of damaged tubular cells in acute tubular necrosis.

The Proximal Tubule
Roughly 80% of the glomerular filtrate is returned to the bloodstream by reabsorption in the proximal tubule. Normally, all glucose and amino acids plus sodium, chloride, phosphate, bicarbonate, magnesium, calcium, other electrolytes, uric acid, water, and a little urea are reabsorbed here. Some urea, creatinine, hydrogen, and ammonia are secreted from the peritubular capillaries into the filtrate by these tubular cells. Some drugs (*e.g.,* para-aminohippuric acid [PAH] and penicillin) are also added to the filtrate by tubular secretion.

At plasma glucose levels of less than 200 mg/dl, all of the filtered glucose is returned back into the bloodstream by active transport. Amino acids, creatine, and some sodium, potassium, phosphate, sulfate, uric acid, and other organic molecules are also actively transported out of the filtrate (where they then diffuse back into the bloodstream).

The *active transport of sodium* is responsible for the osmotic reabsorption of water from the filtrate both here in the proximal and later in the distal tubule. As sodium ions are actively transported out of the cell and into the peritubular fluid, they make the osmotic pressure of this peritubular fluid higher than that of the cell or tubule fluid. Water is thus osmotically "pulled out" of the tubular fluid. Both water and sodium then diffuse into peritubular capillaries and are thus returned to the bloodstream.

The active transport of positively charged sodium ions also creates an electrochemical gradient that draws negatively charged ions — especially chloride — out of the tubular fluid and back into the bloodstream. This electrogenic sodium pump is inhibited by certain diuretics.

Loop of Henle

In the loop of Henle the filtrate (urine) becomes highly concentrated. This part of the nephron is composed of a thin-walled descending portion and a thick-walled ascending portion (see Fig. 15-3). Loops of Henle belonging to juxtamedullary nephrons dip into the medulla of the kidney, which contains a highly concentrated interstitial fluid. (The thin walls of the descending portion are quite permeable.) This permeability, together with the high concentration of the interstitial fluid at this point, causes water to osmose from the filtrate into the interstitial fluid. This makes the filtrate quite concentrated by the time it reaches the ascending limb of the Loop.

The thicker-walled ascending limb is relatively impermeable to water, but it contains ion carriers that actively transport chloride ions out of the filtrate. This creates an electrochemical gradient which "pulls" the positively charged sodium ions out of the filtrate also. This exit of electrolytes without water now makes the filtrate more dilute than before. Indeed, it may even become hypotonic to the blood at this point.

The Distal Tubule

In the distal tubule sodium is again reabsorbed by active transport. Some ammonia diffuses

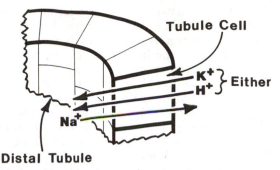

Figure 15-5.
Cation exchange in the distal tubule.

into the filtrate. Also, hydrogen and potassium are added to the filtrate by means of tubular secretion.

The active transport of sodium uses a carrier system that is also involved in the tubular secretion of hydrogen and potassium ions. Figure 15-5 explains this relationship. In this relationship every time the carrier transports sodium out of the tubular fluid, it carries *either* a hydrogen *or* a potassium ion into the tubular fluid on its "return trip." Thus, for every sodium ion reabsorbed, a hydrogen *or* potassium must be secreted, and *vice versa*. The choice of cation to be secreted depends upon the extracellular fluid (ECF) concentration of these ions (hydrogen and potassium).

Knowledge of this cation exchange system in the distal tubule helps us to understand some of the relations these electrolytes have with one another. For example, we can understand why an aldosterone blocker may cause hyperkalemia, or why there can be an initial fall in plasma potassium as severe acidosis is therapeutically corrected.*

Collecting Ducts

Sometimes called collecting tubules, these structures receive the contents of many nephrons (see Fig. 15-2). There is no further electrolyte reabsorption or secretion here, and in the normal

---

*The aldosterone blocker reduces sodium reabsorption. Such reduced reabsorption of sodium also reduces the tubular secretion of either hydrogen or potassium. The hydrogen excess can be buffered, but the potassium simply rises to above normal levels. In severe acidosis, the nephrons have been attempting to compensate by increasing their hydrogen-ion secretion rates. As acidosis is therapeutically corrected (*e.g.,* by sodium bicarbonate administration), one change is secretion of potassium ions (another concerns a shift of potassium into cells). As hydrogen ions no longer need to be secreted, potassium ions become the sole exchange for sodium ions, leading, it is thought, to a reduction in plasma potassium.

well-hydrated person, there is no further water reabsorption either. Should the ECF become more concentrated (*e.g.,* dehydration), osmoreceptors in the hypothalamus respond by stimulating the hypothalamus to secrete antidiuretic hormone (ADH). ADH increases the permeability of the collecting tubule cells to water. This permits the (osmotic) reabsorption of water alone (without electrolytes), which in turn will decrease the concentration of the ECF. Negative feedback loops regulate ADH secretion. This means that as the concentration of the ECF returns to normal, the stimulus to ADH secretion disappears and ADH secretion is stopped.

Juxtaglomerular Apparatus

The nephron is so arranged that the initial portion of the distal tubule lies at the juncture of the afferent and efferent arterioles, which is very near the glomerulus. Here, macula densa cells of the distal tubule lie in approximation to the juxtaglomerular cells of the wall of the afferent arteriole. Both of these cells types plus some connective tissue cells constitute the juxtaglomerular apparatus. The juxtaglomerular cells of this apparatus are believed to secrete renin.

Renin causes plasma angiotensin (made in the liver) to be converted to angiotensin I, which in pulmonary capillaries is converted enzymatically into angiotensin II. This form of angiotensin acts to increase blood pressure, and hence, GFR, by two mechanisms: (1) the constriction of peripheral arteries and (2) the secretion of aldosterone by the adrenal cortex.

Aldosterone stimulates sodium reabsorption by the distal tubule cells. This causes increased water reabsorption, which then increases blood volume. This increase in volume can alleviate renal hypotension and restore the GFR to normal.

Stimulation of the juxtaglomerular apparatus may be varied. One hypothesis states that the macula densa cells are sensitive to the sodium concentration of distal tubule fluid. Sodium concentrations vary with the rate of glomerular filtration. The faster the filtration, the faster the fluid moves through the nephron. This decreases the time for sodium reabsorption, leading to high sodium concentrations in the distal tubule. With slower filtration and movement through the nephron, there is more reabsorption and, consequently, less sodium remaining in the fluid as it arrives at the macula densa. Decreased

sodium concentration (acting as a "proxy variable" for the GFR) can then stimulate the secretion of renin by the juxtaglomerular apparatus. According to another school of thought, the juxtaglomerular cells themselves act as pressure receptors, sensitive to the HP of blood in the afferent arteriole. When these cells note a decrease in HP, they secrete renin. Both of these modalities of stimulation may be correct. In addition, the juxtaglomerular apparatus seems to be stimulated by beta-adrenergics and possibly by the sympathetic stimulation as well (it appears to be enervated by sympathetic fibers).

Clearance

From the foregoing discussion a very important concept in renal function emerges — that of clearance. As the filtrate moves along the nephron, a large proportion of metabolic end products remain in it, unreabsorbed. These products are thus removed (cleared) from the blood and exit the body in the urine. Indeed, of each 125 ml of glomerular filtrate formed per minute, 60 ml leave urea behind in the fluid within the tubules. Stated another way, 60 ml of plasma are "cleared" of urea each minute in normally functioning kidneys. In the same way, 125 ml of plasma are cleared of creatinine, 12 ml of uric acid, 12 ml of potassium, 25 ml of sulfate, 25 ml of phosphate, and so forth each minute.

It is possible to calculate renal clearance by simultaneously sampling urine and plasma. By dividing the quantity of substance found in each milliliter of plasma into the quantity found in the urine, the milliliters cleared per minute can be calculated. This method is used as one means of testing kidney function.

Other methods of assessing renal function involve chemicals that are known to be either filtered only or filtered and secreted. *Inulin,* for example, is only filtered and neither really absorbed nor secreted. Thus, the clearance of inulin provides a measure of glomerular filtration. *Mannitol* can be used similarly. PAH or iodopyracet (Diodrast) are drugs that are secreted in addition to being filtered. As such, their clearance provides an index of plasma flow through the kidneys. They also can be used together with a filtered-only drug in assessing tubular secretion and, hence, the health of tubular cells.

The sodium concentration in the urine can also serve as an index of tubular health in certain situations. For example, in acute renal failure, an increased clearance of sodium can indicate acute tubular necrosis. Accordingly, supernormal blood levels of filtered substances (creatinine and other nitrogenous wastes) indicate a fall in glomerular filtration and, hence, nephron health.

Renal Regulatory Functions

In addition to the excretion of nitrogenous and other wastes, the kidneys can also function in regulating the (1) osmotic pressure, (2) the volume, (3) the electrolyte concentration, and (4) the pH of the ECFs (blood and interstitial fluids) of the body. Let us look at specific mechanisms regarding these.

Osmotic Pressure. A rise in the ECF osmotic pressure stimulates osmoreceptors located in the hypothalamus. Such stimulation causes the hypothalamic supraoptic nuclei to secrete ADH. This hormone is thought to stimulate a sensation of thirst. It also increases the permeability of the collecting tubules to water. This increases water reabsorption, which makes the urine hypertonic and restores homeostasis of ECF osmotic pressure. Increased intake of water (due to thirst) can also serve to dilute the ECF. Conversely, a fall in ECF osmotic pressure serves to decrease the secretion of ADH, thereby enabling the kidneys to excrete a more hypotonic (dilute) urine and thereby increase the ECF to normal.

Volume. Homeostasis of ECF volume is maintained by both the renin-angiotensin mechanism already discussed and the side-effect of the ADH mechanism. Angiotensin also elevates blood pressure directly. Indeed, renin plays a pathologic role in one group of hypertensives.

Electrolyte Concentration. Decreased ECF *sodium* concentrations will directly stimulate aldosterone secretion from the adrenal cortex. Since decreased ECF sodium can also cause a decrease in tubular sodium, it may stimulate the juxtaglomerular secretion of renin, which, indirectly, will increase aldosterone levels. Aldosterone stimulates sodium reabsorption of the distal tubule cells. Thus, sodium homeostasis is restored. A rise in ECF sodium can cause the reverse.

A backup mechanism for *potassium regulation* is also found in renal function. If there are high levels of potassium in the face of normal sodium levels, the distal tubules and collecting ducts actively secrete (reverse of active reabsorption) potassium back into the urine. Similar specific reabsorption mechanisms appear to exist for divalent ions such as calcium, magnesium, and phosphates.

The regulation of the monovalent anions, chloride and bicarbonate, is secondary to sodium-ion regulation. As the positively charged cation, sodium, is reabsorbed, a negatively charged ion is electrochemically carried along. This maintains electroneutrality. Whether the negative ion is bicarbonate or chloride depends upon the pH of the ECF, which is also regulated by buffers and respiratory and renal mechanisms.

pH Regulation. If buffers and the respiratory mechanism for pH homeostasis are insufficient, the kidneys then take part. Remember, the acidity of a solution is directly due to the number of unattached (free) hydrogen ions in it. In *renal compensation for alkalosis,* tubular reabsorption of hydrogen ions is increased and secretion is decreased. This increases the hydrogen-ion concentration of the ECF and thereby decreases the alkalosis.

Renal compensation for acidosis involves an increase in the hydrogen-ion secretion of the tubule cells, especially in the distal tubule cells. Now, bicarbonate and sodium ions are continually being filtered from the glomerulus. And remember, hydrogen-ion secretion by distal tubule cells causes an increase in sodium reabsorption. Such sodium reabsorption can electrochemically increase bicarbonate reabsorption. Thus, as hydrogen ions are being eliminated from the ECF, sodium and bicarbonate ions are being added to it. Both will serve to decrease the acidosis.

Now, the urine can only be acidified (by hydrogen-ion secretion) to a pH level of 4.0 to 4.5. If this mechanism operated alone, only a few hydrogen ions could be secreted before the critical shut-off level of 4.0 was reached because hydrogen would combine with urinary chloride to make hydrochloric acid. Not many of these strong hydrochloric acid molecules are needed to make the urine pH 4.0. This would then stop tubular hydrogen-ion secretion before sufficient compensation for acidosis could be obtained.

Fortunately this does not occur because ammonia (NH_3) is also secreted. The tubule cells deaminate certain amino acids and secrete the nitrogenous radicals from them in the form of ammonia (NH_3). This ammonia combines with hydrogen in the urine to form ammonium (NH_4^+), which in turn can combine with chloride to form ammonium chloride (NH_4Cl).

Since NH_4Cl is a neutral salt, the urine can hold many more secreted hydrogen ions than it otherwise could.

SUMMARY OF RENAL FUNCTION

The total blood flow into the nephrons of both kidneys is estimated to be about 1200 ml per minute. Of this total amount, about 650 ml is plasma. Approximately one-fifth of the plasma filters through the glomerular membranes into the Bowman's capsules, forming 125 ml glomerular filtrate per minute. This filtrate is essentially plasma minus proteins. The pH of glomerular filtrate is equal to that of plasma, or 7.4.

As the glomerular filtrate passes through the proximal tubules, nearly 80% of the water and electrolytes, all of the glucose, proteins, and most of the amino acids are reabsorbed. The glomerular filtrate passes on through remaining tubules where water and electrolytes are reabsorbed, depending upon the need of body fluids and the effectiveness of the regulatory mechanism responsible for maintaining their normal levels.

The pH of the forming urine may rise or fall, depending upon the relative amount of acidic and basic ions that are reabsorbed by the tubule walls. The osmotic pressure of the tubular fluid will depend upon the amounts of electrolytes and water that are reabsorbed. Because of those factors, urine pH may vary from 4.5 to 8.2, and osmotic pressure may vary from one-fourth that of plasma to approximately four times plasma pressure.

The amount of urine delivered to the renal pelvis is usually about 1/125 the amount of glomerular filtrate produced or about 1 ml per minute. This 1 ml of urine will contain nearly one-half of the urea contained in the original 125 ml of glomerular filtrate, all of the creatinine, and large proportions of uric acid, phosphate, potassium, sulfates, nitrates, and phenols.

It should be pointed out that even though all glucose and proteins, nearly all amino acids, and large amounts of water and sodium in the original glomerular filtrate are reabsorbed, a very large proportion of the waste products are never reabsorbed and are found in the urine in highly concentrated form.

In addition to waste excretion, the kidneys function in the regulation of the osmotic pressure, volume, electrolyte concentrations, and pH of body fluids.

BIBLIOGRAPHY

Price SA, Wilson LM: Pathophysiology: Clinical Concepts of Disease Processes. New York, McGraw-Hill, 1978
Stephens G: Pathophysiology for Health Practitioners. New York, Macmillan, 1980

Donald E. Butkus and
Allen C. Alfrey

Renal Failure: Pathophysiology and Management 16

Acute renal failure refers to the sudden (hours to a few days) loss of renal function characterized by an increase in blood urea nitrogen (BUN) and serum creatinine. Although no exact criteria for BUN and creatinine can be set, an increase in BUN from 15 to 30 and in creatinine from 1.0 to 2.0 mg/dl is suggestive of acute renal failure in patients with preexisting normal renal function. In patients with preexisting renal disease, larger variations may be required to suggest the diagnosis, since small changes in renal function, not related to acute renal failure, may be magnified when nephron loss is already present. Early awareness of the diagnosis, however, is critical because of the persistent high mortality rate (60% to 65%) associated with acute renal failure despite the general availability of hemodialysis.

PATHOPHYSIOLOGY OF RENAL FAILURE

The adverse effect of reduced renal perfusion on renal function, as a consequence of various shock states, has been recognized for over a hundred years. However, it was during and following World War II that most of the knowledge in regard to understanding the pathogenesis, physiology, and management of renal ischemia was obtained. Since about 1950 evidence has been accumulated to suggest that early diagnosis of renal failure in association with aggressive treatment of the shock state can reverse functional abnormalities and prevent acute tubular necrosis.

Because of the large amount of renal blood flow required to maintain normal renal function, changes in urinary composition occur early in the shock state when renal perfusion is decreased. Normally the kidneys receive 20% to 25% of the cardiac output (approximately 1200 ml/min). Almost 90% of the blood flow to the kidney is concerned with cortical distribution and, in turn, glomerular filtration. The kidney has an intrinsic ability to regulate blood flow (autoregulation) so that the glomerular filtration rate is kept constant over a blood pressure range of 80 to 180 torr. This is accomplished by variations in the tone of preglomerular and postglomerular arterioles.

However, when renal blood flow is severely compromised as a result of either reduction in effective blood volume, fall in cardiac output, or decrease in blood pressure below 80 torr, characteristic changes occur in renal function. Thus, the capacity for complete autoregulation is exceeded. The glomerular filtration rate falls. The amount of tubular fluid is reduced, and the fluid travels through the tubule more slowly. This results in increased sodium and water reabsorption. Because of the reduced renal circulation, the solutes reabsorbed from the tubular fluid are removed more slowly than normal from the interstitium of the renal medulla. This results in increased medullary tonicity, which in turn further augments water reabsorption from the tubular fluid. Therefore, the urinary changes are typical in the shock state. The urinary volume is reduced to less than 400 ml per day (17 ml/hr), urinary specific gravity is increased, and urinary sodium concentration is low (usually less than 5 mEq/liter). (See Fig. 16-1.)

In addition, substances such as creatinine and urea, which are normally filtered but poorly reabsorbed from the renal tubule, are present in high concentration in the urine as a result of the increased water reabsorption. Because of the characteristic changes associated with renal underperfusion, measurement of urinary volume and specific gravity is a simple method of determining the effect of shock management on renal perfusion.

An increase in systemic blood pressure does not necessarily imply improvement in renal perfusion. This may be especially evident when drugs such as norepinephrine (Levophed) are used to correct the hypotension associated with states of volume depletion. These drugs may be associated with further reduction in renal blood flow as a consequence of constriction of renal arteries. This is manifested by a further fall in urinary volume and rise in specific gravity.

In turn, if the shock state is more appropriately and specifically treated by replacing volume, improving cardiac output, correcting arrhythmias, or by giving isoproterenol (Isuprel), the improved renal perfusion will be manifested as an increased urinary volume and a fall in specific gravity of the urine.

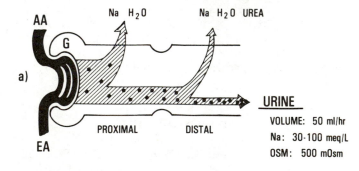

URINE

VOLUME: 50 ml/hr
Na: 30-100 meq/L
OSM: 500 mOsm

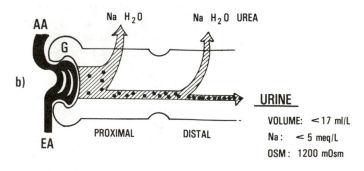

URINE

VOLUME: <17 ml/L
Na: <5 meq/L
OSM: 1200 mOsm

Figure 16-1.
Underperfusion of the kidney *(b)* results in decreased renal blood flow and glomerular filtration, with consequent increase in the fraction of filtrate reabsorbed in the proximal tubule and low urine flow with low sodium content and increased concentration compared with normal *(a)*.

MANAGEMENT OF ACUTE REVERSIBLE RENAL FAILURE

Primary management of renal function impairment is directed at the adequate and specific management of the shock state. The three most common causes for reduced renal perfusion are decreased cardiac output, altered peripheral vascular resistance, and hypovolemia.

Decreased Cardiac Output

Factors such as cardiac arrhythmias, acute myocardial infarction, and acute pericardial tamponade, all of which decrease cardiac output, may be associated with a reduction in renal blood flow. The reversibility of the renal failure is thus dependent upon the ability to improve cardiac function. The specific management has been discussed in earlier chapters.

With the above conditions cardiac output is usually acutely and severely compromised. However, when cardiac output is impaired to a lesser extent over a longer period of time, features of congestive heart failure occur. Again there is reduced renal perfusion, although to a lesser extent. The major feature of this state, from the renal aspect, is avid sodium reabsorption, which results in increased extracellular fluid volume, elevation of central venous pressure, and edema.

Several mechanisms are responsible for the increased tubular reabsorption of sodium (see Fig. 16-2). First, there is a greater reduction in renal blood flow than in glomerular filtration, bringing into play the mechanisms discussed earlier. Second, it has been suggested that blood flow to the superficial cortex is reduced while blood flow to the inner cortical area is increased. It is also thought that the nephrons in the inner cortical region reabsorb a greater percentage of the filtered sodium than the nephrons in the outer cortex of the kidney.

Other factors include increased proximal and distal tubule sodium reabsorption. The mechanisms responsible for the increased proximal tubule sodium reabsorption are poorly understood; however, aldosterone is largely responsible for the increased distal tubule sodium reabsorption. It can be seen that numerous mechanisms are responsible for the increased

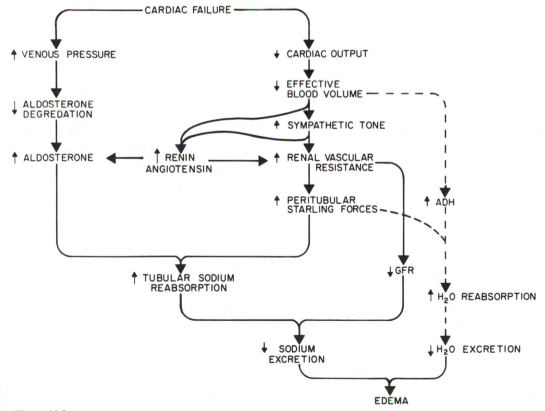

Figure 16-2.
Factors affecting sodium reabsorption with decreased cardiac output.

tubular reabsorption of sodium in congestive heart failure.

Therapy is largely directed at increasing urinary sodium excretion. At times this can be accomplished by improving cardiac output, which in turn increases renal perfusion. This is not always possible, however.

Diuretics are frequently used to increase sodium excretion. These agents directly inhibit sodium reabsorption in the renal tubule. The potency of a diuretic is primarily determined by the site in the renal tubule where sodium reabsorption is blocked.

The two most potent diuretics presently available are furosemide (Lasix) and ethacrynic acid (Edecrin). These agents block sodium reabsorption in the ascending limb of the loop of Henle and in the distal tubule. It is still unclear whether they have an effect in the proximal tubule as well. The thiazide diuretics have their major site of action in the distal tubule and are therefore somewhat less potent than the above agents.

Another diuretic commonly used is spironolactone (Aldactone), which increases urinary sodium by blocking the renal tubular effect of aldosterone.

Aldosterone should be used with caution in patients with severe decreases in cardiac output and renal underperfusion because it decreases potassium excretion and can produce life-threatening hyperkalemia in such patients. The same is true of triamterene, another potassium-sparing diuretic.

Altered Peripheral Vascular Resistance

Renal perfusion is compromised in these states as a result of increased size of the intravascular compartment and redistribution of blood volume. This may be a consequence of gram-negative septicemia, certain drug overdoses, anaphylactic reactions, and electrolyte disturbances such as acidosis.

Management is primarily directed at treating the basic disturbance with appropriate specific therapy plus fluid, electrolyte, and colloid replacement. The controversy in regard to the use of steroids and various pressor agents in gram-negative sepsis is beyond the scope of this discussion.

Hypovolemia

Restoration of extracellular fluid and blood volume is of major importance in the management of any shock state. Evidence for extracellular volume depletion is usually obtained from the history and physical examination.

Historically the patient may give evidence of external sodium and water loss as a result of vomiting, diarrhea, excessive sweating, or surgical procedures. Blood volume may also be compromised as a result of fluid redistribution as seen both with burns and with inflammatory processes in the abdomen, such as pancreatitis or peritonitis. The physical findings associated with extracellular volume depletion are sunken eyes, dry mouth, loss of skin turgor, and tachycardia. Postural hypotension may also be noted.

Therapy is directed at sodium and water replacement. Response to treatment can be judged by changes in urinary volume, specific gravity, central venous pressure, and the above physical findings.

MAINTENANCE OF URINARY FLOW

At times, in spite of adequate treatment of the shock state, urinary volume remains low. This may be a result of either continuing functional impairment in the postshock period or parenchymal renal damage suffered as a consequence of the shock state. Not only is it necessary to differentiate these two states from each other, but a number of authors also feel that prolonged oliguria, if allowed to persist, may eventually lead to acute tubular necrosis. Mannitol and furosemide have been used in this setting for both diagnosis and maintenance of urinary function.

Mannitol is the reduced form of the six-carbon sugar, mannose. It is distributed in the extracellular fluid and is essentially not metabolized. It is freely filtered at the glomerulus and not reabsorbed by the tubule. Because of its small molecular size (180), it exerts a significant osmotic effect and, in turn, increases urinary flow.

Mannitol is usually infused rather rapidly. The more rapid the infusion, the higher the blood level and, in turn, the filtered load. Urine flow is dependent upon the amount of mannitol filtered, and if the infusion is too slow, changes in urinary flow rate will be delayed and less apparent.

The usual test is 12.5 g given intravenously as a 25% solution over 3 to 5 minutes. If urine flow increases to greater than 40 ml per hour, the patient is felt to have reversible renal failure, and his urine volume is then maintained at 100 ml per hour with additional mannitol.

More recently *furosemide* and *ethacrynic acid*

have largely replaced mannitol in the diagnosis of reversible renal failure. A number of patients who fail to develop a diuresis following mannitol will have an acceptable increase in urinary volume following furosemide or ethacrynic acid.

Furosemide in dosages of 200 to 1000 mg is given intravenously. The peak diuresis usually occurs within 2 hours of its administration. If furosemide is effective in increasing urinary volume, it is then repeated at 4- to 6-hour intervals to maintain the urinary flow rate.

In patients failing to respond to furosemide, a diagnosis of acute tubular necrosis is seriously entertained. In patients who respond to furosemide and mannitol, it is important to realize that sodium and water depletion will occur if losses are not replaced. Usually urine volume is replaced by half strength normal saline. In addition, potassium replacement is frequently required.

ACUTE TUBULAR NECROSIS
Although approximately 30% of the cases of acute tubular necrosis occur without a specific etiology being found, some of the more common causes for the development of this syndrome include shock, nephrotoxic agents, and acute renal failure associated with myoglobinuria and hemoglobinuria.

Causes

Shock. There is little doubt that the severity and duration of *traumatic shock* play major roles in predisposing to the development of acute tubular necrosis. Over 40% of a large number of combat casualties in World War II developed acute tubular necrosis. In contrast, acute tubular necrosis was uncommon in Vietnam casualties. This reduced incidence has been attributed to early air evacuation and rapid treatment of shock.

Nephrotoxic Agents. A large number of *chemicals and drugs* have been found to be nephrotoxic. In the hospital patient probably the most common group of nephrotoxic agents is the antibiotics. These include gentamicin, kenamycin, cephaloridine, cephalothin, colistin, polymyxin, and rifampin. In addition, synthetic penicillins, such as methicillin, may produce acute renal failure associated with a hypersensitivitylike reaction.

Acute renal failure is also frequently seen following administration of intravenous contrast agents in pyelography and angiography. This is especially prone to occur with preexisting renal disease, especially in diabetics and patients with multiple myeloma.

Additionally, nonsteroidal anti-inflammatory drugs such as indomethacin and salicylates may produce transitory but severe reduction of renal function, especially in patients whose renal prostaglandin production is compensatorily stimulated, as in congestive heart failure. Because the above agents can adversely affect renal function on a rather frequent basis, especially in patients who are severely ill, renal function should be monitored routinely before and after such therapy. This is especially true with the nephrotoxic antibiotics, which more commonly produce a nonoliguric form of acute renal failure.

Intravascular Hemolysis. A third major category of acute tubular necrosis is that associated with abnormal release of body pigments (myoglobin and hemoglobin). Characteristically the urine is dark in color and positive for hemoglobin. Patients with states associated with *intravascular hemolysis* such as transfusion reactions, malaria, and arsine intoxication may develop acute tubular necrosis. In addition, acute renal failure commonly occurs in patients with myoglobinuria of a variety of etiologies.

Reduced Renal Blood Flow. Numerous investigations have been carried out to define the mechanisms by which nephrotoxic agents and shock induce acute tubular necrosis and oliguria, but to date these have not been clearly defined. Renal blood flow has been found to be reduced to approximately one-third of normal in acute tubular necrosis, whereas the glomerular filtration rate is almost completely suppressed. This is in contrast to other states in which a similar reduction in renal blood flow is accompanied by much better maintenance of glomerular filtration and renal function.

Numerous animal studies have suggested that intratubular obstruction from casts and cellular debris may be involved in the suppression of glomerular filtration. If this obstruction is relieved, renal function returns. Other studies have suggested that there is disruption of the tubule epithelium with excessive back flow of the filtrate out of the tubule lumen, thus explaining the lack of urine formation in the face of

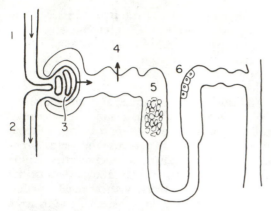

Figure 16-3.
Potential mechanisms causing acute renal failure include decreased filtration pressure because of constriction in the renal arterioles *(1 & 2)*; decreased glomerular capillary permeability *(3)*; increased permeability of the proximal tubules with back-leak of filtrate *(4)*; obstruction of urine flow by necrotic tubular cells *(5)*; increased sodium delivery to the macula densa *(6)*, which causes an increase in renin-angiotensin production and vasoconstriction at the glomerular level.

continuing, although reduced, renal blood flow. (See Fig. 16-3.)

The mechanism responsible for the decreased superficial cortical blood flow in the kidney with acute tubular necrosis has not been defined. However, the recent demonstration of the presence of converting enzyme in the kidney suggests that renin-angiotensin may play a role in this phenomenon.

Manifestations

Classically, patients have oliguria in association with acute tubular necrosis; however, this is not invariably so. A group of patients present with acute nonoliguric (partially reversible) renal failure. This state is especially common in patients receiving nephrotoxic antibiotics. If antibiotics are discontinued before renal function is markedly reduced, the patient frequently sustains moderate functional impairment for 7 to 10 days with gradual return to normal. In general, patients with nonoliguric acute renal failure have few symptoms, and the disease is much less serious than the oliguric form of acute tubular necrosis.

The more classic or oliguric form of acute tubular necrosis begins with an acute precipitating event immediately followed by oliguria (urine volume less than 400 ml/day). The mean duration of oliguria is around 12 days, although it may last only 2 to 3 days or as long as 30 days.

This is accompanied by a usual rise in BUN of 25 to 30 mg per 100 ml per day and creatinine of 1.5 to 2 mg per 100 ml per day. The most common complication in this period is overhydration with resulting cardiac failure, pulmonary edema, and death. In addition, the patient may develop acidosis, hyperkalemia, and symptoms of uremia.

The oliguric phase is followed by gradual return of renal function as manifested by a stepwise increase in urine volume (the diuretic stage). The degree of diuresis is primarily determined by the state of hydration at the time the patient enters the diuretic stage. If the patient is markedly overloaded, urinary volume may eventually exceed 4 to 5 liters per day. This may result in marked sodium wasting, with death resulting from electrolyte depletion.

Because of the slow return of renal function during the diuretic phase, the degree of azotemia may increase during the early part of the diuretic period, and the patient will have similar complications as noted in the oliguric phase. A period of several months is required for full recovery of renal function after the end of the diuretic period.

Differentiating Acute Tubular Necrosis From Decreased Renal Perfusion

During the immediate postshock period, the differentiation between continuing decreased renal perfusion and acute tubular necrosis has to be made. The routine urine analysis is usually of little help in differentiating these two states in that the changes are nonspecific. In both conditions there may be mild proteinuria in association with a moderate number of red blood cells, white blood cells, and granular casts. The major features of the two states are shown in Table 16-1.

The urinary changes present in patients with acute tubular necrosis are largely a consequence of loss of tubule function. Hypertension is uncommon in patients with acute tubular necrosis, and when present suggests fluid and sodium excess.

When the patient presents to the hospital with oliguric renal failure, other causes of acute renal insufficiency must be considered such as lupus glomerulonephritis, periarteritis, rapidly progressive glomerulonephritis, and poststreptococcal glomerulonephritis. In addition, the possibility of chronic parenchymal renal disease exists.

Rarely does the patient with acute tubular ne-

Table 16–1
Use of Lab Values in Differentiating Acute Tubular Necrosis From Decreased Renal Perfusion

Test	Acute Tubular Necrosis	Reduced Renal Blood Flow
Urine		
Volume	< 400 ml/24 hr	< 400 ml/24 hr
Sodium	Between 40 and 10 mEq/liter	< 5 mEq/liter
Specific gravity	1.010	Usually > 1.020
Osmolality	250–350 mOsm/liter	Usually >400 mOsm/liter
Urea	200–300 mg/100 ml	Usually > 600 mg/100 ml
Creatinine	< 60 mg/100 ml	Usually > 150 mg/100 ml
Fe_{Na}	> 3.0%	< 1.0%
Blood		
BUN:Cr	10:1	Usually > 20:1
Response to		
mannitol	None	None or flow increases to > 40 ml/hr
Furosemide	None	Flow increases to > 40 ml/hr

crosis have total anuria. This is an important point in helping to differentiate acute tubular necrosis from obstructive uropathy. However, retrograde urography is frequently necessary to exclude obstruction.

Management

Since acute tubular necrosis continues to carry a high mortality, the major objective is prevention of this complication. The feasibility of preventing the development of acute tubular necrosis in patients with major traumatic injuries by rapid replacement of blood loss and correction of fluid and electrolyte disturbances has been clearly demonstrated.

Similarly, patients receiving potentially nephrotoxic agents should undergo serial determinations to evaluate renal function during the course of the administration of these agents. This can most easily be done by measuring serum creatinine levels on an every-other-day schedule. If the serum creatinine begins to rise, the drug should be discontinued. In the majority of patients, functional deterioration stabilizes, and the patient recovers without the development of severe impairment of renal function.

Drug Therapy.   There is still considerable debate with regard to the effectiveness of *mannitol* and *furosemide* in the prevention of acute renal failure. In fact, some evidence has been accumulated that suggests that furosemide may actually increase the toxicity of certain nephrotoxic

agents. Until this controversy is resolved, it would seem desirable to use these agents sparingly in patients with nonoliguric acute tubular necrosis, especially when it is a consequence of drug intoxication.

Volume Replacement.   After development of acute tubular necrosis, the primary consideration is maintenance of fluid and electrolyte balance. During the oliguric phase, urinary volume is usually less than 300 ml per day. Insensible losses average 800 to 1000 ml per day and are virtually free of electrolytes.

In general, fluid replacement should be approximately 500 ml per day. Additional water will be obtained from the water present in foods plus the water of oxidation from metabolism. Because of the utilization of body proteins and fats, the patient ideally should lose around 1 pound a day in order to maintain water balance. The *danger of fluid overload* with resulting congestive heart failure and pulmonary edema exists throughout the oliguric period. In contrast, during the diuretic phase of acute tubular necrosis there may be extensive *sodium wasting* in association with the increased urinary volumes. It is thus necessary to keep accurate intake and output records as well as daily weights during both phases. This is especially important when there are other avenues of fluid and electrolyte losses such as vomiting, diarrhea, nasogastric suction, and drainages from fistulas. In general, losses occurring as a result of the above should be replaced in full.

Table 16–2
Recommended Dosage for Antibiotics

Group	Antibiotic	Recommended Dose	
		Serum Creatinine 4–10 mg/dl	Serum Creatinine 10 mg/dl
1. Marked reduction in dosage	Tetracycline Oxytetracycline Kanamycin Streptomycin Colistimethate Polymyxin	Loading dose followed by standard doses at intervals of 1 to 2 days	Loading dose followed by standard doses at intervals of 3 to 4 days
2. Modest reduction in dosage		Loading dose followed by:	Loading dose followed by:
	Penicillin G	Standard doses at 4- to 5-hr intervals	Standard doses at 8- to 10-hr intervals
	Lincomycin	Standard doses at 6-hr intervals	Standard doses at 12-hr intervals
	Cephalothin	Standard doses at 12-hr intervals	Standard doses at 24-hr intervals
3. No reduction in dosage	Chloramphenicol Erythromycin Methicillin Oxacillin Novobiocin	Same as in the normal	Same as in the normal

(From Schwartz WB, Kassirer JP: Am J Med, 44:796)

Nutritional Therapy. Outside of adequate fluid and electrolyte replacement, intake is directed at supplying the patient with calories in the form of carbohydrates and fats to decrease the rate of breakdown of body protein. Since 1 g of urea is formed from every 6 g of protein metabolized, protein intake is usually restricted in order to prevent the BUN from rising at too fast a rate.

Drug Precautions. Certain drugs should be avoided or dosage reduced in any patient with markedly impaired renal function. Because of the possibility of magnesium intoxication, *antacids* containing magnesium should be avoided. Because of the reduced renal function, *digitalis* excretion may be reduced. Dosage should be altered to avoid excessively high blood levels. In addition, certain *antibiotics* should be given in much smaller dosages than usually employed (see Table 16-2).

Before administering a drug to a patient with renal failure, it is wise to review the following questions:

- Does the drug depend upon the kidney for secretion?
- Does an excess blood level affect the kidney?
- Does the drug add chemically to the pool of urea nitrogen?
- Does the effect of the drug alter electrolyte imbalance?
- Is the patient more susceptible to the drug because of kidney disease?

For additional information about the modification of drug dosages in uremia, see R. J. Anderson, J. G. Gambertoglio, and R. W. Schrier, *Clinical Use of Drugs in Renal Failure* (Springfield, Illinois: Charles C Thomas, 1978).

Acidosis

Metabolic acidosis of moderate severity is usually present in patients with renal failure. This results from the inability of the kidneys to excrete fixed acids (*e.g.,* H_2PO_4) produced from normal metabolic processes.

The acidosis can usually be easily controlled by giving the patient 30 to 60 mEq of sodium bicarbonate daily.

Hyperkalemia

Hyperkalemia commonly occurs in patients with acute tubular necrosis. This is a consequence of both the reduced ability of the kidneys to excrete potassium and the release of intracellular potassium because of acidosis. The acidosis results in movement of the hydrogen ion into the cell, thus displacing potassium into the extracellular fluid. This maintains electrical neutrality but increases the hyperkalemic state.

An additional mechanism for producing hyperkalemia, often overlooked in acutely ill patients, is caloric restriction, especially glucose restriction. Transport of glucose and amino acids into cells is accompanied by potassium. In acutely ill, catabolic patients, when dietary intake is restricted or intravenous fluid therapy inadvertently disrupted, failure of transport of potassium intracellularly may contribute to hyperkalemia. Because this process requires insulin, insulin deficiency may have the same consequences, and diabetics may therefore be more prone to acute disturbances in potassium balance when renal failure occurs.

Hyperkalemia is manifested clinically by cardiac and neuromuscular changes. Both cardiac conduction disturbances and acute flaccid quadriplegia are life-threatening complications. These hyperkalemic changes are rapidly reversed by giving intravenous calcium gluconate, which has a direct antagonist effect on the action of potassium. Reduction of the serum potassium can be accomplished by treating the acidosis with intravenous sodium bicarbonate. In addition, glucose and insulin are frequently used as an additional method of shifting extracellular potassium to intracellular pools.

Hyperkalemia is usually preventable by avoiding potassium supplements, giving chronic therapy for acidosis, and using sodium polystyrene sulfonate resin (Kayexalate) when serum potassium is even slightly elevated.

Sodium and Water Diuresis

During the oliguric phase of acute tubular necrosis, sodium retention may occur. However, with the onset of the diuretic period, urinary volume and sodium excretion may markedly increase.

Urinary volume is largely determined by the state of hydration at the onset of the diuretic period. Since urinary sodium concentration is relatively fixed, sodium losses are largely determined by urinary volume. Therefore, if the patient is markedly overhydrated at the onset of the

Table 16–3
Common Fluid and Electrolyte Imbalances

Electrolyte Disturbance	Major Symptoms	Major Physical Findings	Etiology
Increased sodium and water	Dyspnea	Edema, anasarca, rales, increased jugular venous pressure	Congestive failure, renal disease, liver disease
Decreased sodium and water	Thirst Weakness	Tachycardia, postural hypotension, sunken eyes, dry mouth, decreased skin turgor	Excessive sweating, vomiting, diarrhea, Addison's disease, renal disease, diuretics without replacement
Decreased sodium and normal water	Headaches Psychological disorder	Hyperreflexia, pathologic reflexes, convulsions, coma	Water without sodium replacement in above states; excess ADH
Normal sodium and decreased water	Thirst	Often no findings or those found in decreased sodium and water	Lack of water intake, diabetes insipidus, excessive sweating, fever
Hyperkalemia	Weakness	Paralysis, ECG changes; spiked T waves	Renal disease, excess potassium replacement
Hypokalemia	Weakness	Paralysis, paralytic ileus, hypoventilation, ECG changes: T waves and prominent U waves	Diuretics, renal disease, diarrhea, vomiting, excess laxatives
Acidosis	Weakness	Kussmaul respiration	Renal disease, diabetic acidosis, certain intoxications
Hypermagnesemia	Weakness	Muscle weakness, hypoventilation, hypotension, flushing	Antacids with renal disease

diuretic phase, sodium losses may be severe. Clinically, sodium depletion is characterized by either extracellular volume depletion, as manifested by tachycardia and postural hypotension, or water intoxication when sodium losses exceed water losses. This latter syndrome is characterized by markedly reduced serum sodium concentrations in association with personality changes, convulsions, coma, and death if allowed to progress untreated.

With acute water intoxication, treatment is directed at raising the serum sodium concentration. This can usually be accomplished by giving hypertonic (3% to 5%) sodium chloride intravenously. Table 16-3 lists common fluid and electrolyte imbalances.

Uremic Syndrome

In addition to the above specific electrolyte disturbances, the patient may develop symptoms associated with any uremic state. Early the patient has nausea, anorexia, and vomiting. Later this progresses to stupor, convulsions, and coma. In addition, the patient may develop bleeding abnormalities, uremic pneumonitis, pericarditis, pleuritis, and so forth.

Dialysis is indicated prior to the development of clinical symptoms of uremia. With the availability of hemodialysis or peritoneal dialysis in most hospitals, there is little reason for the clinical features of uremia to occur in patients with acute tubular necrosis. Most patients having oliguria for more than 4 to 5 days will require dialysis sometime during the course of their acute tubular necrosis. There is little doubt that dialysis has improved survival in patients with acute tubular necrosis.

Prognosis is largely determined by the primary event that led to the development of acute tubular necrosis. Medical causes of acute tubular necrosis such as transfusion reactions, myoglobinuria, nephrotoxic agents, and simple volume depletion are accompanied by a mortality rate of around 25%, whereas cases resulting from trauma and severe surgical complications have a mortality rate of 70% to 80%. Death usually results as a complication of poor wound healing and sepsis.

In view of the continuing high mortality associated with acute tubular necrosis, every effort should be directed toward the prevention of this complication when the patient is seen early during the course of his shock state.

BIBLIOGRAPHY

Anderson RJ, Linas SL, Berns AS et al: Nonoliguric acute renal failure. N Engl J Med, 296:1135–1138, 1977

Bennett WM, Plamp C, Porter GA: Drug-related syndromes in clinical nephrology. Ann Intern Med, 87:582–590, 1977

Cannon PJ: The kidney in heart failure. N Engl J Med, 296:24–33, 1977

Levensky NG: Pathophysiology of acute renal failure. N Engl J Med, 296:1453–1458, 1977

Schrier RW: Acute renal failure. Kidney Int, 15:205–216, 1979

Shin, B, Mackenzie CF, Cowley RA: Changing patterns of post-traumatic acute renal failure. Am Surg, 45:182–189, 1979

Donald E. Butkus

SELECTED TESTS TO MONITOR RENAL FUNCTION

The patient whose condition is serious enough to warrant observation in the critical care unit will frequently manifest abnormalities of renal function, either as the result of impaired ability to excrete nitrogenous waste products or because of an inability to handle water loads efficiently, or both. It is therefore mandatory that certain aspects of renal function be monitored, on an intermittent or a continuing basis, in order that these complications can be detected early and appropriate therapy instituted.

In most circumstances the parameters followed will include the urine output, the urine solute concentration (frequently in relation to the plasma solute concentration), and some parameter of the kidneys' ability to excrete nitrogenous waste products.

Creatinine and Creatinine Clearance

The most commonly used tests of renal function are the serum creatinine and the blood urea nitrogen (BUN), but the most accurate test readily available is the creatinine clearance.

Creatinine is formed as a by-product of normal muscle metabolism and is excreted in the urine primarily as the result of glomerular filtration, with a small percentage secreted into the urine by the kidney tubules. It is therefore a useful indicator of the glomerular filtration rate. The amount of creatinine excreted in the urine of any given individual is related to his muscle mass and will remain quite constant unless muscle wasting occurs.

The actual creatinine clearance is calculated by the formula

$$\text{clearance creatinine} = \frac{UV}{P}$$

where U is the urine creatine concentration, V the urine volume, and P the plasma creatinine concentration. The most important technical aspect of this test is the *accuracy of the urine collection;* it is important to know the exact time it took to form the sample and the exact amount of creatinine present.

The expression UV tells how much creatinine appears in the urine during the period of collection, and this can be readily converted to milligrams per minute, which is the standard reference point. Dividing this by the plasma creatinine concentration (which has to be converted from mg/100 ml to mg/ml) tells the minimum number of milliliters of plasma that must have been filtered by the glomeruli in order to produce the measured amount of creatinine in the urine. The final result is expressed in milliliters per minute, and the normal range varies between 80 and 120, depending on the individual's size and age. The results should be corrected to a standard body size of 1.73 sq m, which can be derived from standard tables if the patient's height and weight are known.

If the kidneys are damaged by some disease process, the creatinine clearance will decrease and the serum creatinine concentration will rise. The urine creatinine excretion will initially decrease until the blood level rises to a point at which the amount of creatinine appearing in the urine is again equal to the amount being produced by the body.

For example, a normal individual with a serum creatinine concentration of 1.0 mg/dl and a creatinine excretion of 1.0 mg per minute has a creatinine clearance of 100 ml per minute. If the individual develops renal disease with 50% loss of renal function, his serum creatinine will rise to 2.0 mg/dl, and he will continue to excrete 1.0 mg of creatinine in his urine per minute. In many

situations in which the patient has rapidly changing renal function and oliguria, as in acute renal failure, the creatinine clearance becomes less reliable until the situation becomes more stable. It is therefore useful to follow the serum creatinine concentration as an indicator of the rate and direction of change until stability occurs.

Blood Urea Nitrogen

The BUN has also been used for many years as an indicator of kidney function, but unlike the serum creatinine, its level tends to be influenced by a great many factors.

Urea, as mentioned in an earlier section, has a clearance less than that of creatinine due largely to the fact that some urea diffuses out of the tubule back into the bloodstream. This is particularly true at low urine flow rates, at which more sodium and water, and consequently more urea, are being reabsorbed. Therefore, in states of relative or absolute volume depletion, the BUN will tend to rise out of proportion to any change in renal function.

In addition, the amount of urea produced per day, unlike creatinine, is quite variable, especially in seriously ill patients. Increased urea production can result from increased protein intake (tube feedings and some forms of hyperalimentation) or increased tissue breakdown as with crush injuries, febrile illnesses, steroid or tetracycline administration, and reabsorption of blood from the intestine in a patient with intestinal hemorrhage. All of these may result in an increased urea production and an increased BUN even though renal function might be normal, and they would also contribute to the rate of rise in BUN in an individual with renal failure.

The opposite is true for patients with decreased protein intake or liver disease (both of which reduce urea production) and for patients with large urine volumes secondary to excessive fluid intake.

The BUN is therefore less useful as a guide to changes in renal function than is the serum creatinine. The BUN is still of significant value, however, especially when looked at in comparison with the serum creatinine concentration. Normally these are present in a ratio of 10:1 (urea:creatinine). Discrepancies in this ratio might point toward a potentially correctable situation as noted in Table 16-4.

Table 16–4
Factors Affecting Serum Urea: Creatinine Ratio

A. Decreased Urea: Creatinine (<10:1)
  1. Liver disease
  2. Protein restriction
  3. Excessive fluid intake
B. Increased Urea: Creatinine (>10:1)
  1. Volume depletion
  2. Decreased "effective" blood volume
  3. Catabolic states
  4. Excessive protein intake

Urinary Concentration and Dilution

As noted earlier, the kidney possesses a considerable capacity to reabsorb filtered water. In individuals with normal renal function, the final concentration of the urine is dependent upon the state of hydration. A patient who is well hydrated will excrete a very dilute urine, and a patient who is dehydrated will excrete a very concentrated urine, as the kidneys attempt to either eliminate or conserve water.

The factor that governs the amount of water excreted, and, therefore, the urine concentration, is the amount of antidiuretic hormone (ADH) secreted by the pituitary gland.

Urinary concentration may be measured by tests for specific gravity or osmolality.

SPECIFIC GRAVITY

The specific gravity of the urine is the time-honored test of the kidneys' ability to concentrate and dilute the urine. The specific gravity measures the buoyancy of a solution compared to water and depends upon the number of particles in solution as well as their size and weight.

Two methods have been used to obtain this measurement in clinical practice, the *hydrometer* and the *refractometer* (or TS meter, as it is frequently called). The hydrometer has been in clinical use for many years and is the less preferred of the two methods because (1) it requires a much larger volume of urine, (2) results are less reproducible, and (3) it requires a greater amount of time.

The refractometer is highly reproducible and requires only a drop of urine for the measurement. In addition, this instrument can be used to measure the total solids of plasma (thus the name TS meter), which are a good indicator of the plasma protein concentration and a useful indicator of the state of a patient's fluid balance, especially when serial determinations are made. The refractometer, because of the above advantages, should replace the hydrometer for specific gravity determinations and should be used in the critical care unit.

The normal kidney has the capacity to dilute the urine to a specific gravity of 1.001 and to concentrate the urine to at least 1.022 (higher values are not unusual). Normally the individual's water balance will determine whether the urine is concentrated or dilute, a dilute urine being an indicator of water excess and a concentrated urine an indicator of water deficit. In many renal diseases the ability of the kidneys to form a concentrated urine is lost, and the specific gravity becomes "fixed" at 1.010, a finding that might be seen in acute tubular necrosis and acute nephritis.

As with many simple laboratory tests, there are limitations in the accuracy of the specific gravity determination. The specific gravity is not always the most accurate indicator of the ability of the kidneys to concentrate the urine because the concentrating ability is a reflection of the concentration of particles in the urine. In addition to the concentration of particles, the specific gravity is also in part dependent upon the size and weight of the particles in solution. Therefore, a falsely high specific gravity determination will be found when high-molecular-weight substances such as protein, glucose, mannitol, and radiographic contrast material are present in the urine. A greater degree of accuracy can be obtained with urine osmolality determinations.

OSMOLALITY

The *osmolality* of a solution is an expression of the total number (concentration) of particles in solution and is independent of the size, molecular weight, or electrical charge of the molecules. All substances in solution contribute to the osmolality to a certain degree. For example, a mol (gram molecular weight) of sodium chloride dissociates incompletely into Na^+ and Cl^- ions and produces 1.86 osmols when dissolved in a kilogram of solvent (such as plasma). A mol of nonionic solute (such as glucose or urea) produces only 1 osmol when dissolved in a kilogram of solvent. The total concentration of particles in a solution is the osmolality and is reported in units of osmols per kilogram of solvent. In clinical situations, because we are dealing with much smaller concentrations, the osmolality is reported in milliosmols (thousandth of an osmol, abbreviated mOsm) per kilogram of solvent (plasma or serum).

The osmolality is generally determined in the

laboratory by measuring the freezing point of the solution, which is directly related to the number of particles in solution. (More recent laboratory methods have taken advantage of another property of solutions, the vapor pressure, as an indicator of osmolality; one advantage is the much smaller sample required to perform the assay.)

The normal *serum osmolality* is made up primarily of sodium and its accompanying anions, with urea and glucose contributing about 5 mOsm each. Therefore, knowing the serum sodium, urea, and glucose concentrations, we can calculate the osmolality of plasma by the formula

$$\text{osmolality} = 2\,Na + \frac{BUN}{2.6} + \frac{glucose}{18}$$

The calculated osmolality will normally be within 10 mOsm of the measured osmolality, which normally averages 290 ± 5 mOsm per kg. The plasma osmolality in normal individuals is quite constant from day to day.

Because water permeates freely between the blood, interstitial fluid, and tissues, a change in the osmolality of one body compartment will produce a shift in body fluids so that the osmolality of the plasma is always the same as that of the other body compartments, except in the most rapidly changing conditions, where a slight lag may occur.

The *significance of the plasma osmolality* lies in the fact that it is the main regulator of the release of ADH. When sufficient water is not being taken in, the osmolality will rise, stimulating the release of ADH, which signals the kidneys to conserve water and produce a more concentrated urine. When excessive amounts of water are ingested, the osmolality decreases, ADH release is inhibited, and the urine becomes more dilute. Under maximum ADH stimulation, the kidneys can concentrate the urine to approximately 1200 mOsm per kg, and with maximum ADH suppression (water load) the kidneys can dilute the urine to approximately 50 mOsm per kg.

Thus, there is no single normal urine osmolality but rather a range in which predicted values might be expected, depending upon the clinical setting. Also, unlike the plasma, the urine osmolality is less dependent upon the urine sodium concentration, and other substances such as urea play a more important role. In renal disease one of the first renal functions to be lost is the ability to concentrate urine. As a reflection of this, the urine osmolality becomes fixed within 50 mOsm of the simultaneously determined serum osmolality. Therefore the osmolality is a useful parameter of renal function.

The *serum and urine osmolalities* are of use in combination in a number of other circumstances. In the patient with diabetes insipidus, which results from neurologic disease or injury, the urine volume would be increased with a low urine osmolality (50 to 100 mOsm), and the serum osmolality would be increased (310 mOsm or greater) unless the fluid loss had been replaced. On the other hand, the patient with carcinoma of the lung, porphyria, or central nervous system (CNS) disease might have an excess production of ADH, or an ADH-like material, and have the opposite picture, with a low serum osmolality and a disproportionately high urine osmolality.

As already indicated, the serum osmolality may be increased or decreased in various states. A decrease in the serum osmolality can occur only when the serum sodium is decreased. An increase in the serum osmolality can occur whenever the serum sodium, urea, or glucose is elevated or when there are abnormal compounds present in the blood, including drugs, poisons, or metabolic waste products that are not usually measured, such as lactic acid. Symptoms due to increased osmolality usually occur when the osmolality is greater than 350 mOsm, and coma occurs when the osmolality is in the 400 range or above (see following section, Serum Sodium Concentration).

The usual close correlation between the measured and calculated osmolality has been mentioned. In certain circumstances the measured serum osmolality might be significantly higher than the calculated osmolality when substances of an unusual nature are present in the blood. Many drugs and toxins such as aspirin and alcohol raise the serum osmolality. In a comatose patient a discrepancy between the measured and calculated serum osmolalities might lead to the appropriate drug screen to provide the correct diagnosis. In patients with heart failure, hepatic disease, or shock, a discrepancy of 40 or more mOsm between the measured and calculated osmolalities, due to unknown metabolites, has been correlated with a mortality rate of 95% or greater.

Serum Sodium Concentration

The serum sodium concentration is generally maintained in a narrow range (135 to 145 mEq/liter) and is dependent upon the body's

Table 16–5
Hyponatremia

Accompanied By	Caused By
Increased total body sodium and edema	Congestive heart failure Decompensated cirrhosis Nephrotic syndrome
Decreased total body sodium and hypovolemia	Diuretics Renal salt wasting Adrenal insufficiency Hemorrhage
Normal total body sodium and hypervolemia	Syndrome of inappropriate ADH release which may accompany CNS and pulmonary disease, tumors, porphyria, drugs, psychiatric disorders, myxedema

state of fluid balance as governed by the release of ADH and water intake.

HYPONATREMIA

In a number of disease states, the serum sodium concentration may be reduced (hyponatremia) because of an inability of the kidneys to excrete free water. This is due to either a persistent release of ADH in response to a decrease in the total or effective intravascular volume or to some inappropriate stimulation of ADH release (not due to volume or osmotic stimuli)*.

Hyponatremia may be associated with an increased total body sodium and edema, a decreased total body sodium and hypovolemia, or a normal or slightly increased total body sodium and increased blood volume, depending upon the clinical disorder that gives rise to the hyponatremia (see Table 16-5).

Volume Depletion.   In patients with edema due to cirrhosis, congestive heart failure, or the nephrotic syndrome, hyponatremia occurs frequently and may be enhanced by the use of diuretics. In these conditions, although there is an overall increase in body sodium and water, ADH release is stimulated because the *effective* blood volume is decreased. As a result the kidneys tend to reabsorb a greater percentage of filtered fluid, which causes further fluid retention and hyponatremia, especially if the patient has unlimited access to water.

Treatment with thiazide diuretics, furosemide, or ethacrynic acid can seriously compound the hyponatremia because these drugs may further decrease the effective blood volume

*A significant decrease in blood volume can override the normal osmotic stimulus to ADH release.

and because they decrease sodium transport in the ascending limb of Henle, which is necessary for the kidneys' ability to excrete free water and maximally dilute the urine.

Patients with volume depletion from sodium or blood loss may also develop hyponatremia when the volume depletion is great enough to stimulate ADH release. In this circumstance, body sodium and blood volume are reduced, and edema is not present. Diuretic administration, renal salt wasting, adrenal insufficiency, and hemorrhage are examples of this type of condition. Because of the decreased blood volume that accompanies these states, ADH release occurs and stimulates water reabsorption in an attempt to restore intravascular volume. If the patient ingests water without salt, or if hypotonic fluids are administered, hyponatremia will result.

In this setting restoration of the blood volume takes precedence over the body's need to maintain its osmotic composition.

Excessive ADH.   Hyponatremia may also occur in a number of conditions that are not associated with a decrease in either effective or absolute blood volume but in which either persistent release of ADH from the pituitary or ectopic production of ADH occurs. This unregulated production of ADH results in what is referred to as *the syndrome of inappropriate ADH release (SIADH)*. This may occur with cerebral disease such as stroke, infection, or trauma; with pulmonary disease such as pneumonia, tuberculosis, or tumor; with systemic disorders such as porphyria and systemic lupus erythematosus; with certain drugs such as morphine and anes-

Table 16–6
Signs and Symptoms Related to Hyponatremia

140–120	*120–110*	*110–100*	*100–95*
Generally none	Headache Apathy Lethargy Weakness Disorientation	Confusion Hostility Lethargy or violence Nausea and vomiting	Dilirium Convulsions Coma Hypothermia Areflexia Cheyne-Stokes respiration Death

thetics; and with psychiatric disorders such as schizophrenia.

When hyponatremia is due to the SIADH, blood volume is slightly increased due to water retention, but edema does not occur. The BUN is generally low normal because of dilution, and the urine is abnormally concentrated in relation to the degree of hypo-osmolality because of the persistent ADH effect.

The urine sodium concentration is frequently high despite the hyponatremia, probably because the mild volume expansion stimulates the kidneys to excrete sodium. The mechanism responsible for the persistent sodium excretion is unknown, but it may be the result of a humoral factor (also called *third factor*) released in response to volume expansion or of altered physical factors that govern tubular sodium reabsorption.

Manifestations. Hyponatremia is important because it can produce a wide range of neurologic symptoms, including death. The severity of symptoms depends upon the degree of hyponatremia and upon the rate at which it has developed. Generally, symptoms do not occur until the serum sodium is below 120 mEq per liter. Table 16-6 depicts the symptoms to be expected in several ranges of hyponatremia, but remember that for each level of sodium concentration, the severity of symptoms encountered will depend upon how rapidly the sodium concentration was lowered.

Treatment. Treatment of hyponatremia depends upon the level of serum sodium, the patient's symptoms, and the cause.

In most cases of mild hyponatremia associated with congestive heart failure or SIADH, fluid restriction to approximately 1000 ml per day is the only treatment necessary. In cases associated with true volume depletion, normal saline will usually correct the volume deficit and restore the sodium concentration to normal. For the most

severe degrees of hyponatremia, with potentially life-threatening symptoms, hypertonic (3%) sodium chloride intravenously may be necessary.

If fluid overload is also a problem, water restriction and intravenous furosemide or ethacrynic acid, both of which cause water loss in excess of sodium, may be the therapy of choice.

For patients with chronic hyponatremia due to SIADH, demeclocycline, which blocks the ADH effect, may be the preferred treatment.

HYPERNATREMIA

Hypernatremia results from primary water deficits in such situations as restricted intake, intestinal losses, and excessive insensible loss, or from nephrogenic or pituitary diabetes insipidus. Hypernatremia due to primary water loss results in a concentrated urine, whereas hypernatremia due to either form of diabetes insipidus is associated with a dilute urine.

Symptoms of hypernatremia are generally the same as those of hyperosmolality and result from CNS dehydration. Mental confusion, stupor, seizures, coma, and death may occur, in addition to other signs of dehydration such as fatigue, muscle weakness and cramps, and anorexia. The serum osmolality is generally above 350 mOsm per liter before significant symptoms are noted. This corresponds to a serum sodium of 165 to 170 mEq per liter.

Treatment consists of administration of free water (without salt), and vasopressin (Pitressin) in those cases due to pituitary diabetes insipidus.

Regulating Urinary Sodium Excretion

The normally functioning kidney has a considerable capability of adapting *urinary sodium excretion* to the individual's needs. In normal circumstances the amount of sodium appearing in the urine in a 24-hour period will exactly equal sodium intake, minus a small amount that is excreted in the feces or in the sweat.

When excess sodium is ingested, adaptation begins within 24 hours to rid the body of excess sodium. When sodium intake is restricted, urinary sodium excretion decreases to match intake. This may take 3 to 4 days to occur, during which a total sodium deficit of mild degree will occur. With extreme sodium restriction, the kidneys can reduce urinary sodium excretion to virtually zero to prevent further deficits in body sodium. Therefore, no absolute value for urinary sodium excretion is "normal," but rather a range of normal exists depending upon the body's state of sodium balance.

Likewise, there is no normal value for *urinary sodium concentration* but rather a range of normal that depends upon the amount of sodium excreted as well as the amount of water that is simultaneously excreted. A low urinary sodium concentration might result from a low sodium intake or might reflect extreme dilution of the sodium concentration by a large amount of ingested or administered fluids. In addition to states of decreased sodium intake, the urinary sodium concentration may be reduced by factors that reduce renal blood flow and result in excessive retention of sodium (and water) to maintain absolute or effective intravascular volume. This would be seen in hypotension or shock from any cause, in congestive heart failure, or in decompensated cirrhosis, all of which might be associated with very low concentrations and absolute amounts of sodium in the urine. (Administration of diuretics might artificially increase the urine sodium in these states.)

Urinary Sodium Excretion Test. In differentiating the oliguria of acute renal failure from that due to prerenal causes, the urinary sodium excretion is frequently used as one indicator of intact renal function. As noted above, states of underperfusion of the kidney are associated with a decrease in urinary sodium concentration (usually < 10 mEq/liter), whereas in acute renal failure, because of damage to the tubular transport mechanisms, urine sodium concentration is generally above 30 to 40 mEq per liter despite oliguria.

Fractional Excretion of Sodium Test. Another test of renal function, used for the same purpose as the urine sodium concentration, is the fractional excretion of sodium (FE_{Na}). This test gives a more precise estimation of the amount of filtered sodium that remains in the urine and is more accurate in predicting tubular injury than the urinary sodium concentration. It is calculated by the formula

$$(U/P) \, Na \, / \, (U/P) \, Cr \times 100$$

in which U and P are the urinary and plasma concentrations of sodium and creatinine, respectively. (Although volume measurements are necessary to derive the absolute urinary excretion of both sodium and creatinine, these cancel out in deriving this formula.)

The test therefore requires the determination of both serum and urinary sodium and creatinine concentrations on simultaneously obtained samples. Values less than 1.0 indicate prerenal azotemia, or underperfusion. Values greater than 3.0 are indicative of acute renal failure.

This test appears to be a little more discriminating in picking up cases of acute renal failure than is the measurement of urinary sodium concentration alone, especially in those patients who have borderline urinary sodium concentration values, and it is being used more frequently as a diagnostic tool.

The Anion Gap

In order to maintain chemical neutrality, the total concentration of cations and anions in the blood (as well as other body fluids) must be equivalent in terms of milliequivalents per liter. However, because there are a number of anions and cations present in blood that are not routinely measured, a "gap" exists between the total concentration of cations and anions and the concentration normally measured in plasma:

$$Na + K \text{ vs. } Cl + CHO_3$$

This gap is composed primarily of an excess of unmeasured anions including plasma proteins, inorganic phosphates and sulfates, and organic acids. The unmeasured cations that exist in smaller concentration are primarily calcium and magnesium.

The anion gap is generally calculated by the following formula:

$$Na - (Cl + HCO_3)$$

and has a normal mean of approximately 12 mEq per liter (range: 8 to 16 mEq/liter). Potassium is generally, but not always, omitted from the formula because of its relatively low concentration and narrow range of fluctuation. Departures from this "normal" anion gap may have important diagnostic significance in acid-base disorders, especially metabolic acidoses, and

Table 16–7
Causes of an Altered Anion Gap

Increased Anion Gap	Decreased Anion Gap
Laboratory error	Laboratory error
Increased unmeasured anions	Increased unmeasured cations
Endogenous metabolic acidosis	Normal cations
Lactic acidosis	Hypercalcemia
Ketoacidosis	Hyperkalemia
Uremic acidosis	Hypermagnesemia
Exogenous anion ingestion	Abnormal cations
Ethylene glycol	Increased globulins (myeloma, etc.)
Methanol	TRIS buffer
Paraldehyde	Lithium
Salicylates	Decreased unmeasured anions
Therapeutic agents	Hypoalbuminemia
Paraldehyde	
Penicillin	
Carbenicillin	
Increased plasma proteins	
Hyperalbuminemia	
Decreased unmeasured cations	
Hypokalemia	
Hypocalcemia	
Hypomagnesemia	

may also assist in the diagnosis of other disorders.

The most common abnormality of the anion gap is an increase that is due most frequently to increased concentrations of lactate, ketone bodies, or inorganic phosphate and sulfate that are found in lactic acidosis, ketoacidosis, and uremia, respectively. Other forms of acidosis associated with ingestion of toxins such as ethylene glycol, methanol, paraldehyde, and salicylates may also produce significant increases in the anion gap. Increases in anion gap due to a decrease in unmeasured cations is rare but can be observed.

Decreases in the anion gap are less common but equally important and can occur because of increases in unmeasured cations or because of decreases in unmeasured anions, such as hypoalbuminemia. Causes are listed in Table 16-7.

Alterations of the anion gap may also be caused by laboratory error in measuring the electrolytes and must always be verified to avoid confusion and diagnostic error. Simultaneous occurrences of two disorders having opposite effects on the anion gap could also obscure any potential diagnostic change. Disorders affecting the anion gap are listed in Table 16-7.

Summary

The knowledgeable use and interpretation of the laboratory determinations described in the preceding paragraphs are of major importance in the assessment of the renal complications of the seriously ill patient. Their value lies in the prevention as well as in the diagnosis of these complications. They are not cited to the exclusion of the usual parameters of close and accurate fluid and electrolyte balance, which are equally important to the understanding of the renal status of the patient.

BIBLIOGRAPHY

Duarte CG (ed): Renal Function Tests: Clinical Laboratory Procedures and Diagnosis. Boston, Little, Brown & Co, 1980

Espinel CH: The Fe$_{Na}$ test: Use in the differential diagnosis of acute renal failure. J Am Med Assoc 236:579–581, 1976

Friedler RM, Koffler A, Kurokawa K: Hyponatremia and hypernatremia. Clin Nephrol, 7:163–172, 1977

Harrington JT, Cohen JJ: Measurement of urinary electrolytes: Indications and limitations. N Engl J Med, 293:1241–1243, 1975

Kokko JP: Renal concentrating and diluting mechanisms. Hosp Pract, February 1979, pp 110–116

Miller RT, Anderson RJ, Linas SL et al: Urinary diagnostic indices in acute renal failure. Ann Intern Med, 89:47–50, 1978

Oh MS, Carroll HT: The anion gap. N Engl J Med, 297:814–817, 1977

Papper S: Sodium and water: An overview. Am J Med Sci, 272:43–51, 1976

Schrier RW, Berl T, Anderson RJ: Osmotic and non-osmotic control of vasopressin release. Am J Physiol, 236:F321–332, 1979

Anne T. Bobal

Management Modalities and Assessment Skills for the Nurse: Renal System* 17

MONITORING FLUID BALANCE

Body fluid equilibrium is based on intake and output—the amount of fluid taken in and the volume excreted. Water is lost through the kidneys, gastrointestinal tract, skin, and lungs and is replaced by water from fluids and solid foods (which are 60% to 90% water), and from the oxidation of food and body tissues. Under normal circumstances and in the presence of adequate renal function, the losses equal the intake, and the net balance is zero. Table 17-1 summarizes water gains and losses.

VARIABLES

A review of the variables that interfere with normal fluid balance may assist the nurse in evaluating fluid problems in the clinical setting.

Fluid imbalances may be the result of

- Inadequate intake
- Excessive losses without adequate replacement
- Impaired renal function

Inadequate Intake

Inadequate fluid intake in the conscious patient may be the result of anorexia, apathy, lethargy,

*The author wishes to thank Pamela Balzer, R.N., Staff Nurse, Home Dialysis Training Unit, University of Colorado Health Sciences Center, Denver, Colorado for her contribution to the peritoneal dialysis portion of the chapter and Roseanne Garner, R.N., Staff Nurse, Hemodialysis Unit, Veterans Administration Unit, Veterans Administration Medical Center, Denver, Colorado for reviewing the hemodialysis portion of the chapter.

Table 17–1
Ways in Which Water and Electrolytes Balance Each Other in Health

Gains	Range in ml	Losses	Range in ml
Water from fluids	500–1700	Water vapor loss through lungs and skin	850–1200
Water from solid food	800–1000	Water loss through urine	600–1600
Water from oxidation of food and body tissues	200–300	Water loss through feces	50–200
Total	1500–3000	Total	1500–3000

The chief sources of fluid gain in health are
Water present in liquids,
Water present in solid food, and
Water derived from oxidation.

These gains equal the losses caused by
Water lost via insensible perspiration,
Water lost through urine, and
Water lost through feces.

Travenol Laboratories, Inc.

and difficulty in swallowing. Weak and feeble patients and infants are especially vulnerable simply because they cannot make their need for water known. In central nervous system disturbances the sense of thirst may be impaired, while in unconscious states the patient is entirely dependent upon nursing personnel for fluid administration.

Excessive Losses

Circumstances that increase losses include the following:

- Fever and increased respiratory rate. A patient with a temperature of 104°F (40°C) and a respiratory rate of 30 to 40 breaths/min can lose as much as 2500 ml in a 24-hour period
- Environment—hot and dry climates
- Activity—increased metabolic rate
- Hyperventilation
- Tracheostomy
- Increased gastrointestinal losses due to vomiting, diarrhea, gastric suction, fistulas, and ileostomies
- Burns. Fluid loss through the skin may amount to 1000 to 2000 ml/day
- Perspiration. With mild sweating a patient may lose up to 500 ml/day, with profuse sweating up to 1000 ml/day
- Diuretic phase of acute tubular necrosis (see Chapter 16)

Decreased Renal Function

The kidneys play an essential role in regulating water and electrolyte balance. Providing renal function is normal, a minimum of 400 ml of fluid must be excreted as urine to prevent the accumulation of metabolic wastes. However, this minimum urinary volume is markedly influenced by the osmotic load excreted.

In certain states such as hyperalimentation the increased urea production will necessitate a larger urinary volume. This also occurs in uncontrolled diabetes in which marked glycosuria requires increased excretion.

NURSING ASSESSMENT

The nurse's role in the evaluation, correction, and maintenance of fluid balance includes accurate recording of intake-output, weight, and vital signs. The most sensitive indices of changes in body water content are serial weights and intake-output patterns, while trends in vital signs provide important supporting data. Assessment of fluid imbalance is based on observation and recognition of pertinent symptoms, and nursing action involves replacement or restriction of fluids.

Intake and Output

An accurate intake-output record will provide valuable data in evaluating and treating fluid imbalances. It is important that all nursing personnel, the patient, and the patient's visitors are involved and instructed. Circumstances will dictate how exact the record should be and what data will be included. For example, in an uncomplicated postsurgical situation, fluid replacement may be projected on estimated and actual losses for a 24-hour period.

All measurable intake and output are recorded and totaled at the end of every shift. However, in the presence of excessive losses or deteriorating cardiac and renal function, more detailed recording of every source of fluid intake and output is necessary. Calculations are often done on an every 1- to 4-hour basis.

Intake includes not only pure liquids such as water and juices, but also those foods which are high in water content such as oranges, grapefruit, and those which become liquid at room temperature such as gelatin and ice cream. Ice chips and cubes must also be measured. It is useful to keep a list of fluid equivalents for fruits, ice cubes, and other sources of fluids.

In severe electrolyte and fluid imbalances the time and type of fluid intake and the time and amount of each voiding should be recorded. This becomes important because it may be useful baseline data during tests for renal function.

A record of *losses* should also include emeses, stools, and drainages. When dressings are saturated with drainage, they should be weighed before and after changing. Other data such as temperature, pulse, respiratory rate, and degree of perspiration should be available for estimating insensible losses.

Weight

Rapid daily gains and losses in weight are usually related to changes in fluid volume. Because of the difficulties in obtaining accurate figures for intake and output records, serial weights are often more reliable. In addition, weight changes will usually pick up imbalances before symptoms are apparent.

As with intake and output records, the weighing procedure should be consistent. The patient should be weighed on the same scale with the same attire, preferably in the morning before breakfast and after voiding. Variations in the procedure should be noted and made known to the physician.

A kilogram scale provides for greater accuracy because drug, fluid, and diet calculations use the metric system, and conversion from pounds to kilograms may lead to discrepancies.

Normally, a patient with a balanced nutritional intake will maintain his weight. A patient whose protein intake is limited or who is catabolic will lose about a pound a day. A weight gain of more than 1 pound per day suggests fluid retention. A generally accepted guide is that a pint of fluid is reflected in one-half kilogram of weight gained.

Assessment of Hypovolemia and Hypervolemia

The diagnosis of extracellular volume depletion or overload is seldom made on the basis of one parameter. The first clue to the nurse may be the patient's general appearance, after which more specific observations are noted.

Symptoms will vary with the degree of imbalance, some symptoms being seen early in imbalance states and others not being evident until severe imbalances are reached. Table 17-2 lists the physical assessment and symptoms of fluid imbalance and can be used as a guide for nursing assessment.

Other guidelines used to evaluate fluid states are hematocrit, central venous pressure (CVP), urine specific gravity, osmolality, and chest roentgenograms. CVP readings and specific gravity have been discussed in Chapters 10 and 16.

In fluid overload, a chest roentgenogram may show the following changes: prominent vascular markings, increased heart size, pleural effusion, infiltrates, or frank pulmonary congestion.

The hematocrit may be elevated in depletion states and decreased in overload, but other factors must be considered. For example, the hematocrit with hypovolemia may be low when significant blood loss has taken place. All data should be evaluated in the light of other influences. Trends are usually more significant than isolated values.

For example, when the nurse notes a decrease in urine output, a systematic assessment should follow in order to determine why this is happening and what nursing interventions are most appropriate. Any system of assessment will work when it is consistent and thorough. After a review of the intake and output records for both the current and the previous day and an assessment of the symptoms and parameters just discussed, a decision to increase or decrease fluid intake can be made. In the absence of symptoms of fluid retention, when intravenous fluids are behind schedule and intake is inadequate for the patient's condition, missed fluids should be given. The patient's fluid status, especially his urine output, should be watched closely for the

Table 17-2
Physical Assessment and Symptoms of Imbalance

Assessment of	Hypovolemia	Hypervolemia
Skin and subcutaneous tissues	Dry, loss of elasticity	Warm, moist, pitting edema over bony prominences, wrinkled skin from pressure of clothing
Face	Sunken eyes (late symptom)	Periorbital edema
Tongue	Dry, coated (early symptom), fissured (late symptom)	Moist
Saliva	Thick, scanty	Excessive, frothy
Thirst	Present	May not be significant
Temperature	May be elevated	May not be significant
Pulse	Rapid, weak, thready	Rapid
Respirations	Rapid, shallow	Rapid dyspnea, moist rales
Blood pressure	Low, orthostatic hypotension, small pulse pressure	Normal to high
Weight	Loss	Gain

next few hours to evaluate whether or not the increase in fluid intake corrected the patient's fluid balance. If, however, urine output is zero or diminished in the presence of adequate fluid intake, no further fluids are given and the physician is called immediately. If a patient presents any of the symptoms of fluid overload discussed earlier, all fluid intake is restricted and the physician is notified immediately.

Fluid replacement, as stated previously, may be calculated for any given period of time, depending on the severity of the situation. For example, a 24-hour calculation of intake for a patient who is oliguric with normal insensible losses could be

Previous 24-hour urine output	100 ml
Insensible loss replacement	500 ml
Total 24-hour fluid allowance	600 ml

While the physician will specify the total amount and kind of fluid replacement, the details of distribution are often decided by the nurse. Priority is given to requirements for administration of drugs, both intravenous and oral. Distribution of the remaining fluid is then made according to patient preference. The nurse guides the patient in his selection to help him avoid using up the entire day's allowance early in the day. Because sodium and potassium may be restricted in the patient with renal failure, fluids such as ginger ale, 7-Up, and Kool Aid, which are low in sodium and potassium, are given.

HEMODIALYSIS

Principles of Operation

Dialysis refers to the diffusion of dissolved particles from one fluid compartment to another across a semipermeable membrane. In *hemodialysis,* the blood is one fluid compartment and the dialysate is the other.

The semipermeable membrane is a thin, porous cellophane. The pore size of the membrane permits the passage of low-molecular-weight substances such as urea, creatinine, and uric acid to diffuse through the pores of the membrane. Water molecules are also very small and move freely through the membrane. Most plasma proteins, bacteria, and blood cells are too large to pass through the pores of the membrane. The difference in the concentration of the substances in the two compartments is called the *concentration gradient.*

The blood, which contains waste products such as urea and creatinine, flows into the dialyzer or artificial kidney where it comes into contact with the dialysate containing no urea and creatinine. A maximum gradient is established so that movement of these substances is from the blood to the dialysate. Repeated passages of the blood through the dialyzer over a period of time (4 to 6 hours) reduces the level of these waste products to a near normal state. Hemodialysis is indicated in acute and chronic renal failure, drug and chemical intoxications, severe fluid and electrolyte imbalances, and hepatorenal syndrome.

The functions of the artificial kidney system are summarized as follows:

- Removes the by-products of protein metabolism such as urea, creatinine, and uric acid
- Removes excess water (ultrafiltration) by changing osmotic pressure. This is done by adding a high concentration of dextrose to the dialysate, or effecting a pressure differential between the blood and fluid compartments by mechanical means
- Maintains or restores the body buffer system
- Maintains or restores the level of electrolytes in the body

Major Components of the Artificial Kidney System

The Dialyzer or Artificial Kidney. This apparatus supports the cellophane compartments. Dialyzers vary in size, physical structure, and efficiency. The efficiency of a dialyzer refers to its ability to remove water (ultrafiltration) and waste products (clearance).

There are advantages and disadvantages to each dialyzer that must be considered in dialyzer selection. Whether the dialyzer will be used primarily for acute or chronic dialysis is one consideration. A highly efficient, shorter-run dialyzer may be more appropriate for use in drug intoxications or in acutely ill patients in whom a long dialysis is undesirable. Since some dialyzers have a greater propensity for clotting, a dialyzer requiring larger doses of heparin may be contraindicated for a patient with active or potential bleeding problems.

Fluid overload may dictate using a dialyzer with maximum ultrafiltration capability. Rapid fluid and electrolyte changes, characteristic of an efficient dialyzer, are often avoided in the chronic patient. A low-blood volume dialyzer is advantageous in dialyzing children and small adults. Economy may dictate the selection of a shorter-run dialyzer to prevent higher personnel costs. Sometimes the final selection depends solely upon the training and philosophy of personnel in charge of the hemodialysis unit.

Dialysate or Dialyzing Solution. The dialysate or "bath" is a solution composed of water and the major electrolytes of normal serum. It is made in a clean system with filtered tap water and chemicals. It is not a sterile system, but since bacteria are too large to pass through the membrane, contamination from this source is not a major problem. Dialysate concentrates are usually provided by commercial manufacturers. A "standard" bath is generally used in chronic units, but variations may be made to meet specific patient needs.

Dialysate Delivery System. A single delivery unit provides dialysate for one patient; the multiple delivery system may supply up to twenty patient units. In either system, an automatic proportioning device along with metering and monitoring devices assures precise control of the water–concentrate ratio.

The single delivery unit is usually used in acute dialyses. It is a mobile unit and dialysate requirements are easily tailored to meet individual patient needs.

Accessory Equipment. This includes a blood pump, infusion pumps for heparin delivery, and monitoring devices to detect unsafe temperatures, dialysate concentration, pressure changes, air, and blood leaks.

The Human Component. Expertise in the use of highly technical equipment is accomplished through theoretic and practical training in the clinical setting. The operation and monitoring of dialysis equipment will differ, however. Reference to the manufacturer's instruction manuals will give the nurse guidelines for the safe operation of equipment. Although the technical aspects of hemodialysis may at first seem overwhelming, they can be learned fairly rapidly.

A more critical aspect, one that takes long to achieve, is the understanding and knowledge that the nurse will use in caring for patients during dialysis. Because hemodialysis is a dynamic changing process, alterations in blood chemistries and fluid balance can occur. The nurse's observation skills, assessment of symptoms, and appropriate actions can make the difference between a smooth dialysis with a minimum of problems and one fraught with a series of crises for the patient and the nurse.

Predialysis Assessment

The degree and complexity of problems arising during hemodialysis will vary from patient to patient and will depend on many factors. Important variables are the patient's diagnosis, stage of illness, age, other medical problems, fluid and electrolyte balance, and emotional state.

An essential first step in the hemodialysis procedure is a review of the patient's history, the clinical records, laboratory reports, and finally the nurse's observation of the patient.

After reviewing the data, and in consultation with the physician, the dialysis nurse will establish objectives for the dialysis treatment. The objectives will vary from one dialysis to the next in the acute renal failure patient whose condition may change rapidly. For example, fluid removal may take precedence over correcting an electrolyte imbalance or vice versa. Bleeding problems, actual or potential, will determine the degree of anticoagulation with heparin.

The patient's emotional state should be included in this initial evaluation. Anxiety and apprehension, especially during a first dialysis, may contribute to change in blood pressure, restlessness, and gastrointestinal upsets. The security provided by the presence of a nurse during the first dialysis is probably more desirable than giving the patient a drug that might precipitate changes in vital signs.

Risk Factors: Prevention, Assessment, and Nursing Intervention

FLUID IMBALANCES

Evaluation of fluid balance is desirable prior to dialysis so that corrective measures may be initiated early in the procedure. Parameters such as blood pressure, pulse, weight, intake and output, and the presence of certain symptoms will assist the nurse in estimating fluid overload or depletion.

The term *dry* or *ideal* weight is used to express the weight at which a patient's blood pressure is in a normal range for him and he is free of the symptoms of fluid imbalance. The figure is not an absolute one, but it provides a guideline for fluid removal or replacement. It requires frequent review and revision, especially in the newly dialyzed patient in whom frequent changes in weight are taking place due to fluid removal or accumulation and to tissue gains or losses.

HYPERVOLEMIA

The presence of some or all of the following may suggest fluid overload: blood-pressure elevation, increased pulse and respiratory rate, dyspnea, moist rales, cough, edema, excessive weight gain since last dialysis, and a history or record of excessive fluid intake in the absence of adequate losses.

A chest roentgenogram to assess heart size or pulmonary congestion may confirm the diagnosis of fluid overload but may not be essential in the presence of overt symptoms. Increase in abdominal girth will suggest accumulation of fluid in the abdominal cavity. If ascites is present, measuring the abdominal girth will provide another useful tool in estimating correction of the problem.

Treatment of fluid overload during dialysis is directed toward the removal of the excess water. Care must be taken to avoid too rapid volume depletion during dialysis. Excessive fluid removal may lead to hypotension, and little is gained if intravenous fluids are given to correct the problem. Thus, it is better to reduce the volume overload over a period of two or three dialyses, unless pulmonary congestion is life-threatening.

An analysis of the causes of the fluid overload is necessary to prevent recurrences. The intake and output record may provide a clue. For example, the patient may have been given excessive intravenous fluids in a "keep open" IV, or fluids used as a vehicle for intravenous medications may not have been calculated in the intake. The patient may not have adhered to his fluid restriction or may have had a decrease in his fluid losses. For example, gastric suction may have been discontinued. Often, after the institution of chronic dialysis, urinary output decreases. If the patient continues his normal fluid intake, he will become fluid-overloaded. In the chronic hemodialysis patient, fluid overload may be related to the intake of high-sodium foods. Moderate restriction is necessary for all patients to prevent extracellular fluid overload. Change in weight provides an indication of water load; an acceptable weight gain is 0.5 kg for each 24 hours between dialyses.

HYPOVOLEMIA

Assessment of hypovolemia is also made on the evaluation of trends in vital signs and symptoms. Clues to hypovolemia include falling blood pressure, increasing pulse and respiration rates, loss of skin turgor, dry mouth, a falling CVP, and a decreasing urine output. A history of excessive fluid loss through profuse perspiration, vomiting, diarrhea, and gastric suctioning with resulting weight loss will further substantiate the diagnosis.

Treatment is directed toward the replacement of previous losses and the prevention of further losses during dialysis.

It is usual practice to phlebotomize the patient at the onset of dialysis. The patient's blood is pumped through the dialyzer, displacing the priming normal saline solution. In the hypovolemic patient the nurse can connect the venous return blood line immediately and infuse the normal saline into the patient. This 200 ml of solution might be sufficient to restore balance or at least prevent further hypotension. Ultrafiltration will be avoided in the hypovolemic patient, and he may even require additional fluids.

Normal saline is the solution used most frequently to replace volume depletion during dialysis because small volumes usually produce the desired effect. Replacement in increments of 50 ml is suggested, with frequent monitoring of blood pressure.

Blood-volume expanders such as albumin are sometimes used in patients with a low serum protein. The treatment is expensive when the underlying cause of the hypoproteinemia is not corrected and repeated infusions become necessary.

HYPOTENSION

Hypotension during dialysis may be caused by preexisting hypovolemia, excessive ultrafiltration, loss of blood into the dialyzer, and antihypertensive drug therapy. Hypotension at the beginning of dialysis may occur in patients with a small blood volume such as children and small adults. Using a small-volume dialyzer or starting dialysis at a slower blood flow rate may avoid or minimize problems.

Hypotension later in dialysis is usually due to excessive ultrafiltration. This may be confirmed by weighing the patient and estimating fluid loss. Keeping the patient in a horizontal position, reducing the blood-flow rate, and discontinuing ultrafiltration may return the blood pressure to normal. If hypotension persists, saline or other plasma expanders may be administered. Intravenous fluids should be kept to a minimum and discontinued as soon as the patient is normotensive. Salty liquids or foods may be given, but their effect is slower than intravenous administration. If hypotension persists in spite of adequate fluid replacement, other medical causes for hypotension should be considered.

Blood loss due to technical problems such as membrane leaks and line separations may lead to hypotension. The use of blood leak detectors and other monitoring devices has reduced the risk of excessive blood loss due to these causes, but they do occur. If separation of blood lines occurs, clamping the arterial blood line and stopping the blood pump immediately will minimize further blood loss. In a membrane leak the dialysis is discontinued and the dialyzer replaced. Although small leaks may seal over, they may progress to gross leaks, and dialysate may cross the membrane into the blood compartment. In this situation, the blood may be returned to the patient, but he should be observed for pyrogenic reactions. If the patient's hematocrit is low, the risk of blood loss may be greater than the possibility of dialysate contamination. Some units have standing policies to cover this contingency; however, decisions may be made according to individual circumstances.

The use of *antihypertensive drugs* in the dialysis patient may precipitate hypotension during dialysis. To avoid this, it is standard practice in many units to omit antihypertensive drugs 4 to 6 hours before dialysis. Fluids and sodium restrictions are more desirable controls for hypertension. *Sedatives* and *tranquilizers* may also cause hypotension and should be avoided if possible.

HYPERTENSION

The most frequent causes of hypertension during dialysis are fluid overload, disequilibrium syndrome, and anxiety.

Hypertension during dialysis is usually caused by sodium and water excesses. This can be confirmed by comparing the patient's present weight to his ideal or dry weight. If fluid overload is the cause of hypertension, ultrafiltration will usually bring about a reduction in the blood pressure.

Some patients who may be normotensive before dialysis become hypertensive during dialysis. The rise may occur either gradually or abruptly. The cause is not well understood, but may be the result of increased cardiac output as fluid overload is corrected.

Hypertension is a common finding in dialysis disequilibrium syndrome and will usually respond to correction of that condition. If the diastolic blood pressure is over 120 or the patient has symptoms, small doses of hydralazine (Apresoline) may be given intravenously into the venous blood line. An initial dose of 10 mg may bring about a favorable response. Hydralazine is preferred to methyldopa (Aldomet) because its effect is more rapid. Blood pressure is monitored at frequent intervals following the administration of antihypertensive drugs.

Anxiety, fear, and apprehension, especially during the first dialysis, may cause transient and erratic hypertension. Sedatives may be necessary, but confidence in the staff and a smooth, problem-free dialysis will help reduce anxiety during subsequent treatments.

DIALYSIS DISEQUILIBRIUM SYNDROME

Dialysis disequilibrium syndrome is manifested by a group of symptoms suggestive of cerebral dysfunction. Symptoms range in severity from mild nausea, vomiting, headache, and hypertension to agitation, twitching, mental confusion, and convulsions. It is thought that rapid efficient dialysis results in shifts in water, pH, and osmolality between cerebrospinal fluid and blood, causing the symptoms.

Disequilibrium syndrome in the acutely uremic patient may be avoided by dialyzing the patient slowly for short periods daily for two or three treatments. Phenytoin (Dilantin) is sometimes used prior to and during dialysis in the new patient to reduce the risk of central nervous system symptoms.

Restlessness, confusion, twitching, nausea, and vomiting may suggest early disequilibrium. Reduction of the blood flow rate and administration of sedatives may prevent more severe symptoms, but it may be necessary to discontinue dialysis if symptoms persist or worsen.

ELECTROLYTE IMBALANCE

With the trend toward early and adequate dialysis, the severe extremes of electrolyte imbalances are not seen with the same frequency as before the widespread use of hemodialysis. Critical electrolyte changes and their management have been discussed in Chapter 16.

Maintenance and restoration of electrolyte balance in the dialysis patient are accomplished primarily with dialysis and to a lesser degree with dietary controls. With the exception of potassium, very few changes in the standard concentration of electrolytes in the dialysate are necessary.

Laboratory tests to evaluate electrolyte status are done before and after each dialysis in acute renal failure. The nurse's role includes knowing normal values, recognizing symptoms of imbalance, and evaluating probable causes. In many institutions nursing intervention also includes taking the necessary corrective measures as defined by the policies of the critical care unit. For example, a patient complains of extreme muscle weakness. The nurse notes excessive amounts of gastric drainage during the previous 24-hour period. The situation suggests hypokalemia, and the nurse orders a stat serum K^+ level. If the result is low, the nurse increases the potassium level in the dialysate from the standard 2.0 mEq per liter to 3.5 mEq per liter. She also monitors the patient for possible cardiac arrhythmias during the procedure.

The electrolytes of main concern in dialysis, which are normally corrected during the procedure, are sodium, potassium, bicarbonate, calcium, phosphorus, and magnesium.

Serum Sodium.   Serum sodium concentration normally varies between 135 mEq per liter and 145 mEq per liter and is a reflection of water volume.

A low serum sodium usually indicates water intake in excess of sodium and is characterized by an increase in body weight. A high serum sodium usually indicates water loss in excess of sodium and is reflected in weight loss. Serum sodium extremes do not, as a rule, become a problem unless the values fall below 120 or rise above 160 mEq per liter. The rate of change is probably more important than the absolute value (see Chapter 16).

Although serum sodium extremes are not usually seen in the adequately dialyzed patient, nevertheless thirst may indicate sodium excess. The patient who is thirsty because of excessive sodium intake will drink excessive amounts of water, which can lead to hypertension and fluid overload. Evaluation of sodium intake should be made in the patient who gains excessive amounts of fluid between dialyses. Again, the recommended weight gain is approximately 1 pound for each day between dialysis. Shifts in sodium and water during hemodialysis may lead to muscle cramping. This can be alleviated by reducing the flow rate and ultrafiltration.

Potassium.   Both hypokalemia and hyperkalemia occur in renal failure. Normal serum concentration is between 3.5 and 5.0 mEq per liter. Levels below 3.0 and above 7.0 mEq per liter may lead to generalized muscle weakness and cardiac arrhythmias (see Chapter 10).

Extremes in the serum potassium level are seen more frequently in the acute patient and may result from either the disease or the therapy. Crushing injuries with extensive tissue destruction, blood transfusions, potassium-containing drugs, and acidosis all contribute to hyperkalemia. Vomiting, diarrhea, and gastric suction may lead to hypokalemia. Rapid correction of serum potassium in either direction should be avoided. Patients on digitalis are of special concern because a low serum potassium potentiates the effects of digitalis. Therefore, rapid lowering of the potassium level during dialysis can lead to hypokalemia, to increased effects of digitalis, and possibly to serious and sometimes fatal arrhythmias (see Chapter 10).

The potassium level in the bath is kept at 3 to 3.5 mEq per liter, whichever is more appropriate for the individual patient. Patients with overt or potential problems should be monitored for cardiac function during dialysis.

Bicarbonate.

Bicarbonate protects the body from excessive acid loads. Normal concentration varies between 25 and 30 mEq per liter.

In uremia, the bicarbonate is depleted because it has been used to buffer the acidosis resulting from the inability of the kidneys to excrete acids. Acidosis in the uremic patient who has not been started on dialysis is corrected by giving sodium bicarbonate.

During dialysis, acidosis is corrected by adding acetate to the dialysate. Acetate diffuses into the blood, where it is metabolized to form bicarbonate.

Calcium.

Normal serum calcium levels range between 8 and 10.3 mg/dl, although this will vary among laboratories. Disturbances in calcium metabolism that result in hypocalcemia occur in renal failure and are thought to involve impaired absorption of dietary calcium and resistance to the action of vitamin D.

The dialysate calcium is kept at 3 mEq per liter to prevent the loss of calcium from the blood to the dialysate. Dialysis, however, does not seem to correct the bone problems that occur in the chronic patient as a result of calcium–phosphorus imbalances (see Chapter 18).

Phosphorus.

In chronic renal failure antacids are used to bind phosphorus in the intestinal tract and prevent its absorption. The lowered serum phosphorus reduces the risk of soft-tissue calcifications.

Antacids are usually given during or after meals; however, because of the medication's unpleasant taste and consistency, patients often omit taking antacids. A high serum phosphorus is an indication to the nurse that the patient is not adhering to the prescribed dose. Some patients save their meager amounts of fluids to wash away the unpleasant taste. Rinsing the mouth with water or a mouthwash may also help.

Magnesium.

The normal plasma level of magnesium is 1.5 to 1.7 mEq per liter. Magnesium accumulates in the serum, bone, and muscle in the presence of renal failure. It is thought to be involved, along with calcium and phosphorus, in the bone problems accompanying chronic renal failure. Although magnesium is removed by the artificial kidney, high levels remain in the bone. It is also difficult to reduce magnesium intake in the diet and provide palatable and nutritious meals.

The regular use of magnesium-containing drugs should be avoided. This applies particularly to antacids that are taken regularly by patients on chronic dialysis. Acceptable non-magnesium antacids include aluminum hydroxide gel (Amphojel), dihydroxyaluminum aninoacetate (Robalate), and basic aluminum carbonate gel (Basaljel).

INFECTION

The uremic patient has a lowered resistance to infection, which is thought to be due to a decreased immunologic response. Therefore, all possible foci of infection should be eliminated. Indwelling urinary catheters and intracaths should be removed as soon as possible, or their use should be avoided altogether. Strict aseptic technique is essential in catheterizations, venipunctures, wound dressings, and tracheal suctioning.

Pulmonary infections are a leading cause of death in the acute uremic patient. Contributing factors include depression of the cough reflex and respiratory effort due to central nervous system disturbances, increased viscosity of pulmonary secretions due to dehydration and mouth breathing, especially in the unresponsive patient, and pulmonary congestion due to fluid overload. Fluid in the lungs not only acts as a medium for growing bacteria but also impedes respiratory excursion.

Nursing techniques that prevent or minimize pulmonary complications cannot be overlooked during the hemodialysis procedure. They include frequent turning, deep breathing and coughing, early ambulation, adequate humidification, hydration, tracheal aspiration, use of intermittent positive pressure machines, and oxygen therapy.

Oral hygiene is important because bleeding from the oral mucous membrane and the accumulation of dry secretions promote growth of bacteria in the mouth, which can lead to a pneumonia.

BLEEDING AND HEPARINIZATION

Bleeding during dialysis may be due to an underlying medical condition such as an ulcer or gastritis or may be the result of excessive anticoagulation. Blood in the extracorporeal system, such as the dialyzer and blood lines, clots rapidly unless some method of anticoagulation is used. *Heparin* is the drug of choice because it is simple to administer, increases clotting time rapidly, is easily monitored, and may be reversed with protamine.

Specific heparinization procedures vary, but the primary goal in any method is to prevent clotting in the dialyzer with the least amount of heparin. Two methods are commonly used: intermittent and constant infusion. In both cases an initial priming dose of heparin is given, followed by smaller doses either at intervals or at a constant rate by an infusion pump. The resulting effect is *systemic heparinization*, in which the clotting times of the patient and the dialyzer are essentially the same.

Absolute guidelines are difficult to give because methods and dialyzer requirements vary. The normal clotting time of 6 to 10 minutes may be increased to the range of 30 to 60 minutes. The effect of heparin is monitored by the modified Lee White method, which measures the length of time it takes for 1 ml of blood to form a solid clot in a clean standard Lee White tube, tipped at 1-minute intervals. More recently, activated partial thromboplastin-time and activated coagulation-time methods have come into use. These have the advantage of providing results in seconds, which gives the dialysis nurse the opportunity to make rapid adjustments in heparin administration.

Systemic heparinization usually presents no risk to the patient unless he has overt bleeding such as gastrointestinal bleeding, epistaxis, or hemoptysis, is 3 to 7 days postsurgery, or has uremic pericarditis. In these situations, *regional heparinization* may be employed. In this technique the patient's clotting time is kept normal while that of the dialyzer is increased. This is accomplished by infusing heparin at a constant rate into the dialyzer and simultaneously neutralizing its effects with protamine sulfate before the blood returns to the patient.

As with systemic heparinization, there is no standard heparin-protamine ratio. Frequent monitoring of the clotting times is the best way to achieve effective regional heparinization. Because of the rebound phenomenon that has been reported following regional heparinization and the use of activated coagulation-time methods, many dialysis units have switched to low-dose heparinization even in the presence of overt bleeding. In this method, minimal heparin doses are used throughout dialysis. Although some clotting may take place in the dialyzer, the small blood loss is preferable to the risk of profound bleeding.

Bleeding problems occasionally occur because of accidental heparin overdose. This may be caused by infusion pump malfunction or carelessness in setting the delivery rate. Because of the hazards, the importance of careful, frequent monitoring of heparin delivery cannot be overemphasized.

ULTRAFILTRATION

Excessive water is removed from the vascular compartment by the process of ultrafiltration. This is accomplished by applying negative pressure to the effluent dialysate. This creates a "siphoning" effect on the dialysate, and water molecules are forced across the membrane into the dialysate. As much as 10 pounds (or 4 to 5 kg) of water may be removed in a 4 to 6 hour period. The amount of negative pressure that is applied is based on the ultrafiltration capability of the dialyzer, the amount of fluid that needs to be removed, and the individual patient's tolerance.

Symptoms of excessive ultrafiltration are similar to those of shock, that is, hypotension, nausea, vomiting, diaphoresis, dizziness, and fainting.

DIAFILTRATION

Aggressive ultrafiltration for the purpose of relieving or preventing hypertension, congestive heart failure, pulmonary edema, and other complications associated with fluid overload is often limited by the patient's tolerance of manipulations of intravascular volume.

Observation by several investigators suggests that there is a significant increase in patient tolerance to large and rapid fluid volume removal when the ultrafiltration process occurs in the absence of diffuse mass transfer. This has resulted in a mode of therapy in which the removal of body fluid is separated from the total dialysis procedure. This is accomplished by (1) initiating dialysis without a dialysate flow, (2) maintaining negative pressure in the dialysate compartment, and (3) resuming the usual dialysis procedure following a predetermined amount of diafiltration time.

PROBLEMS WITH EQUIPMENT

One of the major objectives of a dialysis unit is the prevention of complications resulting from the treatment itself. Hemodialysis involves the use of highly technical equipment. The efficiency of the dialysis, as well as the patient's comfort and safety, is compromised if both the patient and the equipment are not adequately monitored. Mechanical monitors provide a margin of safety but should not replace the observations and actions of the nurse.

Monitoring devices are designed to monitor many parameters, the most important of which are flow, concentration, and temperature of the dialysate, flow and leakage of blood, and air leaks. The design and operation of dialysis equipment and monitoring devices vary greatly; however, they have a common purpose.

Dialysate Flow. Inadequate dialysate flow will not harm the patient, but it will compromise dialysis efficiency. Flow is maintained at the rate recommended for each particular dialyzer. The nurse usually checks the flow at least every hour and makes adjustments as necessary.

Dialysate Concentrate. Sudden or rapid changes in dialysate concentrate may result in red blood cell hemolysis and cerebral disturbances. Mild symptoms include nausea, vomiting, and headache. In severe cases, convulsions, coma, and death may ensue. If several patients in a unit develop similar symptoms simultaneously, dialysate concentrate imbalance should be thought of immediately. If a patient is accidentally dialyzed against water, the first symptom may be sudden severe pain in the returning vein. Because of hemolysis, blood will immediately turn dark brown to black. Dialysis is discontinued at once.

In a single delivery, proportioning system, monitoring devices are built into the system, and the concentrate is monitored continuously. If the concentrate exceeds the predetermined limits, dialysate automatically bypasses the dialyzer until the problem is corrected. The problem may have been caused by an interruption in the water or concentrate delivery. Inflow lines should be checked for kinking and the concentrate container checked for quantity.

In a central delivery system the electrolyte concentration is also checked continuously by a meter that measures the electrical conductivity of the solution. If the solution exceeds the limits, the transfer valve is automatically closed so that no solution in unsafe concentrations is delivered

to the bedside. The solution is bypassed, and a system of visual and audible alarms alerts dialysis personnel to problems. This alarm condition should not be reset to function unless the problem has been corrected.

In a batch system, the bath may be checked in a number of ways. The test for chloride ion is commonly used. It is done before dialysis commences and any time the bath is changed.

Temperature. Most dialysate delivery systems use a heating element to maintain dialysate temperature at optimal levels (98°F to 101°F or 36.7°C to 38.3°C). Some systems include alarms; others require visual observation of the temperature gauge.

Cool temperatures may cause chilling and vessel spasm. Sometimes chilling in the patient is the first indication of a drop in dialysate temperature. High temperatures (over 101°F or 38.3°C) may produce fever and discomfort in the patient, while extremely high temperatures (of 110°F or 43.3°C) will cause hemolysis. Corrections should be made as soon as the temperature reaches 101°F (38.3°C).

Blood Flow. Monitoring adequate blood flow rate throughout dialysis is essential to dialysis efficiency. Factors that influence blood flow rate are blood pressure, shunt and fistula function, and the extracorporeal circuit. A manometer connected to the drip chamber is used to measure the pressure in the blood lines. Changes in blood line pressures are transmitted to the drip chamber and register on the manometer as high- or low-pressure alarms.

A high-pressure alarm indicates a problem in the venous blood line, vessel spasm, or a clotted vein. Vessel spasm is seen in new shunts or with chilling, and a heating pad over the shunt may help to relax the vessel. If a clot is suspected, the vein is irrigated with a heparinized saline solution.

A low-pressure alarm reflects an obstruction to blood flow from the patient. Arterial spasm, clotting, displacement of a fistula needle, and a drop in blood pressure are possible causes. Correction is again directed to the cause.

Blood Leaks. A blood leak detector is invaluable when outflow dialysate is not visible, as in a single-pass delivery system. One type of blood leak detector is a color-sensitive photocell that picks up color variations in the outflow dialysate. Any foreign material such as blood will be detected and an alarm set off. Since false alarms are sometimes set off by air bubbles, the nurse will check the dialysate visually for a gross leak and with a hemostix for smaller leaks.

Dialysis is usually discontinued immediately with a gross leak. Whether or not the blood is returned to the patient is either a matter of unit policy or an individual determination. If the patient is severely anemic, the risk of losing the blood in the dialyzer may outweigh the risk of a reaction to dialysate-contaminated blood. Sometimes minor leaks, in which there is no visible blood in the dialysate and only a small hemostix reaction, seal over, and dialysis is continued.

Air Embolism.   The risk of air embolism is one of the most serious patient safety problems in the hemodialysis unit. Air can enter the patient's circulation through defective blood tubing, faulty blood line connections, vented intravenous fluid containers, or accidental displacement of the arterial needle.

The use of air leak detectors and plastic fluid containers has minimized air embolus risks, but the prevention of potential problems by strict attention to technical details and visual monitoring cannot be overemphasized.

Access to Circulation

Successful repeated hemodialysis depends upon access to the patient's circulation. Methods commonly used are the external arteriovenous (A-V) shunt, the internal arteriovenous fistula, bovine and Gortex grafts, and the femoral vein catheter.

ARTERIOVENOUS SHUNT

The A-V shunt consists of two soft plastic (Silastic) cannulas, one of which is inserted into an artery and the other into a vein. Between dialyses, the cannulas are joined by a hard, plastic (Teflon) connector, and blood flows freely between the two vessels. At the time of dialysis the two cannulas are separated and attached to the blood tubing of the dialyzer.

Cannulation is a surgical procedure performed in the operating room under local anesthesia. The cannula is usually inserted in the forearm of the nondominant arm, although circumstances may dictate placement in other extremities.

Presurgical care should include avoiding venipunctures, intravenous administrations, tourniquets, and blood-pressure cuffs in the affected limb. Nursing care is directed at maintenance of good function and prevention of clotting and infection beginning in the immediate postsurgical period.

General recommendations for promoting shunt life are

- *Limiting activity in the postoperative period.* Shunt functioning can be promoted by elevating the affected extremity for 2 to 3 days to reduce swelling and discomfort, and avoiding weight bearing in a leg shunt for at least a week.
- *Cleanliness.* The shunt site should be kept clean and dry. Good aseptic technique is essential in dressing changes and handling of the shunt. Daily dressing changes are not recommended unless infection with drainage is present. Cleansing at the time of dialysis is usually sufficient and should be done from the exit sites outward. Separate guaze and applicators are used for each exit to prevent cross-contamination. Picking at crusts should be avoided.
- *Proper alignment.* Misalignment may occur if the cannulas are twisted during either the hookup procedure or the reconnection at the end of dialysis. Distortions should be corrected immediately because tension at the exits may lead to small tears in the epithelium, which in turn contribute to clotting and infection. An outer dressing such as Kling, which conforms to the contours of the extremity, is recommended because it prevents the shunt and other dressings from slipping around with normal motions.
- *Gentleness.* Careful, gentle handling of shunt parts is important in extending shunt life. Therefore, jerking and pulling on the cannulas during dialysis procedures should be avoided.
- *Frequent observation.* Early detection and attention to symptoms may lead to the prevention of more serious problems. Clotting and infection are the two major complications.
- *Preventing clotting.* A clue to good blood flow through the shunt is a sound or burst heard with a stethoscope. The sound has been likened to the sound of rushing water. Sometimes the bruit is so strong it can be palpated with the fingers. This is called a thrill. If the bruit is faint or absent, the dressing is removed in order to observe the shunt. The color of the blood should be uniformly red and the shunt warm to the touch. If the shunt is clotted, the blood is quite dark and the red cells and serum may have already separated. Declotting may or may not be successful, depending on the length of time that has elapsed between clotting and detection. The routine declotting pro-

cedure consists of evacuating the clots by irrigating each cannula with a weak heparinized saline solution. Aseptic technique is again emphasized. Once flow has been re-established, the shunt is reconnected and observed closely. It has been the experience of dialysis personnel that once clotting occurs, it will recur unless the cause has been determined and corrective measures taken. A history of trauma, obstruction to flow caused by sleeping with a limb bent or legs crossed, hypotension, and infections is often found. The patient, however, may have an intrinsic clotting problem that may indicate the use of an anticoagulant such as sodium warfarin (Coumadin). This will necessitate the usual observations and precautions taken with anticoagulation therapy. The patient will also need a readjustment in heparin dosage during dialysis.

• *Preventing infection.* The shunt is routinely inspected at the time of dialysis. It is also inspected when the patient develops any unusual symptoms, such as pain or bleeding at exits, between dialysis. Any of the signs of inflammation, such as redness, swelling, tenderness, and drainage are cause for concern and require prompt attention. Cultures are routinely done by the nurse if drainage is noted. Each exit site is cultured separately. Some physicians will treat the infection without cultures, assuming that most shunts are infected with *Staphylococcus aureus.* However, *Pseudomonas* and *Escherichia coli* are sometimes cultured out. Aside from the possibility of further shunt surgery, the most serious complication of a shunt infection is septicemia. To forestall this possibility, some physicians choose to remove an extremely infected shunt immediately. Whether this is done or not, the patient should be observed closely, especially during the hemodialysis procedure when contamination of the bloodstream from an infected shunt is a strong possibility. The development of chills, fever, and hypotension in a patient with an infected shunt should be regarded as a serious sign. Blood cultures should be drawn immediately and the physician notified promptly.

A complication that occurs rarely but one that requires immediate nursing intervention is accidental separation of the cannulas or displacement of the arterial cannula. The appearance of large amounts of bright red blood on the shunt dressing constitutes an emergency and should be investigated without hesitation. If the cannulas have become separated, they should be clamped immediately and then reconnected. For this reason it is essential that shunt clamps be attached to each person who has an A-V shunt. If the arterial cannula has slipped out of the vessel, direct pressure is applied over the artery until medical assistance is available.

ARTERIOVENOUS FISTULA

The arteriovenous fistula technique was developed in response to the frequent complications encountered with the A-V shunt.

In this procedure the surgeon anastomoses an artery and a vein, creating a fistula or artificial opening between them. Arterial blood flowing into the venous system results in marked dilatation of the veins, which are then easily punctured with a large bore 14-gauge needle. Two venipunctures are made at the time of dialysis, one for a blood source and one for a return.

The arterial needle is inserted toward the fistula to obtain the best blood flow, but the tip should not be placed closer than 1 to 1½ inches from the fistula. A traumatic puncture might lead to damage and closure of the fistula. The venous needle is directed away from the fistula in the direction of normal venous flow. It may be placed in either the same vessel, another vein in the same arm, or even in another extremity.

If both needles are inserted into the same vessel, the tip should be at least 8 to 10 cm apart to avoid mixing of the blood, which would result in inadequate dialysis. If it is necessary to place the needles close to each other, a tourniquet is applied between the two needles.

Care of the arteriovenous fistula is less complicated than with the A-V shunt. Normal showering or bathing with soap provides adequate skin cleansing. Traumatic venipunctures or repetition in the same site should be avoided because these lead to excessive bleeding, hematoma, and scar formation. Excessive manipulation and adjustment of the needles should also be avoided for the same reasons. Postdialysis care includes adequate pressure on the puncture sites after the needles are removed.

BOVINE AND GORTEX GRAFTS

The bovine and Gortex grafts were developed in response to a need for blood access in those patients with inadequate blood vessels of their own. A bovine graft is a segment of selected bovine carotid artery that is processed and sterilized for human use. A Gortex, or polytetrafluoroethylene, graft is a prosthetic material manufactured from an expanded, highly porous form of Teflon. Experimental studies in animals showed this to be a suitable vascular replacement. Either type is anastomosed between an artery and a vein. After a suitable healing period, the vessel is used in the same manner as an arteriovenous fistula.

The procedures for preventing complications are the same as those for arteriovenous fistula; however, more frequently seen complications include thrombosis, infection, and aneurysm formation.

FEMORAL CATHETERS

Femoral catheters (also called Shaldon catheters) are used for hemodialysis when other means of access to the bloodstream are not available. This method is used primarily in acute dialysis, but may also be used for chronic dialysis patients because of shunt or fistula failure. It should be considered a temporary measure.

The procedure involves inserting one or two Teflon catheters into the femoral veins. If an arm vein can be used for blood return, only one catheter is used. When two catheters are needed, the lower one is used for the blood supply, the higher one for the return.

Femoral catheterization trays are standard equipment in dialysis units and in critical care units that perform acute dialysis.

The femoral catheters must be secured to the leg to prevent accidental slipping and observed frequently for bleeding during hemodialysis. The catheters are usually removed after dialysis but may be left in place if the patient is scheduled for another dialysis within 24 hours.

Leaving femoral catheters in place over 24 hours may lead to infection. Catheters left in place are irrigated periodically with a weak heparinized saline solution to prevent clotting. The usual dilution is 1000 units of heparin to 30 ml of normal saline, and 4 to 5 ml are instilled into the catheter every 2 to 4 hours.

If the catheters are removed at the end of dialysis, pressure is applied to the puncture sites until complete clotting occurs. The site is checked for several hours thereafter to detect any renewal of bleeding.

PERITONEAL DIALYSIS

Peritoneal dialysis accomplishes the same functions and operates on the same principles of diffusion and osmosis as hemodialysis. In this instance, however, the peritoneum is the semipermeable membrane.

Peritoneal dialysis is an effective alternate treatment when hemodialysis is not available or when access to the bloodstream is not possible. It is sometimes used as an initial treatment for renal failure while the patient is being evaluated for a hemodialysis program.

The advantages of peritoneal dialysis over hemodialysis include use of less complicated technical equipment, less need for highly skilled personnel, availability of supplies and equipment, and minimizing of adverse symptoms of the more efficient hemodialysis. This may be important in patients who cannot tolerate rapid hemodynamic changes.

On the other hand, peritoneal dialysis requires more time to adequately remove metabolic wastes and to restore electrolyte and fluid balance. In addition, repeated treatments may lead to peritonitis, while long periods of immobility may lead to such complications as pulmonary congestion and venous stasis. Because fluid is introduced into the peritoneal cavity, peritoneal dialysis is contraindicated in existing peritonitis, recent or extensive abdominal surgery, the presence of abdominal adhesions, or impending kidney transplantation.

Materials Used in Peritoneal Dialysis

- Solutions. As in hemodialysis, peritoneal dialysis solutions contain "ideal" concentrations of electrolytes but lack urea, creatinine, and other substances that are to be removed. Unlike dialysate used in hemodialysis, solutions must be sterile. Solutions vary in dextrose concentrations. A 1.5% or 4.25% dextrose solution can be used. The use of a 4.25% solution is usually reserved if more fluid removal is needed. Peritoneal dialysate usually contains no potassium, so potassium chloride may have to be added to the dialysate to prevent hypokalemia.

  Close monitoring of the patient's serum potassium is necessary to regulate the amount of potassium to be added.
- Peritoneal dialysis administration set
- Peritoneal dialysis catheter set, which includes the catheter, a connecting tube for connecting the catheter to the administration set, and a metal stylet.
- Trocar set of the surgeon's choice
- Ancillary drugs:
  a. Local anesthetic solution —2% lidocaine (Xylocaine)

b. Aqueous heparin—1000 units/ml
c. Potassium chloride
d. Broad-spectrum antibiotics

Preliminary Procedures

1. The bladder should be emptied just prior to the procedure to avoid accidental puncture with the trocar.
2. The patient may receive a preoperative medication to enhance relaxation during the procedure.
3. The dialyzing fluid is warmed to body temperature or slightly warmer.
4. Baseline vital signs, such as temperature, pulse, respirations and weight, are recorded. If possible, an in-bed scale is ideal so that the patient's weight can be monitored frequently. Moving a lethargic or disoriented patient to a scale may create problems such as catheter displacement.
5. Specific orders regarding fluid removal, replacement, and drug administration should be written by the physician prior to the procedure.

Procedure

Under sterile conditions, a small midline incision is made just below the umbilicus. A trocar is inserted through the incision into the peritoneal cavity. The obturator is removed and the catheter secured.

The dialysis solution flows into the abdominal cavity by gravity as rapidly as possible (5 to 10 minutes). If it flows in too slowly, the catheter may need repositioning. When the solution is infused, the tubing is clamped, and the solution remains in the abdominal cavity for 30 to 45 minutes. Then the solution bottles are placed on the floor, and the fluid is drained out of the peritoneal cavity by gravity. If the system is patent and the catheter well placed, the fluid will drain in a steady forceful stream. Drainage should take no more than 20 minutes.

This cycle is repeated continuously for the prescribed number of hours, which varies from 12 to 36, depending upon the purpose of the treatment, the patient's condition, and the proper functioning of the system.

Automated Peritoneal Dialysis Systems

Automated peritoneal dialysis systems are comparable to hemodialysis systems in that they mix water and dialysate in proper dilution, have built-in monitors, and a system of automatic timing devices that cycle the infusion and removal of peritoneal fluid.

Automated peritoneal delivery systems are more appropriately used for chronic peritoneal dialysis using a permanent, indwelling peritoneal catheter. Less sophisticated devices that minimize the necessity for manual bottle exchanges are more appropriate for the unit that may do an occasional peritoneal dialysis.

Essential Features of Nursing Care

- *Maintenance of accurate intake and output records as well as accurate records of weights* using the same scale are essential in assessing volume depletion or overload.
- *Frequent monitoring of blood pressure and pulse.* Orthostatic blood pressure changes and increased pulse rate are valuable tools in assessing the patient's volume status.
- *Early detection of signs and symptoms of peritonitis.* Low grade fever, abdominal pain, and cloudy peritoneal fluid are all possible signs of infection.
- *Maintenance of the sterility of the peritoneal system* is essential. Use of masks and sterile gloves when doing the abdominal dressing change is mandatory.
- *Early detection and correction of technical difficulties* before they result in physiological problems. Slow outflow of the peritoneal fluid may indicate early problems with the patency of the peritoneal catheter.
- *Prevention of the complications of bedrest* and provision of an environment that will assist the patient in *accepting bedrest* for prolonged periods of time.
- *Constipation should be avoided* because it will decrease the clearance of waste products and cause the patient more discomfort and distention.

Complications of Peritoneal Dialysis and Nursing Intervention

TECHNICAL COMPLICATIONS

Incomplete Recovery of Fluid. The fluid removed should at least equal or exceed the amount inserted. Commercially prepared dialysate contains approximately 1000 or 2000 ml. If after several exchanges the volume drained is less (by 500 ml or more) than the amount inserted, an evaluation must be made.

Signs of fluid retention include abdominal distention or complaint of fullness. The most accurate tool in assessing the amount of unrecovered fluid is weight.

If the fluid drains slowly, the catheter tip may be buried in the omentum or clogged with fibrin. Turning the patient from side to side, elevating the head of the bed, and gently massaging the abdomen may facilitate better drainage.

If fibrin or blood exists in the outflow drainage, heparin will need to be added to the dialysate. The specific dose is ordered by the physician but will be in the range of 500 to 1000 units per liter.

Leakage Around the Catheter. Superficial leakage may be controlled with extra sutures and decreasing the amount of dialysate instilled into the peritoneum. A leaking catheter should be corrected because it acts as a pathway for bacteria to enter the peritoneum. It is important to check the abdominal dressing frequently to detect leakage.

Blood-tinged peritoneal fluid is expected in the initial outflow but should clear after a few passes. Gross bleeding at any time is an indication of a more serious problem and should be investigated immediately.

PHYSIOLOGICAL COMPLICATIONS

Peritonitis. This is a serious but manageable complication of peritoneal dialysis. Early detection and initiation of treatment will lessen the patient's discomfort and prevent more serious complications.

Signs of peritonitis include low-grade fever, abdominal pain when fluid is being inserted, and cloudy peritoneal drainage fluid.

Treatment should begin as soon as a sample of peritoneal fluid is obtained. The specimen should be sent to the laboratory for culture and sensitivity. The patient should then start on a broad-spectrum antibiotic, which is usually added to the dialysate solution but which can also be given intravenously. Depending upon the severity of the infection, the patient's condition should improve dramatically within 8 hours of initiating antibiotic therapy.

Catheter Infection. During the daily dressing change, the exit site should be examined closely for signs of infection such as tenderness, redness, or drainage around the catheter. In the absence of peritonitis, a catheter infection is generally treated with an oral, broad-spectrum antibiotic.

Hypotension may occur if excessive fluid is removed. Vital signs are monitored frequently, especially if a hypertonic solution is used. Lying and sitting blood pressure readings are especially useful in evaluating fluid status. A progressive drop in blood pressure and weight should alert the nurse to potential problems.

Hypertension and fluid overload may occur if all the fluid is not removed in each cycle. An increase in weight requires an assessment of the catheter and dialysate solutions. The exact amount in the bottles should be noted. Some manufacturers add 50 ml to a 1000 ml bottle. Over a period of hours this can make a considerable difference.

Observe the patient for signs of respiratory distress, which may indicate pulmonary congestion. In the absence of other symptoms of fluid overload, hypertension may be the result of anxiety and apprehension. Reassuring the patient and promptly correcting problems are preferable to the administration of sedatives and tranquilizers.

BUN and Creatinine. Close monitoring of the serum BUN and creatinine will assist in the evaluation of the effectiveness of the dialysis. Inadequate clearance of waste products needs prompt attention.

Hypokalemia is a common complication of peritoneal dialysis. Close monitoring of the serum potassium will indicate the need for adding potassium chloride to the dialysate as well as the amount.

PAIN

Mild abdominal discomfort may be experienced at any time during the procedure and is probably related to the constant distention or chemical irritation of the peritoneum. If a mild analgesic doesn't provide relief, inserting 5 ml of 2% lidocaine (Xylocaine) directly into the catheter may help.

The patient may be less uncomfortable if nourishment is given in small amounts, when the fluid is draining out rather than when the abdominal cavity is distended.

Severe pain may indicate more serious problems of infection or paralytic ileus. Infection is not likely in the first 24 hours. Aseptic technique and the use of prophylactic antibiotics minimize the risk of infection. Periodic cultures of the outflowing fluid will assist in the early detection of pathogenic organisms.

COMPLICATIONS FROM IMMOBILITY

Immobility may lead to hypostatic pneumonia, especially in the debilitated or elderly patient. Deep breathing, turning, and coughing should be encouraged during the procedure. Leg exercises and the use of elastic stockings may prevent the development of venous thrombi and emboli.

PSYCHOLOGICAL ASPECTS

Because peritoneal dialysis is a slower and more gradual clearance of waste products, disequilibrium associated with hemodialysis is rarely seen. However, because the treatment is more lengthy, boredom is a frequent problem.

Nursing measures are directed toward making the patient as comfortable as possible. Diversions such as having visitors, reading, or watching TV should be encouraged. Educating the patient about peritoneal dialysis and involving him in his care may reduce some of the anxiety and discomfort.

BIBLIOGRAPHY

Brundage DJ: Nursing Management of Renal Problems. St. Louis, C.V. Mosby, 1976

Dolan P, Greene H Jr: Renal failure and peritoneal dialysis. Nursing 75 5:40–49, 1975

Forland M: Nephrology: A Review of Clinical Nephrology. Garden City, Medical Examination Publishing Company, 1977

Gutch CF, Stoner MH (eds): Review of Hemodialysis for Nurses and Dialysis Personnel, 3rd ed. St. Louis, C.V. Mosby, 1979

Harrington J, Brener ER: Patient Care in Renal Failure. Philadelphia, W.B. Saunders, 1973

Kubo W et al: Fluid and electrolyte problems of tube-fed patients. Am J Nurs, June 1976, pp 912–916

Lancaster LE: The Patient with End-Stage Renal Disease. New York, John Wiley & Sons, 1979

Leb DE: An introduction to hemodialysis. Dial Tranplant 9, No. 6:571–574, 1980

Legut JA: A review of vascular access management. Dial Transplant 4, No. 1:20–31, 1975

Metheny NA, Snively WD: Perioperative fluids and electrolytes. Am J Nurs, May 1978, pp 840–845

Nursing 79 Skillbook Series: Monitoring Fluid and Electrolytes Precisely. Horsham, Intermed Communications, 1978

Oreopoulos D: Peritoneal dialysis is reinstated. J Dial, 2(3): 295–310, 1978

Pflaum SS: Investigation of intake-output as a means of assessing body fluid balance. Heart Lung 8, No. 3:495–498, 1979

Reed G, Sheppard V: Regulation of Fluid and Electrolyte Balance: A Programmed Instruction in Clinical Physiology. Philadelphia, W.B. Saunders, 1977

Roberts SL: Renal assessment: A nursing point of view. Heart Lung 8, No. 1:105–113, 1979

Schrier RW: Renal and Electrolyte Disorders. Boston, Little, Brown & Co, 1976

Shapiro WB et al: Low-dose heparin in the high-risk bleeding hemodialysis patient monitored by activated partial thromboplastin time. Dial Transplant 9, No. 4:322–408, 1980

Stark JL: BUN/creatinine: Your keys to kidney function. Nursing 80 10:33–38, 1980

Stroot V et al: Fluid and Electrolytes. Philadelphia, F.A. Davis, 1977

Tenckhoff H: Peritoneal dialysis today: A new look. Nephron 12:420, 1974

**Karen Choate Robbins and
Ann Marie Powers***

Renal Transplantation 18

Transplantation research began in the early 1900s, although it was not until the early 1950s that transplantation became a realistic and therapeutic approach for chronic renal failure in humans.

Originally, kidneys were grafted into the thigh using the femoral vessels for vascularization. Experience with this procedure was limited to a very few patients. Since this site was obviously not practical for long-term graft survival, surgeons began grafting kidneys into the iliac fossa in the mid 1950s, the site still used today.

Since that time, many centers in the country are performing renal transplants as definitive therapy for *endstage renal disease* (ESRD)†. As more centers evolved, so too have a multitude of approaches and philosophies, with the major differences revolving around the immunosuppressive therapy.

This chapter does not encompass all possible management approaches but will, however, discuss the major points of transplantation and care that are common to all centers and that are well-documented in the literature. It will provide the

*The authors wish to acknowledge the help of Laurine S. Bow, B.S., in preparing the material on tissue typing.

†The recognized federal terminology for chronic renal failure is endstage renal disease (ESRD). As of July 1, 1973, patients with ESRD became eligible for Medicare coverage regardless of age. As a result, no one is denied replacement therapy due to lack of funds. This coverage extends for 3 years from the month of transplant procedure and includes the donor's medical expenses. Coverage for dialysis therapy is for the duration of treatment.

critical care nurse with sufficient information to provide competent care for the transplant recipient.‡

ENDSTAGE RENAL DISEASE
Renal failure is rarely an "all or none" phenomenon but instead is a gradual loss of function involving either part or all of the nephrons, depending upon the basic disease process.

When a patient has minimal renal damage, the body may compensate for certain lost functions, and the patient will have few symptoms. If the process is acute and reversible, the effects of long-term failure (*e.g.,* anemia, osteodystrophy) will not be seen. For many patients, however, the process is a long and exhausting one that affects all body systems.

It is not until irreversible damage to the majority of nephrons (approximately 2 million) occurs and the glomerular filtration rate decreases to 10 ml per minute that a patient is considered to have ESRD (see Chapters 15 and 16).

TRANSPLANT OR DIALYSIS: THE PATIENT'S CHOICE
Once a patient has reached ESRD, he has three options: no treatment and death, chronic dialysis (either peritoneal dialysis or hemodialysis), or transplantation (see Fig. 18-1).

Although the option of no treatment and death is considered and occasionally chosen by the patient, the focus here will be on the treatment options of hemodialysis and transplant (two forms of *replacement therapy*). Intermittent peritoneal dialysis and continuous ambulatory peritoneal dialysis are two other forms of replacement therapy that will not be discussed in this chapter but that are covered in Chapter 17.

‡If further information is desired please refer to *Standards of Clinical Practice. Section II: Transplantation,* available from the American Association of Nephrology Nurses and Technicians, Box 56, North Woodbury Road, Pitman, New Jersey 08071.

Hemodialysis and transplantation are presented here because they are the most prevalent therapeutic approaches. Although dialysis and transplant are separate options, each of these therapies is an integral part of the other. Transplantation cannot be done without the support of dialysis, and if the transplant fails, dialysis is resumed.

Both ESRD and replacement therapy cause symptoms. Therefore, the patient needs to consider the effects of the disease as well as the risks of therapy and recognize that the complications accompanying his underlying disease will still be present post transplant. Table 18-1 outlines the effects of dialysis and transplantation on patients with ESRD.

Renal Filtration
In ESRD, the glomerular filtration rate (GFR) and urinary output are grossly diminished. Therefore, hemodialysis must be done on a regular basis to provide the vital process of renal filtration. With a well-functioning renal graft, however, renal filtration is constant.

Nutrition
Diet is severely restricted in the majority of dialysis patients. These restrictions, which include protein, sodium, potassium, and fluid, are necessary because the equivalent of renal filtration occurs for only a limited number of hours per week.

When the diet is followed, it changes lifetime eating habits and poses severe limits on the patient's social activities. Gross abuse of the diet can result in malignant hypertension, congestive heart failure, pulmonary edema, hyperkalemia or, potentially, cardiac arrest.

After transplantation, the only dietary restriction sometimes imposed upon the patient with good renal function is sodium. Rather than a fluid restriction, the patient is encouraged to drink at least 2 liters per day. Therefore, following successful transplant, the diet more closely

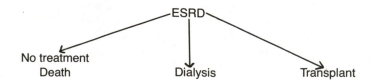

FIGURE 18-1.
Options facing a person with endstage renal disease (ESRD).

Table 18–1
Effects of Endstage Renal Disease Treated by Hemodialysis or Well-Functioning Renal Graft

Effect on	With Hemodialysis	With Well-Functioning Transplant
Renal filtration	Only during dialysis	24 hours/day
Nutrition	Na, K, protein and fluid restrictions	Possible Na restriction for up to 1 year after transplant
Hematologic system	Anemia, fatigue Shortened RBC survival	Normal red blood cells and hematocrit
	Prolonged clotting time	Normal clotting time

Skeletal system	Renal osteodystrophy:
	  osteomalacia
	  osteoporosis
	  osteitis fibrosa cystica
		No further bone resorption

		Steroid-induced osteoporosis Possible tertiary hyperparathyroidism Avascular/aseptic necrosis
Nervous system	Peripheral, gastrointestinal, and genitourinary neuropathy	Neuropathy will not progress, and may improve
	Autonomic nervous system neuropathy	
Sexuality	Decreased libido	Improved libido
	Frequent impotence	Impotence may persist
	Amenorrhea	Ovulation and menses may resume
Liver	Increased risk of hepatitis from recurrent extracorporeal circulation and transfusion	10% incidence of hepatitis due to azathioprine therapy
		Increased susceptibility to viral hepatitis
Cardiovascular system	Risk of vascular access infection, clotting, exsanguination, and frequent site changes	No need for vascular access
	Accelerated atherosclerosis	Effect on atherosclerotic process uncertain
	Hypertriglyceridemia	Increased cholesterol levels
	Ventricular hypertrophy, heart failure	Ventricular size sometimes returns to normal
	Uremic pericarditis	
	Cardiac tamponade	
Muscular system	Decreased muscle mass due to dietary limits	Myopathy that improves when steroid dosage decreases and patient's activity increases
	Decreased exercise tolerance	
Gastrointestinal tract	Increased gastric acid production	Increased risk of ulceration
	Increased incidence of diverticulosis	Diverticulosis predisposes to perforation
	Constipation	Increased incidence of ischemic colitis
Immune system	Increased susceptibility to infection from uremia	Increased susceptibility to infection from immunosuppressive drugs
		Increased incidence of malignancy (especially skin, lymph, and cervix)
Lungs	Risk of pulmonary edema, congestive heart failure	Pulmonary infections secondary to immunosuppressive therapy
Dependence	Dependent on machine to support life	Dependent on medications

approaches a normal one and is much more conducive to socialization.

Hematologic System

Anemia is common to all patients with ESRD. Because the kidney is no longer able to produce adequate amounts of erythropoietic stimulating factor, red blood cell production is low. This, along with shorter red blood cell survival in the uremic patient, causes hematocrits one-half that of normal. This anemia is thought to cause the fatigue that is one of the most frustrating problems for the ESRD patient.

If the diet has been severely limited in protein, then iron and vitamin B_{12} intake will be diminished, thereby reducing the amount of iron that can be absorbed from the intestines. The use of iron and androgen therapy has been of benefit to many patients, although normal hematocrits are rarely seen in spite of such therapy. Increased blood losses in the hemodialysis patient further contribute to low hematocrits. Ruptures and clotting of the dialyzer, residual blood in the dialyzer following termination of the dialysis, and routine laboratory tests constitute sources of significant and chronic blood loss.[1]

The use of blood transfusions prior to transplantation has helped alleviate anemia-related problems. Several months after the transplant, anemia is seldom a problem, and the patient will have a near normal, if not normal hematocrit. Although the kidney was denervated when transplanted, this does not affect the erythropoiesis of the graft. While blood loss from laboratory tests is appreciable immediately following the transplant, it is markedly reduced following hospital discharge. The patient has a normal protein intake, an increased ability to absorb iron, and normal red blood cell survival time, all increasing the ability to maintain the hematocrit at a higher level.

Skeletal System

The kidneys play a major role in maintaining calcium-phosphorus balance in the body. They do this by excreting these elements and also by converting vitamin D to an active form. Loss of nephron (kidney) function, therefore, is accompanied by gross disturbances in calcium metabolism and the development of a complex set of comorbidity problems that are commonly referred to as *renal osteodystrophy*. Renal osteodystrophy refers to three bone disease processes that are caused by the malfunctioning kidneys as opposed to other etiologies: osteomalacia, osteoporosis, and osteofibrosa cystitis.

The ESRD patient may exhibit one or all three processes concurrently. The first process is called *osteomalacia*, which is defined as a softening of the bones. This process can cause bones to become flexible and brittle and can eventually result in spontaneous fractures. The second process is *osteoporosis*, which is defined as increased porosity of the bone and which occurs as bones continue to lose calcium.

Both osteomalacia and osteoporosis are caused by the lack of activated vitamin D to assist in maintaining calcium hemostasis. Activated vitamin D or D_3 acts by increasing renal calcium reabsorption and intestinal transport of calcium into the bloodstream as well as by assisting in calcium mobilization from the bone in conjunction with parathyroid hormone (PTH). Vitamin D is acquired from sunlight or dietary sources, but requires a functioning renal mass for complete activation.

In renal failure, dietary calcium is restricted, lessening the availability of this element to maintain serum calcium values. In addition, the continued serum phosphorus elevation is thought to shut off vitamin D conversion and to increase skeletal resistance to the effect of PTH. The long-term effect of this skeletal resistance is that the parathyroid gland enlarges to secrete enough PTH to increase serum calcium.

The enlargement of the parathyroid causes hyperplasia, or secondary hyperparathyroidism, and *osteitis fibrosa cystica,* the third bone disease process. Symptoms may include itching, metastatic soft tissue calcifications around joints and tendons, vascular calcifications of the large and small blood vessels, and diffuse or local skeletal pain. Continued gland enlargement can lead to tertiary or autonomic hyperparathyroidism diagnosed by hypercalcemia.

Medical management of these problems should be provided early in the course of renal failure through dietary restriction of phosphorus or administration of phosphate binders before initiation of dialysis or transplantation. Normal serum phosphorus is required before vitamin D or calcium supplements can be safely added to the management protocol; otherwise, calcium deposits can occur.

Once the patient is on dialysis, binders are given at mealtime. Calcium supplementation and vitamin D therapy can be initiated as needed. Even with adequate therapy, bone disease may continue, and a subtotal parathyroidectomy may be required to halt the progression of bone changes.

A successful renal transplant stops many of the osteodystrophic changes produced by ESRD because the kidney can again take an active role in calcium metabolism. Occasionally, the parathyroids continue to enlarge, causing *tertiary hyperparathyroidism.* In addition, the catabolic nature of the steroid medication contributes to the development of osteoporosis as well as of *aseptic necrosis of major joints.*

Nervous System

Although the mechanism is poorly understood, *neuropathies* may develop in the presence of severe or chronic uremia. The neuropathies cause muscle weakness, which sometimes requires the use of braces, walkers, or crutches for ambulation. Functions of the autonomic nervous system may be impaired to the extent that the gastrointestinal (GI) tract may be affected and blood pressure control is poor. Patients may actually have chronic hypotension from autonomic nervous system neuropathy.

Neuropathy should not increase in severity following transplantation, and, depending upon the severity of the neuropathy, there may be partial or total reversal following successful transplantation.

Sexuality

Impotence is prevalent among the dialysis patient population. While women may be physically capable of engaging in sexual intercourse, libido is often markedly decreased, lowering their desire for sexual activity.

Most male patients are impotent, perhaps because of their disease or because of antihypertensive medications. The etiology of this complication is probably physiological as well as psychological. Marriages and other comparable relationships can be adversely affected, and the long-term effects can be devastating.

Some patients remain impotent following transplantation, although this is most frequently associated with antihypertensive medication and steroid therapy. The libido, which is decreased while the patient is on dialysis, seems to return to normal following transplant.

Women usually cease to have menstrual periods while on dialysis, and following transplant will once again ovulate and menstruate. Therefore, some means of contraception should be used for 2 years post transplant when renal function is stable and immunosuppression is at a minimum dosage. There is additional risk for the mother and fetus if pregnancy occurs with unstable renal function and higher doses of immunosuppressive medications.

Liver

Problems associated with the dialysis treatments alone are considerable. *Hepatitis* is an ever-present threat due to the frequent extracorporeal circulation. If the transplant recipient receives blood transfusions prior to transplantation, there is an added risk of hepatitis acquired from the transfusions.

Once they are over the initial postoperative period, transplant recipients rarely receive transfusions. However, noninfectious hepatitis associated with the use of the immunosuppressive azathioprine occurs occasionally among transplant recipients. This is usually resolved by discontinuing azathioprine and replacing it with cyclophosphamide.

Cardiovascular System

Vascular access must be maintained in the hemodialysis patient, and loss of sites can sometimes pose life-threatening problems.

Shunts, arteriovenous fistulas, and polytetrofluoroethylene (PTFE) grafts may be used in various combinations to gain permanent access to the circulation. Infections, clotting, high-output cardiac failure, and exsanguination are persistent threats with any type of access. With each access failure, the number of potential sites is reduced until finally all possible sites are exhausted. Access problems account for a significant number of hospital admissions of hemodialysis patients. For the peritoneal dialysis patient, the surgically placed peritoneal catheter is left in place, but the potential for peritonitis is ever present.

The transplant patient need not maintain a vascular access site; in fact, the greatest problem of access is simply to find blood vessels from which to draw blood for laboratory studies to monitor renal function.

Perhaps the most dramatic complication of ESRD is the rate of accelerated *atherosclerosis.* The etiology is not understood, but the greatest cause of mortality in long-term dialysis patients is cardiovascular accidents.

Some of the most advanced atherosclerosis seen at postmortem examination has been in long-term dialysis patients. Because of protein restrictions, most calories are taken in the form of carbohydrates, which leads to an increased level of cholesterol. In addition, there is a hypertriglyceridemia thought to be due to increased synthesis by the liver and decreased clearing by the kidney of lipoprotein and lipase.

The effect of transplantation on atherosclerosis is uncertain but is under investigation. It is thought, however, that cholesterol levels increase after transplant. The return to a normal diet can decrease the dietary contributions to atherosclerotic changes.

Because the dialysis patient usually has little or no fluid output, an increased intake of sodium or fluid will cause *hypervolemia,* which, because the vascular system has difficulty accommodating this fluid excess, can lead to congestive heart failure. Some patients lose as much as 15 pounds of fluid with a single dialysis treatment.

Hypervolemia can occur in the transplant recipient when decreased urinary output occurs as the result of rejection episodes or acute tubular necrosis and is managed by either diuretic therapy or dialysis support.

The specific mechanism causing *uremic pericarditis* is unclear. Depending upon the severity and chronicity of pericarditis, a pericardial window or a pericardectomy is sometimes necessary to control this problem. If the patient has fluid overload, a pericardial rub may not be heard due to the fluid contained in the pericardial sac. What seems to be an appropriate therapy, dialyzing to remove excess fluid, can actually increase the patient's pain because the fluid is removed and the friction is increased. At this point a rub is very prominent. Conservative management of pericarditis varies greatly and may include anti-inflammatory agents.

A patient with uremic pericarditis may develop *cardiac tamponade*. The treatment for the ESRD patient is the same as for any other patient: an attempt to remove the blood from the pericardial sac before an arrest occurs. Cardiac tamponade is an ominous complication with high mortality.

Muscular System

A *loss of muscle mass* is not uncommon in the ESRD patient. Limited dietary intake and inability to exert oneself due to the fatigue associated with anemia are probably the major contributing factors.

The transplant recipient will frequently experience *myopathies* due to steroid therapy. This loss in muscle mass can be recovered with exercise, particularly when the steroids are reduced. In an attempt to avoid severe myopathies, the transplant recipient is encouraged to walk, climb stairs, and exercise as much as possible.

GI Tract

Gastric acid production is increased in many ESRD patients. High levels of parathormone and decreased degradation of gastrin by the diseased kidneys both contribute to this.

While these dysfunctions can be reversed by replacement of normal renal function, there is an increased risk of ulceration post transplant. This risk has been reported to be greatest during a period of compromised renal function, that is, during a rejection episode, when the patient is also receiving higher doses of corticosteroids.[2] It has not been observed during periods of normal renal function and lower-dosage corticosteroid therapy.

The presence of diverticulosis pre transplant has been shown to predispose the person to *perforation* post transplant and should be treated by a colon resection prior to transplantation to reduce the risk of this serious problem.[3] *Constipation* is a problem for the dialysis patient that is contributed to by a limited fluid intake and the use of phosphorus binders. This can actually

lead to development of an antacid bezoar causing impaction, possible perforation, and possible death.[4] GI complications are discussed in more detail later in the chapter.

Immune System

It is known that both dialysis and transplant patients are more susceptible to *infections,* the former from uremia and the latter from medications that lower immunity.

There is a known increased incidence of *malignancy* among transplant patients, especially skin, lymph, and cervix, but the data for the dialysis population are obscure and controversial. The dialysis population is increasingly an elderly one, and comparison with the normal population should consider the age factor. In addition, patients with malignancies at the time of initiation of dialysis are increasing in number, so that the data have not been clearly segregated.

Lungs

Hypervolemia as the result of ESRD can cause congestive heart failure, pulmonary congestion, and pulmonary edema. After transplantation, the risk of congestive heart failure and pulmonary edema diminishes because fluid balance can be maintained by the functioning kidney graft. However, after transplant there is greater risk of pulmonary infection as the result of immunosuppressant therapy (see discussion later in this chapter).

Dependence

Patients with ESRD need dialysis to live, and therefore are physiologically dependent upon a machine. The average hemodialysis patient spends approximately 15 hours per week attached to the machine, while a peritoneal dialysis patient spends even greater lengths of time dialyzing.

Because of the life-sustaining value of dialysis, as well as the time devoted to the procedure, patients have varying degrees of emotional dependence upon the treatment. Some patients keep their dependence in perspective by looking on dialysis as a necessary but not exclusive part of their lives and make an effort to keep the rest of their lives as fulfilling as possible. Others adapt to the dependency by having all their emotional energy revolve around the treatment and the personnel who provide care.

Conversely, the transplant recipient is no longer dependent upon a machine, but rather on medication to support the function of the graft. Patients usually find dependence upon the medication far more acceptable than dependence upon a machine.

Mortality

It is currently accepted that the mortality associated with both forms of replacement therapy, dialysis and renal transplantation, is the same. The range of the mortality rate per patient year is generally acknowledged to be between 5% and 20%, depending upon the institution or expert quoted.

A major problem in nephrology treatment today is that there are no accurate, nationwide, valid statistics to use when comparing mortality rates. Prior to the federal government's involvement in nephrology treatment, national dialysis and transplantation registries existed on a voluntary basis. The 13th and final report of the *Transplant Registry* was published in 1975.

When Congress passed Public Law PL 92-603, which funds all types of kidney disease treatment, it was decided that these national voluntary registries were unnecessary. In its place a federal data system called the *Medical Information System (MIS)* was established. Facilities are now required to submit their patient data to the government at regular intervals. The MIS system, however, has had problems in collecting and reporting accurate data, including mortality rates. Because of this, many dialysis and transplantation centers either continue to use data from the now defunct registries or report data from their own institution.

In view of these problems and the fact that mortality rates are similar for either type of replacement therapy, patients choose transplantation for reasons other than mortality figures, such as freedom from a machine, more control over their lives, or a chance to be "normal."

Recently, another agency of the federal government, the *Network Coordinating Councils*, have started to collect data within their geographic locations. Under PL 92-603, Network Coordinating Councils were created to monitor and improve the quality of care given to ESRD patients. It is hoped that in the future the MIS, in conjunction with the regional data base of the Coordinating Councils, can provide reasonable, accurate statistics for both mortality and morbidity in all ESRD replacement forms so the *patient* can make a wise, informed choice.

Summary

Endstage renal disease is chronic and complex and presents a multitude of problems for the patient, his family, and the health-care team, whether the decision is continued dialysis or transplantation. Many patients will choose transplantation. One of the next steps, then, is tissue typing to find a suitable donor.

FINDING A DONOR FOR RENAL TRANSPLANT

Just as red blood cells can be typed for both donor and recipient to prevent reaction between them, tissue can also be typed, which may reduce the potential for reactions between donor and recipient when organs are transplanted. Antigens that denote an individual's tissue type are coded by the major histocompatibility complex genes (MHC). These genes contain the genetic information to make antigens that are on the surface of all tissue cells. The antigens enable the body to differentiate self from nonself. Therefore, the greater the compatibility between donor and recipient, the better the chances for acceptance of an organ. This compatibility must also include ABO typing, although Rh factor compatibility is unnecessary.

The MHC establishes codes for four major allelic systems, A, B, C, and D loci, of which A and B code for the classic human leukocyte antigen (HLA) system. These antigens are found on the surface of lymphocytes and are used to determine an individual's tissue type. Any peripheral blood sample can be used to determine tissue type. There are more than 60 known HLA antigens and thousands of combinations of antigen types. Each person has two A-locus and two B-locus antigens. These are inherited as a pair or "haplotype," each of which consists of one A- and one B-locus antigen. Additionally, the D locus, which is part of the MHC, is inherited as part of the haplotype. The C locus is apparently insignificant in transplantation.

A test used to identify compatibility of the D locus of the MHC is the *mixed lymphocyte culture (MLC)* or *mixed lymphocyte response (MLR)*. An MLC is a complex test that measures the reaction between donor and recipient when their lymphocytes are grown together in a culture. This test is not suitable for selection of cadaver kidney recipients because the test requires 5 to 7 days for cellular stimulation and division to occur.

A further test, called a *crossmatch,* is set up to

screen the potential recipient for antibodies that he might have against the donor. This crossmatch takes 6 to 8 hours to complete and involves mixing serum from the potential recipient with donor lymphocytes. A positive crossmatch means that the recipient has antibodies against the donor. This response can be thought of as "in vitro" rejection. Thus a "negative" crossmatch is necessary for recipient selection. Occasionally a crossmatch is negative when, in fact, the recipient has antibodies against the donor in insufficient titers to elicit a positive test. A number of other screening tests are being studied but are still research endeavors without clear-cut clinical application for predicting graft survival.

There has been an increasing trend to administer *blood transfusions* to potential recipients prior to transplantation. While the mechanism of action of the transfusions on the immune system is under study, improvement in graft survival in such patients has been observed by many centers.

One should note that the use of new terminology (*e.g.,* MHC) is reflective of new knowledge in immunology. MHC is broader than HLA and actually includes the HLA system as well as other antigen systems. Thus, an awareness of the complexity of the immune system should create an awareness of the complexity of organ transplantation. These mysteries of the immune system represent the thrust of transplantation investigation in the 1980s.

Living Related Donors

As the name indicates, a living related donor is a donor from within the family. The possibility of a compatible donor from within the family should be explored for every potential recipient.

If donor and recipient have inherited the same haplotypes, they are MHC identical, that is, they share the same A, B, and D locus antigens, and this offers the greatest potential for a successful transplant. This match exists only among siblings. If only one haplotype is shared, they are compatible for only one-half the MHC antigens. This "half-antigen match" is the most common match that can exist between parents and children or among siblings. A "no haplotype match" is considered a complete mismatch and is not a desirable situation in which to perform a transplant because no similarity exists between the tissues.

Once a potential living related donor is identified, he has a thorough medical evaluation to determine that he is free of underlying disease, that he has two kidneys, and that donation could in no obvious way jeopardize his well-being. Once this evaluation is successfully completed, a living related transplant may be performed.

Currently under investigation is the use of blood transfusions from the identified donor to the recipient prior to transplantation. This pretreatment protocol, "donor-specific transfusion," has yielded promising results in selected cases.[5]

Cadaver Donors

Approximately one-fourth of the people who are in need of a transplant have a suitable living donor, which means three-fourths of all potential recipients must wait for a suitable cadaver donor.* A potential cadaver kidney donor is a person who dies from a problem not involving the kidneys.

Some illnesses which exclude a person from becoming a donor are malignancy (except primary brain tumors), long-standing diabetes mellitus, chronic hypertension, hepatitis, tuberculosis, and sepsis. Patients with persistent hypotension resulting in oliguria or anuria are not acceptable donors.

Age is not necessarily a limiting factor, and donors have been less than 1 year old and more than 60 years old. Many donors are trauma victims, while others die from cerebral aneurysms and surgery.

CRITERIA FOR DETERMINING DEATH

Historically, death was acknowledged when irreversible cardiac or respiratory arrest occurred. In the mid 1960s, however, the concept of *brain death* came into existence and is now medically accepted as an additional way in which death can be diagnosed. There is an increasing number of states that have passed legislation that acknowledges brain death as a means of determining death. Brain death, or electrocerebral silence, refers to the cessation of total brain activity at both cortical and lower levels even though heart and respiratory functions can be maintained mechanically.

The acknowledgement of brain death is important in obtaining kidneys from cadaver donors because the kidneys should be removed

---

*The 1979 MIS Report stated that of 4309 transplants performed that year in the U.S., 1230 or 28.5% were from living related donors and 3079 (71.5%) were from cadaver donors. There was a 98% response from transplant centers to the federal survey form.[6]

within 30 minutes after respiration and circulation cease. This time limit ensures viable organs for transplant.

As a result of technologic advances that sustain life, and because both physicians and the public want to be protected against premature diagnosis of death, various groups have tried to refine criteria that indicate death.

The most widely accepted criteria for defining death are referred to as the *Harvard criteria*.[7] All criteria must be met on two separate occasions, 24 hours apart, without any change in the findings, unless it is not possible to maintain respiratory and cardiac function.

The Harvard criteria include

- Complete unresponsiveness: total unawareness of external stimuli, *i.e.,* irreversible coma.
- No spontaneous muscular movements, including respiration.

    If the patient has been on a mechanical respirator, it can be turned off for 3 minutes to observe whether the patient breathes spontaneously. For this criterion to be valid, the patient must have a normal carbon dioxide tension and must breathe room air for at least 10 minutes before the test.

- Absent reflexes, spontaneous or elicited, except those which are spinal cord reflexes, *e.g.,* knee jerk.
- A flat electroencephalogram for at least 10 and preferably 20 minutes is a confirmatory rather than an essential criterion.
    - There are further procedural criteria for the way the test should be done.
    - Electroencephalogram results are not valid when there is hypothermia or central nervous system depression from drugs.

Alternate means of determining total and irreversible brain damage include intracranial blood flow studies performed by arteriography or isotope scan. It should be noted that the criteria for determining electrocerebral silence differs in patients under 14 years of age.

The issue of determining death is included in this chapter because of the increasing numbers of patients awaiting cadaver organs for transplant. The role of a new member of the transplant team, *the coordinator,* has evolved from this need for more organs.

The role of the coordinator varies throughout the country and may include grief counseling for the potential donor's family and a resource for the health-care team. The coordinator should be a liaison between the transplant program and the critical care area. Cooperation between the critical care staff and the transplant program will help ensure the availability of organs for transplantation. So that no conflict of interest exists, the physician(s) caring for the potential donor and pronouncing death cannot be involved in the removal or transplantation of organs.

Once kidneys are removed, they can be temporarily maintained for as long as 3 days by a preservation machine or a variety of preservation solutions. Recipient selection and preparation for transplantation are possible because of this time period. In addition, this time interval permits the transportation of kidneys so that a recipient has a greater chance to receive a well-matched graft. Increased sharing of kidneys among centers throughout the country ensures that kidneys will be transplanted even when there is no well-matched recipient locally.

THE NURSE'S ROLE

When a patient meets the criteria and becomes a potential donor, it is necessary to maintain the blood pressure as near normal as possible to provide adequate perfusion of the organ.

At that time there is also the need to support a family who may be troubled not only by the donor's impending death, but also by ambivalence about the decision to donate organs. The chaplain or member of the clergy with whom the family has been associated can be an invaluable support for the family during this very stressful time. The clergy person can also be a positive influence in the decision to make an organ donation. Simmons has found that donation is often a positive experience for the donor's family and in many instances, even helped in the grieving process.[8]

On the one hand, keeping an organ viable may be frustrating for the staff, particularly when the vigilant monitoring and regulation of blood pressure are viewed as taking care away from other patients who will survive. On the other hand, these efforts can be viewed as giving two people a chance at a longer and better life.

Visiting a transplant recipient, particularly one who has received a cadaver organ from a patient they cared for, has helped nurses realize that donation of an organ and the help needed to keep it viable are indeed worthwhile.

CARE OF THE TRANSPLANT RECIPIENT

The transplant recipient is usually cared for in a specially designated area throughout both acute and convalescent phases of recovery. This not only allows for highly proficient nursing care but also eliminates patient transfer, decreases fragmentation of care, and reduces exposure to infection for the newly immunosuppressed patient. In addition, the transplant recipient is usually not critically ill and hence many times does not fit the criteria for admission to a critical care area. Nevertheless, there may be times when transplant patients will be cared for in a critical care area, especially during the acute postoperative phase or when complications occur.

Postoperative Phase of Transplant Recipient Care

Immediately after surgery, the transplant recipient is cared for in a closely monitored area until his condition stabilizes. As the patient arrives in this recovery or intensive care area, the following assessment can be made:

1. Check the patient's level of consciousness and degree of pain.
2. Check the number of intravenous lines present, noting the site, type of solution, and flow rate.
3. Observe the abdominal dressing for drainage, noting whether a Hemovac or drain is present.
4. Check for the presence of Foley and ureteral catheters and observe the patency and urinary drainage of each.
5. Locate the vascular access site and determine its patency by placing either fingers or a stethoscope directly over the access site and feeling or listening for a characteristically loud pulsating noise called a *bruit*.
6. If the patient has been maintained on peritoneal dialysis, check the peritoneal dialysis catheter for closure and maintain sterility.
7. Check the blood pressure, apical pulse, respirations, temperature, and central venous pressure.

    Blood pressure should be taken on the extremity that does *not* have a functioning vascular access site because even momentary interference with arterial blood flow may lead to access malfunction.
8. If a nasogastric tube is present, attach it to an appropriate drainage system.
9. Obtain a baseline weight within 24 hours of surgery.
10. Measure abdominal girth at the iliac crest.

    This is baseline information used at a later time for assessment of complications, *e.g.*, ureteral leak, lymphocele, or bleeding.
11. In the case of a child, monitor more frequently than in an adult because of the dynamic nature of a child's fluid and cardiovascular status (*i.e.*, blood pressures, weights, and central venous pressures).

Answers to the following questions will provide additional baseline information.

- Are the patient's own kidneys present in addition to the graft, and if so, how much urine do they produce daily?

    This information will help determine how much of the urine produced is from the transplanted kidney. If the chart does not provide answers, the patient and family can. In addition, flank scars usually indicate nephrectomy.
- When was the last dialysis treatment?

    The nurse should pay particular attention to the metabolic status if the patient has not been dialyzed within 24 hours of surgery.
- What are the preoperative results of laboratory tests (serum electrolytes, urea nitrogen, creatinine, liver function, calcium, phosphorus, complete blood count with differential and platelet counts, urine electrolytes, specific gravity, creatinine clearance)?
- How much and what kind of intravenous fluid has the patient received?
- Did the patient receive a loading dose of immunosuppressive drugs preoperatively? What is the present dose schedule?
- Was methylprednisolone (Solu-Medrol) given in the operating room, and what is the ongoing dose schedule?
- Is the patient to receive antilymphocytic globulin or other immunosuppressive drugs?

    This drug information helps not only to clarify the regimen, but also to estimate the degree of immunosuppression.
- What preoperative teaching has been done?

    Patients who have received some teaching tend to be less anxious and more cooperative because they know what to expect. A cadaver donor recipient who receives a graft shortly after being placed on the waiting list might be poorly informed because preoperative teaching was not done. In this case, additional explanation is needed. (See Chapter 4 for a more complete discussion of the effects of stress and anxiety on learning.)
- Which physician is to be called—how, where, and when—for ongoing medical care?

    Clarifying and recording this information may enhance communication and efficiency, especially in case of emergency.

Many nursing responsibilities revolve around observing the function of the transplanted kidney, monitoring fluid and electrolyte balance, helping the patient avoid sources of infection, picking up early signs of complications, and supporting the patient and family through recovery phases.

MONITORING RENAL GRAFT FUNCTION

The transplanted kidney may function immediately after revascularization and produce large amounts of urine (200 to 1000 ml/hour), small amounts of urine (<20 ml/hour), or no urine at all.

Ischemic Time. The amount of urine produced is related to the length of time the donor kidney was ischemic. The ischemic time tends to be shorter in the living related transplant situation than in the cadaver transplant situation. Therefore, the living related donor kidney has less ischemic damage and tends to produce more urine in the initial recovery phase.

However, the hourly production of large amounts of urine is called *post transplant diuresis* and is thought to be the result of a proximal tubular defect. The proximal tubule is responsible for 80% reabsorption of water, electrolytes, and glucose, and interference with its function allows more filtrate than normal to be excreted. This is a reversible state in which tubular reabsorptive functions are temporarily lost or greatly diminished because of an ischemic time period that begins with clamping the renal artery in the donor and concludes with the end of the venous revascularization of the recipient.

Preservation Time. The ischemic time is prolonged in the cadaver donor situation because it may take hours to find a suitable recipient after the donor has expired and the graft has been harvested. In this situation the graft is placed on an organ preservation machine or in a preservation solution until a suitable recipient is found.

Acceptable time of preservation is under 50 hours. This preservation time, added to the extreme hypotensive period in cadaver donor patients, points out how long the ischemic period may be and why there is renal tissue damage and low output. Nevertheless, this damage is usually reversible.

The graft, in this situation, may produce either a small quantity or no urine at all for up to 4 weeks after the transplant operation. This output phase is referred to as *acute tubular necrosis.*

Lab Values. The quantity of urine does not have to correlate with the quality of graft function. Renal function is assessed by periodic serum urea nitrogen and creatinine levels and perhaps a beta$_2$–microglobulin test (B$_2$m). B$_2$m is a low molecular weight globulin that is readily filtered by the glomerular basement membrane and almost completely reabsorbed and metabolized by the proximal renal tubules.[9]

A renal scan is a radioisotope test used to determine renal perfusion, filtration, and excretion. It is frequently done in the first 24 hours as a baseline and periodically in the postoperative phase depending upon the patient's recovery and the presence of complications.

Drainage Problems. When a change in urinary output occurs, such as a large volume one hour to a diminished amount the next, mechanical factors that interfere with urinary drainage should be suspected. Clotted, kinked, or compressed tubing in the urinary drainage system may be the cause of the decreased output. When the catheter is occluded by a clot, the patient may complain of pain, feel an urgency to void, or have bloody leakage around the catheter. Milking is the preferred way to dislodge clots because irrigation, even under aseptic conditions, increases the risk of infection.

Urinary Leakage. Urinary leakage on the abdominal dressing and severe abdominal discomfort or distention may indicate retroperitoneal leakage from the ureteral anastomosis site.

Decreased urinary output or severe abdominal pain in the presence of good renal function and adequate pain medication should be reported because technical and surgical complications account for loss of graft function.

Two major types of graft anastomoses are performed. In the first type, the donor kidney is anastomosed at the ureteropelvic junction to the recipient ureter. A Foley catheter is commonly used with this anastomosis. In the second type, which is more commonly used, the donor ureter is implanted into the recipient's bladder and a Foley or ureteral catheter may be used to provide drainage.

The urinary drainage from the ureteropelvic anastomosis tends to be bloody initially but turns pink in a few hours. The urinary drainage from the second type of anastomosis tends to be bloody for the first few days, and clotting is more problematic. The urine is bloody because the bladder is very vascular and tends to bleed after being sutured. With urine outflow, some clots are carried down the catheter while others occlude the lumen.

MAINTAINING FLUID AND ELECTROLYTE BALANCE

Maintaining fluid and electrolyte balance follows the same principles outlined in Chapter 17. Intake is provided intravenously while the patient is unable to take fluids by mouth.

Flow Rate. A standard maintenance solution of 1200 ml per 24 hours for an adult is based on insensible water losses, while replacement solution is calculated for each patient according to such things as urine output, gastric and wound drainage, and central venous pressure (CVP) readings. When urinary output is high, as in post transplant diuresis, replacement will be large, while in oliguric or anuric states replacement will be small. The solutions used most often include 0.9% normal saline, 5% dextrose in water, 0.45% saline, and 2.5% dextrose in water.

Infusion Site. The slow maintenance intravenous solution may be infused through a CVP line, but large amounts of fluid, such as 500 ml, should not be infused directly into the heart. Replacement intravenous solution is generally infused through a peripheral site on the extremity that does *not* have a vascular access site. It is highly unlikely to have an infusion into a vein that has an access because if the renal graft does not function immediately, the patient will need to be dialyzed within the first few days. For this the patient will need a healthy access site.

Electrolyte Values. Serum electrolytes are drawn shortly after the patient arrives in the unit. The frequency of these tests usually depends on graft function. If the patient has a large volume of output, laboratory tests may be done every 4 or 6 hours for the first 24 to 36 hours. If the patient is anuric but otherwise stable, tests for electrolytes are done daily except for potassium, which may be ordered more frequently.

Excessive blood drawing should be kept to a minimum because the recipient is anemic in the initial recovery phase due to ESRD.

The most frequent electrolyte disturbance in the acute postoperative phase is *hyperkalemia.* Most transplant recipients are dialyzed within 24 hours before surgery and therefore have a normal serum potassium in the operating room. If the graft functions and excretes a high volume of urine, it is also generally able to excrete the

excessive serum potassium created by surgical tissue damage. If the patient is oliguric or anuric after surgery, serum potassium will increase to unacceptable levels and will need to be lowered initially by sodium polystyrene sulfonate (Kayexalate) enemas and then possibly by dialysis. Short-chain amino acid preparations (*e.g.,* Nephramine) are also used in some centers to control hyperkalemia.

PREVENTING INFECTION

Life-threatening infections are infrequent, but when present, they may compromise graft survival.

Immunosuppressive drugs are discontinued in the presence of a severe infection, allowing the patient to mobilize his immune response. Consequently, the graft may be sacrificed to save the patient. The immunosuppressive drugs decrease the patient's defense system as they work to prolong graft survival (see discussion below).

The detrimental effect of immunosuppressive therapy is that patients are more susceptible to organisms, even those normally found in the environment. Since most infections are endogenous, strict isolation technique has been abandoned in the postoperative phase. It not only creates psychological problems for the patient, but compliance by all team members is difficult to enforce. Nevertheless, visitors, nurses, and other personnel who have upper respiratory or any other type of infection should not visit or give care to the patient.

General Preventive Measures.

- Cleansing the catheter and perineal area around the urethral meatus with an antiseptic solution every 8 hours will decrease urinary tract infections.
- Changing intravenous tubing daily as well as when it is contaminated will also decrease the risk of sepsis.
- Changing wet dressings frequently will remove an excellent media for organism growth.
- Thorough handwashing before and after patient care is a simple and effective way to decrease organisms in the recipient's environment.

Avoiding Pulmonary Infections. Because pulmonary infections are high on the list of transplant recipient complications, enhancing ventilation and promoting drainage of secretions is paramount. Observing the rate and character of respirations and listening to breath sounds will help determine how often the patient should turn, deep breathe, cough, walk, use blow bottles or tubes, or need postural drainage. Transplant patients can turn to the operative side; in fact, doing so promotes wound drainage and decreases the incidence of hematomas and lymphoceles.

COMPLICATIONS OF RENAL TRANSPLANTATION

Immunity and the Rejection Phenomenon

The most frequently occurring and poorly understood noninfectious complication is *graft rejection*. This process can be confusing because just as renal failure is rarely an "all or none" phenomenon, neither is graft rejection.

Rejection can vary in degree from mild to severe reversible rejection (*i.e.,* rejection episode) to complete or irreversible rejection. Rejection episodes are reversible when treated with a variety of antirejection therapies discussed in the next section.

Antigen-Antibody Reaction. To begin to understand the rejection phenomenon, one needs to understand antigen-antibody reaction. There are two basic types of acquired immunity — humoral and cellular — and both are involved in the rejection process.*

Humoral immunity refers to the system responsible for antigen-antibody reactions. Antigens are large protein complexes that invade the body and elicit an antibody response. Antibodies are globulin molecules that are made in response to a specific antigen. Once formed, these antibodies are capable of attacking the antigen any time after the initial exposure.

Cellular immunity develops when lymphocytes become specifically sensitized against a foreign agent. Lymphocytes, which constitute about 1% of the total number of leukocytes, "bind antigen and then release a host of pharmacological factors called lymphokines which produce a specific inflammatory response that leads to the elimination of antigen."[10]

The transplanted kidney is a foreign antigen implanted in a recipient. Eventually, the recipient's body will recognize the kidney as a foreign

*For an in-depth explanation of the immune system and antigen-antibody reaction, see John Stobo's article in the bibliography.

antigen and mobilize its defense system to try to rid itself of this foreign substance. This process is called *rejection*.

It is important to realize that all transplant recipients' defense immune systems eventually see the kidney as foreign and in some way respond to it. Exceptions to this are recipients who are nonresponders. Such persons either do not respond to any foreign antigen stimulation or respond poorly to stimulation. The nonresponders, however, are few in number; therefore, what becomes important is observing how strongly the immune defensive system responds. Rejection can be broken down into four basic categories: hyperacute, accelerated, acute, and chronic.

Hyperacute rejection can occur within minutes to hours following transplantation. This may occur either because of a major blood group incompatibility or, more commonly, because preformed antibodies existed in titers too low to be detected in the tissue typing tests. There is no treatment for hyperacute rejection, and it always results in loss of the graft, which must be removed.

Accelerated rejection is a slower form of hyperacute rejection, occurring within a few days to approximately one week following the transplant. This, the second most infrequent form of rejection, is probably a function of preformed antibodies and does not respond to any form of therapy. It destroys the kidney, which must then be removed. Both hyperacute and accelerated rejection are results of humoral immunity.

Acute rejection occurs after the first postoperative week. It is the most frequently seen form of rejection and fortunately the type that responds best to therapy. During an acute rejection episode, the patient may experience any, all, or none of the following:

- Decrease in urine output
- Weight gain
- Edema
- A temperature of 100°F (37.8°C) or greater
- Tenderness over the graft site with possible swelling of the kidney itself
- General malaise
- Increased blood pressure

Other findings indicating an acute rejection episode include

- Increased serum creatinine
- Decreased urine creatinine and creatinine clearance

- Possible decrease in urine sodium
- Increased BUN
- Increased serum B_2m
- Increased urine B_2m
- Decreased blood flow as demonstrated on renal scan

Chronic rejection is a gradual deterioration of kidney function and is the result of repeated insults from acute rejection episodes. The symptoms are similar to those of acute rejection except that fever and graft enlargement may not occur.

Chronic rejection results in scarring of renal tissue and infarction of renal vessels from the vasculitis accompanying acute rejection. Therefore in chronic rejection the inflammatory signs are absent.

Laboratory findings are similar in both acute and chronic rejection, but chronic rejection also includes those changes consistent with chronic renal failure, including declining hematocrit, calcium-phosphorus imbalance, and so forth. The rate of deterioration in chronic rejection can vary, and the patient may have adequate renal function from a few months up to a year before replacement therapy is indicated.

There is no effective therapy known to treat this type of rejection. Unlike other forms of rejection, a transplant nephrectomy is not always necessary with chronic rejection because the kidney does not always become necrotic and cause a life-threatening situation.

Immunosuppression Therapy

DRUGS

As the term implies, immunosuppression is the use of drug therapy to suppress the immune response in order to permit acceptance of transplanted organs, most often with a type of tissue at least partially different from that of the recipient. The difficulty of this therapy is in providing enough suppression to prevent rejection without rendering the recipient grossly susceptible to opportunistic infections.

The drugs given to control the immune response are methylprednisolone (Solu-Medrol), prednisone, azathioprine (Imuran), cyclophosphamide (Cytoxan), and antilymphocytic globulin. Major points about these drugs are summarized in Table 18-2.

Methylprednisolone is the parenteral steroid used in the initial postoperative period, and prednisone is the most commonly used oral steroid. *Prednisone* may be given in a variety of schedules and doses, and the philosophy varies from center to center, just as it does with the use of methylprednisolone in the treatment of rejection episodes.

Treatment of rejection episodes may include

Table 18-2
Immunosuppressive Drugs Used In Renal Transplantation

Drug	Adverse Reactions	Dosage	Comments
Methylprednisolone (Solu-Medrol) (IV) Prednisone (PO)	Increased susceptibility to infection	Initial: 2–3 mg/kg of body weight, tapered to an adequate oral maintenance dose	Methylprednisolone is given up to one week post transplant and when patient is not tolerating liquids.
	Masks symptoms of infection Peptic ulcer, GI bleeding		An antacid is taken while patient is on steroids to reduce the risk of gastric irritation and ulceration. Cimetidine may also be used to decrease ulcerogenic tendencies.
	Increased appetite, weight gain		
		During rejection, methylprednisolone may be given in IV boluses up to 1 g/dose	Cardiac arrest can occur if IV bolus of 1 g is given rapidly.

Table 18–2 *(Continued)*

Drug	Adverse Reactions	Dosage	Comments
	Increased sodium and water retention which exaggerate hypertension		Sodium restriction may be necessary when steroid dosage is high or when fluid retention increases.
	Delayed healing Negative nitrogen balance Adrenal gland suppression Behavior and personality changes Diabetogenic effect Muscle weakness Osteoporosis with long-term therapy Skin atrophy, striae Easy bruising Glaucoma, cataracts Hirsutism Acne Avascular/aseptic necrosis		
Azathioprine (Imuran) (IV or PO)	Bone marrow suppression: leukopenia, thrombocytopenia, anemia, pancytopenia Rash Alopecia Liver damage, jaundice Increased susceptibility to infection	Regulated to keep WBCs 5,000 to 10,000. Drug usually stopped when WBCs 3000 or less Initial: 5–10 mg/kg of body weight Maintenance: 2–3 mg/kg of body weight During rejection: maximum of 3 mg/kg of body weight	Lower doses are given when 1. Renal function is poor 2. Given concurrently with allopurinol, which delays metabolism of azathioprine (allopurinol and azathioprine are synergistic)
Cyclophosphamide (Cytoxan) (PO)	Leukopenia, thrombocytopenia Increased susceptibility to infections Metabolites are direct irritants to bladder mucosa and may cause hemorrhagic cystitis Alopecia	1–2 mg/kg (or ½ to ⅔ of Imuran dosage)	Given in place of azathioprine when it causes hepatotoxicity Suggest administration upon awakening to avoid accumulation of metabolites while sleeping Observe for hematuria Encourage fluid intake to dilute metabolites
Antilymphocyte globulin (ALG) Antithymocyte globulin (ATG) (IV, IM, or deep SC)	Anaphylactic shock due to hypersensitivity to animal serum Fever (up to 105°F or 40.6°C) and chills Increased susceptibility to infections due to decreased lymphocytes IM or deep SC injection site may be swollen, red, and painful, with abscess formation Difficulty walking if IM or SC injection given in thigh	Dosage may vary	Skin test for hypersensitivity to animal serum before giving initial dose Lymphocytes or platelets decrease sharply with drug administration; therefore, draw bloodwork for lymphocyte and platelet counts before infusion is started

intravenous injections of methylprednisolone in boluses up to 1 g per dose. It is recommended that it be administered over 20 to 30 minutes. This is particularly important because several cardiac arrests have been reported following the administration of 1 g of methylprednisolone delivered by intravenous push.

Azathioprine, an antimetabolite, is the mainstay of immunosuppression. The patient's ability to consistently tolerate 2 to 3 mg per kg dosage is important for long-term graft survival. Azathioprine cannot be increased to treat rejection because of its bone marrow suppression effects and its cumulative effects in the presence of little or no renal function.

Cyclophosphamide, an alkylating agent is used only in the presence of hepatotoxicity from whatever source. It has been shown to be inferior to azathioprine in prolonging graft survival but represents the most viable alternative to azathioprine therapy. The development of hemorrhagic cystitis increases the risk for later development of cancer of the bladder and also necessitates discontinuation of therapy.

Antilymphocyte or *antithymocyte globulin* is used in a number of centers in an effort to prevent rejection by providing the patient with antibodies against lymphocytes or thymocytes, which are the cells responsible for rejection. These antibodies are produced by injecting human lymph or thymus cells into an animal (horse, rabbit, or goat), which then produces antibodies against these cells.

RADIATION

Radiation therapy given locally to the graft is sometimes used as an adjunct to conventional immunosuppressive therapy during a rejection episode. This therapy has been used since the 1960s, and reports of its efficacy have ranged from beneficial to ineffective. It continues to be used in some centers.

THORACIC DUCT DRAINAGE

Thoracic duct drainage (TDD) has been used since the 1960s by a diminishing number of centers. TDD involves cannulation of the left thoracic duct to remove lymph fluid. The purpose of lymph removal is to reduce the number of lymphocytes available that could become involved in the rejection process. The procedure is usually carried out for several weeks to one month prior to transplantation depending upon the amount of lymph fluid removed.

TDD requires hospitalization for the duration of drainage because the patient's physiological status must be carefully monitored. Fluid and protein replacement are required, and thus, close monitoring of the fluid and electrolyte balance is necessary; some patients may drain as much as one liter per hour.

Inclusion of TDD as part of the immunosuppressive protocol has been disappointing in that improved graft survival has not been consistently demonstrated. Furthermore, it is costly, increases risk to the patient, and prolongs the patient's hospital course.

NEWER APPROACHES

Newer approaches to immunosuppression in the 1980s include Cyclosporin A (CyA) and sublethal levels of total lymphoid irradiation (TLI).

CyA was discovered in Europe and has seen only limited use in controlled clinical trials in the United States. It is a potent immunosuppressive drug that has been studied as the sole immunosuppressive agent as well as in conjunction with other immunosuppressive drugs. Major known side-effects to date include nephrotoxicity, hepatotoxicity, marked hirsutism, tremors, and gum hypertrophy. Its immunosuppressive effects are greatly potentiated when used in combination with other immunosuppressive drugs.[11]

TLI has been used by very few centers and predominantly in massively sensitized patients. Early results with TLI in kidney transplantation suggest that it is most effective when bone marrow from the renal donor is also transplanted.

TLI and CyA have both been associated with an increased incidence of lymphomas. While both remain investigational, CyA seems the most promising agent to alter the immune system to allow for prolonged graft survival.

Infection

One of the greatest crises for the recipient is sepsis because it is still one of the greatest threats to recipient survival. The origin of sepsis may be the blood (septicemia); a single organ, such as the liver, lungs, or pancreas; or the entire body (*i.e.,* a disseminated infection) may be involved.

The pathogens vary from the more commonly seen bacterial organisms to fungal, viral, or even protozoan organisms. The latter organisms are referred to as *opportunistic pathogens.* These organisms, normally found in humans and in the environment, are generally considered harmless. However, the patient with a compromised immune system, such as a transplant recipient, is susceptible to infections from these organisms: thus the term *opportunistic,* since the microorganisms take advantage of the decreased host defenses. Specific examples of these opportunistic infections include herpes simplex, herpes zoster, *Candida albicans,* Aspergillus, Cryptococcus, Nocardia, pneumocystis carinii, and cytomegalovirus (CMV). The presence of any of these infections should be monitored closely because they could pose life-threatening crises.

Oral monilial infections are common, and precautions should be taken to prevent the development of or progression to monilial esophagitis, a serious infectious complication. Precautions should include daily observation of the mouth. Appearance of oral moniliasis should be treated with oral Mycostatin.

If immunosuppressive therapy is reduced or discontinued in the presence of a life-threatening situation resulting from an opportunistic infection, the emphasis *must* be on the patient's life rather than on the graft. Therefore, rejection of the graft is permitted in an effort to save the patient's life. If the graft is totally rejected, the patient is supported with dialysis therapy, and once the infectious process is resolved, the patient can then be considered for retransplantation.

Another problem that contributes to loss of renal function is the antibiotic therapy necessary to control the infection. Amphotericin B, a drug used to treat the fungal infections, is nephrotoxic in that it decreases renal perfusion. The use of mannitol in the amphotericin B solution can counteract the problem of decreased perfusion because it increases renal perfusion. Because many antibiotics and antifungal agents are nephrotoxic, treatment of infections can pose difficult management problems.

Cardiovascular Complications

Although cardiovascular accidents can occur in the acute postoperative period, more frequently they occur a year after transplant and are considered late complications of transplantation. Should the complications occur in the early postoperative period, graft survival and vascular problems are of concern. However, if they occur as late complications of transplantation, graft function has usually stabilized, and vascular complications are the major concern. Patients with a functioning graft may succumb to this type of complication. As stated earlier, it is unclear what the effects of transplantation are upon the atherosclerotic process and subsequent cardiovascular complications.

Since the early 1970s, higher risk patients, such as those with diabetes, vasculitis, systemic lupus erythematosus, and those 50 to 70 years old, have had transplants. In fact, patients with cardiac disease treated by coronary bypass surgery have later received renal transplants. Perhaps these higher risks have contributed to an increase in death from vascular complications. Since there is an increasing patient population 10 years or more post transplant, there is more opportunity to study the etiology of the long-term cardiovascular complications.

GI Complications

GI complications may pose serious and even life-threatening situations for the recipient.

Ischemic bowel disease has been observed in the early post transplant period, but the appearance of this problem and its association with transplantation are uncertain.

Massive GI bleeding may occur as the result of steroid therapy, stress, and the decreased viability of tissues due to earlier protein restrictions.

GI complications most often will occur in the acute postoperative phase, at the point when graft survival is still of major concern. Again, forfeiture of the graft may be necessary in an effort to save the patient's life.

Other serious GI complications include acute pancreatitis, obstruction from bowel adhesions, and ulcerative colitis. Should the patient have an intestinal perforation, then not only is the GI complication a threat, but so is infection.

It should therefore be stressed that a transplant recipient may have one or more of these complications simultaneously, increasing the complexity of both medical and nursing care. The following patient situations point out how interwoven complications may become and how necessary it is to observe for their subtle clues.

Patient Situation No. 1

A 54-year-old recipient of a cadaver kidney was admitted with a fever of 102°F (38.9°C) and lethargy. Diagnostic tests showed chronic rejection with azotemia and bowel obstruction. Laparotomy and a temporary colostomy were performed. The patient returned to hemodialysis three times per week. The abdominal incision became infected with *Escherichia coli,* while pulmonary atelectasis in the postoperative period progressed to infectious pneumonia. Within one week, the patient required intubation and ventilatory support. She was placed in a critical care area. She then developed secondary iatrogenic diabetes mellitus as another complication of steroid therapy. Within a few weeks, she died from disseminated intravascular coagulation and overwhelming, irreversible lung infection.

Patient Situation No. 2

A 50-year-old man was the recipient of a cadaver transplant. The patient was known to have renin-dependent hypertension and was receiving propranolol four times per day. Throughout the immediate post transplant period, the patient complained of "gas pains." Due to this chronic complaint, an evaluation was undertaken but with negative findings. Approximately 3 weeks post transplant, a duodenal ulcer perforated. Because of steroid therapy, the symptoms of perforation were masked to the extent that none of the classic signs of peritonitis were present. In addition, the myocardial effects of propranolol therapy prevented the patient's heart from responding to the sympathetic drive, and as a result his apical rate never varied from approximately 60, in spite of his perforation. About 8 hours following the perforation, the patient's blood pressure began to drop, and bowel sounds were no longer heard. The diagnosis of perforation was made. Thus, the combination of drugs markedly masked the otherwise classic symptoms the patient might have demonstrated.

The need for nurses to be aware of drug actions such as those described above cannot be overemphasized. Constant and thorough evaluation is mandatory in caring for this very complex group of patients. Detailed information concerning the infectious complications, cardiovascular problems, and GI complications of the transplant recipient is not within the scope of this chapter, and the reader is referred to the bibliography.

Hypertension

Hypertension is a common but often transitory complication following renal transplantation. Many patients requiring chronic antihypertensive therapy are hypertensive before the transplant, and their hypertension is made worse by posttransplant steroid therapy. Various factors are responsible for posttransplant hypertension.

STEROID-INDUCED HYPERTENSION

Transplant recipients are placed on steroids, usually prednisone or methylprednisolone. Although these are glucocorticoids, they are converted into mineralocorticoids and cause sodium and water retention. While patients may be on a sodium-restricted diet, drug therapy is often necessary. Spironolactone, an aldosterone-blocking agent, is often useful in treating steroid-induced hypertension, along with the diuretic, hydrochlorothiazide. Nurses must monitor for potential electrolyte imbalances (specifically, hyponatremia and hypokalemia) and instruct the patient and his family about the signs and symptoms of these imbalances and what to do should they occur.

The effect of these drugs does not occur immediately, and therefore electrolyte imbalances are usually not seen until several days after the medications are started. At this time, a brisk diuresis may follow, increasing the potential for both hypovolemia and electrolyte imbalances. Because rapid fluid loss will result in weight loss, the patient's weight should be carefully recorded.

RENIN-DEPENDENT HYPERTENSION

While steroid treatment is one mechanism that causes post transplant hypertension, a second mechanism, renin-dependent hypertension, is seen rather frequently.

Immediately following the transplant procedure, the recipient may have markedly elevated blood pressure. Due to the ischemic injury to the organ between time of removal and time of implantation, excessive amounts of renin may be released. Once adequate circulation has been established within the organ, this mechanism should "turn off," resulting in a return of the pressure to the preoperative level within a few days following the transplant.

While renin itself is not a potent vasoconstrictor, its conversion to angiotensin I and angiotensin II causes vasoconstriction. The immediate postoperative period is not the only time in the progress of the transplant recipient's course that renin-dependent hypertension can occur.

Hypertension may be one of the first clinical manifestations of rejection. The basis of this hypertension is excessive renin production. Since rejection is an inflammatory response, vasculitis within the kidney impedes normal circulation and results in elevated renin levels. Renin levels are elevated in virtually all patients who have hypertension during an acute rejection episode. This phenomenon occurs in chronic rejection as well. Therefore, the nurse should pose the question of ensuing rejection when first detecting an elevated blood pressure.

Renal artery stenosis can also result in renin-dependent hypertension. The stenosis may cause a decrease in renal perfusion leading to increased renin production. When this occurs, an abdominal bruit may be auscultated lateral to the midline and medial to the kidney. The sudden appearance of a bruit or an increase in an abdominal bruit previously present is strongly suggestive of a renal artery stenosis. Surgical correction of the stenosis is almost always successful, and there is rarely loss of renal function as a result of the surgery. In fact, loss of renal function is more likely to occur when surgery is not performed.

Drug Therapy. Metoprolol tartrate (Lopressor) and propranolol (Inderal) are often used to treat renin–dependent hypertension because they act as renin inhibitors. Because these drugs are cardiac depressants, congestive heart failure may result from prolonged use. The use of a diuretic may help to avoid this complication. However, the use of catecholamine–depleting agents such as reserpine is unwise because the patient is unable to respond to a sympathetic drive, owing to the adrenergic blocking effects.

Minoxidil has been effective in treating renin–dependent hypertension that does not respond to therapy with a sympathetic blocker alone. A potent vasodilator, it is usually given with a diuretic such as furosemide because of the sodium and fluid retention it causes. A sympathetic blocker is also advisable to offset the tachycardia minoxidil creates. Hirsutism, the major obvious side effect of minoxidil, can be very distressing to the patient and may actually affect compliance with this therapeutic regimen.

VOLUME-DEPENDENT HYPERTENSION

Volume-dependent hypertension is another problem for the transplant recipient. During rejection episodes or periods of acute tubular necrosis, the patient may become fluid-overloaded due to inadequate fluid output from the kidney.

If the patient does not respond to diuretic therapy, the use of dialysis may be indicated to further control the hypervolemic and hypertensive state until renal function recovers. The development of malignant hypertension precipitating hypertensive crisis is managed as with any other patient.

DRUG PRECAUTIONS

The antihypertensive medications mentioned above are by no means an inclusive list. Many other drugs are appropriate and useful, and those mentioned only represent examples. However, problems associated with antihypertensive therapy are not unique to the transplant patient. Lethargy, impotence, and orthostatic hypotension are just some of the untoward effects of such therapy. However, once renal function has become stable, the patient's steroid dose has been reduced, and his urine output is satisfactory, the need for antihypertensive medications is markedly reduced.

A PATIENT'S VIEW

How do patients who have experienced many complications view their decision to have a renal transplant? One patient received a cadaver transplant that chronically rejected after 3½ years, underwent bilateral total hip replacements for aseptic necrosis, and had impaired vision due to cataracts. When asked if it had been worth it to him to be off dialysis and whether he would like to receive a new kidney graft, he responded without question or hesitation with an emphatic, "Absolutely!"

People who have had successful renal transplantation, even in the face of complications, state unequivocally that they would not alter their decision to have received a renal graft. It is the success of such patients and their appreciation of new lives that makes transplantation a challenging and richly rewarding field.

REFERENCES

1. Hodgson S: Anemia associated with chronic renal failure and chronic dialysis. Nephrol Nurse 2:43–46, 1980
2. Schweizer R, Bartus S: Gastroduodenal ulceration in renal transplant patients. Conn Med 42:85–88, 1978
3. Archibald S, Jirsch D, Bear R: Gastrointestinal complications of renal transplantation, II: The colon. Can Med Assoc J 119:1301–1305, 1978
4. Welch J, Schweizer R, Bartus S: Management of antacid impactions in hemodialysis and renal transplant patients. Am J Surg 139:561–568, 1980
5. Cochrum KC, Hanes D, Potter D, et al: Donor-specific blood transfusions in HLA-D-disparite 1-haplotype-related allograft. Transplant Proc 11:1903–1907, 1979
6. ESRD Office of Special Programs, Department of Health and Human Services: Facility Survey Report. Baltimore, Health Care Financing Administration, Office of Special Programs, 1979
7. A Report by the Task Force on Death and Dying of the Institute of Society, Ethics and the Life Sciences: Refinements in criteria for the determination of death: An appraisal. JAMA 221:48–53, 1972
8. Fulton J, Fulton R, Simmons R: The cadaver donor and the gift of life. In Simmons R, Klein S, Simmons R (eds): The Social and Psychological Impact of Organ Transplantation, pp 338–376. New York, John Wiley & Sons, 1977
9. Vincent C, Revillard JP, Pellet H, et al: B$_2$—Microglobulin in monitoring renal transplant function. Transplant Proc 11:438, 1979
10. Dwyer JM: Understanding modern immunology: I. The development of the human immune system. Conn Med 39:170–174, 1975

11. Calne RY, Rolles K, Thiru S, et al: Cyclosporin A initially as the only immunosuppressant in 34 recipients of cadaveric organs: 32 kidneys, 2 pancreases and 2 livers. Lancet 2:1033–1036, 1979

BIBLIOGRAPHY

Anderson RJ, Gambertoglio JD, Schrier RW: Clinical Use of Drugs in Renal Failure. Springfield, Charles C. Thomas, 1976

Blount M, Kinney AB: Chronic steroid therapy. Am J Nurs, 74:1623–1631, 1974

Campbell J, Campbell A: The social and economic costs of end-stage renal disease. N Engl J Med, 299:386–392, 1978

Chatterjee S: Immunology of infections in transplant recipients. Dial Transplant, 9:135–138, 1980

DeLuca H: Vitamin D metabolism. Clin Endocrinol, 7(suppl):15–17s, 1977

Friedman B, Newmark K: Orthopedic problems in renal patients. Dial Transplant, 4:71–72, 1975

Harrington JD, Brener ER: Patient Care in Renal Failure. Philadelphia, W. B. Saunders, 1976

Haynes RC, Larner J: Adrenocorticotropic hormone; adrenocortical steroids and their synthetic analogs; inhibitors of adrenocortical steroid B_{10} synthesis. In Goodman L, Gilman A (eds): The Pharmacological Basis of Therapeutics, 5th ed, pp 1472–1498. New York, Macmillan, 1975

Jonasson O: Emergencies in renal transplantation. Surg Clin North Am, 52:257–264, 1972

Lamb J: Organ transplantation: Recognizing the donor. Am J Nurs, 80:1600–1601, 1980

Lancaster L (ed): The Patient with End-Stage Renal Disease. New York, John Wiley and Sons, 1979

Lazarus JM: Uremia: A clinical guide. Hosp Med, 15:52–73, 1979

Mandell GL, Hook EW: Opportunistic infections. Hosp Med, 4:40–48, 1968

Opelz G, Terasaki PI: Improvement of kidney graft survival with increased numbers of blood transfusions. N Engl J Med, 299:799–803, 1978

Robbins KC: Hypertension in the renal transplant recipient. J Am Assoc Nephrol Nurses Technicians, 2:171–177, 1975

Sachs B: Renal Transplantation: A Nursing Perspective. Flushing, Medical Examination Publishing Company, 1977

Salvatierra O, et al: The advantages of ^{131}I-orthoidohippurate scintophotography in the management of patients after renal transplantion. Ann Surg, 180:336–342, 1974

Stobo JD: Basic mechanisms of immunity. Hosp Med, 16:22–32, 1980

Strobele B: How to counsel patients on cortisone. RN 38:57–60, 1975

Taylor J, Sadler B, Turk M: Thoracic duct lymph drainage as an adjunct to renal transplantation. Nephrol Nurse, 1:12–16, 1979

Thomas FT, Lee HM: Factors in the differential rate of arteriosclerosis (A.S.) between long surviving renal transplant recipients and dialysis patients. Ann Surg 184:342–351, 1976

Veith FJ: Brain death and organ transplantation. Ann NY Acad Sci, 315:417–441, 1978

Wolf ZR: What patients awaiting kidney transplant want to know. Am J Nurs, 76:92–94, 1976

Section D   Nervous System

Barbara Fuller

Normal Structure and Function of the Nervous System 19

With the evolutionary advent of multicellularity, two needs arose: internal transport and communication-coordination of the parts. The first need is met by the circulatory system and the second need by the nervous system. The latter is the topic of this chapter.

The nervous system traditionally is discussed in both anatomic and functional divisions. Anatomic components are the central nervous system (CNS) (brain and spinal cord) and the peripheral nervous system (spinal and cranial nerves). Functional divisions are the sensory, interpretive, and motor (somatic and autonomic) divisions.

First, let us examine the cells; then we will look at the (1) CNS, (2) sensory pathways, (3) motor division, including the autonomic, and (4) reflexes. This organizational pattern is chosen because it hopefully affords minimal repetition and maximal integration.

CELLS OF THE NERVOUS SYSTEM

The cellular units are the *neuron* — the basic functional unit — together with its attendant cells, the *neuroglias* and *Schwann cells*. It may, perhaps, be easier to treat the attendant cells first and then proceed to neuronal functioning.

Neuroglial Cells

The neuroglial cells are the supportive tissue that lies within the CNS around the neurons. There are three types of glial cells: microglia, astrocytes, and oligodendroglia. These last cells are thought to produce the myelin that covers nerve fibers within the CNS.

While neurons lose their ability to undergo mitosis early in the life of the individual, neuroglial cells seem to retain mitotic abilities throughout the individual's life span. Because of this, nonmetastatic CNS lesions involve glial cells rather than neurons. As the glian tumor enlarges, however, it does adversely affect adjacent neurons early by exerting pressure and later by promoting an inflammatory reaction along with the pressure. The counterpart of the myelin-producing oligodendroglial cell in the peripheral nervous system is the cell of Schwann.

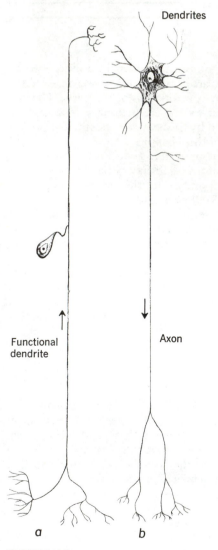

FIGURE 19-1.
(a) Unipolar neuron; *(b)* multipolar neuron.

Neurons

As stated earlier, the basic functional unit of the nervous system is the *neuron,* and all information and activity, whether sensory, motor, or integrative, is processed by it.

The precise characteristic of individual neurons is determined by their specific function. Some are extremely large and may give rise to extremely long nerve fibers. Transmission velocities in the long fibers may be as high as 100 m per second, while smaller neurons with very small fibers demonstrate velocities of 1 m per second. Some neurons connect to many different neurons in a "network," and still others have few connections to other cells of the nervous system.

It has been estimated that there are 12 billion neurons in the CNS. Three-fourths of these neurons are located in the cerebral cortex, where information transmitted through the nervous system is processed. This processing, as indicated above, includes not only the determination of appropriate and effective responses, but also the storage of memory and the development of associative motor and thought patterns.

Neuron Structure.   The neuron is also termed a *nerve cell.* It consists of a nerve cell body that contains nuclear and cytoplasmic material and processes arising from this. These processes are functionally differentiated into axons and dendrites (see Fig. 19-1). *Axons* normally carry nervous impulses away from the cell body, whereas *dendrites* conduct the impulse toward the cell body. Axons and dendrites may be merely microscopic knobs or areas on the cell body surface or they may be cylindrical processes that can, in certain cases, extend up to 4 ft in length.

Neurons do not connect to one another. There are spaces between the axon(s) of one neuron and the dendrite(s) of another. This space is termed the *synapse.* Axons and dendrites may branch, enabling the axon of one neuron to synapse with dendrites of more than one other neuron. Similarly, a neuron may synoptically receive axons from several neurons. The former is an example of *divergence;* the latter exemplifies *convergence.*

Transmitter Action.   One neuron may stimulate or inhibit another by chemical transmission across the synapse. This involves the synthesis of the transmitter by the first neuron. Transmitter packets are then stored in the end(s) of its axon(s). As a nervous impulse passes down the axon, it triggers the release of a certain number of transmitter packets. These chemicals then diffuse across the synapse, where they temporarily attach to receptor binding sites on the dendrite surface.

While the transmitter is bound to the receptor site, the dendritic area is either stimulated (depolarized or hypopolarized) or inhibited (hyperpolarized). Most chemical transmitters are stimulators. Only one, gamma-aminobutyric-acid (GABA), is known to hyperpolarize a neuron.

Within an extremely short interval, millionths of a second, the transmitter detaches from the binding site. It may then reattach or be inactivated. The latter occurs in two basic ways, depending upon the chemical.

One transmitter, *norepinephrine,* diffuses back into the axon to be reused another time. Another transmitter, *acetylcholine,* is destroyed by the chemical, *cholinesterase,* which is normally found at the binding site. In either case, the availability of a transmitter that can attach to the binding sites is temporally restricted. This enables rapid, repetitive, discrete stimulation (or inhibition) of neurons, a necessary factor in the functioning of the nervous system. From this picture we can see that synaptic transmission is a one-way street — that is, from the axon across the synapse to the dendrite of the next neuron. It cannot proceed in the opposite direction.

Sodium Pump in Nerve Impulses.

Now, let us examine the nervous impulse that causes the release of transmitter and that is the essence of neuronal activity in itself. It is essentially the same as that described in the chapter dealing with the normal physiology of the heart.

Briefly, the neuronal membrane contains sodium pumps that keep the inside of the neuron more negatively charged than the outside interstitial fluid. As in cardiac tissue, the cytoplasm of the neuron contains anions (negatively charged particles) that are too large to leave the cell. These electrochemically attract, in part, positively charged potassium ions (potassium is also pumped into the neuron) and positively charged sodium ions as well. If this were all that happened, the influx of positively charged ions would counterbalance the negatively charged ones, electroneutrality would be established within the neuron, and nothing further could occur. However, the active transport enzyme system within the neuronal membrane pumps sodium out of the cell almost as fast as it enters. Even though potassium is pumped into the cell, this is insufficient to counterbalance the anions.

Thus, the inside of the neuron remains negative with respect to the outside as long as the sodium pumps are operating. This, then, is the *resting polarity* of the neuron; it is typically -85 mv.

A stimulus acts locally to turn off sodium pumps. This causes a local influx of sodium and a consequent local *depolarization*. If enough pumps are temporarily inactivated, this can result in a depolarization that is large enough to inactivate sodium pumps in adjacent areas.

A depolarization of such self-propagating magnitude is termed an *action potential*. It is the essence of a nervous impulse. An action potential is a discrete temporary event because the sodium pump can be only temporarily inactivated. Once it turns back on, the electrical events reverse, and the resting potential is once again restored.

The electrical activity embodied in the action potential can be monitored in certain clinical situations. For example, the electroencephalogram depicts multiple action potentials from surface neurons of the brain.

Neuronal Thresholds.

The stimulus that initiated depolarization may be threefold: (1) an action potential traveling to that area from elsewhere on the cell; (2) a sensory receptor potential; and (3) the binding of a synaptic transmitter with the past synaptic binding sites. The last two categories of stimuli possess the property of *additivity*. A small degree of such stimulation will not be sufficient to cause an action potential. It can only cause a state of local depolarization. The extent of this stimulus is therefore termed *subthreshold*. The additivity occurs when two or more subthreshold stimuli occur close enough together in time to trigger an action potential.

In addition to this principle, chemical transmitters can interact in the following way. A certain amount of an inhibitor transmitter (*e.g.,* GABA) can counteract a given amount of a stimulating transmitter. This could occur when neuron A receives both an inhibiting stimulus from neuron B and a stimulating one from neuron C. In this case neuron A would not be activated. If, however, it received twice the stimulus from C as it did from B, it would be stimulated, but only half as much as it would be if C acted alone on A.

These principles underlie much of the normal functioning of cord internuncials and spinal reflexes. For example, certain descending fibers from the brain stem deliver a low-level subthreshold stimulation to certain cord neurons.

This stimulation, while insufficient to activate cord neurons, is enough of a background stimulus to make it easier for other input to fully excite these neurons. Such subthreshold stimuli would be said to be *facilitatory*. When the cord is severed, the distal portion is also separated from receipt of such facilitatory brain stem influences. As a result, it takes greater stimuli to cause action potentials in the neurons in this part of the cord than before. Indeed, when initially separated from the brain, these cord neurons do not function noticeably at all for a few weeks. Such a condition is termed *cord shock*. In it, no reflexes are possible.

Neuronal thresholds can also be influenced by hormones. *Thyroxin* lowers thresholds of certain neurons, and one sign of hyperthyroidism is exaggerated cord reflexes such as the knee jerk and ankle jerk.

Now let us look at the often times confusing terminology concerning the nervous system. A nerve cell is called a *neuron*. A *nerve fiber* is a nonspecific term referring to either a single axon or dendrite. A *nerve* means a bundle of nerve fibers. Thus, a nerve will not contain any nerve cell bodies. *Ganglion* is a term denoting a collection of nerve cell bodies.

CENTRAL NERVOUS SYSTEM

More details can be found in other textbooks devoted solely to this system. The reader is referred to these sources for in-depth discussions. The purpose of this section is to briefly treat major functions so that their abnormalities can be associated with specific brain damage in other chapters.

The CNS comprises the brain and spinal cord. It receives sensory input by way of sensory fibers (dendrites) within spinal and cranial nerves and sends out motor impulses by way of axons in these same nerves. The CNS also contains large numbers of neurons that are entirely contained within it. These neurons are termed *internuncial neurons* or *interneurons* and may exist within brain and cord or connect the one with the other. Let us briefly treat each of the seven major parts of the brain and then the spinal cord.

Cerebrum

Each of the two (left and right) cerebral hemispheres contains a layer of cortex, six cells deep, covering the surface. Underneath this is white matter (nerve fibers). Deep within each hemisphere are several collections of nerve cell bodies

termed the *basal ganglia* and a lateral ventricle containing cerebrospinal fluid. The left and right hemispheres are connected and communicate with each other by a transverse band of nerve fibers termed the *corpus callosum*. Each hemisphere has four lobes named for and generally underlying each of the following skull bones: frontal, parietal, temporal, and occipital. For the most part, each hemisphere serves the contralateral side of the body (fibers cross over in the CNS).

One notable exception is Broca's speech area. This area of cortex subserves all motor speech functions and is located in a posterolateral area of the left frontal lobe for all right-handed and many left-handed persons. Damage to this area in an adult produces motor aphasia.

Cortex. The cortex is thought to operate in all higher mental functions such as judgment, language, memory, creativity, and abstract thinking. It also functions in the perception, localization, and meaning of all sensations, as well as governing all voluntary and especially discrete motor activities (see Fig. 19-2). Various areas of the cortex have been identified as having different motor and sensory functions, but some of these areas are being implicated in other functions as well (*e.g.,* the occipital area is now known to function in some learning processes of blind individuals). Many areas of the cerebrum operate together to produce coordinated human function. Let us look at communication as an example.

Verbal communication is dependent upon the ability to interpret speech and to translate thought into speech. Ideas are usually communicated between individuals by either spoken or written word. With the spoken word the sensory input of information occurs through the primary auditory cortex. In auditory association areas the sounds are interpreted as words and the words as sentences. These sentences are then interpreted by the common integrative area of the cerebral cortex as thoughts.

The common integrative area also develops thoughts to be communicated. Letters seen by the eyes are associated as words, thoughts, and sentences in the visual association area and integrated into thought in this area also. Operating in conjunction with facial regions of the somesthetic sensory area, the common integrative area initiates a series of impulses, each representing a syllable or word, and transmits them to the secondary motor area controlling the larynx and mouth.

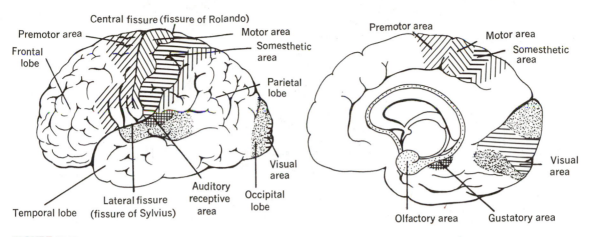

FIGURE 19-2.
Diagram of the localization of function in the cerebral hemisphere. Various functional areas are shown in relation to the lobes and fissures: *(left)* lateral view; *(right)* medial view.

The speech center, in addition to controlling motor activity of the larynx and mouth, sends impulses to the respiratory center of the secondary motor cortex to provide appropriate breath patterns for the speech process.

Basal Ganglia. The basal ganglia function in cooperation with other lower brain parts in providing circuitry for basic and subconscious bodily movements. They provide (1) the necessary background muscle tone for discrete voluntary movements, (2) smoothness and coordination in functions of muscle antagonists, and (3) the basic automatic subconscious rhythmic movements involved in walking and equilibrium maintenance. Lesions of these basal ganglia will produce various clinical abnormalities such as chorea, hemiballismus, and Parkinson's disease.

Diencephalon

Below the cerebrum lies the next brain area, the diencephalon. This area contains the third ventricle and the thalamus. Below is the hypothalamus and above is the epithalamus or pineal gland (see Fig. 19-3). The diencephalon is the most superior portion of what most authors call the *brain stem* (diencephalon, midbrain, pons, and medulla).

The *thalamus* functions as a sensory and motor relay center. It relays sensory impulses, including those of sight and sound, up to the cortex. It also functions in a gross awareness of certain sensations, most notably that of pain. Discrete localization and the finer perceptual details are

cortical functions, but the remaining awareness occurs at the thalamic and even midbrain areas.

It also has other cells, the axons of which travel to association areas of the cortex. The function of these cells and the cortical areas to which they attach is presently unknown.

Lastly, the thalamus possesses some of the fiber tracts of the reticular activating systems that function in promoting consciousness and possibly some aspects of attention.

Hypothalamus

The hypothalamus is the seat of neuroendocrine interaction. It is here that various neurosecretory substances are produced — hormones that were previously attributed to the posterior pituitary (antidiuretic hormone [ADH] and oxytocin) and that stimulate or inhibit the secretion of anterior pituitary hormones.

This area of the brain also contains centers for (1) coordinated parasympathetic and sympathetic stimulation, (2) temperature regulation, (3) appetite regulation, (4) regulation of water balance by ADH, and (5) affecting certain rhythmic psychobiological activities (*e.g.,* sleep).

The hypothalamus is part of another brain subsystem called the *limbic system.* It comprises, in addition to the hypothalamus, the cingulate gyrus of the cortex, the amygdala and hippocampus within the temporal lobes of the cerebrum, and the septum and interconnecting fiber tracts among these areas. The limbic system provides a neural substrate for emotions (terror, intense pleasure, eroticism, etc.). Also, it is here that neural pathways provide a connection be-

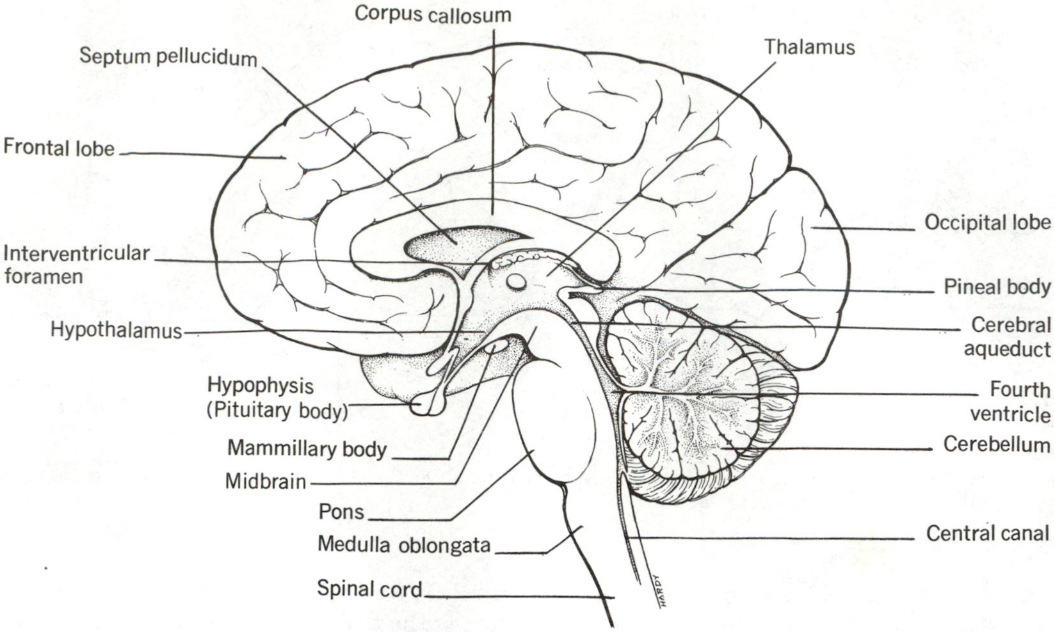

FIGURE 19-3.
Midsagittal section of the brain.

tween higher brain functioning and endocrine-autonomic activities.

Midbrain and Brain Stem

The midbrain lies between the diencephalon and the pons of the brain stem. It contains the aqueduct of Sylvius, many ascending and descending nerve fiber tracts, and centers for auditory and visually stimulated nerve impulses. It is here that the *Edinger-Westphal nucleus* is located. This nucleus contains the autonomic reflex centers for pupillary accommodations to light. It receives fibers from the retina by way of cranial nerve II and emits motor impulses by way of sympathetic and parasympathetic (cranial nerve III) fibers to the smooth muscles of the iris. Impaired pupillary accommodation signifies that either one or more of these inputs or outputs is damaged or that the midbrain itself is suffering insult (often from tentorial herniation or cerebral vascular accident [CVA]). The midbrain also houses fiber tracts of the *reticular activating system* (RAS), a system we will discuss soon.

The *pons varolli* lies between the midbrain and the medulla oblongata of the brain stem and has cell bodies of fibers contained in cranial nerves V, VI, VII, and VIII. It contains pneumotoxic and apneustic respiratory centers and fiber tracts connecting higher and lower centers including the cerebellum.

The *medulla* lies between the pons and the cord. It contains autonomic centers that regulate such vital functions as breathing, cardiac rate, and vasomotor tone as well as centers for vomiting, gagging, coughing, and sneezing reflex behaviors. It also contains the fourth ventricle. Cranial nerves IX to XII have their cell bodies in this area. Impairment in any of these vital functions or reflexes suggests medullary damage.

The brain stem's motor functions also include maintaining bodily support against gravity and maintaining equilibrium. Located within the brain stem is the structural area in which these latter two integrative functions occur, the *bulboreticular formation*. This area receives information from a variety of sources that include all areas of the peripheral sensory receptors via the spinal cord, the cerebellum, the inner-ear equilibrium apparatus, the motor cortex, and the basal ganglia. The bulboreticular area, then, is an integrative area for sensory information, motor information from the cerebral cortex, equilibrium information from the vestibular apparatus, and proprioceptive information from the cerebellum; it also controls many involuntary muscular activities.

Also in the stem are located centers (the raphe

nucleus and the locus ceruleus) responsible for the initiation of sleep and its various stages.

Cerebellum

The cerebellum is located just superior and posterior to the medulla. It receives "samples" of all ascending somesthetic sensory input as well as of all descending motor impulses. Use of these connections enables the cerebellum to match intended motor stimuli (before they reach the muscles) with actual sensory data. This ensures optimal match for voluntary motor "intention" with actual motor action, with time to alter the motor message in case of error. It sends its own messages up to the basal ganglia and cortex, as well as to parts of the brain stem, in order to perform three basic subconscious functions.

The cerebellum functions to (1) produce smooth, steady harmonious and coordinated skeletal muscle actions, (2) maintain equilibrium, and (3) control posture without any jerky or uncompensated movements or swaying.

Cerebellum disease can produce certain symptoms, the most prominent of which are disturbances of gait, equilibrium ataxia (overstability or understability of the walk), and tremors.

Reticular Activating System (RAS) and Levels of Consciousness

The RAS is an ascending fiber system originating in the midbrain and thalamus. Branches extend up to the cortex. In this way, the RAS can stimulate the cortex. The RAS is itself stimulated by the arrival of a variety of sensory impulses and chemical stimuli from various sources. These include input from the optic and acoustic cranial nerves, somesthetic impulses from the dorsal column and spinothalamic pathways, and fibers from the cerebral cortex. In addition, it is stimulated by norepinephrine and epinephrine.

The stimulation of the cortex by the RAS seems to be the major physiological basis for producing consciousness, alertness, and attention to various environmental stimuli. Decreased activity of the RAS produces decreased alertness or levels of consciousness including stupor and coma. Inactivation of the RAS can result from anything that interrupts the entry of a critical amount of sensory input or by any damage that prevents the RAS fibers from sending impulses to the cortex.

Total inactivation of the RAS will produce coma. During sleep, however, the RAS is believed to be inactivated by impulses from certain brain stem nuclei that are responsible for the onset of sleep. Other clinical application derives from the various means of stimulating the RAS. Hence, pain, motor movement, and auditory input can increase a person's level of consciousness, at least temporarily.

Spinal Cord

The spinal cord lies within the neural canal of the vertebral column. It extends down and fills the neural canal to the level of the second lumbar vertebrae. A pair of spinal nerves exits between adjacent vertebrae the entire length of the vertebral column. Below the place where the cord terminates, the neural canal is filled with spinal nerves, extending to their point of exit. Since they occupy less space in the canal at these lower lumbar levels, it is here that spinal taps may most safely be performed. This anatomic fact also explains why injuries to lumbar and lower thoracic vertebrae can produce impairment at disproportionately lower body levels.

Within the cord lie interneurons, ascending sensory fibers, descending motor fibers, and the nerve cell bodies and dendrites of the second order somatic (voluntary) and first order autonomic motor neurons. The cell bodies for sensory neurons lie next to the cord in ganglia of a root (dorsal) of each spinal nerve. Thus we can see that spinal nerves past the roots (just like cranial ones) contain *only* nerve fibers. Some of these fibers can be very long as can be demonstrated by measuring the distance between the lumbar cord and the toes. Also in the cord lies the anatomic circuitry (connections among various sensory and motor neurons) for cord reflexes.

Coverings. The CNS is covered by three layers of tissue called, collectively, the *meninges* and consisting of the pia mater, the arachnoid layer, and the dura mater. The *pia mater* is a cobwebby layer that lies next to the CNS. Next is the *arachnoid layer,* which contains a substantial vascular supply. Last is the *dura mater,* the thickest layer of all, lying next to the base that surrounds the CNS.

Cerebrospinal Fluid (CSF) Circulation. This fluid is a plasma filtrate that is exuded by the capillaries in the roofs of each of the four ventricles of the brain. As such, it is similar to plasma minus the large plasma proteins, which stay behind in the bloodstream. Most of this fluid is made in the lateral ventricles. It moves from there through ducts into the third ventricle of the diencephalon. From here it travels through the aqueduct of Sylvius of the midbrain and enters the fourth ventricle of the medulla. Then most of it passes through holes (foramina) in the roof of this ventricle and enters the subarachnoid space. (A small amount diffuses down into the spinal canal.) In this space the CSF is reabsorbed back into the bloodstream at certain points called the *subarachnoid plexus*.

Impairment of flow reabsorption of CSF leads to hydrocephalus. Various traumatic brain lesions can produce this in the adult.

SENSORY DIVISION

The *sensory system* is the site of origination of most nervous system activities. That is, stimuli received and processed by this system, whether sight, sound, touch, or taste, cause a response somewhere else in the nervous system. The response may be an immediate motor response, or the information may be stored in the brain and then used to determine bodily reactions later.

The sensory system, in general, transmits impulses from the body surface and deep structures into the spinal cord at all levels through the spinal nerves. From here the information is sent to the basal regions of the brain, which include the medulla and the pons, and to the higher brain centers, the thalamus and the cerebral cortex. These are the primary areas of the nervous system for handling sensory input; essentially all other parts secondarily receive and process sensory input.

Even though many sensory activities are responded to and carried out at spinal levels, many sensations from the body *(somesthetic sensations)* are interpreted by the brain. The interpretation of these messages enables us to determine body position and conditions of the immediate external environment, as well as conditions of the internal environment. These are called proprioceptive, exteroceptive, and visceral sensations, respectively.

As indicated above, *proprioceptive sensations* are those sensations that describe the physical position state of the body such as tension in muscle, flexion or extension of joints, tendon tension, and deep pressure in dependent parts like the feet while standing or the buttocks while seated. *Ex-teroceptive sensations* are those that monitor the conditions on the body surface. These include temperature and pain. *Visceral sensations* are like exteroceptive sensations except that they originate from within and monitor pain, pressure, and fullness from internal organs.

Sensory Pathways

Figure 19-4 indicates the possible pathways for processing somesthetic sensations. The fibers ending in the spinal cord initiate the cord reflexes discussed previously. Brain stem fibers initiate reflexes such as those that position the trunk and aid in upright posture. All of these are more complex than spinal reflexes but are still subconscious. As the sensations are transmitted to higher levels, they terminate in the thalamus, where the *general* origin of the sensation and the modality (type) of the sensation are determined. However, the *discrete* localization and modality of the sensations are determined in the cerebral cortex, where information from past experiences is involved in interpretation.

Sensory Receptors

The sensory receptors for somesthetic sensations include both free nerve endings and specialized end organs. Free nerve endings are nothing more than small filamentous branches of the dendritic fibers. They detect crude sensations of touch, pain, heat, and cold. The precision is crude because there are many interconnections between the free endings of different neurons. However, they are the most profusely distributed and perform the general discriminatory functions, whereas the more specialized receptors discriminate between very slight differences in degrees of touch, heat, and cold.

Structurally the special exteroceptive end organs for detection of cold, warmth, and light touch differ from one another and are quite specific in their function as seen in Figure 19-4. The physiological basis for this specific function has not been determined but is presumed to be based upon some specific physical effect on the organ itself.

There are three proprioceptive receptors. Joint kinesthetic receptors are found in the joint capsules and send messages concerning the angulation of a joint and the rate at which it is changing. Information from muscles concerning the degree of stretch is transmitted to the nervous system from the muscle spindle apparatus, while the Golgi tendon determines the overall tension applied to the tendons.

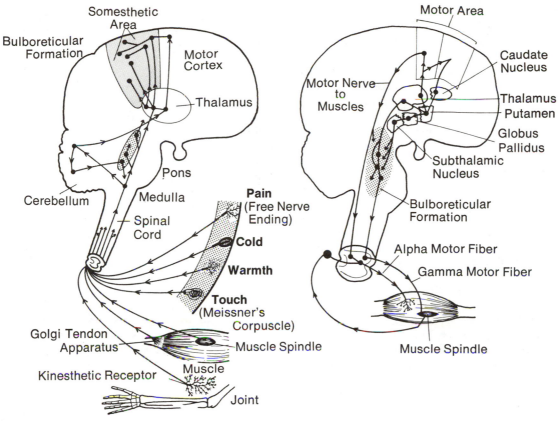

FIGURE 19-4.
General organization of the sensory *(left)* and motor *(right)* divisions of the nervous system. (After Guyton AC: Textbook of Medical Physiology, 5th ed, p 609. Philadelphia, WB Saunders, 1976)

When a sensory effector is stimulated, it responds with an increased frequency of firing. At first there is a burst of impulses; if the stimulus persists, the frequency of impulses transmitted begins to decrease. All sensory receptors show this phenomenon of *adaptation* to varying degrees and at different rates. Adaptation to light touch and pressure occurs in a few seconds, whereas pain and proprioceptive sensation adapt very little if at all, and at a very slow rate. The determination of the intensity of sensation is on a relative rather than an absolute basis and follows a logarithmic response. Therefore, while the intensity of a sensation increases logarithmically, the frequency of response in the nerve ending increases linearly.

Although there are structurally different receptors for detecting each type of sensation, it is the area of the brain to which the information is transmitted that determines the *modality* or type of sensation the individual feels. The thalamus, hypothalamus, and somesthetic area of the cerebral cortex operate together to determine the various sensory qualities. As sensory input arrives at the CNS, the different characteristics such as a pain element or a touch element are determined by the cooperative effort of the areas.

PAIN

The sensation of pain warrants special consideration because it plays such an important protective role for the body. Whenever there is tissue damage, nerve endings are stimulated and the sensation of pain is felt. This sensation is usually felt during the time that tissue is undergoing damage and ceases when the damage ends. This condition is due to the release of chemicals and metabolites such as histamine and bradykinin from damaged cells. Typical damaging stimuli are trauma (cutting, crushing, tearing), ischemia, or intense heat or cold.

In addition to these, acidity of the tissue fluid at the nerve fiber ending is now known to stimulate pain sensations that can be eliminated by making this fluid alkaline.

Variation in pain thresholds both among individuals and within the same individual at different times has been long known. (This is in addition to the wide variation in people's reactions to pain.) It was formerly thought that the sensation of pain depended in large part upon the number of "pain receptor endings" that were simultaneously and continuously stimulated, as well as upon variations in cortical or brain stem thresholds.

Gate Theory.   More recent evidence, however, points to the existence of gating mechanisms in the substantia gelatinosa at all levels of the spinal cord, which are capable of regulating the amount of pain impulses than can enter the spinothalamic tract and travel to the brain. This cord level of pain regulation opens new avenues to the treatment of pain.

Briefly, two types of fibers are involved. One is a small diameter (S) fiber that carries impulses responsible for the sensation of pain (pain impulses). The other is a large diameter (L) fiber that carries impulses responsible for cutaneous tactile sensations. The S and L fibers each synapse with two other cells—a gate cell and a T cell of the spinothalamic tract. The gate cell also synapses with the T cell and acts to *inhibit* (by hyperpolarization) the T cell. L-fiber impulses stimulate the gate cell, thereby hyperpolarizing the T cell to a certain degree. S-fiber impulses inhibit the gate cell and stimulate the T cell. Since the gate cell is inhibited, the T cell is not. Thus, by itself, the S-fiber impulse readily gains access to the spinothalamic tract.

If tactile skin receptors *in the same dermatome* are stimulated simultaneously with S fibers, then the action of the L fibers will (by way of the gate cell) hyperpolarize the T cell and thereby make it more difficult for S-fiber impulses to stimulate the T cell (gain access to the spinothalamic tract). Thus the relative S- to L-fiber activity can determine the degree of pain impulses that can enter the CNS at the level of the cord (see Fig. 19-5).

Rubbing or other tactile sensation such as provided by transcutaneous nerve (skin) stimulation applied to a painful area may reduce the sensation of pain perceived by the patient.

Although much more remains to be learned, we know that primitive sensations of pain occur once the ascending impulses from the spinothalamic tract reach the midbrain, and more refined and somewhat localized perception occurs at the level of the thalamus. Most refined and localized sensations, as well as their significance to the person, occur at the level of the cortex. In no way do we have any neurologic basis for individual variability in reactions to pain.

MOTOR DIVISION

Figure 19-4 depicts the motor division, which is responsible for stimulating the effector organs of the body. Effectors are skeletal and smooth muscles as well as exocrine glands and certain endocrine ones as well. Since we have already discussed most of this system in reviewing the CNS, let us just briefly finish the somatic motor division and turn to the autonomic division.

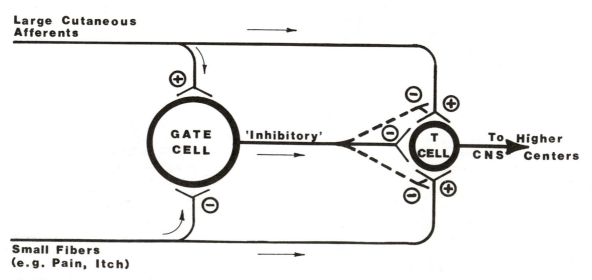

FIGURE 19-5.
Spinal gate theory. (After Melzack R, Wall P: Pain mechanisms: A new theory. Science 150:971–979, 1965)

Intentional, willed actions begin in the contralateral motor cortex. Descending motor fibers (pyramidal and extrapyramidal) cross over either in the medulla or in the cord. The basal ganglia, the bulboreticular system, and the cerebellum all perform their necessary functions that ensure smooth coordinated action of all involved skeletal muscles. These descending fibers then synapse with internuncials that in turn synapse with and stimulate the alpha somatic motor neuron. Discrete willed coordinated activity results.

Reflexes

The nervous system responds to sensory input through motor mechanisms that control bodily function and position. As demonstrated in Figure 19-1, the motor division of the CNS is organized in a hierarchic manner as is the sensory division. That is, a large number of reflexive motor functions are mediated through the spinal cord, while others operate through brain stem centers.

Basically, a reflex is an instantaneous and automatic motor response to a sensory input. It involves a sensory receptor, one or more transmitter interneurons, and an effector organ. The effector is the end organ that receives the motor impulse, such as a skeletal muscle, internal organs such as the gut or heart, or an exocrine or endocrine gland. While perception of the sensation may occur, this is not part of the reflex arc. Similarly, cortical integration and voluntary motor activity are also not involved. An example of a reflex is the almost instantaneous withdrawal of a hand or foot from a painful stimulus.

There are two types of reflexes: those involving the cord and those involving the brain.

Simple cord reflexes include the *axon reflexes* that provide increased blood flow to damaged tissues in the skin. Proprioceptor reflexes that are processed at the spinal cord include the *stretch reflex,* which helps maintain normal muscle tone, posture, and positioning of limbs with respect to the rest of the body. Another proprioceptive reflex mediated at the spinal level is the *tendon protective reflex,* which protects the tendon and muscle against excessive stretch. The *extensor thrust reflex* aids in the support of the body against gravity.

Also included in spinal reflexes is the *withdrawal,* pain, or flexor reflex. The purpose of this reflex is obvious. Operating in association with this reflex is the *crossed extensor reflex.* When one limb flexes in withdrawal from a painful stimulus, the opposite limb extends, pushing the whole body away from the source of the painful stimulus.

An important feature of all reflexes is reciprocal inhibition, which occurs in the antagonist muscle of the one stimulated. For example, when a flexor reflex stimulates the biceps, it also inhibits its antagonist, the triceps, and provides for more efficient performance of motor activities in the upper arm.

Spinal cord activities also include reflex circuits, which aid in the control of visceral functions of the body. Sensory input arises from visceral sensory receptors and is transmitted to the spinal cord, where reflex patterns appropriate to the sensory input are determined. The signals are then transmitted to autonomic motor neurons in the gray matter of the spinal cord, which send impulses to the sympathetic nerves innervating visceral motor end organs.

A most important autonomic reflex is the *peritoneal reflex.* Tissue damage in any portion of the peritoneum results in the response of this reflex, which slows or stops all motor activity in the nearby viscera.

In the presence of transsectional injuries at the brain stem, cord reflexes are also capable of modifying local blood flow in response to cold, pain, and heat. This vascular control by autonomic reflexes in the spinal cord operates as a backup mechanism for the usual brain stem control patterns.

Also included in the autonomic reflexes of the spinal cord are those causing the emptying of the urinary bladder and the rectum. When the bowel or bladder becomes distended, sensory signals are transmitted to the internuncial neurons of the upper sacral and lower lumbar segments of the cord. Motor signals traveling by way of the parasympathetic neurons excite the main portion of the bowel or bladder, at the same time inhibiting the internal sphincters of the urethra or anus. This causes the organ to contract and the sphincter to open, thereby evacuating the organ. Normally these reflexes are overridden by cortical centers until an appropriate time and place for evacuation arises.

BRAIN REFLEXES

Brain reflexes operate in the same way as do cord ones, except that the brain houses the connection, not the cord. Brain reflexes include those involving the cardioregulatory and vasomotor centers of the medulla, plus the pupillary adjustment one that involves the midbrain. Since the sensory and motor arms of the heart rate and vasopressure reflexes are commonly known, let us discuss just the *pupillary reflex.*

Light in the retina causes stimulation of the optic nerve. Fibers in this nerve travel to the

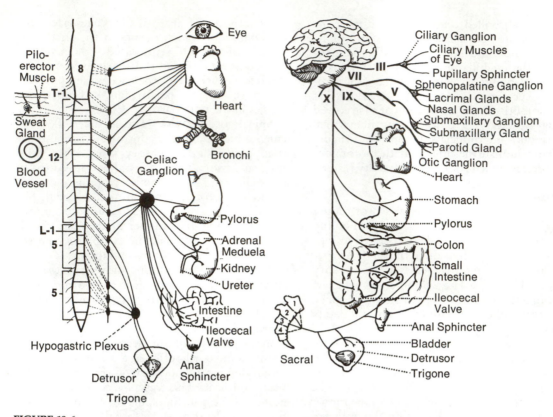

FIGURE 19-6.
Anatomy of the autonomic nervous system. (After Guyton AC: Textbook of Medical Physiology, 5th ed, pp 769–770. Philadelphia, WB Saunders, 1976)

Edinger-Westphal nucleus in the midbrain. Here the sensory fibers synapse with interneurons. The result is outgoing autonomic motor impulses to the smooth muscles of the iris. Increases in parasympathetic (by way of cranial nerve III) or decreases in sympathetic impulses cause pupillary constriction in response to the light. As the light stimulus of the retina decreases, this reflex causes pupillary dilation. Lack of this reflex signifies damage to the midbrain—optic fiber connection or to the oculomotor nerve (cranial nerve III).

Autonomic Division

This division comprises both *sympathetic* and *parasympathetic motor fibers*. They are responsible for contraction and relaxation of smooth muscle, rate of contraction of cardiac tissue, the secretion of exocrine glands, as well as the secretion of the adrenal medulla and islets of Langerhans in the pancreas. Table 19-1 summarizes the actions of both types of fibers.

The sympathetic and parasympathetic sections differ on the basis of (1) the anatomic distribution of nerve fibers, (2) the secretion of two

different neural transmitters by the postganglionic fibers of the two divisions, and (3) the antagonistic effects of the two divisions on the organs they innervate. Figure 19-6 shows the anatomy of the sympathetic and parasympathetic nervous systems.

As seen in Figure 19-6, the sympathetic system is comprised of a chain of prevertebral ganglia receiving fibers from the thoracolumbar region of the spinal cord and distributing postganglionic fibers to the various organs innervated. The parasympathetic system, on the other hand, has rather long preganglionic fibers coming from the craniosacral area of the CNS, which terminate in ganglia that are closely associated with the organ innervated. Short postganglionic fibers then innervate the tissues of the organs directly. Note that cranial nerve X provides for parasympathetic innervation of most of the gastrointestinal tract, even those parts that lie in the abdominal cavity.

Another difference between the two divisions of the autonomic nervous system is the neural transmitters secreted by the postganglionic fibers. Parasympathetic postganglionic nerve fibers secrete acetylcholine and thus are referred to

Table 19–1
Autonomic Effects on Various Organs of the Body

Organ	Effect of Sympathetic Stimulation	Effect of Parasympathetic Stimulation
Eye: Pupil	Dilated	Contracted
Ciliary muscle	None	Excited
Gastrointestinal glands	Vasoconstriction	Stimulation of thin, copious secretion containing many enzymes
Sweat glands	Copious sweating (cholinergic)	None
Heart: Muscle	Increased activity	Decreased activity
Coronaries	Vasodilated	Constricted
Systemic blood vessels:		
Abdominal	Constricted	None
Muscle	Dilated (cholinergic)	None
Skin	Constricted or dilated (cholinergic)	None
Lungs: Bronchi	Dilated	Constricted
Blood vessels	Mildly constricted	None
Gut: Lumen	Decreased peristalsis and tone	Increased peristalsis and tone
Sphincters	Increased tone	Decreased tone
Liver	Glucose released	None
Kidney	Decreased output	None
Bladder: Body	Inhibited	Excited
Sphincter	Excited	Inhibited
Male sexual act	Ejaculation	Erection
Blood glucose	Increased	None
Basal metabolism	Increased up to 50%	None
Adrenal cortical secretion	Increased	None
Mental activity	Increased	None

(Guyton AC: Textbook of Medical Physiology, 5th ed, p. 773. Philadelphia, WB Saunders, 1976)

as *cholinergic fibers,* whereas sympathetic post-ganglionic fibers are called *adrenergic fibers* because they secrete noradrenalin (norepinephrine). The actions of these two antagonistic chemical transmitters are summarized in Table 19–1.

Notice that many (but not all) of the organs innervated by autonomic fibers receive both parasympathetic and sympathetic fibers. These effector organs receive a given amount of stimulation from both subdivisions at all times. This is called a *tonic effect* or *resting frequency.* As the specific action of one subdivision is called for, this division increases its rate of firing to the effector organ while the other decreases its rate. This tonic or resting frequency of stimulation also occurs for effector organs that are innervated by only one type of fiber (*either* sympathetic or parasympathetic).

For example, if sympathetic discharge to a blood vessel was "on" or "off," this would result in constriction of vessels only during "on" periods. But since there is a normal resting frequency, increasing it causes more vasoconstriction and decreasing it results in less vasoconstriction or vasodilatation. This tonic effect persists throughout both the sympathetic and the parasympathetic divisions of the autonomic nervous system and is responsible for the high degree of effectiveness of the system in the regulation of visceral activities.

In addition to the two subdivisions of the autonomic motor division, there are two different actions of adrenergically (sympathetically) stimulated effector organs. These actions are determined by the type of receptor site on the effector organ. Receptor sites may be alpha or beta. Table 19-2 lists the effects of both types of adrenergic receptors. As can be seen, some tissues have both, but most effector organs have only one.

Patterns of autonomic function can be regulated or triggered by centers in the hypothalamus, medulla, and bulboreticular formations. However, autonomic functioning does not seem limited to the stem. Stimulation of certain corti-

Table 19–2
Alpha and Beta Adrenergic Effector Responses

Effector Organ	Receptor	Action
Eye		
Iris muscles	Alpha	Mydriasis
Ciliary muscle	Beta	Relaxation (permission) Meets distance
Salivary glands	Alpha	Thick secretion
Heart		
SA node	Beta	Increased heart rate
Atria	Beta	Increase in contractility and conduction
AV node, bundle, & Purkinje fibers	Beta	Increased velocity of conduction
Ventricles	Beta	Increased contractility and conduction velocity, increased pacemaker rate
Coronary vessels	Alpha	Constriction
	Beta	Dilatation
Blood vessels (all others)	Alpha	Constriction
	Beta	Dilatation
(Renal, pulmonary, skin, and cerebral vessels have only alpha receptors.)		
Lung		
Bronchial muscle	Beta	Relaxation
Bronchial glands	Beta	Inhibition
Liver		
Parenchyma	Beta	Glycogenolysis
Pancreas		
Beta cells of islets	Beta	Insulin secretion
	Alpha	Inhibition of secretion
GI tract		
Muscles	Beta	Increased motility
Sphincters	Alpha	Contraction (closure)
Kidney		
Juxtaglomerular apparatus	Beta	Renin secretion
Urinary		
Detrusor	Beta	Relaxation
Bladder		
Trigone and sphincter	Alpha	Contraction
Skin		
Piloerection muscles and sweat glands	Alpha	Slight secretion Contraction

cal nerves can trigger both discrete and widespread autonomic changes. Exact mechanisms for these interactions await research, but this cortical involvement seems to parallel that for sensory and somatic motor operations.

BIBLIOGRAPHY

Chusid JG: Correlative Neuroanatomy and Functional Neurology, 17th ed. Los Altos, Lange Medical Publications, 1979

Eccles JC: The Understanding of the Brain, 2nd ed. New York, McGraw-Hill, 1977

Eliasson SG et al: Neurological pathophysiology, 2nd ed. Oxford University Press, 1978

Ganong WF: Review of Medical Physiology. Los Altos, Lange Medical Publications, 1977

Hospital Practice, Special Report: Recent studies on the nature and management of acute pain, January 1976

Melzack R, Wall PD: Pain mechanisms: A new theory. Science 150:971–979, 1965

Nathan PW: The gate-control theory of pain: A critical review. Brain 99:213–258, 1976

Stephens G: Pathophysiology for Health Practitioners. New York, Macmillan, 1980

Pathophysiology of the Central Nervous System

20

Robert W. Hendee

ASSESSMENT CONSIDERATIONS

Nurses in a critical care unit caring for individuals who have acute nervous system injury or illness serve as the patient's first line of defense. In order to ensure superiorccare, a multitude of routine supportive acts must be performed in repetition.

Concomitantly, the nurse must carry out frequent neurologic and (in cases of multiple systems injuries) other evaluations with constant vigil for subtle changes in blood pressure, pulse rate and regularity, respiratory activity, sensorial status (level of consciousness), and motor and sensory function. Alterations when they occur may be the initial indication of impending deterioration, leading to rapid demise unless immediate action is taken to alleviate the underlying pathology. An example may be helpful.

Patient Situation

A 19-year-old right-handed female was seen in the emergency room following a vehicular-induced closed head injury. During the initial neurosurgical evaluation her arousal mechanism was moderately depressed, but she responded purposefully and uniformly upon request. No focal or lateralizing signs were evident except for tendency for enlargement of the left pupil (pupillary inequality is termed *anisocoria*). One hour later, following repair of facial lacerations and with stability of sensorial status, she was moved to the critical care unit for further observation. The patient's condition was discussed with the receiving nurse by the neurosurgical resident.

Soon thereafter the nurse noted definite, persistent anisocoria, with diminished reaction to light of the dilating pupil and more difficulty in arousing the patient. Immediately the resident was called, and in the interim mannitol was prepared for intravenous administration. This was begun upon the physician's arrival as a deteriorating situation was apparent. The patient was transferred to the operating room, by which time her respiratory condition required external assistance, both pupils had dilated, and she was unresponsive to painful stimuli. Emergency trephinations revealed an acute subdural hematoma over one cerebral hemisphere and an epidural hematoma over the opposite hemisphere.

Fortunately the young woman recovered with minimal neurologic damage. Her life was undoubtedly saved by the awareness and prompt action of the critical care nurse.

Opportunity for the nurse to discover other interesting and extremely important findings is ever present. Serosanguineous drainage from ears, nose, or scalp wound, even when it has been debrided and repaired but incompletely explored in the emergency unit, will represent cerebrospinal fluid (CSF) leak until proved otherwise. Progressive urinary output of abnormally high levels following injury or certain types of intracranial and facial surgery may represent diabetes insipidus (DI). Neither of these conditions need cause concern about the immediate demise of the patient. If left unobserved too long, however, they may result in unnecessary intracranial infection or hypovolemia and severe electrolyte imbalance. These in turn will lead to new problems of care and worsened condition of the patient, possibly precluding complete recovery or ultimately leading to death.

Experience aids the nurse in sharpening her powers of observation to recognize the slight changes that may be the precursors of the full constellation of signs of increased intracranial pressure or brain herniation. The same holds for alterations in lower-extremity motor and sensory function after incomplete spinal cord injury. Experience also imparts confidence to the nurse, as does knowledge of the more common patterns of deterioration, in assisting her to determine whether additional observation is warranted or whether she should seek the physician's reevaluation immediately.

Physicians rendering quality care in the treatment of critically ill patients should always allocate time to discuss with the nurse, even briefly, the particulars of each new patient upon arrival in the critical care unit. At that time the nurse must establish *precise* baseline information to her own satisfaction and seek clarification if necessary.

In these days of vehicular abuse, exposure to dangerous equipment, and use of complex mechanical recreational devices, many of the patients in any large and active critical care unit are those with acute cranial or spinal injuries. Intracranial abscesses, aneurysms, arteriovenous malformations and tumors, and nontraumatic spinal cord lesions also continue to require neurosurgical care. This section will discuss some of the common problems that may arise in the general neurosurgical population.

NEUROSURGICAL PROBLEMS

Increased Intracranial Pressure

Elevated intracranial pressure may be acute, subacute, or chronic, depending upon the duration, severity, and rapidity with which it develops. The magnitude of the effects is determined by the extent to which the intracranial structures adapt and the time allowed for the process. It then refers to a situation wherein the normal central nervous system contents are obliged to compete for space within the bony confines of the cranium. Additional limitations are imposed by the sensitivity of the brain in general to trauma and of the cranial nerves and vessels to stretch and compression. The fibrous partitions between parts of the brain (falx cerebri, tentorium cerebelli) also act as intrinsic barriers to displacement of the cranial contents and may result in pressure against the nervous and vascular structures.

Competition with the normal intracranial contents may arise extrinsic to the brain—for example, from epidural or subdural hematomas, or tumors arising from the covering of the brain (meningiomas), all of which may exert pressure against any of the brain's surfaces. Intrinsically, hydrocephalus (due to tumors located in the posterior fossa or elsewhere, subarachnoid hemorrhage, or congenital anomalies), intracerebral or intracerebellar hematomas (due, for example, to hemorrhage from aneurysms), malformations, and cerebral edema all may create abnormal intracranial pressure.

A focal or diffuse intracranial lesion of sufficient size, regardless of the etiology or whether extracerebral or intracerebral, imparts a mass effect, the result of which is an obligatory shift of the normal contents. If the pressure is acute and the mass significantly large, dramatically rapid adverse effects will be noted, as in the case of most epidural hematomas. These are usually due to temporal bone fracture and laceration of the middle meningeal artery, implying more rapid hemorrhage than that which is venous in origin, unless large venous structures such as the major venous sinuses are involved. Such structures are the origin of major venous bleeding, which may lead to early tragedy.

The ultimate result, even in the case of long-standing, slowly evolving subdural hematomas, is some degree of impingement upon the superficial cerebral substance and secondary distortion of the cranial nerves, vessels, and brain stem.

Pressure of the medial aspect (uncus) of the medially displaced temporal lobe on the superior part of the third cranial (oculomotor) nerve results in progressive pupillary dilatation on the same side because of interference with the pupilloconstrictor fibers carried by that nerve. Occasionally the opposite oculomotor nerve will be compressed against its ipsilateral cerebral peduncle, with false lateralization of the abnormal (enlarged) pupil.

A sign of early increased intracranial pressure may be seen in injury to the sixth cranial (abducens) nerve, which is manifested by impaired abduction of the appropriate globe. The abducens nerve traverses the greatest distance between sites of origin and function and thereby has the greatest theoretic chance of injury by compression or stretch.

Compression of the cerebral hemispheres or distortion of or injury to the brain stem will result in alterations in arousal. In the latter structure the reticular activating system is involved. Interference with the cardiorespiratory centers will be evidenced by depression and perhaps irregularity of pulse rate and concomitant elevation of blood pressure, as well as abnormalities visible on the cardiac monitor suggestive of primary cardiac disease. In addition there will be abnormalities of respiratory depth, rate, and regularity. Pupillary abnormality, decreased spontaneous movement, and weakness of the opposite limbs, and, where the dominant side of the brain is involved, speech dysfunction (dysphasia) will also be apparent. It should be noted, however, that lateralizing signs (hemiparesis, speech disorders, pupillary changes) may not be present initially; rather, headache, progressively severe nausea, emesis, and sensorial depression leading to obtundation will be the most striking symptoms and findings.

It is helpful for both nurse and physician to have concise understanding of the terminology used for the various pathologic levels of consciousness:

- *Stuporous/very lethargic* — sleepy or trancelike but can still be aroused to respond with volitional, well-defined, and purposeful acts, whether the acts be socially acceptable or not
- *Semicomatose* — does not perform volitional acts upon request but does have individual, purposeful movements (defensive withdrawal) or motor activity that is categorized as
  a. *decerebrate* — extension of lower extremities, extension and inward rotation of upper extremities
  b. *decorticate* — extension of lower extremities, flexion and internal or external rotation of forearms
  c. *opisthotonic* — extension of extremities, neck, and trunk
- *Coma* — implies no spontaneous or induced response except that noted, for example, in the pulse and respiratory rate when nociceptive (painful) stimulation is used

It is burdensome to rely on more categories than those listed above.

Continuous monitoring techniques that allow instantaneous readings of intracranial pressure are becoming universally used in the care of critically ill patients regardless of the cause of the increased pressure. Such monitors may be of the kind that measure surface pressure (epidural or subdural), or they may record central pressure by means of catheters placed within a lateral ventricle. The former generally require insertion in an operating theater environment, whereas the latter may be easily installed via a twist drill hole placed through the calvarium with the patient remaining in the intensive care unit bed. Although the ventricular catheter technique is most invasive, it also allows for removal of ventricular fluid, which at times, even in small quantities, may serve to reduce intracranial pressure significantly. Both devices allow for more rapid therapeutic response to patients having increased intracranial pressure and serve as valuable additions to the total monitoring of the patient (see Chapter 22).

Cerebral Concussion and Contusion

A *cerebral concussion* is the transient stage in which consciousness is lost after a blow to the head. Implied or inherent therein is interruption of normal neural activity. The loss of consciousness is "usually reversible." Retrograde amnesia (loss of memory of events prior to the injury, usually recent rather than remote) occurs, varying in severity depending on the degree of injury.

It is obvious that severe head injuries may be sustained without cerebral concussion by the strict definition—that is, without loss of consciousness, even briefly. Moreover, patients with injuries that consist purely of concussion should be expected to recover without any neurologic sequelae. Individuals who remain unconscious for more than one hour must be suspected of having suffered more than a simple concussion.

It is worth emphasizing that loss of consciousness is not mandatory for a diagnosis of severe head injury, at the same time recognizing that a certain percentage of patients with a clinical diagnosis of "simple" cerebral concussion will upon observation be found to have or develop significant injury.

This is well illustrated in the "classic" case of epidural hematoma, in which the patient is initially rendered unconscious, perhaps only for a minute or so, and appears to recover, refusing medical assistance. A short time afterward the patient becomes drowsy, eventually obtunded, hemiparetic, and develops anisocoria. Unless neurosurgical intervention occurs, virtually all victims will die. This is the reason head-injury patients must be observed so closely in the critical care unit even though they may at the onset and, for the great percentage, later, appear quite normal.

Cerebral contusion *per se* is usually more serious and refers to injury resulting in bruising of the brain. This may be minimal or a widespread, massive, and fatal nerve tissue insult.

Contusions in general carry a higher risk than concussions regarding permanent damage and significant lesions. Contusions may be accompanied by brain lacerations and hematomas and may lead to depressing problems of intractable, fatal cerebral edema. Individuals with focal or lateralizing neurologic signs are evaluated by specific neurodiagnostic procedures (computerized axial tomography [CT] if available and time permits, or cerebral angiography) to differentiate brain contusion, a nonoperative problem, from traumatic space-occupying lesions that may be surgically remediable.

Treatment for contusion without accompanying surgical injury consists of excellent general supportive care and usually steroids to preclude or reduce concomitant cerebral edema.

Cerebral Edema

A fairly frequent and frustrating situation to deal with is that in which significant cerebral edema is present after head injury. Often no concomitant surgical lesion is present that, once removed, might alleviate pressure, and medical therapeutics may be to no avail. The result is that the patient succumbs.

Edema of the brain consists of swelling (excess fluid), which causes increased bulk in which the white matter is more vulnerable than the gray. It may be especially evident in the cerebral tissue surrounding tumors or abscesses or following the removal of a tumor or hematoma from the surface of the brain when significant compression with accompanying vascular stasis has occurred.

Cerebral edema may be associated not only with cerebral contusions related to impact forces but may be present after thrombosis of cortical veins (in overwhelming sepsis or dehydration), hypoxia, water intoxication, vascular inflammation, exposure to cold, tin poisoning, and hormonal imbalance. This has been called "benign" intracranial hypertension or pseudotumor cerebri, wherein presence of a tumor is mimicked.

Therapy directed at relief of cerebral edema consists of both medical and surgical modalities. The latter includes a technique of decompression. Among the former are *adequate respiratory care* (airway and ventilation) to preclude or reduce hypoxia, which may lead to further edema if persistent, and *cerebral dehydrating agents,* which are hyperosmolar in nature (urea, mannitol) and serve to attract fluids into the cerebral vascular space for transport to the kidneys, acting rapidly to create diuresis. However, these agents have the propensity to create a "rebound" phenomenon unless a longer-acting agent is used at the same time.

It is speculated that 4 to 5 hours after administration of *urea* or *mannitol,* plasma osmotic pressure becomes lower than tissue osmotic pressure as a result of the induced diuresis. Consequently, fluid shifts to the interstitial compartment and cerebral edema can again become a problem.

Steroids such as dexamethasone (Decadron), which act to reduce swelling by means as yet not clearly understood but perhaps related to a stabilizing effect on membrane permeability, have a slower onset of action but may reduce the rebound effect when used in conjunction with the cerebral dehydrating agents.

Other methods include relative dehydration of the boby *in toto* by restriction of replacement fluid and use of salt-containing fluids to maintain the patient on the low or dry side of fluid maintenance; hypothermia to decrease the metabolic needs of the injured cerebral tissue; elevation of the head, when feasible, to promote venous return from the brain to the heart; and cautious use, when deemed necessary, of intermittent positive pressure breathing techniques, which, although beneficial to pulmonary care, may increase intracranial pressure.

Experience proves that, in general, younger patients tend to show higher rates of recovery following cerebral contusions and edema than do individuals past the second or third decade.

The signs of cerebral edema are those of any space-occupying situation if the intracranial pressure is sufficiently elevated. Severe, intractable edema may be present from the onset or appear later (by hours or days), even acutely, despite the appearance of a relatively stable course and the use of the entire spectrum of preventive or therapeutic measures.

Because of the importance of observation unaffected by outside influences, sedatives and analgesics are rarely used during periods of neurologic evaluation, even in the face of other injuries (for example, femoral or other long-bone fractures). Paraldehyde seems to be most efficacious in those with head injuries; however, it should be used only when the patient is severely confused or combative, threatening more harm to himself by his thrashing and inability to rest.

Should the patient show more depression in sensorial status at any time, squeezing the trapezius or discreet use of a safety pin in the sole will assist in determining whether arousal is possible, as from an exhausted slumber that is known to occur when a patient is exposed to a critical care unit environment for several days. If the patient is severely ill to begin with, recognition of changes indicative of deterioration becomes more difficult postoperatively or after trauma, for there is less room for physiological change.

CSF Fistula

Fistulas that allow leakage of CSF are dangerous because they may predispose to meningeal infection, cerebritis, and death. They frequently follow injuries causing basilar skull fractures and meningeal tear or depressed skull fractures in which the irregular bone edge interrupts the meningeal integrity. CSF leak may occur spontaneously without antecedent trauma in situations of chronic, progressive elevated intracranial pressure.

Fracture at the base involving the posterior or middle cranial fossae may allow drainage of the bloody or serosanguineous fluid by way of the external auditory canal. Eventually the fluid becomes xanthochromic, then clear, and if infected, may be purulent.

Drainage from the nares by way of the paranasal or frontal sinuses is seen in basilar or low frontal fractures in the frontal fossa. Patients who are sufficiently alert may complain of fluid trickling into the oropharynx when reclining or partially seated. Often discharge through the nares is noted by a spurt or flow of fluid when the patient sits or stands and leans forward.

A specimen of the discharge should be obtained in any case for evaluation by the physician. If the fluid does not contain blood or its disintegration products, a positive glucose test (qualitative) confirms the fluid as CSF.

It is important to be more vigilant for CSF leaks if basilar skull fracture is identified on examination of the skull radiographs, if the patient has Battle's sign (ecchymosis, edema, and tenderness over the mastoid bone), or periorbital or nasal discoloration and edema.

Suspicion should be raised promptly whenever dressings covering a scalp wound become stained with watery, usually serosanguineous, fluid. There may exist a previously undetected fracture with underlying meningeal laceration. Postoperative staining of a craniotomy dressing will indicate inadequate meningeal closure or elevated intracranial pressure decompressing itself by CSF leak through the meningeal suture line.

In any case, it is of utmost importance that prophylactic antibiotics be administered until the fistula heals spontaneously (with the assistance of lumbar punctures to lower the CSF pressure, if necessary) or correction of wounds or operative closure is carried out.

It is usual to maintain as far as possible, with appropriate right- or left-sided dependent posturing, a head-up position to allow better drainage. This lowers the intracranial CSF "pressure head" and precludes pooling of CSF in, for example, the paranasal sinuses, whereby bacterial organisms then have a better chance to congregate for access through the fistula to the intracranial fluid.

In the presence of CSF leak one should not try to clear the nose by blowing because this allows forceful retrograde displacement of organisms into the fistula.

Diabetes Insipidus

DI represents a pathologic state wherein abnormally great quantities of dilute urine are excreted, at times up to 20 liters per day. The kidneys have lost ability to control the amount of fluid output because of absence or deficit in antidiuretic hormone (ADH), which is produced in the supraoptic and paraventricular nuclei of the hypothalamus. The hormone is eventually released by the neurohypophysis (posterior pituitary) and appears to act on the distal renal tubules to promote reabsorption of water. Approximately 85% of the hypothalamic nuclei involved in production of the hormone must be impaired before insufficient ADH is available.

The excessive urinary output is matched by excessive thirst in persons alert enough to recognize it, requiring increased fluid intake. This contrasts with the situation found in psychogenic polydipsia, in which excess water is consumed, resulting secondarily in excess output.

Individuals with depressed arousal and inability to regulate their own intake will eventually lose enough fluid to lead to hypovolemia and death unless replacement in proper amounts is supplied for them. Replacement of water and glucose alone without appropriate electrolytes will result in water intoxication and cerebral edema because electrolytes accompany the water lost by the kidneys.

Control of water balance is more complicated than one may be led to believe based on the preceding information alone. The entire complex mechanism is not fully understood, but it incorporates not only ADH but osmoreceptors and baroreceptors and one additional hormone at least, aldosterone. In general, however, if the water available to the body is decreased, the secretion of ADH is increased, leading to water retention. In states of excess body water, ADH secretion is normally diminished, allowing for loss of the excess fluid.

DI is usually expected, transiently at least, but at times it occurs in florid and permanent fashion following open procedures for pituitary and parasellar lesions (craniopharyngioma) and in transsphenoidal approaches using cryotherapy for pituitary ablation. It is hoped that newer transsphenoidal microsurgical techniques, where applicable, will preclude leaving a postoperative pituitary cripple and reduce the chances for DI.

DI may also be seen in other surgical procedures performed in the region of the hypothalamus and in head injuries with basilar fractures involving the sphenoid bone, gunshot wounds of the head, hypothalamic tumors, hydrocephalus, maxillofacial injuries with displaced fractures, nasopharyngeal tumors invasive of the base of the skull, aneurysms encroaching upon the sellar or suprasellar space, and the like. Of course, some patients without traumatic lesions may have DI among other symptoms or as the sole presenting symptom.

In cases of DI it is essential that evaluation be carried out for concomitant anterior pituitary insufficiency. This is usually manifested initially as adrenal crisis with hypotension, generalized weakness, anorexia, depressed arousal, hypothermia, and psychotic symptoms.

Recognition of DI in the early postoperative period may be difficult if cerebral dehydrating agents have been used before or during surgery because the diuresis created by them may continue for the first postoperative day or so. Use of steroids may also cause increased urinary output. If the patient is awake, however, he will complain of progressively severe thirst if DI is present. Urine output will increase and persist despite the amount of fluid intake (which is usually maintained below normal replacement levels after cranial neurosurgery), and urine specific gravity will fall or remain below about 1.007 to 1.008. Suspicion of the entity is confirmed by serum and urine electrolyte and osmolality determinations (see Chapter 10).

The presence of persistent DI will result in exhaustion of the alert patient, who is unable to rest for long because of the frequent need to micturate and replenish fluids, the replacement fluids consisting of iced juices and other electrolyte-containing liquids. In this case, vasopressin (Pitressin) will eventually be required, just as in severe, continuing DI in patients unable to voluntarily replace their losses.

It should be reemphasized that patients developing florid DI may lose enormous amounts of urine in a relatively short period of time, leading to hypovolemia, unless a diagnosis is surmised or established and treatment undertaken. When the diagnosis is secure, it is most efficacious to allow the patient to satisfy his replacement needs by drinking according to his thirst. It is more difficult in those requiring intravenous therapy, but especially in the latter cases, meticulous quantitation of intake and output is mandatory.

It should also be noted that transient, manageable DI may occur and then undergo spontaneous total remission even after a florid initial course. The use of vasopressin, unless as a short-acting form, coincident with the spontaneous remission might lead to relative renal insufficiency and oliguria until effects of the extrinsic vasopressin are completed.

Intracranial Hemorrhage

Intracranial hemorrhage not related to trauma is encountered most frequently secondary to rupture of cerebral aneurysms. It may also occur from vascular malformation, rupture of weakened vessels under the strain of systemic hypertension, or occasionally in relation to cerebral neoplasms *per se* or leukemic infiltrates or aggregates.

More common than generally recognized are hemorrhages during periods of anticoagulation therapy for previous myocardial infarction, because of vascular insufficiency, and as prophylaxis of pulmonary embolus in phlebitis of the lower extremities. Admittedly there is usually an antecedent minor head injury or episode of severe straining in anticoagulated patients.

Massive, rapid hemorrhages also may occur in diffuse intravascular coagulopathy (DIC) whatever the basic cause. The hemorrhage may be confined to the spaces associated with the meningeal layers or involve the intracerebral substance.

In ruptured aneurysms, unless a space-occupying lesion is present necessitating emergency surgery, such as subdural or intracerebral hematoma, the patient is frequently too ill for immediate surgery because of severe spasm in the cerebral vessels. He generally does not become a candidate for direct attack on the aneurysm unless the neurologic situation improves markedly and repeat arteriography confirms remission of vascular spasms.

This holds true despite the knowledge that a significant percentage may be expected to have a recurrent hemorrhage that could prove fatal in the interval while awaiting sufficient improvement to allow surgery.

Headache (frequently severe), nausea, emesis, stiff and tender neck, and photophobia are common complaints if the patient is adequately alert.

Spinal Cord Injury

Trauma to the spinal cord is not uncommon in automobile, motorcycle, and mountain–climbing accidents. It also occurs from the use of trampolines and sky kites and seems in-creasingly frequent in skiers. Care of the patient with a complete or significant incomplete lesion involves psychological difficulties for both nurse and patient as soon as the permanency of the neurologic deficit becomes apparent to the latter. *Immediate and complete* lesions hold little if any chance of recovery.

Spinal shock is the term used to denote complete loss of voluntary neurologic integrity distal to the level of injury. It is the *fact* of cord sectioning, not the *act,* that produces spinal shock and implies paralysis of the muscles and anesthesia of the tissue below the lesion; that is, sensation and voluntary motion are abolished and are never recovered. The stretch reflexes, although lost initially, do recover and eventually become overactive several weeks after the injury. The mass-reflex response usually appears several months later with exaggerated withdrawal reflexes and spread of the reflex activity to the visceral autonomic outflow. Thus, by merely stroking the sole of the foot a patient may be stimulated to perspire, withdraw extremities, and empty bladder and bowel. The mass-reflex activity may be spontaneous at times.

Return of *spinal reflexes* is noted in the initial 1 to 3 weeks, beginning with withdrawal upon stimulation of the sole. Later in the period, anal and genital reflexes and the presence of a Babinski sign are noted. Progressively vigorous and brisk withdrawal is elicited, and the zone of positive elicitation becomes larger.

Autonomic reflexes remain suppressed following injury longer than somatic reflexes. Thus, the patient's skin is completely dry during the first 4 to 8 weeks, but perspiration later may be severely intense.

Injury to the spinal cord above the cervical levels of 3 and 4 is usually not compatible with survival owing to interruption of the innervation to the diaphragmatic muscles that supply respiratory function when the intercostal musculature is lost by lower cervical injuries. Higher cervical trauma may also contribute to edema, more cephalad, involving important medullary centers.

Because of the initial loss of sympathetic outflow, patients are often hypotensive as a result of loss of vascular tonus below the injury. For the same reason hypothermia may be profound because of loss of heat through the dilated vessels.

Patients with cervical injury often seem to be unstable from the standpoint of regulation of blood pressure and maintenance of respiratory activity when initially turned on their frames, especially in rotating from supine to prone position. It is necessary to be prepared to render immediate respiratory assistance and to return the patient to the supine position if significant cardiac and blood pressure irregularities occur.

Syndrome of Inappropriate Secretion of Antidiuretic Hormone (SIADH)

This phenomenon was initially described by Schwartz and co-workers and further defined by Bartter. The features are hyponatremia and hypotonicity of the plasma in conjunction with excretion of urine, which is hypertonic to plasma and which contains appreciable amounts of sodium. In addition there is absence of hypokalemia and edema, normal cardiac, renal and adrenal function, and normal or expanded plasma and extracellular fluid volumes (*i.e.,* no evidence of dehydration or hypovolemia). The presence of low serum blood urea nitrogen and uric acid levels assists in confirming the diagnosis.

The secretion of ADH (vasopressin) is "inappropriate" in that it continues despite the decreased osmolality of the plasma.

Some neoplastic conditions (carcinoma of the lung, duodenum or pancreas, or thymomas) may produce a chemical substance that is similar or identical to the arginine vasopressin produced in the hypothalamopituitary system but which is independent of normal physiological controls. Thus, an aberrant secretion is the factor in these cases.

In other conditions such as hemorrhage, trauma, central nervous system infection or disease, or pulmonary disease, or in the postoperative period, abnormal secretion of endogenous ADH is the etiology. Use of medications such as vincristine, chlorpropamide, hydrochlorothiazide, and carbomazepine (Tegretol) may also result in the syndrome.

The symptomatology of SIADH is basically that of water retention at one end of the spectrum proceeding to water intoxication at the other end. In this regard, I have seen definite symptoms that subsequently cleared with the usual therapy even with a serum sodium reduced no more than the range of 120 to 125.

Bartter states that water retention (and concomitant dilution of the serum sodium concentration) occurring slowly or when not severe causes headache, asthenia, somnolence, lethargy, and confusion. More rapidly occurring dilution, or water intoxication *per se,* is associated with anorexia, nausea, and emesis, proceeding to delirium, fits, aberrant respirations, hypothermia, and coma. Prior to coma the stretch reflexes may disappear, the presence of Babinski's sign is noted, and pseudobulbar palsy may occur.

Diagnosis can be established by readily available laboratory procedures, although radioimmunoassay of plasma ADH might be the most confirmatory method. The serum sodium concentration and serum osmolality are the best routine indices.

Treatment consists of restriction of fluid intake (even limited to perhaps 500 ml per day maximum in severe cases) and where applicable the treatment of underlying disorders (*e.g.,* administration of cortisone in Addison's disease) or the discontinuation of carbomazepine or other causative medications. Administration of salt (sodium chloride solutions) is usually of only transient benefit but may be considered where water intoxication is severe in order to attempt to acutely increase serum osmolality.

COMPUTERIZED TOMOGRAPHY (CT)

CT or computerized axial tomography is a relatively new radiographic modality that is now vital in diagnosing and treating nervous system abnormalities.

In essence, CT scanning measures densities of the skull, spine, and the deeper soft tissue structures. It has become invaluable in rapid screening of patients for traumatic intracranial hematomas, for example, as well as for abscesses, tumors, and intracerebral hemorrhages due to aneurysms and arteriovenous malformations. In addition, it is extraordinarily helpful in diagnosing hydrocephalus and in follow-up assessment after removal of intracranial lesions, particularly in following the course of a brain abscess after it has been drained or after removal of tumor or clots. Numerous spinal disorders such as syringomyelia, cord tumors, and spinal fractures may be diagnosed by CT.

Although CT scanning has not entirely negated the use of arteriography or air studies, it has substantially reduced the need for these more uncomfortable invasive procedures and will continue to play a progressively important role in the care of critically ill neurosurgical patients.

BIBLIOGRAPHY

Bartter FC: The syndrome of inappropriate secretion of antidiuretic hormone. *Disease-A-Month,* Year Book Medical Publishers, November 1973

Merritt HH: A Textbook of Neurology, 6th ed. Philadelphia, Lea & Febiger, 1979

Rosenberg RN (ed): Neurology. New York, Grune & Stratton, 1980

Schwartz WB, Bennett W, Curelop S et al: A syndrome of renal sodium loss and hyponatremia probably resulting from inappropriate secretion of antidiuretic hormone. Am J Med 23:529–542, 1957

Youmans JR: Neurological Surgery. Philadelphia, WB Saunders, 1972

Marilynn J. Washburn

CEREBRAL VASCULAR ACCIDENTS (CVAs)

Changes in the cerebral vasculature may be due to any of several causes ultimately leading to stroke. The most common immediate cause is the formation of a blood clot, or thrombus, at a given point, usually in the middle cerebral artery or one of its branches.

CLASSIFICATION

Transient Ischemic Attack (TIA)

Onset of the thrombus-caused stroke is usually slow, often occurring over a period of days, with resulting vascular congestion and edema around the infarcted area. This patient often has had TIAs (small strokes). Some of these premonitory symptoms consist of falls or dropping attacks for no reason, blurring of vision or transient monocular blindness, transient paresthesia, ataxia, dysphasia, nerve palsies, disorientation, vertigo or light-headedness, or behavior change noted by the family and friends (see Table 20-1). Sensitivity to these warning signs on the part of the family or nurse and appropriate medical intervention may prevent this particular form of CVA.

Causes of CVA

In contrast, the CVA caused by an embolus may be more rapid in onset and usually occurs during waking hours. The embolus-caused CVA is commonly related to primary heart disease (chronic atrial fibrillation, rheumatic valve disease, or the mural thrombus of a myocardial infarction).

Other causes of embolus may be tumor, bacteria, fat from an associated fracture, or air embolism. Symptoms vary depending upon the site of interference with the blood supply to the brain (see Figs. 20-1, 20-2).

Diagnosis

Noninvasive testing techniques can help to pinpoint the area of infarct resulting from a CVA. CT scans will demonstrate mass effect of the area involved, but postinfarct timing must be considered. CT scans may be inaccurately normal if done too early; findings will become positive after 10 to 14 days. Carotid phonangiography, an electronic auscultation of the carotid artery, will indicate the presence of stenosis or occlusion. Doppler studies and ocular plethysmography assist in detecting impaired cerebral blood flow.

Table 20–1
Symptoms Occurring During Transient Ischemic Attacks (TIAs)

Carotid Occlusion	*Vertebral-Basilar Occlusion*
1. Aphasia	1. Vertigo or dizziness
2. General or focal seizure	2. Hearing loss or tinnitus
3. Contralateral weakness or numbness	3. Visual graying or loss
4. Ipsilateral migraine-type headache	4. Diplopia
5. Transient blurring of vision or blindness in ipsilateral eye	5. Dysarthria
6. Homonymous visual field loss	6. Dysphagia
	7. Hemiparesis
	8. Occipital headache
	9. Homonymous visual field loss

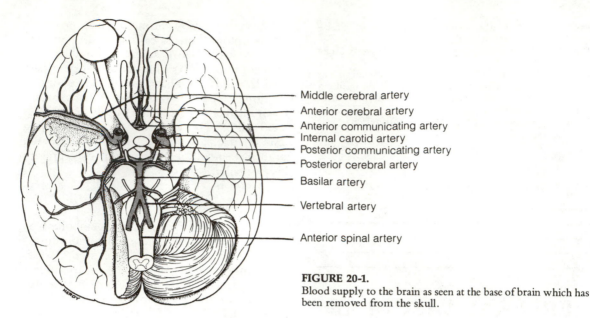

Middle cerebral artery
Anterior cerebral artery
Anterior communicating artery
Internal carotid artery
Posterior communicating artery
Posterior cerebral artery
Basilar artery
Vertebral artery
Anterior spinal artery

FIGURE 20-1.
Blood supply to the brain as seen at the base of brain which has been removed from the skull.

Treatment

Treatment is aimed at prevention of stroke by the use of anticoagulant therapy. Studies are currently in progress to determine the effectiveness of aspirin as an anticoagulant. New surgical techniques such as carotid endarterectomy and cerebral artery anastomoses are being perfected.

Cerebral Hemorrhage

Hemorrhage, while probably less frequent than thrombus- or embolus-caused CVAs, is much more rapid and dramatic in onset and frequently follows exertion.

Hypertension and atherosclerosis are often involved. The patient may have severe headache,

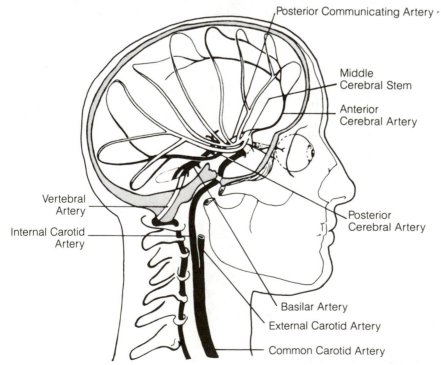

Posterior Communicating Artery

Middle
Cerebral Stem

Anterior
Cerebral Artery

Vertebral
Artery

Internal Carotid
Artery

Posterior
Cerebral Artery

Basilar Artery

External Carotid Artery

Common Carotid Artery

FIGURE 20-2.
Blood supply of the brain.

nausea and vomiting, more severe motor deficit, and frequently may be comatose. If there is blood in the spinal fluid, he will have signs of meningeal irritation (nuchal rigidity, positive Kernig's sign, photophobia).

Recognition of the above patterns will assist the nurse in collecting data for the physician who will make the diagnosis. The point is not for the nurse to make the diagnosis, but in planning appropriate nursing care, the nurse needs adequate data.

The patient with intracranial hemorrhage will be treated so as to avoid any rebleeding. The Valsalva maneuver is avoided, as is anything that might elevate the blood pressure.

Causes of hemorrhage may be a ruptured aneurysm, severe head trauma, blood dyscrasias, or tumor. Surgical removal of the large clot formed by the hemorrhage is indicated in an attempt to avert an often fatal outcome.

Effects of Stroke

The spinal reflex arc (lower motor neurons) when interrupted yields a *flaccid paralysis*. When the efferent nerve in the arc is interrupted, this also prevents stimulation or inhibition from the upper motor neuron (arising in the intracranial central nervous system) for voluntary motor function. When the upper motor neuron is interrupted (as in stroke or traumatic brain damage) the spinal reflex arc remains intact. Thus, whenever the afferent nerve is stimulated in the arc, the corresponding efferent function occurs.

Accordingly, stroke patients develop *spasticity* because of the interruption of the upper motor neuron influence. The pyramidal and extra-

pyramidal systems are also both involved in the control of resultant tonus.

The nurse must recognize that while occasional upper motor neuron lesions may yield a permanent flaccid paralysis, this is relatively rare. The initial flaccid paralysis is caused by a state of "shock" or depressed reflex function that occurs with sudden nerve damage. Soon spasticity will appear.

Exercise will maintain joint range of motion as well as "fatigue out" some muscle spasms. It must be brought to the patient's attention that exercises will maintain muscle tone and joint function and reduce disability, should significant function return. The nurse must also inform the patient that frozen, flexed joints, particularly in the upper extremity (1) are painful, (2) reduce social acceptance when one is unable to wash the axilla, (3) inhibit one's dressing, (4) do not allow for the assistive functions that even a paralyzed limb has to offer, such as stabilizing objects while the other hand works on them. Exercise in controlling spasticity is very important to the patient's maximum rehabilitation.

A stroke patient's *motor deficit* (hemiplegia or hemiparesis) is on the opposite side to the brain damage when the middle cerebral artery is affected because the pyramidal tracts (the voluntary motor nerves) cross at the level of the medulla.

The hemiplegia of the stroke patient is the result of an upper motor neuron lesion. It follows the general rule that upper motor neuron lesions yield spastic paralysis, while lower motor neuron lesions yield flaccid paralysis (see Fig. 20-3).

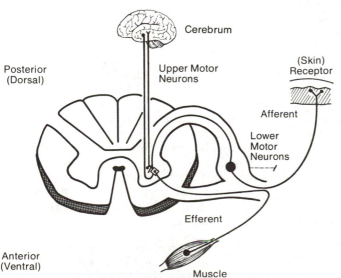

FIGURE 20-3.
Upper motor neurons vs. lower motor neurons (spinal reflex arc). (Courtesy of Sylvia Meeks.)

SEIZURES

The convulsive state is the mode of expression of the nervous system to overwhelming stimuli resulting in sudden, transient alterations of brain function.

Paroxysmal, excessive neural discharge may result from acute cerebral anoxia, hypoglycemia, other metabolic disturbances, overhydration, cerebral vascular accident, intracranial infection, and brain tumor.

Most commonly, the abnormal discharge is due to the presence of an organic lesion, with the irritable focus being in the partially damaged tissue adjacent to the brain tumor, vascular malformation or lesion, or brain abscess. The type of injury and the severity of damage to the brain are significant considerations when one is predicting the occurrence of seizure activity following cranial trauma.

Not all patients with sustained cerebral trauma will develop a seizure disorder. Genetic history and a variety of factors such as hyperventilation, sleep deprivation, fever, emotional stress, and drug therapy, in addition to the trauma, will have an effect on the seizure threshold.

Classification

The variety of physical and psychological characteristics of convulsive activity has led to the establishment of a general classification of seizures. It should be noted that there is no single convulsive type, but certain similar characteristics facilitate the formation of basic categories.

The common factor in all seizure types is the occurrence of dysrhythmic electrical disturbances of characteristic form and voltage found on the electroencephalogram (EEG). The EEG is the most effective tool available for diagnostic appraisal of seizure activity. Seizure activity is classified using the characteristic configuration and spacing of spikes and waves shown on the EEG tracing (see Fig. 20-4).

CT scan provides a noninvasive technique for localizing focal lesions related to seizure activity. Cerebral injury such as cerebral artery infarct, subdural or epidural hematomas, and brain abscesses are readily visible with minimum radiation exposure (4 to 5 rads) or risk to the patient. Seizure disorders not related to cerebral trauma often have CT abnormalities of diffuse cerebral atrophy, metastatic lesions, or hemiatrophy.

Grand Mal. Often the most alarming in terms of physical manifestation, this type of seizure is frequently preceded by an "aura" in the conscious patient. About half of the patients experience this personalized warning, which may be a temporary visual, olfactory, or auditory sensation such as a flash of lights, a particular smell, or a feeling of impending distress.

With abrupt onset, the person may cry out before entering a phase of tonic contraction, lasting about 60 seconds and during which respirations cease and cyanosis occurs. The activity then becomes clonic in nature as the muscles of the face and extremities display jerky movements; breathing is resumed, although irregular and stertorous. Bowel and bladder incontinence may occur, teeth are clenched, and physical injury is often sustained before the body relaxes.

The person may remain unconscious for several minutes, awakening in a confused, drowsy state often followed by sleep. Todd's palsy, which is temporary paresis or paralysis of the extremities following the clonic phase, may or may not occur. Often the person has no recollection of the event upon awakening.

Petit Mal. This type of activity rarely occurs in adults but is common in childhood. Unlike the grand mal type, petit mal seizures have no aura and are much shorter in duration (5 to 30 seconds). Transient clouding of consciousness (a blank stare) is often the only symptom. Eye blinking and minor movements of the head may be noted, but major physical manifestations are not present. This type of seizure may occur several times in a day and frequently goes unnoticed.

Psychomotor (Temporal Lobe). Occurring more commonly in adults than in children, these episodes are at times confused with psychic equivalents of temporal lobe origin such as déjà vu (an abnormal feeling of having lived through a new situation before) and hysteria, owing to the sometimes bizarre physical activity.

Of longer duration than the petit mal, an attack often begins with an inappropriate gesture, followed by a repetitive, seemingly purposeful activity that often does not fit the situation. Automatic behavior may consist of lip-smacking, hand-wringing, or disrobing. Postseizure amnesia follows.

Focal. This seizure results from the focal irritation of a part of the motor cortex, usually in the hemisphere opposite the affected side of the

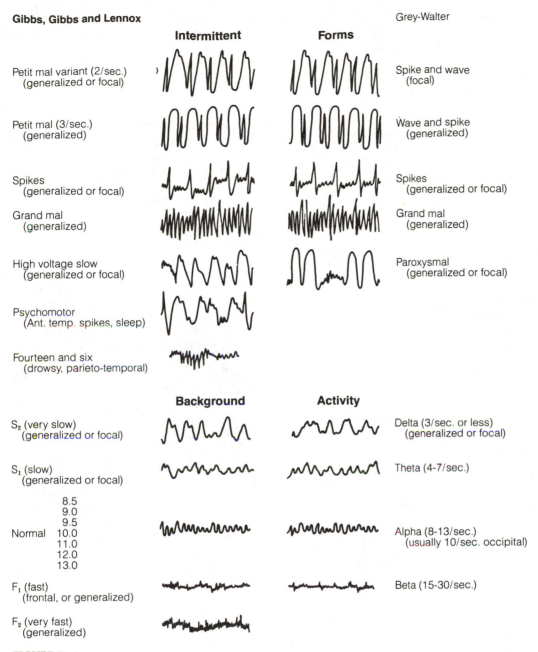

Gibbs, Gibbs and Lennox

Intermittent **Forms**

Grey-Walter

Petit mal variant (2/sec.) (generalized or focal) — Spike and wave (focal)

Petit mal (3/sec.) (generalized) — Wave and spike (generalized)

Spikes (generalized or focal) — Spikes (generalized or focal)

Grand mal (generalized) — Grand mal (generalized)

High voltage slow (generalized or focal) — Paroxysmal (generalized or focal)

Psychomotor (Ant. temp. spikes, sleep)

Fourteen and six (drowsy, parieto-temporal)

Background **Activity**

S_2 (very slow) (generalized or focal) — Delta (3/sec. or less) (generalized or focal)

S_1 (slow) (generalized or focal) — Theta (4-7/sec.)

Normal
8.5
9.0
9.5
10.0
11.0
12.0
13.0
— Alpha (8-13/sec.) (usually 10/sec. occipital)

F_1 (fast) (frontal, or generalized) — Beta (15-30/sec.)

F_2 (very fast) (generalized)

FIGURE 20-4.
EEG classifications. (MacBryde CM, Blacklow RS: Signs and Symptoms, 5th ed, p 684. Philadelphia, J.B. Lippincott, 1970)

body in patients over 10 years of age. Activity may occur in "jacksonian march"-type fashion, beginning in the distal part of an extremity and progressing proximally.

Consciousness is not generally lost unless activity advances to both sides of the body. As in grand mal seizures, Todd's palsy may be present in the postictal state and usually indicates a structural abnormality in the opposite hemisphere.

Status Epilepticus. This refers to a succession of epileptic attacks, either grand mal or petit mal, in which the postseizure phase of one episode overlaps with the discharge of the next, with the patient never fully regaining consciousness. Sustained grand mal activity is an emergency situation with potential lethal outcome, requiring immediate intervention.

Diazepam (Valium), up to 10 mg intravenously, is often administered first to stop the seizure activity, followed by an intravenous infusion of 1 g of diphenylhydantoin (Dilantin).

Dilantin given at a rate of 50 mg/min has been found to be most effective in controlling status epilepticus with the least amount of sedation. This is of primary importance in patients who have sustained head trauma, in whom altered states of consciousness are used as parameters for increased intracranial pressure. Infusion rates of Dilantin faster than 50 mg/min may cause undesired effects on respiration, heart rate, and blood pressure.

Appropriate measures for airway maintenance and physical protection must be taken, and vital signs monitored closely. General anesthesia may be required if other measures are unsuccessful in controlling the seizures.

Anticonvulsant Therapy

Control of seizure activity can usually be achieved with a moderate dosage of one of several anticonvulsants available. Dosage should be regulated to control seizures at nontoxic doses. Blood level tests to determine drug concentration are useful in establishing therapeutic dosages.

Diphenylhydantoin (Dilantin, phenytoin) is one of the most commonly used anticonvulsants. It is most effective for control of grand mal, focal, and psychomotor seizures. Toxic symptoms the nurse must be aware of include nystagmus, slurred speech, ataxia, lethargy, and cerebellar symptoms. Lack of motivation, decreased ability to concentrate, and low energy levels are also mild behavioral symptoms.

Phenobarbital may be effective for all types of seizure control and is commonly used. Primidone (Mysoline) is a barbituratelike compound used to control psychomotor seizures. Carbamazepine (Tegretol), valproate (Depakene) and clonazepam (Clonopin) have recently been introduced in the United States for anticonvulsant therapy.

Nursing Responsibility

A grand mal seizure seldom goes unnoticed and can be a frightening scene when first witnessed. The nurse in the critical care unit must know the measures to institute to protect the patient from injury. Accurate observation is essential. Of primary importance is remaining with the patient and staying calm. Loosen restrictive clothing and be sure there is something soft beneath the patient's head. Remember that the cyanotic state is unpreventable and transient. Position the patient on his side, if possible, to facilitate drainage of mucus and saliva. Do not attempt to open clenched teeth, even with a padded tongue blade. Teeth clenching occurs almost immediately and it is too late to prevent biting of the tongue if it was between the teeth at the onset of the attack. Observations to be made include the seizure pattern and the duration of each phase, the types of movement and the body parts involved, bowel or bladder incontinence, pupil size and eye movement, loss of consciousness, and patient behavior following the episode (*e.g.,* falling asleep, inability to speak, temporary paralysis).

The term *seizure* has a frightening connotation to patient and family alike. Often the patient has no awareness or understanding of his behavior. Accurate observations by the nurse and discussion with the patient following such an event will assist in appropriate assessment and management.

Management Modalities: Nervous System 21

Marilynn J. Washburn

CARE OF THE BRAIN-INJURED PATIENT

Individual Response to Brain Injury
Neurologic damage does not occur without effecting some change in a person's behavior response. His personality and entire characteristic behavior pattern will undergo some changes, either temporary or permanent, depending upon the locus and severity of the injury.

Lesions of the temporal, parietal, and occipital lobes, which comprise the posterior cerebrum, will affect the quality of reception and interpretation of sensory input from the environment. More specifically, each of the principal lobes of the brain can be associated with a particular function. The occipital lobe at the posterior of the skull is crucial for visual perception, while the temporal lobe is associated with auditory reception and interpretation. Visual-spatial perception involving the nonauditory and nonvisual functions of touch, space, and movement are attributed to the parietal lobe. The frontal lobe in the anterior cerebrum plays a major role in integrating emotion with social behavior, me-

349

diating personality. Coordination, balance, and rhythm are functions of the cerebellum.

Frontal Lobe Lesions. Types of maladaptive behavior have been conveniently labeled and can be attributed to injury of various lobes of the brain. One of the most frequently used labels is *frontal lobe syndrome,* describing that behavior which is a consequence of injury to the frontal lobe. The frontal lobe is essential to the planning and carrying out of goals, coordinating the "self-concept" with external social forces, and organizing volitional activity.

"Frontal" patients will display a flat affect and an apathetic response to any situation and will have difficulty in displaying appropriate social behavior. Their "I don't care" attitude may lead to unfounded judgments of "lazy," "worthless," and "indifferent." Involvement in group activities of short duration is useful therapy in this situation.

Temporal Lobe Lesions. Lesions of this lobe elicit particular behavior depending upon whether the right or left lobe is affected. Patients sustaining *left* temporal lobe injury will commonly develop a philosophizing type of personality. Interested in religion and personal destiny, they will often become morbid and over-emphasize negative features. Stress is not handled well, often leading to catastrophic behavior. Confronted with a simple arithmetic problem, the patient may become dazed, agitated, and exhibit temper. Care should be taken to establish a predictable daily routine with any change made very gradually.

An injury with focus in the *right* temporal lobe is often associated with depression, aggressive behavior, and emotional lability. Attempts to point out undesired behavior to the patient often meet with his denial of these aspects of his behavior.

Parietal Lobe Lesions. Damage to the parietal lobes will lead to rather vague symptoms of behavior. The patient may not have an awareness of the deficit he has. A lesion in the dominant hemisphere will involve speech disturbances, while involvement of the nondominant hemisphere results in defective visual-spatial perception. Speech therapy is usually of great benefit to these patients.

EFFECTS OF SEVERE BRAIN TRAUMA

In evaluating patient response and behavior change, it is important to have some idea of what the patient was like prior to injury. Emotional outbursts or consistent behavior responses may be part of the patient's premorbid personality and not a direct consequence of the injury. The patient's family or "significant others" provide a vital link to understanding the patient's behavior prior to injury.

Inappropriate Behavior. Following severe brain trauma, the patient may exhibit an inability to control his emotions. Frequently, he may cry continually or burst into inappropriate paroxysms of laughter. Often the content of his dialogue will not fit the emotion displayed. Such affective lability is due to an impairment of the "fine tuning" ability to control emotional response. Interruption of inappropriate emotional responses helps the patient to gain control and conserve energy.

Prompt feedback following inappropriate behavior may be helpful; angry comments will only perpetuate the behavior. Behavior modification techniques may be successful in some instances if the staff approach is very consistent. For example, if a patient uses abusive language when talking with another person, the staff may modify this behavior by consistently ignoring it or terminating the conversation once the patient becomes abusive. The situation should be discussed with the patient first and then dealt with in a consistent fashion.

Confusion. States of confusion are also common following brain injury. Due to sustained memory impairment, the patient may not be able to state correctly where he is now but may accurately describe an event in his past. He may regress in time, consistently answering neuro exam questions with the same incorrect responses, such as, "It's 1967. Nixon is President." The ability to retain new learning, such as his doctor's name or what he had for breakfast, is impaired, leading to a significant effect on behavior.

Hostile Behavior. Even more difficult to cope with than confusion is the hostile, combative phase common in cases of severe head injury. The patient who displays loud, physically aggressive and verbally abusive behavior is a serious management problem in the critical care unit. This phase is often temporary, lasting days or weeks. Prevention of physical injury, as well as unlimited patience, is of prime importance during this time.

Sensory Impairment. Sensory reception is often significantly impaired following neurologic injury. Compounding this impairment is the environment of the critical care unit, devoid of stimuli having any meaning to the patient. Incapable of verbal response, the comatose patient should be assumed to receive sensory input, and staff and visitors alike should direct conversation *to* him, not *about* him.

Sensory deprivation can be diminished by supplying short, frequent periods of sensory input that is meaningful to the patient. A favorite radio program, tape recording, or 30 minutes of music from the patient's favorite radio station provide more meaningful stimulation than constant radio accompaniment, which becomes as meaningless as the continual bleep of the cardiac monitor.

Brief explanations of nursing actions, such as, "I'm going to take your blood pressure now," provide verbal stimuli and aid in orienting the patient. A calendar with the days marked off and a clock also reinforce orientation.

MANAGEMENT

Tranquilizing agents are contraindicated owing to their effect on the central nervous system of masking or altering changes that may be symptomatic. Paraldehyde is probably the drug of choice when there is no alternative. It has been found to be most effective when administered on a scheduled basis as opposed to prn usage.

Restraints are suggested only as a last resort to prevent physical harm to patient or staff. Soft restraints of wrists and ankles should be released when the nurse is with the patient, to allow for unrestricted muscle movement. The Michelle Craig bed was designed to provide a padded, soft environment in which the patient can move about without risk of physical injury (see Fig. 21-1).

Essential to any treatment of the brain-injured patient is the establishment of *routine*. In addition to the memory impairment and confusion brought on by injury, most brain-injured patients have an impaired ability to transfer learning from one situation to another. The consistency of a schedule of daily activities strengthens learning and memory by repetition and alleviates anxiety. The nurse in the critical care unit can do much to establish a schedule specific to the patient. With information obtained from relatives, a daily routine of activities can be established that incorporates the patient's preinjury preferences and habits.

Mobilizing the patient in a wheelchair and

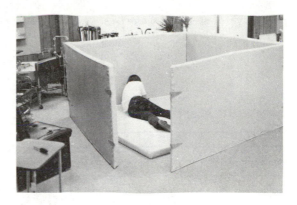

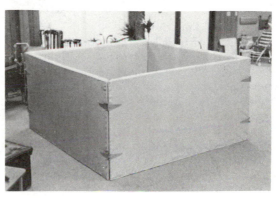

FIGURE 21-1.
The Michelle Craig bed provides a protective environment for the restless brain-injured patient. (Available from Wheelchairs, Inc., 3500 South Corona Street, Englewood, Colorado and through all Abbey Medical locations.)

dressing him in his own clothes, even while comatose, are effective means of stimulation, appropriate even in the critical care unit. Early mobilization and passive range of motion are essential for prevention of contractures and other complications that will impede rehabilitation.

BIBLIOGRAPHY

Carini E, Owens G: Neurological and Neurosurgical Nursing, 6th ed. St. Louis, C.V. Mosby, 1978

Chusid J: Correlative Neuroanatomy and Functional Neurology, 17th ed. Los Altos, Lange Medical Publications, 1979

Gardner H: The Shattered Mind. New York, Alfred A. Knopf, 1975

MacBryde CM, Blacklow RS: Signs and Symptoms, 5th ed. Philadelphia, J.B. Lippincott, 1970

Meador B, White P: The post-op dangers in carotid endarterectomy. RN 43, No. 4:54–57, 1980

Norsworthy E: Nursing rehabilitation after severe head trauma. Am J Nurs, 74:1246–1250, 1974

Pincus JH, Tucker GJ: Behavioral Neurology. New York, Oxford University Press, 1974

Stillman MJ: Stroke! How to care for a recovering patient. RN 42, No. 11:49–56, 1979

Tyler H, Dawson D: Current neurology, Vols. 1 & 2. Boston, Houghton Mifflin, 1979

Cary Lou Martinson

Respiratory Function

Respiratory distress is a common component of brain injury. With decreased levels of consciousness, an airway must be maintained. An endotracheal tube can be used for days, but to prevent complications a tracheostomy should be considered.

Since the neurophysiology of respiration is so complex, the neurologic insult could produce problems at any of a number of levels. The highest level of respiratory control is found in the brain-stem structures of the pneumotaxic center, the nucleus solitarius, and the medulla oblongata. These brain-stem centers can be injured by increased intracranial pressure and hypoxia, as well as by direct trauma or interruption

of blood supply. When the brain-stem centers are affected, the patient becomes dependent on an external source of control and thus becomes ventilator dependent.

BREATHING PATTERNS

Different respiratory patterns can be identified when there is an intracranial dysfunction (see Fig. 21-2).

Cheyne-Stokes breathing is periodic breathing with the depth of each breath increasing to a peak and then decreasing to a state of apnea. The hyperpneic phase usually lasts longer than the apneic phase. Cheyne-Stokes respiration usually indicates bilateral lesions located deep in the cerebral hemispheres. With traumatic brain injury, the onset of Cheyne-Stokes breathing might be due to herniation of the cerebral hemispheres through the tentorium, indicating a deteriorating neurologic condition. This herniation can also cause compression of the midbrain, and *central neurogenic hyperventilation* will be observed. This hyperventilation is sustained, regular, rapid, and fairly deep. It is usually caused by a lesion of the low midbrain or upper pons.

Apneustic breathing indicates respiration with a pause at full inspiration and full expiration. The etiology of this pattern is usually occlusion of the basilar artery, causing infarction of the lateral portions of the brain stem.

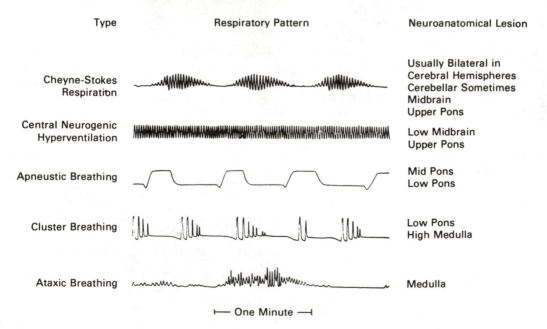

FIGURE 21-2.
Abnormal respiratory patterns associated with coma. (Gifford RRM, Plaut MR: Abnormal respiratory patterns in the comatose patient caused by intracranial dysfunction. J Neurosurg Nurs 7, No. 1:58, 1975)

Cluster breathing may be seen when the lesion is high in the medulla or low in the pons. This pattern of respiration is seen as gasping breaths with irregular pauses.

The real centers of inspiration and expiration are located in the medulla oblongata. Any rapidly expanding intracranial lesion, such as cerebellar hemorrhage, can compress the medulla, and *ataxic breathing* will result. This is totally irregular breathing with both deep and shallow breaths associated with irregular pauses. When this pattern of respiration occurs, a ventilator should be made available to the patient because there is no predicting respiratory rhythm or continuation of respiration.

Interference with some cranial nerves can also influence respiration. The brain-stem centers receive information from chemoreceptors in the carotid artery and aorta and from stretch receptors in the lungs by way of the glossopharyngeal (IX) and the vagus (X) nerves. Outgoing information from the brain stem then travels by way of the phrenic nerve, which leaves the spinal cord with the third cervical nerve and activates the diaphragm. The intercostal muscles that expand the chest wall are activated by the intracostal nerves of the thoracic spinal cord. Even if the brain-stem centers, the cranial nerves, and the thoracic nerves are all intact, the patient may still develop respiratory problems if pulmonary hygiene is inadequate.

MANAGEMENT

The majority of brain-injured patients will have perfectly normal respiratory rates and adequate oxygen exchange but still may not tolerate closing of an open tracheostomy because of the inability to handle their secretions. Pulmonary hygiene then becomes the responsibility of the nurse.

It is important to observe the patient for spontaneous coughing. Also note if he takes occasional deep breaths (sighs). Coughs and sighs are essential to keep the lungs fully expanded and to prevent pooling of secretions that lead to infection.

Preventing atelectasis and pneumonia is the goal in the immobile patient with a decreased level of consciousness. Atelectasis and pneumonia can be prevented by frequently stimulating the cough reflex and suctioning secretions by means of either the nasopharyngeal route or an open tracheostomy. Turning the patient frequently not only helps prevent skin sores but also mobilizes secretions and decreases pooling in the dependent lobes. Actually, any movement

of an inactive patient helps the pulmonary status. By getting a brain-injured patient up in a chair or on a tilt table or even doing range of motion, you are stimulating the patient to do some deep breathing.

Without nursing stimulation and vigilant suctioning, respiratory complications can easily be fatal to a brain-injured patient.

Urinary Control

In the acute brain-injured patient, fluid management is essential, and a Foley catheter is necessary to accurately measure urinary output. Too often the Foley catheter is forgotten as a source of irritation as well as of potential infection. Even though a brain-injured patient has lost voluntary control of his bladder, the reflexes for normal voiding may be intact. With the brain-injured patient the neurologic insult is upper motor neuron, leaving the lower motor neuron reflexes intact and uninhibited. This means most brain-injured patients will empty their bladders because of a reflex arc at the spinal cord level. Therefore, a Foley catheter can be avoided if the nursing staff can manage the incontinence problem.

For the male patient, an indwelling catheter can be removed and an external (condom-type) collector used. Care must be taken to monitor the patient's voiding to ensure that the bladder does not become overdistended or that a high residual volume is not left in the bladder. When a Foley catheter is removed, a straight catheter should be used to measure the postvoid residual volume. If the volume is below 100 ml for at least three residual checks, the patient may remain catheter free. Residuals above 100 ml indicate the presence of constant static urine, which increases the possibility of bladder infection.

Of course, if the patient does not void within a reasonable period of time as indicated by fluid intake, a catheter should be used to prevent distention. Limit fluids to 600 ml in a 6-hour period. If the fluid intake is 600 ml and the patient has not voided, a straight catheter should be used to empty the bladder. Continue this intermittent catheterization program until the patient starts to void spontaneously with low residual checks, or until it can be assessed that the bladder is flaccid with no reflexive emptying.

Unfortunately, external collectors are not available for female patients, but success can be obtained by transferring the patient to the toilet on a regular schedule when she is at least partially responding to the environment, and her condition permits. Environmental cues such as sitting on a toilet and being in a bathroom might be adequate to stimulate the patient to void even though she is unable to communicate needs.

Many brain-injured patients with motor control involvement develop very *spastic bladders* and have painful bladder spasms. To the brain-injured patient with decreased ability to understand his situation and to communicate his difficulties, an uncomfortable Foley catheter and painful bladder spasms are a source of great irritation. As a result, the patient may become more agitated and preoccupied with discomfort and less able to focus on more important environmental stimuli. Therefore, removing the Foley catheter can aid in reorientation of a brain-injured patient, as well as decrease the complication of bladder infection.

Bowel Control

Many complications can be avoided if a good bowel program is started in the critical care unit. Straining to evacuate stool can increase intracranial pressure causing neurologic deterioration. Thus, it is important to give adequate stool softeners and to facilitate evacuation on a regular basis.

The actual mechansim of emptying the bowel is basically a reflex activity at the spinal cord level. With brain injury, the voluntary control of stimulating or inhibiting the reflex is impaired. The reflex may be stimulated by the nurse on a routine basis to establish a predictable, controlled bowel program. The stimulation may be digital, a small-volume enema, or a chemical stimulant such as a Dulcolax suppository.

A *digital stimulation* consists of inserting a gloved, lubricated finger into the external rectal sphincter. With a slow circular motion against the sphincter the spinal cord reflex will be initiated. Both internal and external rectal sphincters will open, peristalsis will increase, and a normal evacuation can occur. If done too vigorously, a digital stimulation can cause discomfort. Some patients are too alert to tolerate this procedure, and then an enema or suppository may be preferable.

All of these methods enable the nurse to control evacuation. Establishing a regular routine for daily bowel movements prevents constipation and impaction, accidental bowel movements or continuous small stools, and avoids embarrassment for the patient and visiting family members.

Bed Positioning

With damage at the brain-stem level, there is a release of tonic reflexes that result in the assumption of abnormal postures. Abnormal muscle tone is reinforced by these reflexes and, in time, can create complications such as increased spasticity, scoliosis, contractures, and hip subluxation. It is easier to "mold" a patient's posture and muscle tone early post injury. Proper positioning helps to inhibit abnormal tone and allows for easier handling by the physical and occupational therapists and nurses who are helping the patient maintain full range of motion.

Countering Abnormal Posturing. Most common in the brain-injured patient is *opisthotonic posturing*. This is a forward arching of the back and hyperextention of the head with all extremities rigid and straight or hyperextended. This posturing is exaggerated when the patient is supine. Trunk rotation and flexion of the lower extremities will help break up this posturing (see Fig. 21-3). If the patient is left flat on his back with legs out straight, you will see an increase in extensor muscle tone. Turning the hips to a side-lying position and flexing the knees will relax the tone.

Head positioning is important because of an *asymmetric tonic neck reflex*. This reflex is demonstrated when the extremities on the same side to which the head is turned extend, and the opposite extremities flex. Therefore, to do range of motion on a tightly drawn up arm, try turning the head to that side and see if the muscle tone decreases.

Each brain-injured patient will have different reflexive posturing, and the nurse must evaluate what positions can be accomplished. The goal of effective positioning is to break up reflexive patterns and decrease abnormal muscle tone.

Preventing Contractures. *Passive range of motion* is used to stretch muscles and to maintain joint mobility. With the immobile patient, the nurse should move each joint through its normal range of motion on a regular basis. The activity is accomplished easily during a bath. When tightness does occur, splinting may help regain lost range of motion.

An easy and effective way to splint an extremity is with pillow splinting. Put one or two pillows along the outstretched arm and secure them tightly with an Ace bandage. The pillow splint can be left in place for approximately an hour at a time if skin pressure points are not a problem. With proper use of pillow splints,

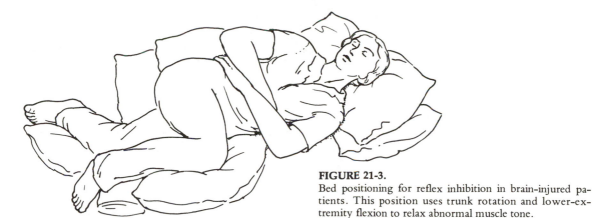

FIGURE 21-3.
Bed positioning for reflex inhibition in brain-injured patients. This position uses trunk rotation and lower-extremity flexion to relax abnormal muscle tone.

range of motion in the elbow joint can be increased and maintained.

With a tight hand grip, either voluntary or involuntary, a cone can be used to decrease the development of hand contractures. Pressure on the insertion of a muscle inhibits muscle contraction; thus, the use of a hand cone as opposed to a soft wash cloth can actually cause relaxation of the hand and maintain normal functioning.

Preventing Pressure Sores.   With loss of sensory and motor function, the brain-injured patient is left vulnerable to skin breakdown, and bed positioning becomes an important concern from this aspect. There is one simple rule to follow to prevent pressure sores: prevent pressure.

With current technology, there are numerous tools to help achieve this goal. There are beds designed to constantly change pressure areas by keeping the patient in continual motion from side to side (Roto Rest Bed). There are beds designed to facilitate turning while maintaining body alignment, such as the Stryker frame, the circle electric bed, and the Stoke-Edgerton bed. There are also numerous items to be placed on a bed to make pressure less of a problem, such as alternating pressure air mattresses, water mattresses, gel-foam pads, and sheepskins. But the fact remains that an immobile patient who is not turned regularly can develop pressure sores in time, no matter what mattress is used. Each patient must be evaluated individually as to his skin tolerance (how fast his skin turns red without being turned). However, 2 hours is an average skin pressure tolerance time for an acutely ill patient.

Another technique helpful in preventing pressure problems is to pad above and below prominent bony processes. For example, when the patient is on his side, put a rectangular foam pad or small pillow above and below the hip trochanter and above the lateral malleolus of the ankle. Also pad between bony pressure points such as the knees (see Fig. 21-4). The nurse should place her hand under the bony processes to confirm that pressure has been relieved. When the patient is on his back, place a pad above and below the sacrum and above the heels (see Fig. 21-5). Circular pads called "doughnuts" may actually impair circulation by causing circular pressure around the protected area. Use of rectangular pads allows for collateral circulation, while still relieving pressure.

Coma Position.   During initial coma, the patient may be very flaccid, and the "coma position" is recommended to facilitate handling of oral secretions or vomitus to prevent aspiration (see Fig. 21-6).

BIBLIOGRAPHY

Allen N: Prognostic indications in coma. Heart Lung 6:1075–1083, 1979

Chusid J: Correlative Neuroanatomy and Functional Neurology, 17th ed. Los Altos, Lange Medical Publications, 1979

Farber SD: Sensorimotor Evaluation and Treatment Procedures for Allied Health Personnel, p 42. Indiana University Foundation, 1974

Gifford RRM, Plaut MR: Abnormal respiratory patterns in the comatose patient caused by intracranial dysfunction. J Neurosurg Nurs 7, No. 1:57, 61, 1975

Penfield W: The Mystery of the Mind: A Critical Study of Consciousness and the Human Brain. Princeton, Princeton University Press, 1975

Plum F, Posner JB: The Diagnosis of Stupor and Coma, 2nd ed. Philadelphia, F.A. Davis, 1972

Toole JF (ed): Clinical Concepts of Neurological Disorders. Baltimore, Williams & Wilkins, 1977

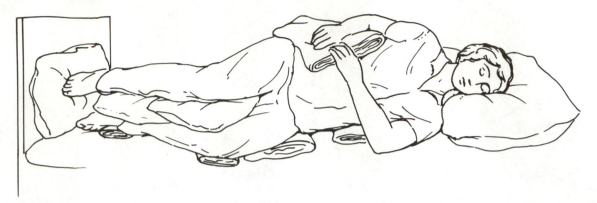

FIGURE 21-4.
Side lying position. Pads are used above and below the trochanter and lateral malleolus to relieve pressure.

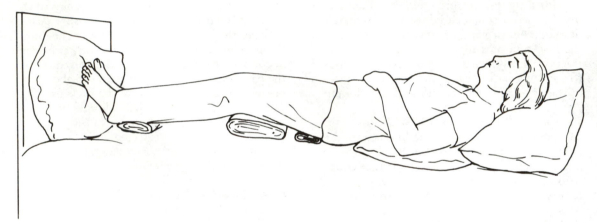

FIGURE 21-5.
Supine position. Pads are used above and below the sacrum and above the heels to relieve pressure. A pad above the knees prevents hyperextension of the knees and relieves pressure on the popliteal space.

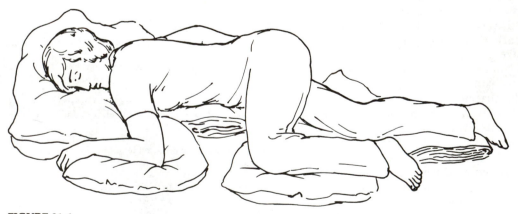

FIGURE 21-6.
Coma position. Shoulders are turned almost prone for better drainage of the oral and nasal passages.

Carole Kravec

COMMUNICATION DISORDERS

Because the brain contains centers for all thought processes, a patient who has sustained brain injury is likely to demonstrate some kind of communication disorder. Areas that may be affected include speech, language, memory, visual perception, cognitive abilities, problem-solving, concentration, and thought organization. The site of the injury and etiology determine the type of problem, its severity, and prognosis.

Aphasia

Patients who have sustained injury to certain areas of the dominant cerebral hemisphere may evidence aphasia. The left hemisphere of the brain is usually dominant for speech regardless of handedness. Specific areas of the left hemisphere which have been defined as most important for speech and language function are (1) the posterior temporoparietal region (Wernicke's area), (2) the three gyri anterior to the precentral face area (Broca's area), and (3) the superior, supplementary area, which appears to be dispensable but is probably important if other areas of speech are destroyed (see Fig. 21–7).

Aphasia is a term used to describe an acquired loss of language, with reduction of available language in all modalities. It is important to understand the difference between speech and language. Language is the entire system of symbols that we learn as children to communicate efficiently with one another. This language system is comprised of our ability to interpret what sounds we hear as words, of the letters and numbers we learn to read and write to communicate without drawing detailed pictures of our environment, and of our ability to produce certain sounds to convey thoughts to other people.

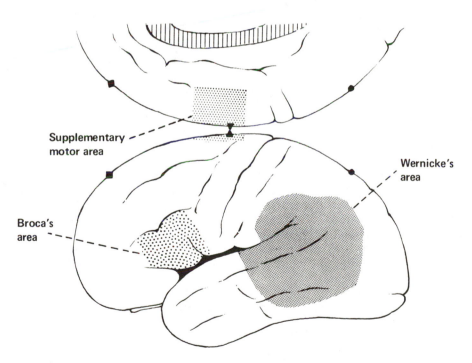

Supplementary motor area

Wernicke's area

Broca's area

FIGURE 21–7.
Three speech areas of dominant cerebral hemisphere: (1) the posterior, or parietotemporal area (Wernicke's area), is most important; (2) the anterior, or Broca's area, is next most important but is dispensable in some patients at least; (3) the superior, or supplementary motor area, is dispensable but may be important after damage to other speech areas. (Redrawn after Fig. IV-8 in Penfield W, Roberts L: Speech and Brain-Mechanisms, p 80. Princeton, Princeton University Press, 1959. Reprinted by permission of Princeton University Press)

Speech is merely the sounds we make with our mouths to convey language.

Language encompasses all aspects of the learned symbols we use to communicate — listening, reading, writing, numbers. An aphasic patient may have difficulty thinking of the correct word or may say inappropriate or meaningless jargon words. He is usually not aware of his errors. Since all language modalities are usually about equally impaired, an alphabet board or language board will not be helpful to this type of patient because he will have difficulty recognizing letters and words also.

When communicating with an aphasic patient, it is best to use simple language and ample gestural and environmental cues. Pointing to the desired object, tone of voice, facial expression, time of day, and hospital routine all contribute to the patient's understanding. Use pantomime and encourage the patient to do the same to aid communication.

Aphasic patients quickly become adept at "filling-in the blanks" when they do not understand completely. It is easy to overestimate their level of auditory comprehension and to assume that the aphasic patient understands everything that is being said. It is important to check this level of understanding fairly. Ask the patient to point to objects in the room, being careful not to nod or point in the correct direction. This is often difficult for a tester to do, because we all use gesture naturally. Modify what questions are asked of the patient because he will learn quickly what responses are expected of him. Getting a clear picture of the patient's level of understanding is not only important clinically but will alleviate frustration and confusion for the staff. The patient may be labeled as uncooperative, cross, or irrational when the staff believes he understands, but he behaves as if he does not.

Speak in a normal tone of voice. Aphasic patients are not deaf (unless they were pre onset), but merely have difficulty understanding the meaning of what they hear. Use short sentences; the patient may forget the beginning of a long sentence by the time you finish saying it. Avoid useless chatter that may confuse him.

Apraxia

Apraxia is the inability to carry out, on request, a complex or skilled movement that cannot be accounted for by muscle weakness or paralysis, sensory deficits, or lack of understanding. *Ideational apraxia* is the inability to formulate the ideational concept to perform complicated motor acts, even though the patient knows what he wants to do. *Ideomotor apraxia* is the state in which the patient can perform an act spontaneously or habitually but not on command. *Limb-kinetic* or *motor apraxia* is the loss of memory patterns needed to perform a movement. *Oral* and *verbal apraxia* refer to apraxia affecting the volitional positioning of the oral musculature to speak or perform oral movements.

Performance of an apraxic patient is inconsistent and variable. In speech, he may be able to say words spontaneously but cannot repeat them when he wants to. He may spontaneously pick up his spoon to eat his soup but cannot demonstrate its function when the soup is removed. Apraxia may be seen in any voluntary movement such as pointing, swallowing, talking, walking, or dressing.

If apraxia is present, avoid giving the patient a command to follow. Instead of saying, "Take a drink of water," simply give him the glass and let him perform the act automatically.

Dysarthria

Dysarthria is a group of speech disorders resulting from disturbances in muscular control of the speech mechanism (weakness, slowness, poor coordination, or altered muscle tone) due to damage to the central or peripheral nervous system. Motor processes of speech that may be affected include respiration, phonation, resonance, articulation, and prosody. Specific types of dysarthria have been defined and can be a valuable diagnostic tool to determine the site of the neurologic lesion.

Patients who are difficult to understand due to slurred, dysarthric speech should be encouraged to reduce their rate of speaking and to "overemphasize" speech movements. These patients are likely to have swallowing difficulties, also, because of muscle weakness or poor coordination.

Visual Perception Deficits

The right hemisphere of the brain is the center of visual-spatial functions. It controls the ability to judge distance, size, position, rate of movement, form, and the relation of parts to wholes. A patient who has sustained right hemisphere damage, usually resulting in left hemiplegia, is likely to speak in complete sentences but evidences problems in visual perception and spatial planning. Even with concentration, he may be unable to roll over in bed, feed himself, or discriminate the inside or outside of his clothes. He may have difficulty judging distances from an object or determining when he is sitting upright or leaning. This type of patient often has difficulty reading because he "loses his place" continually.

These difficulties often go undiagnosed because the patient is highly verbal and appears to be functioning normally. Because of his behavior, it is easy to overestimate this patient's abilities. He acts as if his deficits are not present. He tends to make excuses for his errors, such as, "I never was much of a reader." "I have a calculator to add and subtract." "My husband does all of the driving; he could push this wheelchair." The left hemiplegic is often a poor judge of his own abilities and safety.

These patients respond best to verbal cuing. Excess visual input, such as cluttered room, large number of people, gesturing to patient, may be more confusing than helpful. Try talking a patient through an activity and encourage him to describe each step himself at the same time. These patients benefit from repetition for new learning.

Visual Field Deficits

Homonymous hemianopsia is a visual field deficit that often occurs with cerebral vascular accident (CVA). Since neural pathways for vision cross at the chiasm, lesions occurring in the occipital area (visual cortex) produce blindness in half of both eyes on the opposite side of the lesion (see Fig. 22-2 in Chapter 22).

Most right hemiplegics who have right field cuts learn to compensate for this deficit quickly by turning their heads slightly. This enables them to use the intact visual field of both eyes. Formal testing can be performed when the patient can understand testing directions and can maintain his focus on a midline point. However, visual field deficits can be picked up clinically by observing functional activities such as eating, response to staff and visitors approaching from both sides, and personal hygiene activities.

Left hemiplegic patients typically have more difficulty compensating for left visual field deficits because their visual perception is also impaired. These patients may deny that objects exist to their left even when attention is called to them. This left ignoral generally makes the rehabilitation process difficult.

Left *aversion, neglect,* or *ignoral* can be observed in reading. Typically a patient can spell a word aloud but does not see all the letters when asked

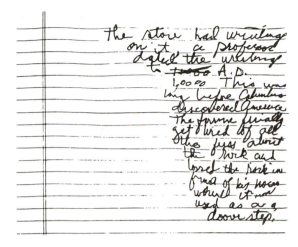

FIGURE 21-8.
Example of patient's writing demonstrating left visual ignoral.

to read a word. He may mistake the word *women* for *men* because he does not see the letters *wo.* He may mistake numbers by omitting the left side. Thus he may mistake *$24.99* for *$4.99.* When writing, the patient typically writes only on the right side of the page (see Fig. 21-8). Because the spatial organization center is also affected, this patient has difficulty recognizing these deficits, much less compensating for them.

Cognitive Deficits

Patients who sustain brain injury from trauma are likely to exhibit language disorders that are symptoms of generalized cognitive disorganization. Basic speech and language skills may be intact but may reflect problems in short-term memory, thought organization, concentration, initiation, and orientation. Coma or decreased level of response may persist for several weeks or months. Patient responses may be limited in nature (reflex movements, increased gross body movement, opening eyes) and may be noted only when stimulation is present. When left alone, the patient may remain quiet and still. As level of awareness increases, he may begin to respond to discomfort by pulling at his nasogastric or tracheostomy tube or by becoming restless or agitated. Although he is apparently unresponsive to environmental stimulation, he does respond to his own internal agitation and stimulation, often in a nonpurposeful manner.

With increased awareness, the patient begins

to respond to things around him, although he has difficulty maintaining selected attention for any length of time. Short-term memory is extremely impaired, although long-term memory may be intact. The patient may begin to wander with the intention of going home. Agitation may persist but is more goal-directed and aimed at external stimuli. The patient may be able to tolerate irritations (catheter, nasogastric tube, etc.) once they have been explained to him.

As the patient's ability to concentrate increases, improvements in short-term memory and learning will be evident. He will begin to show carry-over for old learning tasks (dressing, hygiene, etc.); new learning tasks show little carry-over. He may have difficulty organizing his thoughts to perform an activity. Since a great deal of retraining is based on language and reasoning, the speech pathologist can often provide guidance in improving the patient's cognitive organization.

BIBLIOGRAPHY

Brown J: Aphasia, Apraxia, and Agnosia. Springfield, Charles C Thomas, 1972

Darley FL, Aronson AE, Brown JR: Motor Speech Disorders. Philadelphia, W.B. Saunders, 1975

Fowler R, Fordyce W: Stroke: Why Do They Behave That Way? Booklet published by American Heart Association (50-035-A)

Hagen C, Malkmus D, Burditt G: Intervention strategies for language disorders secondary to head trauma. Unpublished paper, American Speech-Language-Hearing Association Convention, Atlanta, 1979

Porch B: Communication. In Hirschberg G et al (eds): Rehabilitation: A Manual for Care of the Disabled and Elderly, pp 100–139. Philadelphia, J.B. Lippincott, 1976

Schuell H, Jenkins JH, Jimenes-Pabon E: Aphasia in Adults: Diagnosis, Prognosis, and Treatment. New York, Hoeber, 1964

Cynthia Johnson Dahlberg

REESTABLISHMENT OF ORAL INTAKE

Normal Swallowing Function

Knowledge of normal swallowing function is essential before initiating an oral intake program with a brain-injured patient. Swallowing is primarily a reflexive action and is usually described in three stages.

In the oral stage, the tongue controls a bolus of food or liquid by pressing it against the soft palate and forming a seal around it. There is a respiratory pause on inspiration as the larynx moves up and forward to close and protect the airway. The seal around the bolus is broken as the soft palate elevates and closes the nasopharynx to prevent nasal regurgitation. The oral stage may include some volitional tongue movements but is primarily a reflexive action.

In the pharyngeal stage, with the soft palate elevated and the airway occluded, the tongue propels the bolus back against the posterior pharyngeal wall with anterior to posterior rippling motions. The muscles of the pharynx then contract sequentially to move the bolus down through the pharynx. The cricopharyngeal sphincter relaxes and opens in the esophageal stage as the bolus of food enters the esophagus. Peristaltic waves carry the bolus down the esophagus and into the stomach.

The swallowing reflex can be initiated by sensory stimulation of three cranial nerves. The glossopharyngeal nerve (IX) innervates the posterior tongue, the mucosa of the oropharynx, the soft palate, and the tonsillar area. The vagus nerve (X) provides sensory innervation to the mucosa of the larynx above the level of the vocal cords, the epiglottis, portions of the pharynx, and the esophagus. The trigeminal nerve (V) provides sensory innervation to the mucosa of the palate, the uvula, and the tonsillar area. Sensory stimulation to initiate a swallow is conveyed to the cranial nuclei in the medulla of the brain stem, which coordinates the simultaneous inhibition of respiration and the motor act of swallowing.

Over 20 different muscle pairs are involved in

the swallowing process, and they are innervated by six cranial nerves and the motor neurons of the first three cervical levels of the spinal cord. The cranial nerves involved include the hypoglossal (XII) for tongue movements; the vagus (X) for movement of the larynx, pharynx, and esophagus; the glossopharyngeal (IX) for pharyngeal muscle contractions and elevation of the soft palate; the facial (VII) for portions of the laryngeal action; and the trigeminal (V) to activate the tensor muscle of the soft palate. Swallowing is the most complex "all-or-none" reflex that results in an integrated, synchronized pattern that is individually constant and occurs below the level of consciousness.

Factors to Consider Before Initiation of Oral Intake

Medical Condition.   The patient's medical condition should be stable before oral intake is initiated. Conditions that contraindicate oral intake include fever (which may mask signs of aspiration pneumonia), the necessity of frequent suctioning, respiratory insufficiency, or other acute medical problems. Aspiration pneumonia can seriously complicate the patient's condition, especially in the presence of other medical problems.

Level of Consciousness.   The level of consciousness should at least allow for generalized responses to noxious stimulation, such as grimaces, restlessness, or pushing away. The patient's eyes should be open, but maintenance of eye contact or eye tracking is not necessary.

Swallowing Ability.   Swallowing ability should be evaluated and determined to be adequate without danger of aspiration. The most effective evaluation technique is cinefluorography (barium swallow) with the patient in an upright position. Anteroposterior and lateral views of the passage of barium in the swallowing sequence can easily reveal swallowing dysfunctions, such as poor tongue control, difficulty in initiation of the swallow, nasopharyngeal regurgitation, pharyngeal retention, inadequate relaxation of the cricopharyngeal area, or aspiration into the larynx. If cinefluorography demonstrates significant aspiration, an oral intake program is contraindicated.

Swallowing function is evaluated by subjective observation as well, and in some settings this may be the only method available. Many patients can be made to swallow with tactile stimulation around the mouth or larynx, or simply observed when swallowing saliva. The action of the tongue, the upward movement of the larynx, and the respiratory pattern are observed for rate, duration, and sequence, and compared to normal function.

Some patients also demonstrate primitive oral reflexes with stimulation of the oral area. These are the same reflexes that a newborn has, and are usually controlled by higher brain centers by the age of 1 year. The patient's brain injury has removed the inhibitory control mechanisms of the higher brain centers, and, consequently, the primitive brain-stem reflexes are released.

The most easily observed primitive oral reflexes are a suckling pattern (a repetitive forward, up, and backward movement of the tongue usually followed by a swallow), chewing (rhythmical chewing motions without jaw closure), and biting (jaw closure and holding when the area between the teeth or the gums is stimulated).

Respiratory Status.   Another major consideration before the beginning of oral intake is the patient's respiratory status. Respiratory function should be adequate with a small Jackson trach tube (size 4 or below), a Kistner button, or a normal airway.

If the patient's respiratory function is such that a cuffed trach tube or a Jackson, size 5 or larger, is required, the oral intake program should be postponed, since a large tracheostomy gives the patient an artificial airway that alters the normal coordination of respiration and swallowing. The tracheostomy tube can limit up and forward movement of the larynx because the tube itself anchors the trachea to the muscles and skin of the neck. Regurgitation and aspiration into the larynx may result from compression of the cervical esophagus by the tracheostomy tube.

The larger trach tubes with inflated cuffs cause even more compression of the esophagus; food or secretions may overflow and rest above the inflated cuff, and pressures from the swallow itself force liquids and even semisolids around the cuff into the trachea.

Consequently, larger tracheostomy tubes are a negative factor in attempting to reestablish safe swallowing function. The normal nasal-oral airway should be established by plugging the smaller Jackson trach tubes, using a Kistner button, or removing the tracheostomy before a patient is started on an oral intake program.

Cough Strength.   The final consideration is evaluation of cough strength. The patient should demonstrate a cough reflex adequate for protection of the airway. A weak cough will not clear the airway in the event of aspiration, and thus the patient should not be started on oral intake.

Overall Criteria.   The patient is ready to initiate an oral intake program if the above five factors are met: medical condition is stable; at least generalized responses to noxious stimuli are present; swallowing function is present; respiratory function is adequate; and the cough reflex is strong. Most severely brain-injured patients require at least a few weeks to elapse post injury before all these requirements are met.

Procedure

Removal of Nasogastric Tube.   If the patient has a nasogastric tube, it should be removed at least a few hours before food is introduced orally. The nasogastric tube can cause nasal and pharyngeal irritation, esophagitis, and laryngeal edema. The irritation and inflammation produce excessive secretions that are difficult to remove and interfere with the swallowing process. The presence of a foreign object passing through the nasal, oral, pharyngeal, and esophageal areas only interferes with swallowing efficiency.

Positioning.   The patient is best positioned in bed or in a chair from 45° to 90° upright, with the neck slightly flexed. Care should be taken not to extend the neck, as this makes upward movement of the larynx (to protect the airway from aspiration) more difficult. The ideal environment is free from distracting noises and movements for more effective concentration on the swallowing process.

Food Selection.   Often the physician will order clear liquids for the initial oral trial. Thin liquids are easily affected by gravity, and they flow through the mouth and pharynx quickly, before the patient is able to initiate a swallow. Consequently, solids with a clear liquid base, such as gelatin or popsicles, are a better choice as they can more easily be controlled in the mouth.

Food should be chosen to provide maximum stimulation in temperature, taste, color, and texture when possible. Bland tastes and lukewarm temperatures (such as tepid tap water) provide minimal stimulation to the patient and should be avoided in the initial stages, especially for patients with a reduced level of awareness. Milk products and sweets should be avoided as well because they cause excess mucus production.

Pureed foods are introduced if the patient demonstrates adequate control of the clear solids. The diet expands as the patient gains swallowing efficiency and control. From pureed foods, the patient progresses to foods that require minimal chewing, such as finely chopped meat, fruit, and vegetables. As chewing ability and tongue control improve, foods are chopped in larger pieces until the patient is able to tolerate a regular diet. Foods the patient did not enjoy prior to injury are to be avoided. Close contact should be maintained with the dietary department to provide nutritious and attractive meals within the patient's swallowing ability. The dietitian can also be helpful in recommending various protein or caloric supplements if indicated.

Techniques.   Techniques used during an oral intake session depend upon the patient's individual swallowing pattern, but some *general suggestions* apply to most patients. It is important to verbalize the entire process to the patient, even if understanding is questionable. The food or liquid should be described as to taste, smell, and appearance. The swallowing process is emphasized with comments such as "Move your tongue," "Push that food back," "Hold your breath," and "Swallow." The food is introduced as far posteriorly in the mouth as possible with firm pressure from the spoon. Metal spoons should always be used because plastic spoons can easily break and shatter, especially if the patient has a biting reflex.

In *hemiplegic patients* with unilateral sensory or motor impairment of the face, food and liquid should be placed in the mouth on the intact side. Also, swallowing efficiency can be improved if the patient's head is tilted slightly to the intact side so gravity will direct the food or liquid to the area of normal sensory and motor function. "Pocketing" of food in the impaired side of the mouth is characteristic of hemiplegic patients, and they need to be reminded to clear food from the mouth on both sides. Following a meal, it is important to carefully check the oral cavity and clear any residual food that may have lodged in the impaired side.

The *amount per swallow* is initially small, approximately 5 ml or less. Patients with poor tongue control lose food in the sides of the mouth, and large amounts are not completely evacuated after the first swallow. The food remaining in the oral cavity can easily slide down the pharynx after the swallow is completed and cause choking. Many patients have greater difficulty with liquids than with solids; consequently, liquids should initially be given carefully in small amounts.

If the introduction of food or liquid into the mouth fails to set off the reflexive swallow, *additional stimulation* is provided. Firm upward pressure on the floor of the mouth, light upward stroking of the larynx, or light tactile stimulation around the mouth may provide the stimulation necessary to trigger the swallowing reflex.

Staff members who feed the severely brain-injured patient must be carefully observant of the patient's swallowing behaviors. The staff member provides external control of the swallowing process with the introduction of food into the mouth, the amount per swallow, and the stimulation of the swallowing reflex. Too much food given too fast greatly increases the likelihood of aspiration.

Intake Goals. Goals are established for the total amount of fluid and caloric intake needed in 24 hours. All care givers participating in the oral intake program should use a consistent feeding technique and accurately record the amount of fluid and caloric intake.

Supplemental methods of intake are used when the patient is unable to maintain adequate nutrition orally. These supplemental methods may include intravenous feeding or gastrostomy. Reinsertion of the nasogastric tube should be avoided, if possible, due to the irritation of the swallowing mechanism and interference with the swallowing process. In cases of significant swallowing dysfunction with slow improvement in swallowing ability, a gastrostomy is ideal; the patient can continue on a consistent feeding program, and adequate nutrition can be maintained.

Careful monitoring of oral intake to maintain adequate nutrition is essential, especially in the initial stages. Periodic serum electrolytes and nitrogen balance checks are indicated. Weight should be charted on a regular basis.

WHEN TO DISCONTINUE ORAL INTAKE

Oral intake should be discontinued if the patient shows evidence of aspiration pneumonia. A sudden spike in temperature, a chest roentgenogram showing right lower lobe infiltration, or increased right lower lobe sounds after feeding are all indicative of aspiration.

Aspiration pneumonia is most frequently found in the right lower lobe of the lung due to the effect of gravity and the relatively straight downward course of the right bronchus as compared to the more acute angle of the left bronchus. The oral intake program should also be discontinued if the patient develops other complications that require priority treatment or if the tracheostomy tube is increased above a Jackson size 4 or changed to a cuffed trach tube. Any significant decrease in the patient's level of consciousness may indicate neurologic complications, and the oral intake program should again be terminated.

BIBLIOGRAPHY

Beeson PB, McDermott (eds): Textbook of Medicine, 14th ed. Philadelphia, W.B. Saunders, 1975

Best CH, Taylor NB: The Physiological Basis of Medical Practice, 10th ed. Baltimore, Williams & Wilkins, 1979

Bonanno PC: Swallowing dysfunction after tracheostomy. Ann Surg 174, No. 1:29–33, 1971

Donner MW, Silbiger ML: Cinefluorographic analysis of pharyngeal swallowing in neuromuscular disorders. Am J Med Sci, May 1966, pp 134–150

Ganong WF: Review of Medical Physiology, 9th ed. Los Altos, Lange Medical Publications, 1979

Pinkus NB: The dangers of oral feeding in the presence of cuffed tracheostomy tubes. Med J Aust, June 1973, pp 1238–1240

Marilynn Mitchell

CARE OF THE PATIENT WITH SPINAL CORD INJURY

Functional Abilities at Different Levels of Injury

Spinal cord injury is one of the most devastating of all traumatic injuries. Nursing care must be directed toward the concomitant physical, emotional, and social problems. With alertness to changes, close observation, and on-going assessment of these patients by the critical care nurse, many complications of cord injury no longer occur, or at least are recognized early so that appropriate treatment is implemented.

Realistic goal-setting is determined by the level and extent of the injury. The higher the injury is on the spinal cord, of course, the greater the loss of motor activity and sensation. The level of spinal cord injury is defined by the number of the most distal uninvolved segment of the cord.

C1–C4 Lesions. With a C1–C4 lesion, the trapezius, sternomastoid, and platysma muscles remain functional. Intercostal muscles and the diaphragm are paralyzed and there is no voluntary movement (physiological or functional) below the spinal transection. Sensory loss for levels C1 through C3 includes the occipital region, the ears, and some regions of the face. Sensory loss can be illustrated by a diagram of the dermatomes of the body (see Fig. 21-9,A & B).

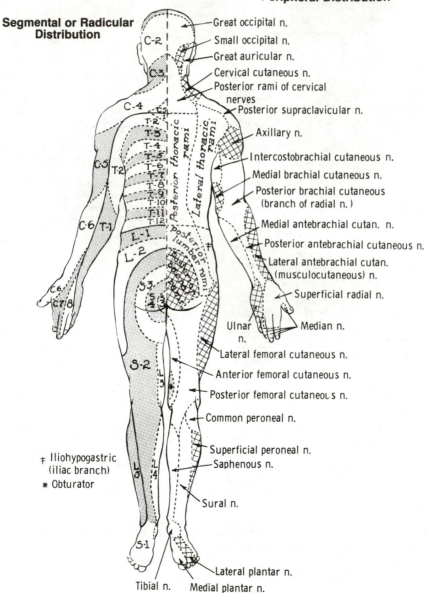

Peripheral Distribution

Segmental or Radicular Distribution

- Great occipital n.
- Small occipital n.
- Great auricular n.
- Cervical cutaneous n.
- Posterior rami of cervical nerves
- Posterior supraclavicular n.
- Axillary n.
- Intercostobrachial cutaneous n.
- Medial brachial cutaneous n.
- Posterior brachial cutaneous (branch of radial n.)
- Medial antebrachial cutan. n.
- Posterior antebrachial cutaneous n.
- Lateral antebrachial cutan. (musculocutaneous) n.
- Superficial radial n.
- Median n.
- Ulnar n.
- Lateral femoral cutaneous n.
- Anterior femoral cutaneous n.
- Posterior femoral cutaneous n.
- Common peroneal n.
- Superficial peroneal n.
- Saphenous n.
- Sural n.
- Lateral plantar n.
- Medial plantar n.
- Tibial n.

‡ Iliohypogastric (iliac branch)
∗ Obturator

FIGURE 21-9.
(A) Cutaneous innervation. (Reproduced, with permission, from Chusid JG: Correlative Neuroanatomy & Functional Neurology, 17th ed, p 206. Copyright 1979, Lange Medical Publications, Los Altos, California)

A patient with a C1, C2, or C3 quadriplegia requires full-time attendance due to dependency on a mechanical ventilator. This person is also dependent in all activities of daily living, such as feeding, bathing, and dressing. A person with this level of injury is able to operate an electric wheelchair (which should have a high back for head support) with chin or breath control. A mouthstick can be used to operate a typewriter or a telephone.

A C4 quadriplegic usually needs a mechanical ventilator too, but may be off of it intermittently. There is usually dependence on others for the activities of daily living, although he may be able to feed himself with the aid of feeding devices. This patient still needs an electric wheelchair, although because of better head control, a high-backed chair is not essential.

C5 Lesions. When the C5 segment of the cord is damaged, the function of the diaphragm is impaired secondary to posttraumatic edema in

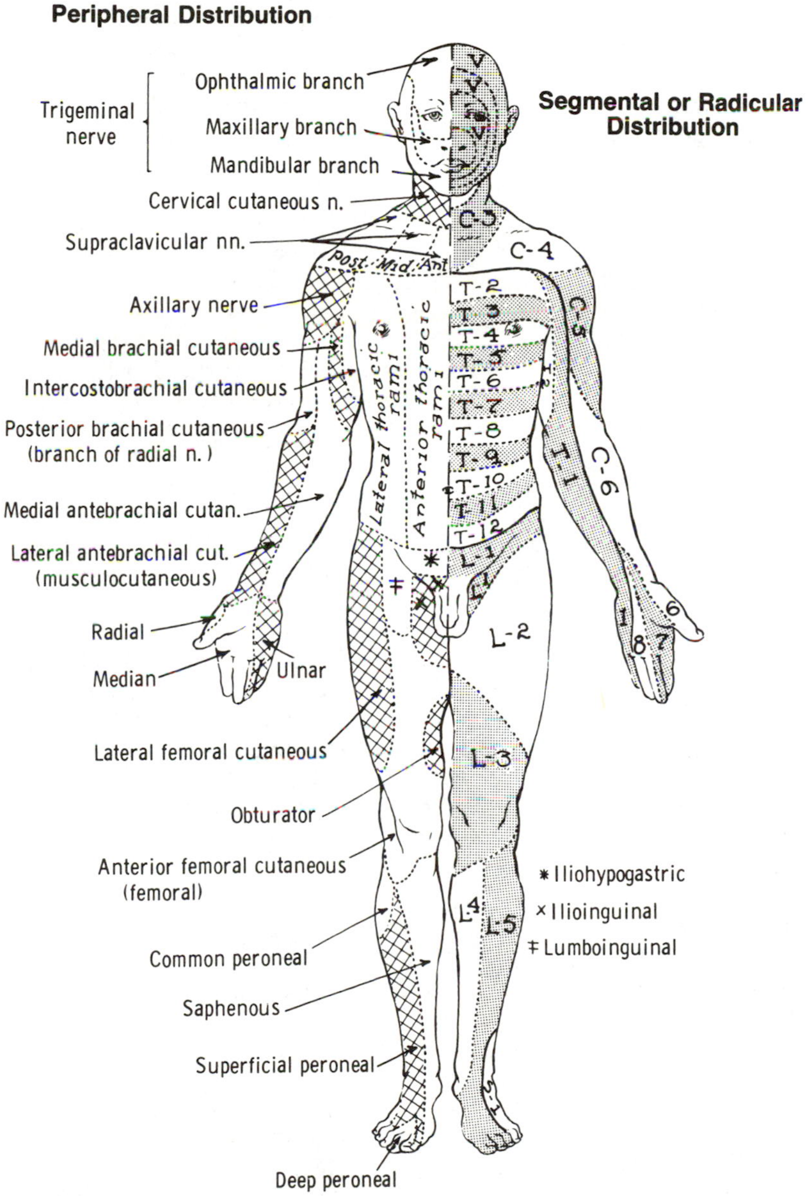

FIGURE 21-9.

(B) Cutaneous innervation. (Reproduced, with permission, from Chusid JG: *Correlative Neuroanatomy & Functional Neurology,* 17th ed, p 205. Copyright 1979, Lange Medical Publications, Los Altos, California)

the acute phase. Intestinal paralysis and gastric dilatation may compound the respiratory distress. The upper extremities are outwardly rotated from impairment of the supraspinous and infraspinous muscles. The shoulders may be markedly elevated due to uninhibited action of the levator scapulae and trapezius muscles. Following the acute phase, reflexes below the level of the lesion are exaggerated. Sensation is present in the neck and the triangular area of the anterior aspect of the upper arms.

A C5 quadriplegic is usually dependent for activities such as bathing, shaving, and combing of hair, but he has better hand-to-mouth coordination, allowing him to feed himself with the aid of a feeder or brace. These aids allow him to brush his teeth and to dress his upper extremities. With the use of mechanical aids, this patient can usually write.

Assistance is needed, as with higher level quadriplegia, in transfers from wheelchair to bed or vice versa. An electric wheelchair is still preferable with a C5 quadriplegic, although a manual wheelchair may be managed if it has quad pegs (projections on the hand rim which allow for greater ease of movement of the wheelchair). A person with this level of injury may find that manual manipulation of a wheelchair is very tiring.

C6 Lesions. In a C6 segment lesion, respiratory distress may occur because of intestinal paralysis and ascending edema of the spinal cord. The shoulders are usually elevated, with arms abducted and forearms flexed. This is due to the uninhibited action of the deltoid, biceps, and brachioradialis muscles. Functional recovery of the triceps is dependent upon correct positioning of the arms (forearm in extension, arm in adduction). Sensation remains over the lateral aspect of the arms and dorsolateral aspect of the forearm.

A C6 quadriplegic is independent in most of his own hygiene and is sometimes successful in lower extremity dressing and undressing. He is independent in feeding with or without mechanical aids. Light housework can be accomplished, and he is able to drive a car with hand controls.

C7 Lesions. Cord lesions at the level of C7 allow the diaphragm and accessory muscles to compensate for the affected abdominal and intercostal muscles. The upper extremities assume the same position as in C6 lesions. Finger flexion is usually exaggerated when the reflex action returns.

A C7 quadriplegic has the potential for independent living without attendant care. Transfers are independent, as are upper and lower extremity dressing and undressing, feeding, bathing, light housework, and cooking.

C8 Lesions. The abnormal position of the upper extremities is not present in C8 lesions because the adductors and internal rotators are able to counteract the antagonists. The latissimus dorsi and trapezius muscles are strong enough to support a sitting position. Postural hypotension may occur when the patient is raised to the sitting position due to the loss of vasomotor control. This postural hypotension can be minimized by having the patient make a gradual change from the lying to the sitting position. The patient's fingers usually assume a claw position.

A C8 quadriplegic should be able to live independently. He is independent in dressing, undressing, driving a car, homemaking, and self-care.

T1–T5 Lesions. Lesions in the T1–T5 region may cause diaphragmatic breathing. The inspiratory function of the lungs increases as the level of the thoracic lesion descends. Postural hypotension is usually present. A partial paralysis of the adductor pollicis, interosseous, and lumbrical muscles of the hands is present, as is sensory loss for touch, pain, and temperature.

T6–T12 Lesions. Lesions at the T6 level abolish all abdominal reflexes. From the level of T6 down, individual segments are functioning, and at the level of T12, all abdominal reflexes are present. There is spastic paralysis of the lower limbs. Patients with lesions at a thoracic level should be functionally independent.

The upper limits of sensory loss in thoracic lesions are as follows:

Level of Lesion	Upper Limit of Sensory Loss
T2	Entire body to inner side of the upper arm
T3	Axilla
T5	Nipple
T6	Xyphoid process
T7, T8	Lower costal margin
T10	Umbilicus
T12	Groin

Bowel and bladder function may return with the reflex automatism.

L1–L5 Lesions. The sensory loss involved in L1 through L5 lesions is as follows:

Level of Lesion	Sensory Loss
L1	All areas of the lower limbs, extending to the groin and back of the buttocks
L2	Lower limbs excepting the upper third of the anterior aspect of the thigh
L3	Lower limbs and saddle area
L4	Same as in L3 lesions, excepting the anterior aspect of the thigh
L5	Outer aspects of the legs and ankles, and the lower limbs and saddle area

Patients with these lesions should attain total independence.

S1–S5 Lesions. With lesions involving S1 through S5 there may be some displacement of the foot. From S3 through S5, there is no paralysis of the leg muscles. The loss of sensation involves the saddle area, scrotum, glans penis, perineum, anal area, and the upper third of the posterior aspect of the thigh.

Adaptive Devices. Paraplegics vary in the amount of adaptive equipment that is useful in helping them be functionally independent; this is dependent upon the level of injury. A T4 paraplegic may be able to stand up and walk with the aid of long leg braces and forearm crutches, although performance of this requires a great deal of physical energy.

T10 paraplegics are often more successful in ambulation with long leg braces and forearm crutches because there is more musculature preserved at this level than at the T4 level. L2 paraplegics can often accomplish ambulation with short leg braces and forearm crutches.

Orthopaedic vs Neurologic Level of Injury

These generalized goals for functioning at the different levels of spinal cord injury are not hard and fast for every patient. Functional performance may vary from patient to patient, depending upon whether one has a complete or an incomplete lesion. When an injury to the spinal cord is incomplete, there may be segments distal to the lesion that are still intact, although the orthopaedic level of injury is higher. For instance, the orthopaedic level of injury may be a C5 fracture, but the patient may be neurologically intact to C6. Since it is important to know what level of performance a patient can achieve, the neurologic level to which he can perform is really more significant than knowing where the orthopaedic injury is.

When speaking of a complete cord injury, the orthopaedic level of injury may be the same as the neurologic level of injury. No segments distal to the injury are preserved. This person will closely follow the dermatome chart for his level of sensory loss.

Acute Phase of Spinal Cord Injury

ASSESSMENT

During the initial assessment of a spinal cord-injured patient, a *digital rectal exam* is important in the determination of whether the injury is incomplete or complete. The lesion is incomplete if the patient can feel the palpating finger or if he can contract the perianal muscles around the finger voluntarily. Sensation may be present in the absence of voluntary motor activity. Sensation is seldom absent when voluntary perianal muscle contraction is present. In either case, the prognosis for further motor and sensory return is good.

Rectal tone by itself, without the criteria of voluntary perianal muscle contraction or rectal sensation, is not evidence of an incomplete cord injury. Some rectal tone may be accounted for by local reflexes.

SPINAL SHOCK

Spinal shock can be seen with either complete or incomplete motor and sensory deficits. Spinal shock differs from traumatic shock in several ways. In cord lesions above the sympathetic outflow (T5), there is an initial fall in blood pressure. This *hypotension* is more pronounced in cervical injuries. The blood pressure returns to normal a few days after the injury, but the reflex depression remains for a long period.

The reduced peripheral resistance and consequent pooling of blood in spinal shock is due to the vasomotor paralysis that occurs in spinal injury above the level of T6 and produces hypotension. In this instance the hypotension is like that of neurogenic shock. The low blood pressure in uncomplicated cord injury is accompanied by bradycardia due to reflex vagal

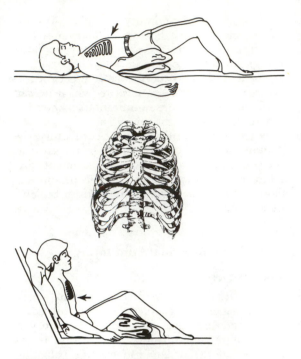

FIGURE 21-10.
Quad coughing technique. These positions are for diaphragmatic quad coughing only. *(Top)* To push the diaphragm, place one hand flat in the middle of the torso above the stomach and below the ribs. *(Middle)* Front view of the ribs; diaphragm indicated by heavy line. *(Bottom)* To compress the chest, place both hands flat and position on both sides of the chest. Do not move on top of the rib cage, because this could cause damage.

activity. When other injuries are present, there may be hypovolemia and tachycardia. Cardiac arrest is a potential danger in spinal shock due to this vasomotor instability. There is also the potential for deep vein thrombosis in the spinal shock phase due to venous pooling of blood, but it is more likely to occur after reflex activity has returned.

Hypothermia and absence of sweating below the injury level may also be seen in the spinal shock stage. Initially, flaccid paralysis is seen below the level of injury with bowel and bladder atony. Sacral reflexes and priapism may be present in patients with upper motor neuron lesions.

The appearance of involuntary spastic movement indicates that the spinal shock is resolving. Reflex activity returns over several days in patients with upper motor neuron lesions. Reflex perianal muscle contraction often returns before the deep tendon reflexes (DTRs). One can test for the reflex perianal muscle contraction during a digital rectal exam by pinching the glans or the base of the penis (bulbocavernous reflex) or by pulling on the Foley catheter.

In a female, squeezing of the clitoris will stimulate the reflex, if present. Absence of this spinal reflex arc implies that there is no physiological continuity between the lower spinal cord and supraspinal centers.

Nursing Care Considerations

RESPIRATORY CARE

Hypoventilation from inadequate innervation of respiratory muscles is a common problem after spinal cord injury. It is important to assess whether the intercostal muscles are functioning or whether the patient has only diaphragmatic breathing. The diaphragm, the major respiratory muscle, is innervated by the phrenic nerve, which travels through the third, fourth, and fifth cervical segments of the cord.

Any time a patient has a cervical cord injury, *respiratory failure* should be anticipated. Even though initially the patient may have what appears to be adequate diaphragmatic breathing (the intercostals would not be functioning because they are innervated from the thoracic region of the cord), cord edema can act like an ascending lesion and may compromise function of the diaphragm. Frequent checks of tidal volume and vital capacity and frequent auscultation of breath sounds should be routine.

The spinal cord-injured patient may have further respiratory compromise because of preexisting pulmonary disease or coexistent chest injuries. Alveolar ventilation may be directly affected by the pulmonary collapse or by consolidation from *retained secretions* or aspiration of vomitus. *Pulmonary edema* may also result from incorrect management of intravenous fluids. Paralytic ileus and gastric dilatation may increase the pressure on the diaphragm and cause further respiratory embarrassment. Interference with the cough reflex and fluid imbalance may combine to obstruct the airways.

Assisting the patient with the *"quad" coughing technique* may help him to more effectively clear his airways, despite weakness or loss of the respiratory muscles that produce the automatic cough reflex. With this quad coughing technique, the sides of the patient's chest (if on his side or abdomen) or the diaphragm (if supine) are compressed during exhalation (see Fig. 21-10). This technique is often most helpful following postural drainage or clapping of the chest.

When turning a patient to a *prone position* on a Stryker frame, the nurse needs to remain at the bedside for the first few turns to evaluate the patient's respiratory tolerance of the turn. High quadriplegics can experience respiratory arrest in the prone position because movement of the diaphragm is compromised. Bradycardia in the prone position is also common.

METABOLIC CONSIDERATIONS

The patient with spinal cord injury demonstrates a surprisingly florid metabolic response to an injury that is usually associated with little tissue damage. If the injury is uncomplicated, the metabolic derangement reaches a peak within 48 to 72 hours post injury. A return to normal may be anticipated between 10 and 14 days post injury.

When the spinal injury is complicated by other factors such as surgical intervention or other medical problems, the metabolic response is greater and more prolonged. This metabolic response is characterized by a marked retention of sodium and water, increased potassium excretion, breakdown of body protein, and an oliguric period followed by diuresis. A reduced glomerular filtration rate secondary to hypotension compounds the sodium and water retention.

Starvation is also a factor in the metabolic disturbance since the majority of cord-injured patients are unable to tolerate oral food or fluid for at least a week following the injury. This can lead to a negative nitrogen balance in the body.

Since it may be difficult to ascertain the patient's state of hydration on admission due to the vasodilatation, *monitoring of fluid intake and output* is necessary to prevent pulmonary edema, tubular necrosis, electrolyte imbalance, and congestive heart failure.

The intravenous caloric intake should be approximately 2000 calories per 24 hours. It may be necessary to give the patient *hyperalimentation* to accomplish this. Patients with spinal cord injury tend to lose weight easily because of the increased catabolic activity.

GASTROINTESTINAL CONSIDERATIONS

Cord-injured patients often have gastrointestinal difficulties. This complication is seen most frequently in the patient whose lesion is in the cervical or thoracic region of the cord. The pathophysiology of this complication is thought to involve an imbalance between parasympathetic and sympathetic innervation of the bowel caused by interruption of the supraspinal control of sympathetic centers in the thoracic and upper areas of the spinal cord.

The cessation of smooth muscle function lasts for about 5 to 7 days. There is an accumulation of fluid in the stomach and intestines with vomiting and *abdominal distention*. Acute gastric dilatation frequently occurs in patients with high cord lesions with or without paralytic ileus. When the distention compresses the vena cava or elevates the diaphragm, there may be an exacerbation of the hypotension or hypoventilation associated with cervical cord injury.

Acute gastrointestinal *hemorrhage* may also occur secondary to a stress ulcer. Signs of a *stress ulcer*, which is due to an abnormal release of catecholamines, often occur between day 6 and 14 after injury. The problem may be aggravated by steroid therapy. The nurse should be alert if the quadriplegic patient complains of sudden unexplained shoulder pain. It may be referred pain from the gastrointestinal tract. A small amount of antacid medication may be instilled into the patient's stomach whenever the *p*H of the gastric aspirate is below 3.0 in order to prevent the complication of stress ulcer.

The combination of starvation and gastrointestinal and metabolic changes may precipitate ketosis, dehydration, and other electrolyte and acid–base imbalances. Because of the gastrointestinal complications, a nasogastric tube should be inserted and bowel sounds monitored. The *nasogastric tube* prevents vomiting and probably aids in earlier resolution of the ileus. *Oral fluids* may be started at 25 to 50 ml per hour after bowel sounds have returned. If there is no evidence of residual gastric aspirate, oral fluids may be gradually increased. Food intake may begin when the patient can tolerate 75 to 150 ml of fluid per hour. Chances are great that the patient initially will have a poor appetite, partially due to depression and partly due to the fact that he has suffered sensory loss.

SKIN CARE

Pressure is a common cause of structural damage to a muscle and its peripheral nerve supply. There is a definite time/pressure relationship in the development of *pressure sores*. Skin can tolerate minute pressure indefinitely, but great pressure for a short time is disruptive. Microscopic tissue changes secondary to local ischemia occur in less than 30 minutes. Pressure interferes with arteriolar and capillary blood flow.

When the pressure is prolonged, there is a definite superficial circulation and tissue damage. The damage may be associated with congestion and induration of the area or blistering and loss of superficial epidermal layers of skin. As the pressure continues, the deeper skin layers are lost, leading to necrosis and ulceration. Serous drainage from such an ulceration can constitute a continuous protein loss of as much as 50 g per day. Prolonging the pressure results in deep penetrating necrosis of the skin, subcutaneous tissue, fascia, and muscle. The destruction may progress to gangrene of the underlying bony structure. Pressure necrosis can begin from within the tissue over a bony prominence where the body weight is greatest per square inch.

A *turn schedule* for the patient is obviously important. It should be carried out at least every 2 hours. Use of an air mattress does not preclude the need to turn. The condition of the skin should be checked before and after the position change. Patients should be encouraged to check their own skin condition with a mirror, when possible, to recognize their skin's tolerance to pressure, that is, the amount of time one can lie or sit in the same position without redness that does not fade within 15 minutes.

Patients should also be taught how to do *weight shifts,* especially when they are getting up in their wheelchair for long periods during the day. A weight shift is a means of relieving pressure from any bony prominence. When in the sitting position, the main bony prominences are the ischial tuberosities and the sacrum.

There are several methods of accomplishing a weight shift. There is a *full recline,* in which the patient is reclined in his wheelchair to relieve the ischial pressure, and the weight is thereby distributed throughout his entire dorsal surface. The *side to side* weight shift is accomplished when the patient hooks his forearm around one push-handle of the wheelchair and then leans sideways over the opposite wheelchair tire. The *half push-up* weight shift relieves pressure from one ischium by leaning on one elbow and pushing off the opposite wheelchair tire or armrest. This process is repeated in the other direction to relieve pressure from the opposite ischium. The *full push-up* weight shift relieves ischial pressure by pushing up with the arms from the tires or armrests of the wheelchair. Which of these weight shifts a patient can accomplish will of course depend on the motor ability of the individual.

To avoid skin breakdown, the skin should be protected from perspiration, stool, and urine. Use of incontinence pads tends to hold the perspiration next to the skin and thus should be avoided. A bedpan does not work well with a spinal cord-injured person. It is so hard that it can cause a pressure area over the coccyx, it does not allow access to the anus for digital stimulation, and it can upset the spinal alignment necessary for proper healing.

CONTRACTURES

Prevention of contractures should be initiated upon admission. Muscle shortening from disuse of an extremity can occur within 3 days. A paralyzed extremity is more likely to contract to a flexed position because the muscles used to flex an extremity are stronger than those used to extend it. If contractures are allowed to develop, the patient's recovery cannot be optimal. He will not be able to recover full motor use of a contracted extremity.

CARDIOVASCULAR INVOLVEMENT

During the spinal-shock phase, vasomotor tone is lost and blood pools in the periphery, lowering blood pressure because of the decreased circulating volume. *Orthostatic hypotension* may also occur because the patient is unable to compensate for changes in position. The vasoconstricting message from the medulla cannot reach the blood vessels because of the cord lesion.

Deep vein thrombosis is a silent complication in spinal cord-injured patients and carries with it the hazard of *pulmonary embolism.* The development of a thrombosis is influenced by stasis in the venous system, local trauma, continuous contact of the patient's calves and thighs with the bed, prolonged immobilization, and the patient's inability to sense pain.

With the development of venous thrombosis, there is swelling of the involved limb, local redness, increased skin warmth, and a slight systemic temperature rise (which may be masked if the patient is receiving steroids).

The *routine turn schedule* for skin maintenance mobilizes the patient sufficiently to help prevent venous thrombosis. Thigh-high *elastic stockings* or bandages properly applied also have prophylactic value. They should be removed for about 30 minutes each 8-hour period.

Other preventive measures include *determining the patient's leg circumference* 20 cm above and below the upper border of the patella on admission, for a baseline, and then daily thereafter. *Passive range of motion* exercises to lower extremities should be carried out at least twice a day. *Anticoagulant therapy* may also be considered. If there is no contraindication, such as concomitant head injury, the patient should be placed in *Trendelenberg position* (about 15°) for a minimum of 1 hour every 8 hours to help the blood return to the heart from the lower extremities.

BOWEL PROGRAM

Smooth muscle peristalsis begins as soon as the paralytic ileus secondary to spinal shock resolves. Keep in mind that bowel impaction frequently occurs during the period of ileus. The defecation reflex remains intact with lesions above the sacral segments. The reflex is interrupted with lower motor neuron lesions, but the autonomous bowel has an intrinsic contractile response. Bowel training is based on a fixed time pattern that takes the place of the cerebrally monitored urge. For the patient with a lower motor neuron lesion, continence is assured by regularly evacuating the bowel.

Peristalsis should be stimulated as soon as bowel sounds are present. This is safely done with stool softeners, mild laxatives, or suppositories. Enemas, other than the oil-retention type, should be avoided because the risk of intestinal perforation is high.

The actual bowel program may be based on bowel habits prior to the injury. The time of day should be established in relation to the patient's future social needs. A bowel program can be used in conjunction with digital stimulation.

Once a pattern is established, *digital stimulation* may be used alone. While the pattern of evacuation is being established, digital stimulation should be used after any involuntary bowel movement to assure complete evacuation of the rectum. There may be patients who will not tolerate digital stimulation without having an episode of autonomic dysreflexia. Nupercainal ointment can be used to insert the suppository or for digital stimulation in those patients prone to this phenomenon.

A bowel program may be modified according to individual need, as determined by stool consistency. A high fluid intake should be maintained.

URINARY MANAGEMENT

Acute tubular necrosis may occur during the first 48 hours post injury as a result of hypotension. In the acute phase of injury, the urine output should be measured hourly. An indwelling catheter is necessary to accomplish this. The urine should be tested for specific gravity, blood, protein, bile, and sugar to help monitor electrolyte balance.

The long-range objective of bladder management, regardless of the level of the lesion, is to achieve a means whereby the bladder consistently empties, the urine is sterile, and the patient remains continent. The ultimate goal is to have the patient catheter free, with consistent low residual urine checks, no urinary tract infection, and no evidence of damage to the upper urinary tract structures.

Intermittent Catheterization. One method of bladder management is accomplished by intermittent catheterization, and it may begin in the early recovery phase after the spinal shock has resolved. The purpose of this program is to exercise the detrusor muscle, with the goal again being to have the patient catheter free. The advantage of this method is that no irritant remains in the bladder; consequently, the risk of urinary tract infection, periurethral abscess, and epididymitis is reduced.

To initiate this program the patient is catheterized every 4 to 6 hours. A record is kept of voided amounts and residual amounts. If there is a residual of over 500 ml, the frequency of catheterization should be increased until residuals are under that amount. A urine specimen is obtained for culture and sensitivity at the start of the program. The fluid intake between catheterizations is limited to 600 to 800 ml. The number of catheterizations can be decreased as voided amounts increase or as residual amounts decrease. When a male patient begins to void between catheterizations, an external collector can be used to maintain continence.

Prior to the catheterization procedure the patient should be assisted to empty the bladder by Crédé, Valsalva, anal dilatation, or any other method that will trigger voiding for the individual. These methods stimulate the sacral reflex arc. The objective is to achieve a repeatable residual urine volume of 10% of the voided volume. The catheterizations may be stopped when the residuals become less than 150 ml.

Factors that may hinder efforts to achieve urinary continence include bowel impactions, cystitis, bladder stones, pressure sores, systemic infections, and anxiety.

Indwelling Catheter. Another urinary protocol that can be followed involves an indwelling bladder catheter. This catheter can be a urethral catheter or a suprapubic catheter. The catheter is attached to a gravity drainage system at all times. High fluid intake is encouraged. The catheter insertion site should be washed once or twice daily with soap and water. Betadine swabs may also be used to cleanse the insertion site. These catheters should not be changed routinely but only if they become plugged or develop granulation inside. Male urethral catheters should be taped up on the abdomen to prevent urethral-scrotal fistulas. Female urethral catheters should be taped to the inside of the thigh.

A male urethral catheter should not be larger than a size 16, 5 ml inert catheter. A female urethral catheter should not be larger than a size 20, 5 ml inert catheter. A suprapubic catheter should not be larger than a size 24, 5 ml inert catheter.

The method of clamping an indwelling catheter with intermittent release and drainage of the bladder is no longer used in many spinal cord rehabilitation facilities. If the patient should have a large residual volume between the times the bladder is drained, the urine has nowhere to go except to reflux back into the kidneys. This situation can be very detrimental to the patient's kidneys. Overdistention also destroys the detrusor muscle's ability to contract, thereby jeopardizing the return of automatic functions.

MEDICATIONS

Some medications are commonly used in patients with spinal cord injuries while others are contraindicated. *Cortisone* (dexamethasone MSD) may be used initially for a short period to relieve the physiological stress phenomenon. Intravenous therapy *(hyperalimentation)* may be indicated during the spinal-shock phase or possibly for longer periods depending upon coexistent complications. The intravenous site of choice is the subclavian vein, as there is less chance of thrombosis secondary to the vasomotor paralysis. For this reason, the veins of the lower extremities should never be used for intravenous administration. Low-dose *heparin* may be used prophylactically against venous thrombosis, although there is much contradictory literature regarding its worth.

Subcutaneous and intramuscular injections are not absorbed well because of the lack of muscle tone. Sterile abscesses may result, causing autonomic dysreflexia or an increase in spasms. *Injection sites* are the deltoid area, the anterior thigh, and the abdominal area. These sites should be rotated, and the volume injected should not exceed 1 ml at any one site.

As a rule, sensation in cord-injured patients is limited. Intractable pain may be present after spinal shock and is due to nerve root damage. Abnormal sensation may occur at the level of the lesion in injuries causing diverse nerve root

damage, such as with gunshot wounds or knife wounds. Narcotics are not favored because of the high probability of addiction. Attention to position and other comfort measures, along with the use of mild analgesics such as aspirin or acetaminophen, is a more acceptable approach.

Tranquilizers can be used to dull the environment during the initial stage following cord injury; however, behavioral problems are not relieved by tranquilizers. The psychological stages of the recovery process must be resolved, and this cannot be accomplished if the patient remains sedated. As reflex automatism returns, relief of spasms has been achieved with *diazepam.*

PHYSICAL THERAPY

A program of physical therapy and rehabilitation should be organized shortly after the patient's hospital admission. Realistic short- and long-term goals must be set jointly with the patient. Rehabilitation is often a very protracted process. The patient must be aware that results from the program will not be seen overnight. Thus, it is important that the patient and his family be part of the rehabilitation conference when goals are discussed.

A myriad of problems can surround the patient with a spinal cord injury. Each person responds differently and adjusts to his injury in different ways. When his whole life must be changed because of a spinal cord injury, the emotional and social problems, as well as the physical ones, can seem overwhelming. Patients need the support of the family and significant others at this time. The critical care nurse assumes a major role in helping both patient and family to cope with the problems. Rehabilitation of cord-injured patients can be slow and tedious and psychologically draining for the nurse, but it also offers great rewards in terms of the personal satisfaction that comes from meeting the challenges.

SEXUALITY

After a cord injury, patients are concerned about their ability for sexual function, although many may not verbalize this concern for quite awhile. When the questions do come, it is helpful if the nurse can respond in an informed way instead of telling the patient to ask the physician.

Most male cord-injured patients believe their total sexuality is tied to erection and ejaculation. There are three general types of erection in males. A *psychogenic erection* can occur by simply thinking sexual thoughts. The area of the cord responsible for this type of erection is between T11 and L2. Therefore, if the lesion is above this level, the message from the brain cannot get through the damaged area. *Reflexogenic erections* are a direct result of stimulation to the penis. Some patients may get this type of erection when changing their catheter or pulling the pubic hairs. The length of time the erection can be maintained is variable; thus, its usefulness for sexual activity is variable. Reflexogenic erections are better with higher cervical and thoracic lesions. Damage to lumbar and sacral regions may destroy the reflex arc.

The third type of erection is *spontaneous*. This may occur when the bladder is full, and it comes from some internal stimulation. How long the spontaneous erection lasts will determine its usefulness for sexual activity. The ability to achieve a reflexogenic or spontaneous erection comes from nerves in the S2, S3, and S4 segments of the cord. Male penile implants are now available for patients whose erections are very brief or not present at all.

Not many males with a complete cord injury have ejaculations. Sometimes retrograde ejaculation into the bladder will occur. Some male patients remove their urethral catheter prior to intercourse. Others leave their catheter in place and fold it back over the penis. Despite the physical side-effects of the spinal cord injury, the patient's sex drive should not change from what it was before the injury.

Women with spinal cord injury may find they need to use a lubricating jelly such as KY jelly (water soluble) prior to intercourse. If the woman was practicing birth control before the injury, it should still be a concern after the injury. Fellatio and cunnilingus are practices many patients find satisfying.

The sexuality of an individual involves the total person, not just sexual behavior. It includes what one thinks about himself in general. Cord-injured patients need to be made aware that meaningful, loving relationships are still attainable. Sexual counseling is often needed to communicate these messages.

AUTONOMIC DYSREFLEXIA

Autonomic dysreflexia or hyperreflexia is a syndrome that sometimes occurs in patients with a spinal cord lesion at T7 or above and constitutes a medical emergency. The syndrome presents quickly and can precipitate a seizure or a stroke. Death can occur if the cause is not relieved.

The syndrome can be triggered by bladder or intestinal distention, spasticity, decubitus ulcers, or stimulation of the skin below the level of the injury. Ejaculation in the male can initiate the reflex, as can strong uterine contractions in the pregnant female.

These stimuli produce a sympathetic discharge that causes a reflex vasoconstriction of the blood vessels in the skin and splanchnic bed below the level of the injury. The vasoconstriction produces extreme hypertension and a throbbing headache.

Vasoconstriction of the splanchnic bed distends the baroreceptors in the carotid sinus and aortic arch. They in turn stimulate the vagus nerve, and that results in a bradycardia, which is the body's attempt to lower the blood pressure. The body attempts to reduce the hypertension also by superficial vasodilatation of vessels above the cord injury. As a result of this, there is flushing, blurred vision, and nasal congestion. Because the spinal cord injury interrupts transmission of the vasodilatation message below the level of the lesion, the vasoconstriction continues below the level of the lesion until the stimulus is identified and interrupted. The vasoconstriction results in pallor below the level of the lesion, while flushing occurs above the lesion.

When autonomic dysreflexia is recognized, there are several things the alert nurse can do quickly and can teach the patient to do. The head of the bed should be elevated and frequent checks of the blood pressure should be made. The bladder drainage system can be quickly checked for kinks in the tubing. The urine collection bag should not be overly full. Some protocols for checking the patency of the urinary drainage system include irrigating the catheter with 10 to 30 ml of irrigating solution. The nurse should make sure absolutely no more than that amount is used because the addition of the fluid may further aggravate the massive sympathetic outflow already present. If the symptoms persist after these checks are made, the catheter should be changed to allow the bladder to empty. If the patient did not have a catheter in place when the hyperreflexia began, one should be inserted.

If the urinary system does not seem to be the cause of the stimulus, the patient should be checked for *bowel impaction*. The impaction should not be removed until the symptoms subside. Nupercainal or xylocaine ointment can be applied to the rectum to anesthetize the area until symptoms subside. Patients prone to autonomic dysreflexia use these ointments routinely with their bowel program.

If the patient's blood pressure does not return

to normal, the use of a *sympathetic ganglionic blocking agent,* such as atropine sulfate, guanethidine sulfate (Ismelin), reserpine (Serpasil), or methyldopa (Aldomet) may be used. Hydralazine (Apresoline) and diazoxide (Hyperstat) are also sometimes used.

PSYCHOLOGICAL PROCESSES

Different authors have different names for the stages of loss and grief a patient with spinal cord injury goes through on the road to rehabilitation. The psychological adjustment to the loss of one's previous physical abilities is unique to each individual. The rate at which a person works through this process varies, and none of the stages are static. A person can move back and forth between stages. The emotions felt and displayed by a patient with a cord injury are no different from the emotions felt by all of us at one time or another, and recognition of that fact may be a helpful guideline in empathizing with the patient's feelings.

Whatever names we give to the stages of grief, there are certain emotions that are felt by the patient following a cord injury.

Stage I—Shock and Disbelief. During this phase the patient does not request an explanation of what has happened to him. He is overwhelmed by the injury. There may be more concern with whether he will live than with whether he will walk again. This period may result in extreme dependence on the staff members. Staff members at the same time may feel the patient doesn't understand the ramification of his injury. The staff may identify with his feelings of being overwhelmed because they themselves are often overwhelmed with the acute medical management of this catastrophic illness.

Stage II—Denial. The process of denial is an escape mechanism for the patient. Generally the whole disability is not denied, but particular aspects of it are. For instance, the patient may say he cannot walk now, but in 6 months he will be able to. Bargaining, instead of being a separate stage, can be considered a form of denial. Bargains with God may be in the form of offering Him the legs if He will just return function of the arms. Staff often find it difficult to deal with patients in this stage.

A helpful approach is to focus on the here and now instead of trying to break down the denial. For instance, when a patient refuses to go to physical therapy or refuses certain aspects of his care because this is not a permanent disability, the staff can say that *today* he cannot walk; hence, these treatments are necessary.

Focus on the present problems. This is not the stage to talk to the patient about long-term changes, such as ordering a wheelchair or making modifications on his home. More appropriate matters to deal with would be bladder training, skin care, or range of motion exercises.

Stage III—Reaction. During this stage, instead of denying the impact of the injury, the patient expresses this impact. There may be severe depression and loss of motivation and involvement. Previous hobbies or interests lose their meaning. There is great helplessness during this period, and there may be suicidal statements.

Staff members can help at this stage by listening to the patient as he works through his feelings. The staff should avoid setting up failure situations, which could happen if they push the patient too fast. Because the patient tends to withdraw during this stage, staff may help by introducing diversional activities.

Another type of reaction seen is *acting out,* which may include anger or sexual, drug, or alcohol abuse. Anger may be expressed verbally or physically. The patient feels no one can do anything right—including family or staff. This kind of behavior makes staff want to avoid contact with the patient. Some limits do need to be set with the patient to protect himself and the staff if he becomes truly abusive.

Stage IV—Mobilization. Problem-solving behavior can be seen during this stage. The patient is looking toward the future and wants to learn about his self-care. In fact, he may become very possessive of his therapist or nurse and resent the time she spends with other patients. This is a time of sharing and planning between patient and staff.

Stage V—Coping. It is felt by some in the field of rehabilitation that people do not accept the disability *per se,* but instead, learn to cope with it. Disability is still an inconvenience, but it is no longer the center of their lives. Life is again meaningful to the person, and he is again involved with others.

BIBLIOGRAPHY

Baxter R: Sex counseling and the SCI patient. Nursing 78, September 1978, pp 46–51

American Association of Neurosurgical Nurses: Core Curriculum for Neurosurgical Nurses, Maryland, 1977

Carol M, Ducker T, Byrnes D: Acute care of spinal cord injury: A challenge to the emergency medicine clinician. Crit Care Quart 2, No. 1:7–21, 1979

Feustel D: Autonomic hyperreflexia. Am J Nurs, January 1976, pp 228–230

Guttman L: Spinal Cord Injuries: Comprehensive Management and Research. London, Blackwell, 1973

Kahn E, et al: Correlative Neurosurgery, 2nd ed. Springfield, Charles C Thomas, 1969

Mooney T, Cole T, Chilgren R: Sexual Options for Paraplegics and Quadriplegics. Boston, Little, Brown & Co, 1975

Pires M: Spinal cord injuries. In Coping with Neurologic Problems Proficiently, Nursing Skillbook Series, pp 99–123. Pennsylvania, Intermed Communications, 1979

Taggie J, Manley MS: A Handbook of Sexuality After Spinal Cord Injury. Denver, Craig Hospital, 1978

Tyson G et al: Acute care of the spinal cord injured patient. Crit Care Quart 2, No. 1:45–60, 1979

Wilson S: Neuro-Nursing. New York, Springer, 1979

Carolyn M. Hudak

HYPOTHERMIA

The use of hypothermia (lowered body temperature) in clinical situations ranges from treating gastric hemorrhage to attempting to prevent irreversible cerebral damage. Decreased body temperature reduces cellular activity and consequently the oxygen requirement of tissues. Hypothermia is therefore induced in situations involving interrupted or reduced blood flow to vital areas to minimize tissue damage due to diminished oxygen delivery. This is the rationale for using hypothermia during open heart and neurosurgical procedures.

The presence of fever (hyperthermia) in any patient produces greater cellular oxygen requirements because of the increased rate of metabolism. Each degree of temperature elevation above normal increases metabolism approximately 7%. This fact becomes especially significant in the patient whose vital centers may already be compromised because of cerebral edema surgically induced or resulting from another form of insult such as hypoxia from cardiac arrest. It is to provide some margin of safety in these situations until injured tissue can recover that the body temperature is lowered or maintained at normothermic levels. Current emphasis is on preventing marked elevations in body temperature as opposed to markedly lowering the temperature. Physiological responses to cold remain the same, and there are occasions when actual hypothermia is desirable.

Since the critical care nurse is usually responsible for inducing the hypothermic state and monitoring the patient during this therapy, it is important to be aware of the physiological manifestations of the various phases of body cooling.

Phases of Hypothermia

1. COOLING PHASE

For the conscious patient, lowering body temperature is at best a most unpleasant experience. It goes without saying that adequate explanation and support for the patient and his family are integral parts of nursing care.

Methods. Although the method of inducing hypothermia will depend upon the situation and the equipment available, there are essentially two ways to proceed—surface cooling or the more direct method of bloodstream cooling. *Bloodstream cooling* is the method employed during open heart surgical procedures when the blood passes through the cooling coils in the cardiopulmonary bypass machine.

Surface cooling with the use of blankets circulating a refrigerant is the method usually employed in critical care units. The cooling blanket may be placed directly against the patient, or more esthetically, a sheet can cover the blanket and be tucked under the mattress to hold the blanket in place. (This should not negate turning the blanket with the patient to maintain skin contact with the cooling device.) The important point here is to avoid placing any degree of thickness between the patient and the blanket, as this will serve as an insulator and impede the cooling process.

When cooling is initiated, one blanket may be placed under the patient and another placed on top to hasten the cooling process. If a top blanket is used, care must be exercised in observing the patient's respiratory status because the weight of the cooling blanket may limit chest excursion. Keeping the blanket in contact with areas of superficial blood flow such as the axilla and groin will also expedite cooling. In the event that a cooling device is not available, ice bags can be used to initiate the cooling process, using these same principles.

Physiological Reactions. The body's initial reaction to cold exposure is an attempt to conserve body heat and to increase heat production. *Skin pallor* that occurs is due to a vasoconstrictor response that limits superficial blood flow and thus loss of body heat. Intense activity in the form of *shivering* occurs to maintain body heat. The effects of these compensatory responses will be reflected in the vital signs, and it is important that the nurse understand these transient variations and consider them in evaluating the patient.

During the first 15 to 20 minutes of hypothermia induction, all *vital signs* increase. Pulse and blood pressure rise in response to the increased venous return produced by vasoconstriction. Respiratory rate increases to meet the added oxygen requirements of increased metabolic activity produced by shivering and to eliminate the additional carbon dioxide produced. If the patient hyperventilates with shivering, respiratory alkalosis can develop. The initial rise in temperature is a reflection of this increased cellular activity.

Since the patient requiring hypothermia usually has an existing cellular oxygenation problem, the increased oxygen consumption induced by shivering is undesirable. For this reason, chlorpromazine (Thorazine) may be given at the beginning of induction to reduce hypothalamic response. *Hypoglycemia* is a potential occurrence during vigorous shivering because increased glucose is required for the increased metabolic activity.

After approximately 15 minutes, the vasoconstrictor effect is broken by means of a negative feedback loop, and warm blood flow to the body surface is reestablished. This accounts for the reddened skin color following initial skin pallor. This same phenomenon can be demonstrated by holding an ice cube in the hand for a short period of time.

As Temperature Decreases. As superficial warm blood flow is reestablished, body heat is lost and body temperature begins to drop. The temperature can be monitored by a rectal probe taped in place, which allows for frequent or continuous readings. Fecal material should be removed before the probe is inserted. Because blood cooled at the body surface continues to circulate through the body core, "downward drift" of the temperature usually continues for approximately 1° after the cooling blanket is turned off. In the obese patient, a greater degree of drift may be experienced. For this reason, the cooling device should be turned off before the desired hypothermic level is actually attained. Close temperature monitoring will be necessary to determine if the trend remains downward or whether an increase in temperature occurs, requiring use of the blanket again.

Skin care becomes particularly crucial owing to the presence of cold and its circulatory effects. Position can be changed to eliminate pressure points, taking care to move the blanket with the patient so that body contact is maintained with the cooling device. Experience has indicated that the skin can be protected by applying a thin coating of lotion followed by talcum powder; this does not appear to impede the cooling process. The application can be repeated in accordance with the skin care program, but the skin should be gently washed at least every 8 hours to remove the accumulated coating.

2. HYPOTHERMIA

When the desired level of hypothermia is achieved, usually around 32°C (89.6°F), a number of other physiological changes become apparent. The vital signs at this stage are all diminished. The development of respiratory acidosis is a real possibility, since at deeper levels of hypothermia, ventilation falls off more rapidly than does reduced carbon dioxide production. Also, with increasing hypothermia the oxygen dissociation curve shifts to the left, and at lower tensions oxygen is not readily released by hemoglobin to the tissues. Because of the developing circulatory insufficiency and increased metabolic activity due to shivering, metabolic acidosis is also a possibility.

Secretion of antidiuretic hormone is inhibited, and an increase in urine output may be noted with a drop in the specific gravity. During hypothermia, water shifts from the intravascular spaces to the interstitial and intracellular spaces. This results from sodium moving into the cell in exchange for potassium and taking water with it. This fluid shift produces hemoconcentration, and nursing measures must be taken to prevent embolization. Such measures would include passive range of motion exercises and frequent change of position.

In hypothermic states, for every degree of temperature below normothermic levels, cerebral metabolism is decreased 6.7%. At 25°C (77°F) the brain volume is reduced 4.1%, and extracellular space increases about 31.5%. The sensorium fades at 34° to 33°C (93° to 91.4°F). For the neurologic patient who already has a depressed sensorium, other measures to evaluate changes in the patient's level of response must be relied on, such as evaluating purposeful or non-purposeful movements in response to painful stimuli and the degree of painful stimuli necessary to elicit a response.

Because all cellular activity diminishes with hypothermia, cerebral activity decreases and hearing fades at approximately 34° to 33°C (93° to 91.4°F) due to reduced cochlear response. At 18° to 30°C (82° to 86°F) there is no corneal or gag reflex, and pulse irregularities may be noted due to myocardial irritability, which probably occurs as a result of potassium moving into the cell.

Ventricular fibrillation is a common occurrence at this level, and consequently the patient is usually maintained at a hypothermic level around 32°C (89.6°F) to avoid cardiac problems.

Drugs tend to have a cumulative effect in the hypothermic patient. Decreased perfusion at the injection site and decreased enzyme activity result in slower chemical reactions. Therefore the intravenous route is preferred, and intramuscular or subcutaneous injections should be avoided. If a drug must be given hypodermically, it should be given deeply intramuscularly and vigilance maintained during the rewarming phase for cumulative effects.

Another potential occurrence in hypothermia is that of *fat necrosis.* This results from prolonged exposure to cold and decreased circulation, which allows crystals to form in the fluid elements of the cells, leading to necrosis and cellular death. Nursing measures that can minimize fat necrosis include turning the patient frequently, massaging the skin to increase circulation, and avoiding prolonged application of cold to any one area.

When the patient has reached the desired hypothermic level, vital signs will also level out at reduced values. Changes in vital signs must therefore be evaluated in light of the patient's hypothermic state. For example, if you are caring for a neurosurgical patient cooled to 32°C (89.6°F) and if his vital signs have decreased as you would normally expect, an increase in pulse, respirations, or blood pressure to "normal levels" must be interpreted in view of the hypothermic state. Is an infectious process present? Are changes occurring in the patient's neurologic status? Is intracranial pressure increasing?

If the patient is to be maintained at the hypothermic level for a prolonged period of time, this can be accomplished in a number of ways. The patient (after his temperature has risen several degrees) may need to be placed on the cooling blanket periodically and returned to the desired level.

Nursing measures should be carried out gently, with a minimal degree of activity to the patient to prevent an increase in body heat, such as providing passive range of motion exercises. Bathing of the patient should be done with tepid or cool water to avoid increasing temperature in this manner.

It cannot be overemphasized that prevention of pulmonary problems in the hypothermic patient is almost entirely dependent upon nursing care. Change of position allowing for postural drainage, measures to promote adequate ventilation, and suctioning to remove accumulated secretions are all extremely important in this patient.

3. REWARMING

Once it is determined that the patient no longer requires the hypothermic state, rewarming can be accomplished by a number of methods. These methods include surface rewarming, bloodstream rewarming, or rewarming naturally. Allowing the patient to rewarm naturally is the preferred method. The cooling device is removed. Blankets may be used to cover the patient but no artificial heat is used, and the patient is allowed to warm at his own rate. As the patient approaches normothermic levels, it is to be anticipated that vital signs will return to precooling levels due to reversal of the physiological events.

One of the hazards of artificially inducing rewarming is that of warming the skin and muscles before the heart. The heart remains in a cooled state and is unable to pump sufficient blood to meet the oxygen demands of the superficial areas. Further warming increases the dilatation of peripheral vessels and blood pools, resulting in decreased circulating volume, decreased venous return, and therefore decreased cardiac output. This sequence of events can be avoided if the heart is warmed first, as in the bloodstream method, or by allowing the body to rewarm naturally.

Other complications that may occur during the rewarming process are hyperpyrexia, shock (for reasons just cited), and acidosis. The acidosis occurs as a result of the increase in metabolic activity in those areas already warmed and an insufficient circulation to meet the metabolic requirements of this increased activity. Oliguria may also result, probably due to antidiuretic hormone secretion.

During this rewarming phase the patient must

be monitored closely for indications necessitating recooling. Using the patient's normothermic status as a baseline, these indications would include a fading sensorium, greater increase in pulse and respirations than would normally be expected with the warming process, and a drop in the blood pressure.

Another important facet to be monitored is the cumulative effect of drugs given previously.

The necessity for interpreting clinical changes in the patient on the basis of the physiological changes brought about through cooling and then rewarming cannot be overemphasized. The nurse must anticipate changes and findings based on the patient's pathology and other variables present that would alter those findings. When those findings that are anticipated do not occur, and when there is a deviation from the anticipated, the critical care nurse must be prepared to ask the question *Why?* and go about systematically determining why the anticipated change is not present. Only when the nurse is able to do this can optimum nursing care be rendered.

BIBLIOGRAPHY

Bender HW Jr et al: Reparative cardiac surgery in infants and children: Five years experience with profound hypothermia and cardiac arrest. Ann Surg 190(4):437–443, 1979

Chiv RC et al: The importance of monitoring intramyocardial temperature during hypothermic myocardial protection. Ann Thorac Surg 28(4):317–322, 1979

Levy LA: Severe hypophosphatemia as a complication of the treatment of hypothermia. Arch Intern Med 140(1):128–129, 1980

Southwick FS et al: Recovery after prolonged asystolic cardiac arrest in profound hypothermia: A case report and literature review. JAMA 243(12):1250–1253, 1980

Assessment Skills for the Nurse: Nervous System 22

Corinne A. Cloughen

NEUROLOGIC NURSING ASSESSMENT

Nursing care of the neurologic patient must be approached with the attitude that the patient can resume a useful life and be an asset to society. Nursing assessment must be done completely and systematically to establish a baseline of function and to identify when change has occurred. Understanding the physiology involved in change allows for proper nursing judgments and the appropriate intervention. Certainly a proportion of head-injured and stroke patients die or function at less than their potential, not because of pathophysiology, but as a result of nurse-allowed or nurse-induced disability. Assessment will be discussed so that disability is abolished as far as possible and not induced (or allowed to occur).

The objectives for neurologic crisis care are

- To maintain and support life
- To prevent complications and further neurologic deficit
- To help the patient to accept and adjust to his limitations

The first things the nurse should notice upon admission are the patient's general appearance, age, sex, general health, and symmetry of appearance. Check for any bruising, lacerations and involuntary movement. While examining the patient, ascertain any complaints he may have (*e.g.*, headache, pain, seizure, dizziness, visual problems, loss of balance). Ascertain the time of occurrence and duration of the symptoms that the patient mentions. This may help you and the physician in pinpointing specific areas of dysfunction that may deserve special attention when neurologic checks are made.

A medical history is important in order to ascertain evidence of vascular disease, diabetes, renal disease, anemia, cancer, and other metabolic dysfunctions that can complicate the neurologic picture. The patient's mental and emotional status as well as general intelligence should be noted. These aspects of the assessment may be delayed if the patient is in need of immediate medical attention.

There should be a standard neurologic check sheet that is used by the nursing staff to note any changes in the patient's condition. It should include vital signs, level of consciousness, extremity movement, and comments relative to the patient's condition. The terms used in describing the levels of consciousness should be clearly defined and used by all care givers (*e.g.*, stuporous to one person may mean lethargic to another).

Level of Consciousness

Level of consciousness is the most reliable index for determining neurologic status. Since numerous terms exist for describing levels of consciousness, and these may not have the same meaning for everyone, it is better to describe the patient's actions and state of awareness.

- Does he arouse to verbal stimuli?
- Is he oriented to time, place, person, and recent events?
- Are his actions and responses appropriate?
- Is he confused?
- Can he answer simple questions and follow simple commands?

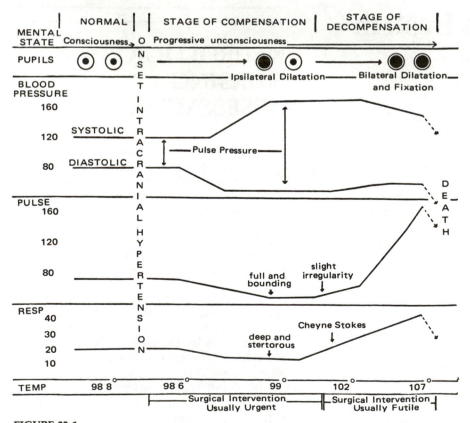

FIGURE 22-1.

Chart showing changes in mental state, pupils, blood pressure, pulse rate, respiratory rate, and temperature before and after the onset of fatal increase of intracranial pressure.

• If the patient does not respond to verbal stimuli, does he respond to noxious stimulation by purposeful withdrawal or primitive reflexes, or is there no response to painful stimuli?

Note what stimulus is used to issue a response, beginning with light touch and progressing to deep pain. Progressive restlessness and agitation should not be interpreted as an improvement in the level of consciousness, as it may be an indication of increased intracranial pressure (IICP). Sedation should therefore be avoided in cases of agitation.

Vital Signs

Classic signs of *increased intracranial pressure* (IICP) include an elevated systolic pressure in conjunction with a widening pulse pressure, slow bounding pulse, and respiratory irregularities.

Following any emergency treatment that may be indicated, such as maintenance of the airway for adequate ventilation, vital signs should be taken immediately and followed frequently. Any indication of shock should alert one to search for signs of thoracic and intra-abdominal injuries. It must be remembered that vital signs are only signs and are not infallible in determining the patient's neurologic status (see Fig. 22-1).

Hypoventilation following cerebral trauma can lead to respiratory acidosis. As the blood CO_2 increases and blood O_2 decreases, cerebral hypoxia and edema can result in secondary brain trauma. *Hyperventilation* following cerebral trauma produces respiratory alkalosis with increased blood O_2 and decreased blood CO_2 levels. This causes vasoconstriction of cerebral vessels and decreases oxygen consumption, resulting in cerebral hypoxia.

Since temperature elevation increases cellular metabolism, measures should be implemented to maintain temperature in the normal range, or hypothermia may be induced if indicated.

Pupillary Changes

In conjunction with checking the level of consciousness and vital signs, pupils must be checked frequently. Pupils are best checked in a darkened room for size, shape, equality, and reaction to light. Light directed into one eye should constrict the pupil in both eyes (consensual pupillary reflex). *Anisocoria* (unequal pupils) may be normal in a small percentage of the population or may be an indication of neural dysfunction. Ipsilateral dilation (dilation of the pupil on the same side as the injury) can be an indication of increasing ICP. Severe central or bilateral pressure may cause dilation and fixation of both pupils. Bilaterally constricted pupils may be due to damage to the pons and midbrain, which paralyzes the sympathetic fibers to the oculomotor nerve.

Extremity Movement and Strength

Extremity movement and strength should also be evaluated frequently. The upper extremities can be checked by having the patient push away from and pull against your resistance. Grasp is not a reliable index for testing upper extremity strength because a weak grasp may be indicative of peripheral neuropathy alone. If weakness is noted, have the patient hold his arms straight out with eyes closed and observe for any drift of an extremity. The lower extremities are checked by having the patient raise his legs against your resistance. Weakness noted in any of these tests indicates damage to the pyramidal tracts or within the pyramidal system, which controls voluntary movement.

Size, tone, and muscle strength should be tested throughout the major muscle groups of the body. Careful observation for a resting or intentional tremor should be included at this time.

Superficial and deep reflexes are tested on symmetric sides of the body and compared in relation to the strength of contraction elicited. Pathologic reflexes should be noted, including the presence of a Babinski sign (dorsiflexion of the big toe and fanning of the toes when the sole of the foot is stroked). This indicates pyramidal tract disease in a person over 2 to 3 years of age. (See Table 22-1.)

Cranial Nerves

I. Olfactory. The first cranial nerve contains sensory fibers for the sense of smell. This test is usually deferred unless the patient complains of an inability to smell. The nerve is tested, with eyes closed, by placing aromatic substances near the patient's nose for identification. Each nostril is checked separately. Loss of smell may be caused by a fracture of the cribriform plate or a fracture in the ethmoid area.

II. Optic. Gross visual acuity is checked by having the patient read ordinary newsprint. The

Table 22–1
Tests for Reflex Status

Deep Reflexes

Reflex	Site of Stimulus	Normal Response	Pertinent Central Nervous System Segment
Biceps	Biceps tendon	Contraction of biceps	Cervical 5 & 6
Brachioradialis	Styloid process of radius	Flexion of the elbow and pronation of the forearm	Cervical 5 & 6
Triceps	Triceps tendon above the olecranon	Extension of the elbow	Cervical 6, 7, & 8
Patellar	Patellar tendon	Extension of the leg at the knee	Lumbar 2, 3, & 4
Achilles	Achilles tendon	Plantar flexion of the foot	Sacral 1 & 2

Superficial Reflexes

Reflex	Normal Response	Pertinent Central Nervous System Segment
Upper abdominal	Umbilicus moves up and toward area being stroked	Thoracic 7, 8, & 9
Lower abdominal	Umbilicus moves down	Thoracic 11 & 12
Cremasteric	Scrotum elevates	Thoracic 12 & lumbar 1
Plantar	Flexion of the toes	Sacral 1 & 2
Gluteal	Skin tenses at gluteal area	Lumbar 4 through sacral 3

Pathologic Reflexes

Reflex	How Elicited	Response
Babinski	Stroke lateral aspect of sole of foot	In pyramidal tract disease, an extension or dorsiflexion of the big toe occurs — in addition to fanning of the toes
Chaddock	Stroke lateral aspect of foot beneath the lateral malleolus	Same type of response
Oppenheim	Stroke the anteromedial tibial surface	Same type of response
Gordon	Squeeze the calf muscles firmly	Same type of response

(DeJong RN, Sahs AL et al: Essentials of the Neurological Examination, pp 39–47. Philadelphia, Smith Kline Corporation, 1976)

patient's preinjury need for glasses should be noted. Visual field testing should be done by having the patient look straight ahead with one eye covered. The examiner will move a finger from the periphery of each quadrant of vision toward the patient's center of vision. The patient should indicate when he sees the examiner's finger. This is done for both eyes and the results compared with the examiner's visual fields, which are assumed to be normal. Damage to the retina will produce a blind spot. An optic nerve lesion will produce partial or complete blindness on the same side. Damage to the optic chiasm results in bitemporal hemianopsia, blindness in both lateral visual fields. Pressure on the optic tract can cause homonymous hemianopsia, half blindness on the opposite side of the lesion in both eyes. A lesion in the parietal or temporal lobe may produce contralateral blindness in the upper or lower quadrant of vision respectively in both eyes (this is known as *quadrant deficit*). Damage in the occipital lobe may cause homonymous hemianopsia with central vision sparing (see Fig. 22-2).

An ophthalmoscopic examination should be done, with close observation of the optic disc, the vessels, and the periphery of the retina.

III. Oculomotor; IV. Trochlear; VI. Abducens.

These cranial nerves are checked together because they all innervate extraocular muscles. The parasympathetic fibers of the oculomotor nerve are responsible for lens accommodation through control of the ciliary muscle and regulation of the iris and pupillary change. The motor fibers of the oculomotor nerve innervate the muscles that elevate the eyelid as well as those that move the eyes up, down, and medially, including the superior rectus, inferior oblique, inferior rectus, and medial rectus muscles. The trochlear nerve innervates the superior oblique muscle to move the eyes down and out. The lateral rectus muscle moves the eyes laterally and is innervated by the abducens nerve. Diplopia, nystagmus, conjugate deviation, and ptosis may indicate dysfunction of these cranial nerves. These nerves are tested by having the patient follow the examiner's finger

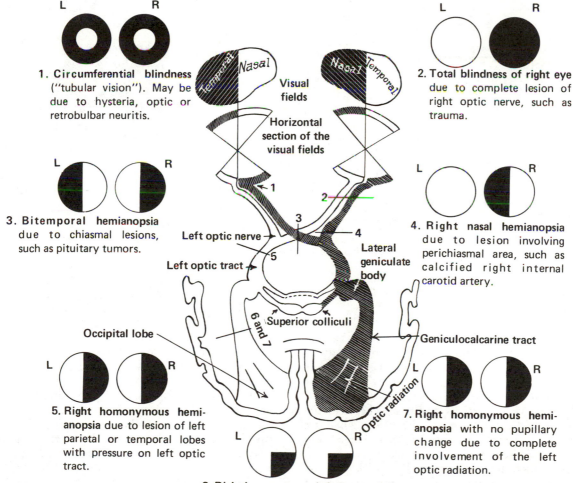

1. **Circumferential blindness** ("tubular vision"). May be due to hysteria, optic or retrobulbar neuritis.

2. **Total blindness of right eye** due to complete lesion of right optic nerve, such as trauma.

3. **Bitemporal hemianopsia** due to chiasmal lesions, such as pituitary tumors.

4. **Right nasal hemianopsia** due to lesion involving perichiasmal area, such as calcified right internal carotid artery.

5. **Right homonymous hemianopsia** due to lesion of left parietal or temporal lobes with pressure on left optic tract.

6. **Right homonymous inferior quadrantanopsia** due to partial involvement of optic radiations (upper portion of left optic radiation in this case).

7. **Right homonymous hemianopsia** with no pupillary change due to complete involvement of the left optic radiation.

FIGURE 22-2.
Visual field defects associated with lesions of visual system. (Reproduced, with permission, from Chusid JG: Correlative Neuroanatomy & Functional Neurology, 17th ed, p 91. Copyright 1979, Lange Medical Publications, Los Altos, California)

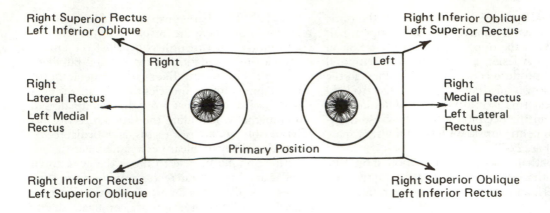

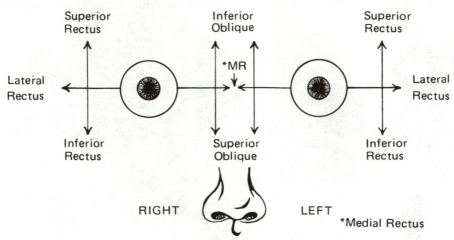

FIGURE 22-3.
(Top) Muscles used in conjugate ocular movements in the six cardinal directions of gaze. *(Bottom)* Diagram of eye muscle action. (Reproduced, with permission, from Chusid JG: Correlative Neuroanatomy & Functional Neurology, 17th ed, p 94. Copyright 1979, Lange Medical Publications, Los Altos, California)

with his eyes as it is moved in all directions of gaze (see Fig. 22-3).

V. Trigeminal. The trigeminal nerve has three divisions: ophthalmic, maxillary, and mandibular. The sensory portion of this nerve controls sensation to the face and cornea. The motor portion controls the muscles of mastication. This nerve is partially tested by checking the corneal reflex; if it is intact, the patient will blink when the cornea is stroked with a wisp of cotton. Facial sensation can be tested by comparing light touch, temperature, and pinprick on symmetric sides of the face. The ability to chew or clench the jaw should also be observed.

VII. Facial. The sensory portion of this nerve is concerned with taste on the anterior two-thirds of the tongue. The motor portion controls

muscles of facial expression. With a central (supranuclear) lesion, there is muscle paralysis of the lower half of the face on the side opposite the lesion. The muscles about the eyes and forehead are not affected. In a peripheral (nuclear or infranuclear) lesion, there is complete paralysis of facial muscles on the same side as the lesion.

The most common type of peripheral facial paralysis is Bell's palsy, which consists of ipsilateral facial paralysis. There is drooping of the upper lid with the lower lid slightly everted, and facial lines on the same side are obliterated with the mouth drawn toward the normal side. Artificial tears as well as taping the eye closed may be indicated to prevent corneal abrasion and irritation.

VIII. Acoustic. This nerve is divided into the cochlear and vestibular branches, which control hearing and equilibrium, respectively. The vestibular nerve is not routinely evaluated but can be checked by doing a caloric test, which should stimulate the vestibular ocular reflex. The test consists of irrigating the ear canal with ice water until the patient complains of nausea or dizziness or until nystagmus is noted, which usually takes 20 to 30 seconds. If no reaction occurs within 3 minutes, the test is discontinued.

The cochlear nerve is tested by air and bone conduction. A vibrating tuning fork is placed on the mastoid process; after the patient can no longer hear the fork, he should be able to hear it for a few seconds longer when it is placed in front of his ear (Rinne's test). The patient may complain of tinnitus or decreased hearing if this nerve is damaged.

IX. Glossopharyngeal; X. Vagus.

These cranial nerves are usually tested together. The glossopharyngeal nerve supplies sensory fibers to the posterior third of the tongue as well as the uvula and soft palate. The vagus innervates the larynx, pharynx, and soft palate, as well as conveys autonomic responses to the heart, stomach, lungs, and small intestines. Autonomic vagal functions are not usually tested because they are checked on the general physical exam. These nerves can be tested by eliciting a gag reflex, observing the uvula for symmetric movement when the patient says "ah," or observing midline elevation of the uvula when both sides are stroked. Inability to cough forcefully, difficulty swallowing, and hoarseness may be signs of dysfunction.

XI. Spinal Accessory.

This nerve controls the trapezius and sternocleidomastoid muscles. It is tested by having the patient shrug his shoulders against resistance.

XII. Hypoglossal.

This nerve controls tongue movement. It can be checked by having the patient protrude his tongue. Check for deviation from midline, tremor, and atrophy. If deviation is noted secondary to damage of the nerve, it will be to the side of the lesion.

Higher Intellectual Function Tests

Intellectual performance should be evaluated within the context of the patient's educational and socioeconomic background. The quality of language production can be ascertained by the patient's ability to speak, read, write, and comprehend. Deficiency in any of these language functions is known as *aphasia*. Depending upon the type of aphasia noted, different areas of damage in the brain can be located.

Abstract reasoning is often evaluated by having the patient explain simple proverbs and slogans, such as, "A rolling stone gathers no moss." Keep in mind that many "normal" people have difficulty with this exercise. Subtraction of serial 7's from 100 is a test of calculation and attention span.

The inability to recognize objects by sight, touch, or sound is termed *agnosia*. The ability to recognize and identify objects by touch is called *stereognosis* and is a function of the parietal lobe. Identification of an object by the sense of sight is a function of the parieto-occipital junction. The temporal lobe is responsible for identification of objects by sound. Each of these senses should be tested separately. For example, a patient may not be able to identify a whistle by its sound but may recognize it immediately if he holds it or looks at it.

Sensory Tests

The primary forms of sensation are evaluated first. These include light touch, superficial pain, temperature, and vibration. With the patient's eyes closed, multiple areas of the body are tested, including the hands, forearms, upper arms, trunk, thighs, lower legs, and feet.

Note the patient's ability to perceive the sensation; compare distal areas to proximal areas and compare right and left sides at corresponding areas. Note if sensory change involves one entire side of the body. Abnormal results may indicate damage somewhere along the pathways of the receptors in the skin, muscles, joints and tendons, spinothalamic tracts, or sensory area of the cortex.

Cortical forms of sensation should also be tested. Disturbances of these forms, when the primary forms of sensation are intact, indicate damage to the parietal lobe. Cortical forms of sensation include

- *Graphesthesia* —the ability to recognize numbers or letters traced lightly on the skin. Bilateral sides are compared.
- *Point localization* —the ability to locate a spot on the body touched by the examiner.
- *Two-point discrimination* —tested by using two sharp objects and determining the smallest area in which two points can be perceived.
- *Extinction phenomenon* —the inability to recognize that two areas have been touched when the examiner simultaneously touches two identical areas on opposite sides of the body.
- *Texture discrimination* —the ability to recognize materials such as cotton, burlap, and wool by feeling them.

All tests are done with the patient's eyes closed.

Cerebellar Function Tests

The cerebellum controls balance and coordination, and there are many tests of function. Some of the more common ones follow:

- *Romberg test* —done by having the patient stand with his feet together, first with his eyes open, then with eyes closed. Observe for sway or direction of falling and be prepared to catch the patient if necessary.
- *Tandem walking* —done by having the patient walk heel to toe.
- *Finger to nose test* —done by having the patient touch his finger to the examiner's finger, then touch his own nose. Overshooting or past pointing the mark is called *dysmetria.* Both sides are tested individually.
- *Heel to shin test* —done by having the patient run the heel of one foot down the shin of the other leg. This is done on both sides.
- *Rapidly alternating movements (RAM)* — checked on each side by having the patient touch each finger on one hand to his thumb in rapid succession, or by performing rapid pronation and supination of his hand on his leg. Observe for accuracy and smoothness of action in these tests. Ataxia and tremor are common manifestations of cerebellar dysfunction. Inability to perform RAM is termed *adiadokokinesia.*

Other Observations

- *Battle's sign,* bruising over the mastoid area, is suggestive of basal skull fracture.
- *Raccoon's eyes* or periorbital edema is suggestive of fronto-basilar fracture.
- *Rhinorrhea,* drainage of cerebral spinal fluid (CSF) via the nose, is suggestive of fracture of the cribriform plate with herniation of a fragment of the dura and arachnoid through the fracture.
- *Otorrhea,* drainage of CSF from the ear, is usually associated with fracture of the petrous portion of the temporal bone.
- *Decorticate posturing* occurs when the cortex of the brain is nonfunctioning (supratentorial damage). The arms are abducted and in rigid flexion, with the hands internally rotated and fingers flexed. The legs are in rigid extension.
- *Decerebrate rigidity* indicates damage to the midbrain. Full extension of the arms and legs occurs, with internal rotation at the shoulder, flexed fingers, and internally rotated toes.
- *Meningeal irritation* can be detected by the presence of nuchal rigidity in conjunction with pyrexia, headache, and photophobia. A positive *Kernig's sign,* pain in the neck when the thigh is flexed on the abdomen and the leg extended at the knee, may also be present.

Throughout the neurologic assessment, the examiner should note the patient's behavior for appropriateness, emotional status, cooperativeness, attention span, and memory.

Following the neurologic exam, the nurse should record her findings, with particular emphasis on the abnormalities. Frequent reevaluation is necessary to ascertain change in the patient's condition.

Nursing care is directed toward returning the patient to maximum functioning, preventing complications and further neurologic deficits, and helping the patient adjust to his limitations. Rehabilitation begins as soon as the patient enters the hospital. Adequate assessment of the neurologic patient can not only prevent unnecessary complications and disability but is the first ingredient for optimum rehabilitation.

BIBLIOGRAPHY

Chusid JG: Correlative Neuroanatomy and Functional Neurology, 17th ed. Los Altos, Lange Medical Publications, 1979

DeJong RN: The Neurological Examination, 4th ed. Hagerstown, Harper & Row, 1979

Nursing Skillbook, Coping with Neurological Problems Proficiently. Nursing '79 Book. Horsham, Intermed Communication, 1979

Parsons LC: Respiratory changes in head injury. Am J Nurs, November 1971, pp 2187–2191

Plum F, Posner JB: Diagnosis of Stupor and Coma, 2nd ed. Philadelphia, F.A. Davis, 1972

Rosenberg RN (ed): Neurology. New York, Grune & Stratton, 1980

Strub RL, Beack FW: The Mental Status Examination in Neurology. Philadelphia, F.A. Davis, 1977

Walton JN: Essentials of Neurology, 4th ed. Philadelphia, J.B. Lippincott, 1976

Corinne A. Cloughen

ASSESSMENT OF THE COMATOSE PATIENT

Many patients who would never have made it to the emergency room 10 years ago are now being cared for in critical care units and are returning to useful and productive lives. Caring for the comatose patient, who frequently is on life-support equipment, is a definite nursing challenge. The critical care nurse must be aware of subtle changes in the patient's condition and must assess and manage nursing care accordingly.

Stimuli Response

Evaluating the comatose patient often entails a more extensive neurologic examination than what has been previously discussed under neurologic nursing assessment. This patient does not respond to verbal stimuli. There may be little or no response to noxious stimuli. It is important to note what, if any, stimuli initiate a response and to describe the type of response obtained. If the patient withdraws and groans to painful stimuli, he is considered *semicomatose.* Motor response in the comatose patient may be appropriate, inappropriate, or absent (see Fig. 22-4A,B,C,D). Appropriate responses, such as withdrawal, mean that the sensory pathways and corticospinal pathways are functioning (see Fig. 22-4A). There may be monoplegia or hemiplegia, indicating that the corticospinal pathways are interrupted on one side.

Inappropriate responses include decorticate rigidity and decerebrate rigidity. *Decorticate* rigidity results from lesions of the internal cap-

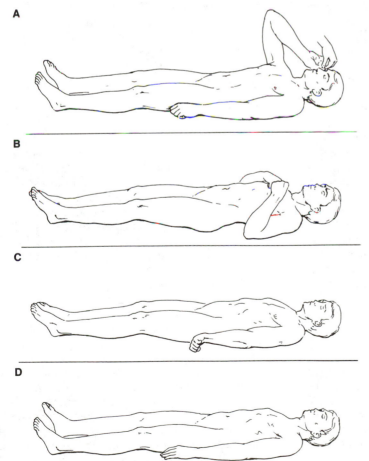

A

B

C

D

FIGURE 22-4.
Motor responses to pain. When you apply a painful stimulus to your unconscious patient's supraorbital notch, he'll respond in one of these ways: *(A)* Localizing pain. An appropriate response is to reach up above shoulder level toward the stimulus. Remember, a focal motor deficit such as hemiplegia may prevent a bilateral response.

As brain stem involvement increases, your patient may respond by assuming one of the following postures. Each one shows more advanced deterioration. *(B)* Decorticate posturing. One or both arms in full flexion on the chest. Legs may be stiffly extended. *(C)* Decerebrate posturing. One or both arms stiffly extended. Possible extension of the legs. *(D)* Flaccid. No motor response in any extremity. An extremely ominous sign.

sule, basal ganglia, thalamus, or cerebral hemisphere that interrupt corticospinal pathways. It is characterized by flexion of the arms, wrists, and fingers and adduction of the upper extremities and by extension, internal rotation, and plantar flexion of the lower extremities (see Fig. 22-4B).

Decerebrate ridigity consists of extension, adduction, and hyperpronation of the upper extremities and extension of the lower extremities, with plantar flexion of the feet (see Fig. 22-4C). Many times the patient is also opisthotonic, with teeth clenched. Injury to the midbrain and pons results in decerebration. At times the inappropriate responses of decortication and decerebration may switch back and forth. If there is no response to noxious stimuli or very weak flexor responses, the patient probably has extensive brain-stem damage. Seizure activity and tremors must also be noted and reported.

Pupils

Careful examination of the pupils is also important in evaluating the comatose patient. Note the size, shape, equality, and reaction to light (both direct and consensual responses). Check the position of the eyes. Are they deviated upward or downward? Are both eyes looking in the same direction or are they dysconjugate?

An important test of brain-stem function is the oculocephalic reflex, also known as *doll's head phenomenon.* This is a reflex ocular movement that can only be elicited in patients with a decreased level of consciousness. To check this reflex, hold the patient's eyes open and quickly but gently turn the head from side to side. If the reflex is present, the eyes will move in the direction opposite from which the head is being turned. Repeat this test by moving the head up and down. Again, the eyes will move in the opposite direction if the reflex is intact. These observations frequently can help pinpoint the area of brain dysfunction.

Corneal Reflex

Check for the presence of a blink and corneal reflex. If these reflexes are absent or if the patient doesn't keep his eyes closed, eye care should be given. Artificial tears should be instilled every 2 hours, and the eyes should be taped closed, making sure that the eyelashes are not against the cornea. If the eyes look irritated, an ophthalmic antibiotic ointment may be indicated.

Gag and Cough Reflex

Check the patient for a gag and cough reflex. Brain-stem damage could abolish these reflexes. If the gag reflex is absent, the patient should never be left on his back because aspiration is always a possibility. The patient should be suctioned at least every 2 hours, unless ordered otherwise, to prevent possible respiratory complications.

Other observations to be noted include changes in rate, depth, and pattern of respirations. Frequent and prolonged hiccoughs may also be a sign of brain-stem irritation. Damage to the hypothalamus can destroy the temperature-regulating mechanism of the body, causing excessively high body temperatures. Cooling measures may be indicated, but care should be taken that the body temperature remains normothermic unless hypothermia is specifically indicated.

Close observation of the patient's neurologic status, as well as vital signs and intake and output, is essential in adequately assessing the patient. At times the physician may determine the need for monitoring ICP (see section on ICP later in this chapter). Medications may be ordered according to the patient's ICP. Routine calibration of the transducer should be performed to assure accuracy. If a patient has an ICP device in place, it should be kept as aseptic as possible.

Glasgow Coma Scale

The Glasgow Coma Scale (also known as the Glasgow Responsiveness Scale) has been gaining acceptance in recent years as a tool for assessing the comatose patient. This scale is based on the study of 700 patients with severe head injuries.

One of the major advantages of this tool is that it provides a rigorous definition of coma, thus eliminating the ambiguity associated with terms such as *levels, unresponsive,* and *unarousable.* Use of the scale is valuable in establishing a baseline for individual patients and monitoring their progress so that impending complications can be quickly identified and proper treatment instituted.

The originators of the Glasgow Scale define coma as the inability to obey commands, to speak, or to open the eyes. Thus, the parameters that the scale evaluates are eye opening, best motor response, and verbal response. The scale appears in Table 22-2.

The patient's score is recorded as an eye, motor, verbal (EMV) sum, with a possible range of 3 to 15. A score of 3 to 5 is considered low, while anything above 8 is interpreted as high. The reliability of the scale has been established, and it appears to have some value as a predictor of outcome. For example, the outcome at 6 months for a group of patients *with* eye opening was considerably better both in terms of mortality and in the numbers making a moderate or good recovery than for a group of patients *without* eye opening.

Several different scales place high emphasis on the reactivity of pupils. Supposedly, bilateral unreactive pupils are indicative of extreme brain dysfunction. However, when unreacting pupils are associated with a relatively high EMV score (*i.e.*, high responsiveness), the cause is most likely found to be local damage to the second or third cranial nerves or to the globe or to the effect of drugs being used in the treatment of the patient.

Brain Death
The patient's condition may be so severe that brain death ensues. It is important to be able to identify the signs and symptoms of this situation. The criteria for brain death are as follows:

- No spontaneous respirations for 4 minutes without ventilatory support
- No spontaneous movement, even to painful stimuli
- No brain-stem function:
  Dilated and fixed pupils
  No corneal reflexes
  Absent doll's head eye movements
  Absent vestibular ocular reflex
  Absent pharyngeal reflex
- Absent cerebral blood flow determined by either cerebral flow scan or arteriogram
- The patient must not be hypothermic or have a recent history of ingestion of central nervous system depressants.

The final pronouncement of brain death must be made by two physicians, one a neurosurgeon or neurologist and the other a physician participating in the patient's care; neither physician can be part of an organ-transplant team.

BIBLIOGRAPHY
Finklestein S et al: The diagnosis of coma: Its pitfalls and limitations. Heart Lung 8, No. 6:1059–1064, 1979
Jennett B, Teasdale G: Aspects of coma after severe head injury. Lancet 1, Pt 2:878–881, 1977

Table 22–2
Glasgow Coma or Responsiveness Scale

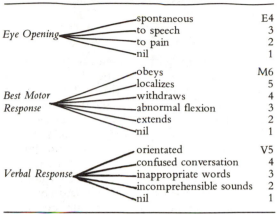

Eye Opening	spontaneous	E4
	to speech	3
	to pain	2
	nil	1
Best Motor Response	obeys	M6
	localizes	5
	withdraws	4
	abnormal flexion	3
	extends	2
	nil	1
Verbal Response	orientated	V5
	confused conversation	4
	inappropriate words	3
	incomprehensible sounds	2
	nil	1

(Adapted from Jennett B, Teasdale G: Aspects of coma after severe head injury. Lancet 1, Pt 2:878, 1977)

Loen M et al: Psychosocial aspects of care of the long-term comatose patient. J Neurosurg Nurs 11, No. 4:235–237, 1979
Winston SR: EMT and the Glasgow coma scale. J Iowa Med Soc 69, No. 10:393–398, 1979

Rae Nadine Smith

INVASIVE NEUROLOGIC ASSESSMENT TECHNIQUES

And men ought to know that from nothing else but from the brain come joys, delights, laughter and jests and sorrows, griefs, despondency and lamentations. And by the brain, in a special manner, we acquire wisdom and knowledge and see and hear and know what are foul and what are fair, what are bad and what are good, what are sweet and what unsavory . . . By the brain we distinguish objects of relish and disrelish and the same things do not always please us. And by the same organ we become mad and delirious, and fears and terrors assail us, some by night and some by day.

Hippocrates C 460–360 B.C.

Harvey Cushing, with his use of blood pressure measurement, is said to be the first neurosurgeon to introduce a form of instrument monitoring. We have progressed from this early, intermittent, and limited pressure monitoring into advanced techniques for continual pressure measurement. In 1951, Guillaume and Janny published the first report on continuous monitoring of ICP. Today, invasive techniques are frequently used to accurately and continuously assess the blood pressure, pulmonary artery pressure (PAP), ICP, and cerebral perfusion pressure (CPP) of the neurologic patient.

Correlating invasive measurements with noninvasive clinical assessment frequently reduces the amount of time required to accurately diagnose the problem, increases the amount of time available for treatment, provides continual feedback on the patient's response to selected treatments, and assists with prognosis. Aggressive management of critically ill neurologic and neurosurgical patients has reduced mortality without increasing the incidence of vegetative or severely disabled patients.

INDICATIONS FOR MEASUREMENT

Blood Pressure
Direct or invasive blood pressure measurements of critically ill patients provide a variety of advantages over indirect or noninvasive techniques. These include (1) accuracy (indirect or cuff pressures are particularly inaccurate during hypotensive episodes because of decreased cardiac output and increased vascular resistance), (2) ability to monitor the mean arterial pressure (MAP), (3) provision of a continual reading with an alarm system, (4) access for blood sampling, and (5) more efficient use of nursing time. Neurologic conditions in which accurate and continual blood pressures are important include

Increased Intracranial Pressure (IICP)
Both hypoxia and hypercarbia contribute to alterations of ICP. An increased PCO_2 results in cerebral vasodilation, thereby increasing blood volume and ICP. Serial blood gases are necessary if PCO_2 is to be regulated by a method such as controlled hyperventilation. The majority of patients with severe head injuries develop hyperventilation with respiratory alkalosis.

Early changes in respiratory patterns are usually too subtle for bedside detection. Serial blood gases obtained by an indwelling arterial cannula provide a safer, more efficient technique of blood sampling and certainly one more comfortable for the patient than repeated arterial punctures. The continual monitoring of the pressure between blood gas samplings protects the patient from the risk of bleedback and clotting of the cannula.

In patients with IICP or the potential to develop it, direct mean blood pressure measurement is compared with the mean ICP to determine the cerebral perfusion pressure (MAP minus mean ICP). A normal CPP is at least 50 to 60 torr.

Vascular Lesions
It is well established that an elevation of blood pressure is a cause of aneurysm rerupture. Aneurysms and subarachnoid hemorrhages are frequently treated by induced hypotension. Just as blood pressure is continuously monitored on a patient in shock being treated with vasopressors to increase pressure, it should likewise be monitored on the patient being treated with hypotensive agents to reduce pressure. In this situation, both hypertension and severe hypotension must be avoided.

Strokes
MAP must be maintained at a level above 60 to 70 torr to prevent the loss of autoregulation mechanisms in areas of focal cerebral ischemia.

Spinal Cord Injury
During a laminectomy, increased blood pressure is often considered a warning sign of pressure on the spinal cord.

Clinically, acute cervical cord injuries are often associated with hypotension. In this situation, blood pressure monitoring is often accompanied by blood volume monitoring, such as pulmonary artery and central venous pressure (CVP) monitoring.

During the hypotensive stage, patients with acute spinal cord injury have a low CVP. As sympathectomized muscles gradually regain tone, the blood-containing space contracts.

If the patient has been receiving vigorous fluid replacement to correct his low blood pressure and low CVP, pulmonary edema may result.

Increased fluid volume causes increased venous pressure on the left side of the heart that frequently is not manifested in CVP readings taken on the right side of the heart. Therefore, PAPs are routinely measured in these patients.

PULMONARY ARTERY PRESSURE

PAP reflects pressures from the left side of the heart and gives an accurate determination of fluid volume as affected by intravenous fluid replacement or diuresis.

Examples of conditions in which accurate blood volume monitoring is indicated include

Cord Injury

Pulmonary edema usually develops within 11 to 24 hours after cord injury. Death from pulmonary edema is not uncommon in acute quadriplegia.

Head Injury

Pulmonary edema develops rapidly after head injury.

Multiple Trauma

The blood volume picture is further complicated in the trauma patient who presents with acute cervical spinal cord injury with associated injury, particularly of the chest. It is often difficult to determine if the patient is hypotensive secondary to the sympathectomy effect or to the blood loss.

IICP (Increased Intracranial Pressure)

Management techniques such as osmotherapy and induced barbiturate coma lead to cardiovascular instability and hypovolemia.

INVASIVE TECHNIQUES OF VASCULAR MEASUREMENT

Determination of pressures requires the use of a transducer and monitor. A transducer can be defined as a device used to change varying pressures into proportionately varying signals that can be displayed on an oscilloscope, meter, or recorder (see Fig. 22-5). The first report of the use of a transducer for human blood pressure measurement was in 1947. Unbonded strain gauge, solid state, differential transformer, and quartz crystal transducers are currently available for clinical application.

Blood Pressure Measurement. The basic system for blood pressure measurement consists of a transducer that is connected by a tubing system directly to the patient's artery, usually the radial or femoral. Other sites include brachial, axillary, superficial temporal, central aorta, and dorsalis pedis arteries. Pressure from the artery is transmitted to the transducer by a column of fluid and converted to a pressure tracing that can be read on a monitor (see Fig. 22-5).

To avoid clotting of the arterial cannula, a mildly heparinized flush solution, such as normal saline or lactated Ringer's, is administered at a continual rate of 3 to 6 ml per hour. To prevent bleeding back, the flush solution is maintained at a pressure higher than the patient's systolic arterial pressure. The complication of sepsis is avoided by maintaining a sterile system between the transducer and the patient.

With a system such as this, Gardner's study

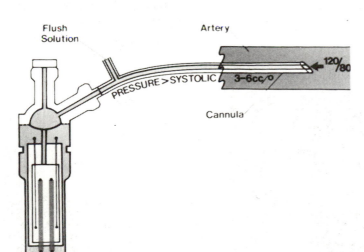

FIGURE 22-5.
Basic principle of blood pressure measurement. The system provides a continual reading with an alarm system as the pressure from the artery is transmitted by the fluid column to the diaphragm of the transducer. In this particular example, the strain gauge wires are activated, converting the pulsating physiological pressure into an electrical signal that is displayed on a monitor.

reported the risk to be 0.2% with a total of 4500 direct arterial lines in over 12,000 intensive care patient days. Other hospitals have published similar statistics.[1]

Pulmonary Artery Pressure Measurement.   To determine PAP and wedge pressures (PAW), a balloon-tipped catheter is inserted at the bedside. The catheter is inserted percutaneously or by venous cutdown into the antecubital, jugular, subclavian, or femoral vein. It is then advanced through the vein into the right atrium, to the right ventricle, and into the pulmonary artery.

The progress of the catheter through the right side of the heart is followed by distinctive waveform changes on the oscilloscope or recorder. With the balloon inflated, the catheter wedges into a distal branch of the pulmonary artery. This PAW reflects the pressure of the left side of the heart. PAWs are taken intermittently; with the balloon deflated, continuous PAPs are obtained.

The basic system for setting up and maintaining the PA catheter is the same as that described for blood pressure measurement, using a continual flush rate of 3 ml per hour.

Intracranial Pressure

ICP monitoring used in conjunction with other invasive and noninvasive assessment techniques has significantly aided in the diagnosis, treatment, and prognosis of the patient with a potential for developing intracranial hypertension.

ICP measurement usually provides an indication of changes in ICP dynamics before such changes are clinically evident, facilitating the initiation of measures to reduce IICP.

The classic syndrome of IICP, which includes increased pulse pressure, decreased pulse, and decreased respirations with pupillary changes, usually occurs only in association with posterior fossa lesions and seldom with the more commonly observed supratentorial mass lesions, such as subdural hematoma. When these classic Kocher-Cushing signs do accompany a supratentorial lesion, they are associated with a sudden pressure increase and usually herald a state of decompensation. Brain damage is usually irreversible at this point, and death is imminent.

Between the onset of IICP and herniation is a stage in which a wide variety of treatments are available to reduce ICP. Measures such as hyperventilation, the drainage of CSF, hypothermia, and the use of corticosteroids, barbiturates, and hypertonic solutions have proved valuable adjuncts to surgery. Since these techniques are usually most effective before the patient becomes clinically symptomatic, the need for pressure-reducing measures is best determined by direct pressure measurement (Fig. 22-6).

INDICATIONS FOR ICP MONITORING

The Monro-Kellie hypothesis states that the volume of the intracranium is equal to the volume of the brain plus the volume of the blood plus the volume of the cerebrospinal fluid (CSF). Any alterations in the volume of any of these components of the cranial vault, as well as the addition of a lesion, will lead to an increase in ICP (see chart that follows).

The brain can accommodate or compensate for minimal changes in volume by partial collapse of the cisterns, ventricles, and vascular systems. During this compensatory period, the ICP remains fairly constant. When these compensatory mechanisms have been fully used, pressure

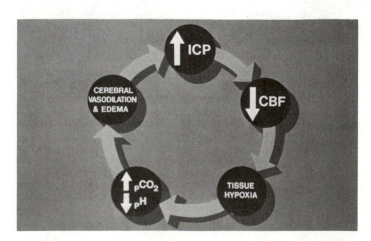

FIGURE 22-6.
Cycle for malignant progressive brain swelling. As the ICP increases, cerebral blood flow (CBF) decreases, leading to tissue hypoxia, a decrease in pH, an increase in PCO_2, cerebral vasodilation, and edema, thus leading to further pressure increases. This malignant cycle continues until herniation occurs.

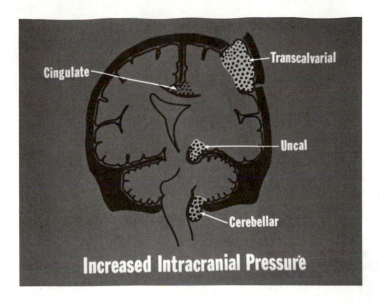

Increased Intracranial Pressure

FIGURE 22-7.
The major types of cerebral herniation are (1) herniation of the cingulate gyrus under the falx; (2) herniation of the uncus of the temporal lobe beneath the free edge of the tentorium; (3) downward displacement of the midbrain through the tentorial notch; and (4) sometimes, with an open head injury, transcalvarial herniation.

increases rapidly until herniation occurs, and the blood supply to the medulla is cut off (see Fig. 22-7). The ability of the intracranial contents to compensate depends upon the location of the lesion and the rate of expansion.

Conditions that may be indications for ICP measurement include

Head Injury

Diagnosis
Patients who develop intracranial mass lesions after head injury almost universally develop intracranial hypertension. ICP monitoring has proved valuable in detecting cerebral edema or hematoma formations. Computerized axial tomography (CT scans) or cerebral angiography are then used to differentiate between the two. ICP monitoring also facilitates differentiating brain-stem dysfunction secondary to increases in ICP from primary brain-stem injury, which is associated with a normal ICP.

In addition, it has been recommended that continued monitoring be carried out for all patients with burr holes, patients who fail to regain consciousness within 48 hours after injury, and patients whose level of consciousness deteriorates, unless the patient has meningitis or a brain abscess.

Treatment
• Diuretics and dehydration:
The amount and frequency of drugs used to treat IICP are titrated by continual monitoring.

Intermittent Positive Pressure Ventilation (IPPV):
The control of PCO_2 levels may require drugs such as chlorpromazine or morphine sulfate to optimize the patient's response to the ventilator. Increases in ICP secondary to muscle tremors may be treated with paralytic agents such as pancuronium bromide (Pavulon), necessitating dependence on artificial ventilation. Since neurologic response is suppressed by these drugs, ICP, blood pressure, PA, and cerebral perfusion pressure (CPP) monitoring become mandatory for safer patient care.

INDICATIONS FOR ICP MONITORING
Increased Volume of Brain
    Cerebral edema
    Trauma
    Surgery
    Stroke
    Tumor
Increased Volume of Blood
    Hematomas
    AV malformations
    Aneurysm
    Stroke
    Increase in PCO_2
Increased Volume of CSF
    Decreased CSF reabsorption
    Congenital hydrocephalus
Lesions
    Tumors
    Abscesses

Iatrogenic increases in pressure secondary to therapeutic measures such as chest physiotherapy, suctioning, and positioning are quickly identified.

Prognosis:
Miller and Sullivan reported on a series of 160 consecutive, severely head-injured patients. They determined that patients with intracranial mass lesions following head injury often develop early, severe intracranial hypertension. Patients with acute subdural hematomas seem to be most prone to IICP. In patients with diffuse brain injury, ICP is usually elevated but not to the same degree. It was reported that patients who maintained ICPs of 45 to 60 torr within the first 48 hours after injury, despite all therapeutic intervention, had a mortality rate approaching 100%.

In patients with diffuse brain injury, any elevation above 10 torr on admission resulted in progressively worsening prognoses. They feel this suggests that the initial level of ICP is to some degree an indication of the extent of diffuse brain damage. Recurrent or persistent intracranial hypertension was more frequently a problem with intracerebral lesions, contusion, hematoma, and brain swelling than with discrete extracerebral hematomas, whether epidural or subdural. Recurrent or persistent intracranial hypertension was associated with a poorer outcome.[2]

Subarachnoid Hemorrhage

Pre-op:
The level of ICP correlates well with the clinical grade of the hemorrhage. The ICP is of value in determining the best time for surgery, predicting and detecting rebleeding, and for determining the etiology of neurologic deterioration. ICP monitoring facilitates the use of diuretics, dehydrating agents, and hyperventilation.

In addition, it can be determined which patients have CSF absorption impairment, indicating the need for continuous ventricular fluid drainage or a permanent shunt.

Pediatrics

Neonates and infants:
Noninvasive anterior fontanel monitoring has proved useful in hyaline membrane disease, intracranial hemorrhage, meconium aspiration syndrome, meningitis, and hydrocephalus.

Head injury:
Children are particularly prone to cerebral edema, but if successfully managed, they have a good prognosis.

Reye's syndrome:
The mortality and morbidity of this disease have been substantially reduced by the measurement of ICP, usually by intraventricular catheter or subarachnoid screw, and the subsequent control of cerebral edema and maintenance of adequate cerebral perfusion. When continuous monitoring is used, the frequent "A" waves seen in these children can be detected and treated. This has proved to be particularly useful in stage three or four coma.

During exchange transfusions, marked alterations in ICP have been observed. In patients with diminished brain compliance or impairment of cerebral vascular autoregulation, exchange transfusion may have an adverse effect on ICP. The use of ICP monitoring reduces this risk.[3]

Brain Tumors

ICP tends to remain normal, with episodic increases seen particularly at night. Elevations in ICP tend to occur when the mass has enlarged to the point where the patient is demonstrating neurologic deterioration with papilledema, headache, and vomiting. Metastatic tumors can cause massive edema. Patients may be monitored preoperatively to determine their response to the preoperative therapeutic regimen and to assist in determining the optimal time for surgery. Postoperatively, they may be monitored to assist with the diagnosis and treatment of diffuse generalized cerebral edema secondary to extensive manipulation of the brain during surgery.

Cardiac Arrest

Of long-term cardiac arrest survivors, 10% to 20% suffer permanent severe brain damage ranging from intellectual changes to vegetative states following global ischemic-anoxic insults. ICP measurement has been of value in the development of new specific neuron-saving therapies for "postresuscitation disease" to assist in the restoration of mentation.[4]

Post End Expiratory Pressure (PEEP)

The use of PEEP can increase ICP or reduce arterial blood pressure, thereby reducing CPP and decreasing cerebral blood flow (CBF). This may be because PEEP causes a rise in intrathoracic pressure, which reduces cardiac filling pressure, leading to a decrease in cardiac output. The circulatory compensation is incomplete and the blood pressure falls, causing a reduction in CPP. ICP may be increased by impedance to cerebral venous outflow. In one study significant increases in ICP occurred in approximately 50% of the patients given PEEP. Patients with baseline ICPs greater than 25 torr showed the most significant increases in ICP.[5]

For optimal titration of PEEP in the patient who may develop intracranial hypertension, it is recommended that ICP and blood pressure be monitored continuously and measurements be made of neurologic status and intracranial and pulmonary compliance. Volume pressure responses (VPRs) and arterial blood gases are, therefore, indicated.

Strokes

Increases in ICP are common with spontaneous intracerebral hemorrhage and routinely present in comatose patients. In ischemic stroke, high ICP is likely after cerebral infarction has progressed to coma with midline brain shift. ICP monitoring has been effective in the initiation and maintenance of therapeutic intervention. It has also provided valuable information for research on the mechanisms and amelioration of focal brain ischemia.

Surgery

During surgery ICP monitoring provides assistance in determining the optimal position for the patient and his responses to various anesthetic agents and ventilatory support.

ICP MEASUREMENT

There are basically three techniques for measuring ICP: (1) intraventricular, (2) subarachnoid (subdural), and (3) epidural (extradural).

Intraventricular Technique. The intraventricular technique of ICP measurement was first reported in 1951 and consists of placing a catheter into the lateral ventricle. A twist drill hole is placed lateral to the midline at the level of the coronal suture, usually on the nondominant side. A catheter is placed through the cerebrum into the anterior horn of the lateral ventricle. On occasion, the occipital horn is used. Connected to the ventricular catheter by a stopcock or pressure tubing is a pressure transducer (see Fig. 22-8). Sterile saline or Ringer's lactate solution is used to provide the fluid column between the CSF and diaphragm of the transducer. A continuous flush device is not used for ICP measurement.

The miniature transducer may be positioned directly on the patient's head. A standard size transducer is mounted at the bedside with the venting port positioned at the level of the fora-

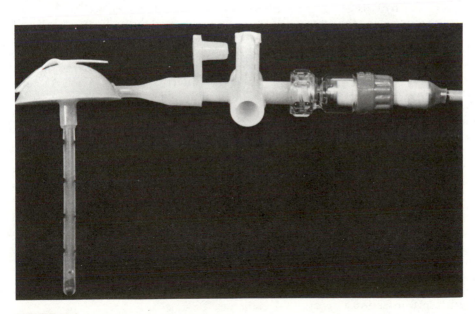

FIGURE 22-8.
Intraventricular cannula with subminiature transducer.

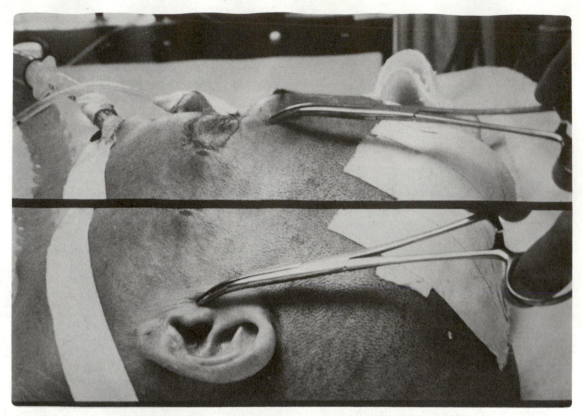

FIGURE 22-9.
Zero reference points for lining up venting port of transducer with the level of the foramen of Monro.

men of Monro (Fig. 22-9). External landmarks for this position are the edge of the brow or the tragus of the ear. For every 1 inch of discrepancy between the level of the transducer and the pressure source, there is an error of approximately 2 torr.

Advantages
• Direct measuring of pressure from the CSF
• Access for CSF drainage or sampling
• Access for determining VPRs
• Access for instillation of drugs

Disadvantages
• Requires puncture of the brain
• Difficulty in locating the lateral ventricle following midline shifting of the ventricle, or collapse of the ventricle as a normal compensatory mechanism for increases in pressure
• Risk of infection. Miller reported no infection in patients monitored 3 days or less, with a 4% infection rate in patients monitored more than 3 days. Sundbärg and co-workers documented a clinically apparent CNS infection rate of 1.1%.[2,6]

Subarachnoid Technique. The measurement of ICP by means of a subarachnoid screw (Figs. 22-10 and 22-11) was first reported in 1973. The screw device is inserted through a twist drill hole and extends into the subdural or subarachnoid space. Although the cerebrum is not penetrated, pressures, as with the intraventricular technique, are measured directly from the CSF. A transducer filled with saline or Ringer's lactate solution may be fastened directly to a stopcock on the screw or connected by pressure tubing. As with any technique for monitoring ICP, a continuous flush device is contraindicated.

An alternate technique for monitoring subarachnoid pressure is the ribbon-shaped cup catheter. The catheter is usually used in conjunction with a craniotomy procedure and is inserted through a subcutaneous tunnel and burr hole. Volume pressure responses have been determined using these techniques. Subarachnoid pressures correlate well with intraventricular pressures.

Advantages
• Direct pressure measurement from CSF

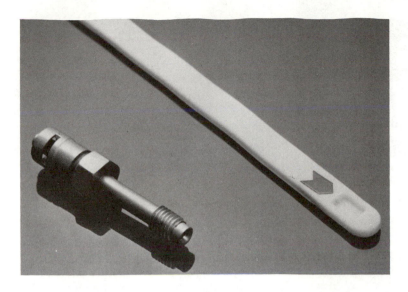

FIGURE 22-10.
Subarachnoid screw *(left)* and cup catheter *(right)*.

- Does not require penetration of cerebrum to locate ventricle
- Access for determining volume pressure responses
- Access for CSF drainage and sampling

Disadvantages
- Risk of infection comparable to intraventricular technique
- Requires closed skull
- More difficult to use for VPR studies and CSF drainage than ventricular catheters
- High ICP may cause blockge of the measuring devices

Epidural Technique.   This technique involves placing an epidural device such as a balloon with radioisotopes, a radio transmitter, or a fiberoptic transducer between the skull and the dura. Some researchers feel that dural compression and surface tension, as well as thickening of the dura during prolonged monitoring, tend to cause inaccuracies in the pressure readings. Although subarachnoid and intraventricular pressures correlate well with each other, there have been inconsistent correlations between direct CSF pressure and pressure measurement using various epidural techniques.

Certain fiberoptic and solid state transducers

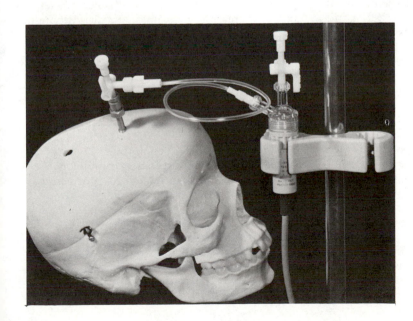

FIGURE 22-11.
Measurement of ICP by means of subarachnoid technique with standard size transducer.

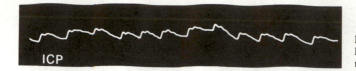

FIGURE 22-12.
ICP waveform demonstrating hemodynamic and respiratory oscillations.

have proved to be of value for noninvasive anterior fontanel pressure monitoring of neonates and infants. A special holder is used to attach the transducer to the anterior fontanel. A normal ICP is less than 10 torr. These pressures have correlated well with intraventricular pressures.

Advantages
• Less invasive
• Selected transducers useful for anterior fontanel monitoring

Disadvantages
• Questionable reflection of CSF pressure. With high ICPs, epidural pressures considerably overread ventricular pressures.
• No route for CSF drainage and sampling
• Volume pressure responses not feasible
• Inability to zero and calibrate some systems after measurement is initiated
• Transducer placement. Transducer must touch but not indent the dura and must be parallel to or coplaner with the dura. If the dura is stretched, the pressure recording will be affected by dural compliance.

PRESSURES

Range. Normal ICP ranges between 0 and 10 torr, with an upper limit of 15 torr. ICP is routinely monitored as a mean pressure. During coughing or straining a normal ICP may increase to 100 torr. In acute situations, patients frequently become symptomatic at pressures around 20 to 25 torr.

The patient's tolerance of changes in ICP varies with the acuteness of its onset. Patients with a slower build up of ICP, such as occurs with certain brain tumors, are more tolerant of elevations in the ICP than patients with rapid development of pressure changes such as that seen in acute subdural hematoma. Most physicians consider 20 to 40 torr a moderate elevation, and pressures greater than 40 torr are considered a severe elevation.

ICP may rise to the level of the MAP. The greater the variations in the mean ICP, the more nearly exhausted are the compensatory mechanisms for intracranial volume increases.

Although protocols vary, measures to reduce ICP are usually initiated if the patient shows neurologic deterioration or when the ICP reaches 20 to 25 torr.

Waveforms. The appearance of ICP waveforms varies according to the technique of measurement being used and the patient's pathology. Hemodynamic and respiratory oscillations can be observed in ICP traces. At times the waveforms closely resemble arterial pressure waveforms and other times CVP waveforms. To varying degrees, oscillations corresponding to the arterial pulsations are seen.

In patients with ICP less than 20 torr, a slower waveform synchronous with respiration, caused by changes in intrathoracic pressure, can be seen (see Fig. 22-12).

Some patients exhibit waveform variations most commonly known as A, B, and C waves. These were originally defined by Lundberg.[7]

"A" waves, also known as *plateau waves,* are spontaneous, rapid increases of pressure between 50 to 200 torr, occurring at variable intervals (see Fig. 22-13). They tend to occur in patients with moderate elevations of ICP, last 5 to 20 minutes, and fall spontaneously. The plateau waves are usually accompanied by a temporary increase in neurologic deficit. Although the mechanism of A waves has not been firmly established, it is felt that they indicate decreased intracranial compliance. In a study involving patients with aneurysm, Nornes correlated an increased frequency of plateau waves with a tendency to rebleed.[8]

"B" waves are small, sharp rhythmic waves with pressures up to 50 torr, occurring at a frequency of 0.5 to 2.0 per minute. They correspond to changes in respiration, providing clues to periodic respiration related to poor cerebral compliance or pulmonary dysfunction. B waves are often seen with Cheyne-Stokes respirations. At times they occur in patients with normal ICP and no papilledema.

"C" waves are small, rhythmic waves with pressures up to 20 torr, occurring at a rate of approximately 6 per minute. They are related to the Traube-Herring-Mayer waves of arterial

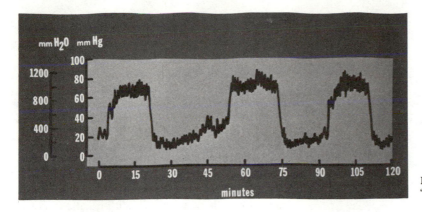

FIGURE 22-13.
"A" or plateau waves.

blood pressure. Like A waves, they indicate severe intracranial compression, with limited remaining volume residual within the intracranial space.

CEREBRAL PERFUSION PRESSURE

CPP is calculated by subtracting the mean ICP from the mean systemic arterial pressure (MAP) (See Fig. 22-14):

$$CPP = MAP - ICP.$$

Normal cerebral blood flow (CBF) is provided by a CPP in the range of 40 to 130 torr. The autoregulation system for maintenance of constant blood flow does not function at pressures less than 40 torr. When the CPP is zero, there is no CBF. In other words, when ICP equals MAP, CPP equals zero and CBF is zero. CBF may totally cease at pressures somewhat above zero.

If CPP decreases secondary to a decreased blood pressure, CBF begins to drop at 50 to 60 torr. If CPP decreases secondary to increased ICP, CBF is maintained until the CPP falls to 40 torr.

When brain damage is severe, as with widespread brain edema or where blood flow has been arrested in the brain, CBF may be reduced at relatively normal levels of CPP. This is due to impedance to the flow of blood across the cerebrovascular bed. CBF may not increase despite increases in CPP if autoregulation is impaired. This condition is referred to as *pressure-flow dissociation*.

VOLUME-PRESSURE CURVE

The volume-pressure curve is the curve that relates supratentorial ICP to the volume of the increasing mass lesion. When the intracranial lesion begins to develop, there is little initial increase in pressure because of the compensatory shifts of blood and CSF. Once these compensatory mechanisms have been fully used, the curve becomes steeper or nonlinear. This usually occurs at approximately 15 torr. Uniform increments of volume now cause progressively larger increases in ICP. This is due to a decrease in intracranial compliance. The cranial contents become stiffer, and free communication of CSF between the lateral ventricles and infratentorium is lost. Drastic increases in ICP may result from hypercarbia, hypoxia, rapid eye movement (REM) sleep, pyrexia, or the administration of certain anesthetics.

Intracranial compliance can be tested by obtaining a volume pressure response (VPR). A technique used by Miller consists of injecting 1 ml of sterile saline into the intraventricular catheter or 0.1 ml into the subarachnoid screw. If the ICP increases less than 2 torr with a 1-ml injection given over an interval of 1 second, the patient is not undergoing compensatory changes. A response of at least 3 torr per ml is considered a sign of altered compensation or compliance. A VPR of 5 torr per ml or more is an urgent indication for repeat study of the patient. It is recommended that VPRs be done by way of an intraventricular cannula. In select

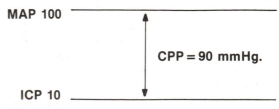

FIGURE 22-14.
Cerebral perfusion pressure.

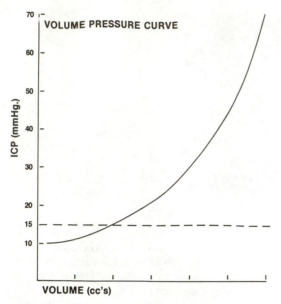

FIGURE 22-15.
Volume pressure curve.

cases, intraventricular fluid is withdrawn after the study. (See Fig. 22-15.)

MANAGEMENT OF THE PATIENT WITH INCREASED INTRACRANIAL PRESSURE (IICP)

Surgical decompression, ventricular drainage, low PCO_2, massive steroids, osmotic diuretics, and induced barbiturate coma are among the measures used to treat intracranial hypertension. Although no one therapeutic regime has been universally accepted, the goals in treatment of the patient with IICP remain the same—

- To reduce ICP
- To improve CPP
- To reduce brainshift and distortion and the systemic effects they induce

The following discussion covers measures currently used in the management of IICP.

Surgical Decompression. Intracranial mass lesions are evacuated as early as possible, usually with replacement of the bone flap.

Ventilation. Endotracheal intubation is usually used with a tracheostomy performed by the third day if ventilation is still required. Intermittent positive pressure ventilation (IPPV) is indicated in head injury patients in coma, patients with ICPs greater than 30 torr after postcranial surgery, with chest injuries, and in patients with decerebrate spasms or uncontrolled seizures secondary to brain damage. Reducing the arterial PCO_2 causes cerebral vasoconstriction, which reduces cerebral blood volume.

Ventilation is usually done at a slow rate (approximately 10 to 12 cycles/min) with a high tidal volume (15 ml/kg body weight) to moderate hypocapnia (25 to 35 torr). If necessary, small doses of chlorpromazine or morphine sulfate are often used to phase the patient with the ventilator. For selected patients, paralyzing agents such as pancuronium bromide are used. When paralyzing or tranquilizing drugs are used, ICP monitoring is mandatory. With normally reacting blood vessels, a drop in PCO_2 from 40 to 20 torr is associated with a reduction in elevated ICP of approximately 30%. Reduction of PCO_2 below 20 torr causes no further vasoconstriction.

Arterial PO_2 is maintained over 70 torr.

PEEP is used at levels up to 10 cm of water and requires ICP monitoring.

Position. The head is elevated 10° to 20° unless contraindicated by limb fractures. Flexion of the knees is contraindicated.

Hypothermia. Although hypothermia decreases the cerebral metabolic rate of oxygen consumption, used alone it may cause a reduction of cerebral blood flow. With the exception of patients in induced barbiturate coma, normothermia is usually used. Temperature elevations are promptly treated.

Hypothermia has been successfully used in conjunction with induced barbiturate coma. The combination may offer synergistic protection, acting through different mechanisms to control IICP.

Blood Pressure Control. *Blood Pressure Reduction.* IICP and neurologic dysfunction can be aggravated by systemic vasodilator drugs such as sodium nitroprusside (Nipride). With a normal PCO_2, Nipride causes a significant increase in ICP with only a slight decrease in blood pressure. The use of hyperventilation attenuates but does not obliterate the ICP effect.

When induced hypotension is needed in the patient with IICP, Nipride administration should be carefully titrated. Ideally, the drug should only be used in surgery after the skull is opened.

Although high arterial blood pressure may be detrimental in patients with IICP, in patients with a very high ICP, a reduction in blood pressure may further reduce cerebral blood flow. Reduction of arterial blood pressure is contraindicated in patients with brain edema when CBF is already reduced.

Blood Pressure Elevation. Postoperative intracranial aneurysm patients with cerebral ischemia secondary to severe intracranial vascular spasm have demonstrated marked clinical improvement following short periods of induced arterial hypertension.

Paralyzing Agents. Since muscle tremors can cause elevations of ICP, paralyzing agents such as curare or, more commonly, pancuronium bromide (Pavulon), are used for muscle relaxation. ICP, blood pressure, and PA monitoring with assisted ventilation are then mandatory.

Steroids. Glucocorticoids such as dexamethasone, betamethasone, and methylprednisolone have proved effective in reducing brain edema and ICP and in improving neurologic status, particularly in brain tumor patients with peritumoral edema. Clinical improvement is usually seen within 24 hours. An elevated resting ICP is not usually reduced until the second or third day of treatment. Steroid therapy has proved to be the most effective in patients with focal chronic lesions. Standard doses of steroids have not been effective in reducing IICP associated with acute head injury, but higher doses of dexamethasone may be of value.

CSF Drainage. In patients with impaired absorption of CSF such as after a subarachnoid hemorrhage, impaired circulation of CSF such as with hydrocephalus and certain brain tumors, or IICP without total collapse of the ventricles, controlled CSF drainage may facilitate a reduction in ICP. Ventricular drainage should always be against a positive pressure of 15 to 20 torr to prevent ventricular collapse. Best results are obtained when there is bilateral dilatation of the ventricles. Decompression should be gradual, particularly in children. Although CSF drainage is routinely done by intraventricular catheter (ventriculostomy), in selected patients CSF can be drained by a subarachnoid screw.

Osmotherapy. Osmotic agents such as mannitol, urea, and glycerol or isosorbide may be used to assist in the management of IICP. At times diuretics are used in conjunction with osmotherapy, requiring even more careful consideration of fluid and electrolyte balance. Although the osmotics have long been considered to introduce the risk of rebound, with ICP returning to or becoming higher than the pressure initially being treated, this phenomenon is now being questioned. Some investigators feel that rebound is unlikely when the drugs are properly managed. Regardless of which agent is used, the optimal dose is the lowest dose that reduces ICP. Since the absolute effect of any drug cannot be determined in advance, continual monitoring of ICP is required to determine the correct dosage for a given patient. By titrating drug administration by means of ICP monitoring, the problem of increased osmolarity resulting from too high or too frequent dosages can be avoided.

The hyperosmotic agent most commonly used is 20% mannitol. Intravenous urea is seldom used because of the problem with severe local reaction if leakage occurs at the injection site. Mannitol therapy is often initiated if the patient's ICP has exceeded 25 torr for at least 10 minutes. A dose of 0.25 to 1.00 g per kg of body weight is administered intravenously over a 10- to 15-minute period. The use of barbiturates reduces the mannitol requirement. Results should be evident within 15 minutes of completion of administration. Osmotherapy may increase CBF even when ICP is not reduced. In extremely ill patients, the administration of mannitol may cause parallel increases in blood pressure and ICP, with clinical deterioration.

Induced Barbiturate Coma. Although somewhat controversial, induced barbiturate coma has been documented as increasing survival and decreasing morbidity, particularly in patients with head injuries and Reye's syndrome.

Mechanism. The mechanism by which ICP is reduced has not been firmly established. The barbiturate appears to have a direct, restrictive effect on cerebral vasculature, diverting small amounts of the blood from well-perfused areas to ischemic areas, thereby improving cerebral pressure and collateral circulation. Vascular spasms are reduced, improving CBF. It lowers the systemic blood pressure, thereby decreasing blood-brain barrier disruption. Effects of noxious stimuli, such as critical care unit noise, are blunted, and patients are more tolerant of positioning and suctioning. The total muscle relaxation and immobilization reduce cerebral venous pressure. Both blood pressure and ICP become less labile.

Table 22–3
Management of Patients in Induced Barbiturate Coma

Problem	Outcome	Management
Uncontrolled IICP (ICP > 20 torr for > 30 min and unresponsive to usual Rx methods)	ICP maintained at less than 15 torr CPP at least 60–70 torr Temperature between 37° and 38° rectally	Monitor ICP continuously Calculate CPP (MAP – ICP) q1h; notify physician if 50 torr or less Fluid restriction of 80 ml/hr or as ordered Administer diuretics (*e.g.,* mannitol, Lasix) as ordered Maintain normothermia with hypothermia-hyperthermia blanket or antipyretic agents
Adequate barbiturate level to control ICP	Serum barbiturate level maintained at about 3.0 mg/dl ICP at less than 15 torr	Administer pentobarbital q1h slowly intravenously as ordered (rate 10 min/100 mg) Daily serum barbiturate levels
Hypotension due to cardiovascular instability and hypovolemia	Arterial systolic pressure maintained above 90 torr Urinary output at least 30 ml/hr CVP and PAP within normal limits Normal sinus rhythm	Continuous monitoring of arterial pressure, PAP, CVP, ECG pattern Check cuff pressure q shift and prn Administer vasopressor (*e.g.,* dopamine if systolic < 90 torr) (One dose of pentobarbital may be held) Urinary output q1h
Respiratory depression (unable to breathe spontaneously, absence of cough reflex)	Arterial blood gases—PCO_2 within normal limits or 22–25 torr PO_2-100/torr Normal breath sounds bilaterally	Maintain on ventilator at 10–14/min and sigh 10:2 ratio or as ordered Endotracheal tube or tracheostomy care Monitor cuff pressure continuously Suction and bag q1h and prn Irrigate tube with normal saline prn Suction nasopharyngeal secretions q2h and prn Arterial blood gases daily and prn Check breath sounds q 1–2h
Fluid and electrolyte imbalance 2° to fluid restriction, diuretics, and GI suction	Serum osmolality <320 mOsm Serum electrolytes within normal limits (*e.g.,* NA,K) Normal sinus rhythm Absence of T-wave depression and U waves BUN, creatinine, and hematocrit within normal limits Absence of clinical signs of dehydration	Serum osmolality bid (hold mannitol, Lasix if > 320 mOsm and notify physician) Electrolytes, BUN, creatinine, Hct daily and prn Monitor PAP and ECG pattern continuously Urinary output and specific gravity q1h Total intake and output q24h and cumulatively Observe skin and mucous membranes for evidence of dehydration
GI depression (absence of bowel sounds, inability to assimilate)	Absence of vomiting Absence of impaction Absorption of tube feedings	Salem-sump or nasogastric tube to gravity drainage or intermittent suction Measure gastric output q shift Auscultate for bowel sounds q shift and prn Palpate abdomen for distention Check for impaction Check gastric contents for assimilation when tube feedings are initiated after bowel sounds have returned
Loss of gag, swallow, and corneal reflexes	Absence of aspiration Absence of trauma to cornea	Suction oropharynx q1h and prn Position on each side, avoid placing on back as much as possible Cleanse eyes and apply liquid tears or Lacri-Lube S.O.P. q4h and prn Tape eyelids closed prn

Table 22–3 (Continued)

Problem	Outcome	Management
Susceptibility to infection	WBC within normal limits Cultures negative	Strict aseptic technique Culture questionable sites prn
Inadequate nutrition due to catabolic state	Minimal weight loss	Multivitamins daily as ordered Parenteral hyperalimentation as ordered
Immobility	Absence of atelectasis Absence of skin breakdown Absence of thrombophlebitis and pulmonary embolism Absence of contractures	Institute appropriate preventive measures (specific details of care are beyond the scope of this chapter)
Inability to cope and lack of understanding by the family/significant others	Verbalize realistic expectations Verbalize an appropriate understanding of the patient's condition and the therapy	Allow the family members to ventilate and ask questions Answer questions Give appropriate information without generating unrealistic expectations

(Reproduced with permission from Ricci M: Intracranial hypertension: Barbiturate therapy and the role of the nurse. J Neurosurg Nurs 11, No. 4:247–252, 1979)

Indications. Criteria vary extensively. In a recently published protocol, barbiturate coma was initiated when the ICP remained greater than 20 torr for more than 30 minutes despite use of the usual therapeutic modalities.[9]

Procedure. Prior to administration of the barbiturate, usually pentobarbital, ICP, blood pressure, PAP, and electrocardiogram (ECG) monitoring with assisted ventilation are initiated. Baseline electroencephalogram (EEG) and brain stem–evoked responses (BAER) recordings are taken. An EEG is taken prior to initiation of barbiturate coma to document spontaneous electrocortical activity, and BAER are recorded to assess brain-stem integrity. Although high serum barbiturate levels will totally suppress electrocortical activity, BAER will remain as long as there is brain-stem function.

Dosage. To place the patient in a light coma, a loading dose of 3 to 5 mg per kg of pentobarbital is given by slow intravenous push. The expected response is a drop in ICP of at least 10 torr within 10 minutes. If the patient responds to the loading dose, a maintenance dose of 1 to 3 mg per kg per hour is given to maintain barbiturate levels of 2.5 to 3.5 mg per dl and to maintain EEG activity at 2 to 5 Hz for several days. Impaired liver or kidney function will affect serum barbiturate levels. If the patient does not respond to the first loading dose, a second loading dose is given 2 hours later. The onset of action of intravenous pentobarbital is 1 minute. It has a half-life of 4 hours. The usual techniques for reduction of ICP continue to be used in conjunction with barbiturates. Mannitol doses are reduced.

Nursing Management. The patient in barbiturate coma becomes dependent. Clinical neurologic evaluation is almost impossible, making extensive, accurate monitoring of physiological responses to therapy mandatory. Artificial ventilation is required, and all vital functions must be maintained by the critical care team. Table 22-3 summarizes the management of the patient in induced barbiturate coma.

Indications for Discontinuing Barbiturate Coma. Barbiturate coma should be discontinued if any of the following exist: an ICP less than 15 torr for 24 to 72 hours; a normal VPR (less than 3 torr/ml); a systolic blood pressure less than 90 torr despite the use of vasopressors such as dopamine; lack of ICP response; progressive neurologic impairment such as deterioration of auditory BAER; abolition of the need for vasodilator therapy to reduce systolic blood pressure below 160 torr; cardiac arrest.

The barbiturates are gradually tapered over a period lasting from 24 hours to several days. Arousal is gradual and prolonged, even after blood levels have been zero for several days. Patients must be weaned slowly and carefully from the respirator because of muscle weakness resulting from the therapy.

Patients have vacuous facial expressions for several days despite normal blood barbiturate levels. Occasionally, during the first 24 hours, they develop slow, abnormal movements that

Table 22–4
Troubleshooting ICP Lines

Problem	Cause	Action
No ICP waveform	Air between the transducer diaphragm and pressure source	Eliminate air bubbles with sterile saline or Ringer's lactate
	Occlusion of intracranial measurement device with blood or debris	Flush intracranial cath or screw as directed by physician: 0.25 ml sterile saline is frequently used
	Transducer connected incorrectly	Check connection and be sure the appropriate connector for amplifier is in use
	Incorrect gain setting for pressure or patient having plateau waves	Adjust gain setting for higher pressure range.
	Trace turned off	Turn power on to trace
False high reading	Transducer too low	Place the venting port of the transducer at the level of the foramen of Monro: for every 1 inch the transducer is below the pressure source there is an error of approximately 2 torr
	Transducer incorrectly balanced	With transducer correctly positioned, rebalance
		Transducer should be balanced q 2–4 hours and prior to the initiation of treatment based on a pressure change
	Monitoring system incorrectly calibrated	Repeat calibration procedures
	Air in system: air may attenuate or amplify pressure signal	Remove air from monitoring line
High pressure reading	Airway not patent: an increase in intrathoracic pressure may increase PCO_2	Suction patient
		Position
		Chest physiotherapy
	Ventilator setting incorrect	Check ventilator settings
	PEEP	Draw arterial blood gases
		Hypoxia and hypercarbia cause increases in ICP
	Posture	Head should be elevated 10°–20° unless contraindicated by other problems such as fractures
	Head and neck	The head should be positioned to facilitate venous drainage
	Legs	Limit knee flexion
	Decerebrate	Muscle relaxants or paralyzing agents are sometimes indicated
	Excessive muscle activity during decerebrate posturing in patients with upper brain-stem injury may increase ICP	
	Hyperthermia	Measures to control muscle movement, infection, and pyrexia
	Excessive muscle activity	
	Increased susceptibility to infection	
	Fluid and electrolyte imbalance secondary to fluid restrictions and diuretics	Draw blood for serum electrolytes, serum osmolality
		Note PAP
		I & O with specific gravity
	Blood pressure: vasopressor responses occur in some patients with IICP	Use measures to maintain adequate CPP
	Low BP associated with hypovolemia, shock and barbiturate coma may increase cerebral ischemia	
False low pressure reading	Air bubbles between transducer and CSF	Eliminate air bubbles with sterile saline or Ringer's lactate
	Transducer level too high	Place the venting port of the transducer at the level of the foramen of Monro. For every 1 inch the transducer is above the level of the pressure source there will be an error of approximately 2 torr

Table 22–4 (Continued)

Problem	Cause	Action
	Zero or calibration incorrect	Rezero and calibrate monitoring system
Low ICP pressure	Collapse of ventricles	If ventriculostomy is being used there may be inadequate positive pressure. Check to make sure a positive pressure of 15–20 torr exists. Drain CSF slowly
	Otorrhea or rhinorrhea	These conditions cause a false low pressure reading secondary to decompression. Document the correlation between drainage and pressure changes.

appear athetoid in nature. Dysarthria is common. Anticonvulsants are used to control withdrawal seizures. Status epilepticus has been reported.

TROUBLESHOOTING ICP

When the monitor indicates a change in ICP, it must first be determined if the reading is accurate. If the reading is accurate, an attempt is then made to determine the reason for the pressure change. Table 22-4 provides a guide to troubleshooting ICP lines.

Clinical Implications

Monitoring ICP, blood pressure, PAP, and CPP and correlating these measurements with noninvasive clinical assessments often reduce the time required to obtain an accurate diagnosis, increase the time available for treatment, and provide continual feedback on the patient's response to selected treatments.

Clinical evaluation alone is not a reliable means of detecting changes in blood pressure, PA pressure, ICP, and the patient's response to treatment. The classic Kocher-Cushing syndrome is usually not a warning, but rather a symptom of brain death. Recognizable clinical signs and symptoms of increased ICP usually occur after the patient has passed the optimal time for treatment, and sometimes not at all.

Routine nursing measures such as suction, positioning, and taking rectal temperatures, as well as interruptions in osmotherapy and ventilator support, have been found to significantly affect CPP. One study associated discussion about the patient's condition at the patient's bedside with an increase in ICP.[10] Invasive neurologic assessment techniques should be used only in critical care facilities with trained personnel. The information obtained must be accurate and reliable and correlated with other clinical assessments to be instrumental in the diagnosis, prognosis, and management of IICP and to be of value in research on intracranial hypertension.

REFERENCES

1. Gardner RM et al: Percutaneous indwelling radial artery catheters for monitoring cardiovascular function: Prospective study of the risk of thrombosis and infection. N Engl J Med 290:1227–1231, 1974
2. Miller JD et al: Severe intracranial hypertension. In Trubohovich R (ed): Management of Acute Intracranial Disasters, International Anesthesiology Clinics, Vol 17. Boston, Little, Brown & Co, 1979
3. Trauner D et al: Treatment of elevated intracranial pressure in Reye syndrome. *Ann Neurol* 4, No. 3:275–278, 1978
4. Safar P: Pathophysiology and resuscitation after global brain ischemia. In Trubohovich R (ed): Management of Acute Intracranial Disaster, International Anesthesiology Clinics, Vol 17. Boston, Little, Brown & Co. 1979
5. Shapiro H et al: Intracranial pressure responses to PEEP in head-injured patients. J Trauma 18, No. 4:254–256, 1978
6. Sundbarg G et al: Complications due to prolonged ventricular fluid pressure recording in clinical practice. In Brock M, Dietz H (eds): Intracranial Pressure. New York, Springer-Verlag, 1973
7. Lundberg N: Continuous recording and control of ventricular fluid pressure in neurosurgical practice. Acta Psychiatr Scand, 36, Suppl. 149:1–193, 1960
8. Nornes H: Monitoring of patients with intracranial aneurysms. In Clinical Neurosurgery: Proceedings of the Congress of Neurological Surgeons, Vol 22. Baltimore, Williams & Wilkins, 1975
9. Ricci M: Intracranial hypertension: Barbiturate therapy and the role of the nurse. J Neurosurg Nurs, 11, No. 4:247–252, 1979
10. Mitchell P et al: Relationship of patient-nurse activity to intracranial pressure variations: A pilot study. Nurs Res, 27, No. 1:4–10, 1978

Specific Crisis Situations

Judith Ives

Disseminated Intravascular Coagulation Syndrome* 23

Disseminated intravascular coagulation syndrome has the singular distinction of being the oldest universally accepted hypercoagulable clinical state known. The many faces of this syndrome have led to such synonyms as *consumption coagulopathy, diffuse intravascular clotting,* and *the defibrination syndrome.* In most "clotting circles," however, the syndrome has become honorably dubbed *"DIC"* and will be referred to by this nickname throughout this chapter.

To understand the pathogenesis of DIC, a working knowledge of the intravascular clotting mechanisms and clotting inhibitors is necessary. Prior to the discussion of DIC, these mechanisms will be sequentially and simply outlined in the pages that follow.

THE BLOOD COAGULATION MECHANISM

In the normal state, the coagulation mechanisms are inactive; when activated they may proceed along either the intrinsic pathway or the extrinsic pathway. *In vivo,* both pathways are necessary for normal hemostatic homeostasis, and both pathways produce thrombin, which catalyzes the conversion of fibrinogen to fibrin, resulting in blood clot formation. However, each of the pathways involves different clotting factors and is initiated by different injuries or stimuli.

*We wish to acknowledge the contribution of John H. Attshuler, M.D., who prepared this chapter in the first and second editions of this text.

Intrinsic Pathway

Disruption of the endothelium membrane that lines the blood vessels activates the intrinsic clotting mechanism by exposing the underlying collagen. Following the initiating injury, changes in clotting factors start immediately. The changes that occur bear the relationship of enzyme (organic catalyst) to substrate (specific substance upon which an enzyme acts). The initiation of change causes molecular alteration in one clotting factor. The unaltered clotting factor, known as a proenzyme, is present in the plasma in very low concentrations and is converted to an altered state — an active enzyme. The product of this enzymatic reaction (the enzyme) activates the next factor (substrate). Thus, one molecule of enzyme acts upon a specific substrate, which is also a proenzyme clotting factor. The single active enzyme molecule is capable of converting not one, but perhaps thousands of specific substrate molecules into other active enzymes. This

is but a single event in what is to become an entire series of enzyme-substrate reactions.

A chain reaction is born whereby activation of a single proenzyme molecule may lead to activation of the entire clotting mechanism. The chain reaction involves at least 9 well-defined clotting factors with 34 others reported as being involved in disputed points along the way. At one place in the chain reaction, the reaction is known to be self-perpetuating so that a vicious cycle of clot activation ensues, causing clot formation to accelerate rapidly. This cascading of events may be paralleled with a waterfall.

Thus, as a result of disruption of the endothelium, blood touches an abnormal surface, traumatizing the blood, and initiating the intrinsic mechanism. This injury converts inactive factor XII (Hageman factor) to the active enzymatic form of XII designated *XIIa*. The enzyme XIIa acts upon the next clotting proenzyme factor — inactive factor XI — converting it to the active

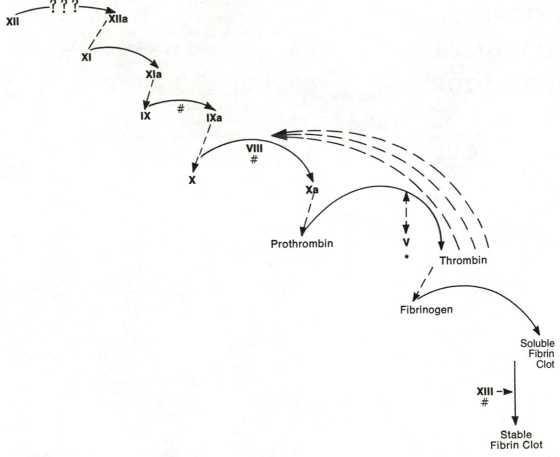

FIGURE 23-1.
Clotting sequence. (#) Calcium ion required; (*) calcium and fat (lipid) substance derived from platelets — both required.

enzyme XIa. Active XIa is responsible for the activation of factor IX and requires calcium ions. The activation of the next factor, factor X, requires factor VIII, and activation of factor prothrombin requires factor V. Furthermore, a fatty (lipid) substance derived from platelets (platelet cofactor 3) must be present at the site of activity of both factors VIII and V.

The self-perpetuating effect in the mechanism takes place by creating the vicious cycle of activation of factor X through the effect of thrombin on factor VIII. *Thrombin* enhances the activity of factor VIII so that it interacts more rapidly with factor IXa and thus catalyzes the activation of factor X. In the clotting sequence thrombin is a very potent enzyme, converting fibrinogen to fibrin clot. The initial fibrin clot is further stabilized by yet another clotting factor, XIII. Diagrammatically, the clotting sequence may be represented as in Figure 23-1. Notice that the activation of factor VIII by thrombin creates the activation of factor X, resulting in the self-perpetuating effect.

Extrinsic Pathway

The triggering mechanism initiating the extrinsic pathway is injury to tissues and vessels that release tissue *thromboplastin* into the circulation. As in the intrinsic pathway, a chain of events occurs leading to clot formation. Tissue thromboplastin catalyzed by factor VII activates factor X and, in the presence of calcium ions and factor V, active factor Xa catalyzes the conversion of prothrombin to thrombin, resulting in clot formation.

Another mechanism providing for the activation of the clotting factors following vascular injury is injury to red cells, leukocytes, or platelets resulting in increased availability of *phospholipid,* a component necessary for the proper functioning of both the intrinsic and extrinsic clotting pathways. It is thought that the release of these phospholipids accelerates blood coagulation.[1]

The result of all these clotting mechanisms is the formation of factor Xa, which converts prothrombin to thrombin and results in fibrin formation. Thus, it can be seen that at factor Xa all these mechanisms merge into a final common pathway to clot formation.

Clot Formation

When a blood vessel lining is injured in the course of normal wear and tear, holes occur through which blood leaks out. The hole, however, is promptly plugged by the adherence of platelets to the hole, thus preventing blood leakage outside of the vessel. The seepage of tissue juice into the rent in the vessel wall attracts more platelets and causes the latter to adhere to the hole, effectively plugging up the leak. This phenomenon is further enhanced by the platelets' own ability to release a chemical, adenosine diphosphate (ADP), which causes platelets to get stickier and attract new platelets to the area. Because platelet plugging may interfere with normal smooth flow (laminar flow) of blood through the vessel, eddy currents are set up that tend to activate the intrinsic clotting mechanism. If there were significant vessel or tissue damage, the extrinsic pathway would also be activated.

Unchecked intrinsic activation would cause clots to form on top of the platelet plug, releasing thrombin in the process of clotting, further attracting platelets to the clot site and causing additional clots to form at the local site of vessel leak. The result of this activation would be total vessel occlusion as depicted in Figure 23-2 if there were no *in vivo* mechanism operating to maintain the blood in a fluid state to prevent intravascular clotting.

Coagulation Inhibitors

Within humans there is a well-controlled balance between clotting and lysis. Through the action of physiological coagulation inhibitors, the blood is maintained in its fluid state. These inhibitors work by limiting reactions that promote clotting and by breaking down any clots that do form. Coagulation inhibitors include the following

- The liver and reticuloendothelial system, which clear activated clotting factors from the blood
- The liberation of antithrombins, which inactivate thrombin in serum or plasma, thus retarding the conversion of fibrinogen to fibrin
- The maintenance of adequate blood flow, which acts to dilute activated clotting factors and assist in their removal
- The interference with thrombin at its site of action on fibrinogen by the fibrinolytic system[2,3]

The fibrinolytic system is the system antagonist to the coagulation mechanism. Similar to the coagulation mechanisms, the fibrinolytic system also involves a chain reaction whereby

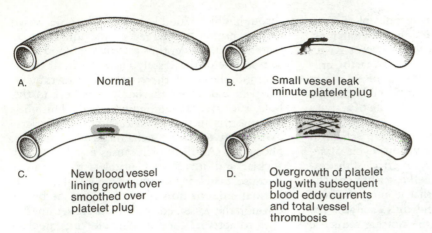

A.   Normal

B.   Small vessel leak
minute platelet plug

C.   New blood vessel
lining growth over
smoothed over
platelet plug

D.   Overgrowth of platelet
plug with subsequent
blood eddy currents
and total vessel
thrombosis

FIGURE 23-2.
Sequence of thrombus formation in blood vessels.

activation of a series of proenzymes results in lytic enzymes capable of dissolving clots. The dissolving or lytic enzyme is called *plasmin* and is derived from the proenzyme plasminogen, which is normally present in whole blood. Plasminogen is converted into plasmin by enzymes called *plasminogen activators*. Plasminogen activator levels are transiently increased in response to exercise, stress, anoxia, and pyrogens.[4]

Activated factor XII, thrombin, and substances in tissues are believed to be involved in the formation of plasmin from plasminogen. Plasmin acts to lyze fibrin and attacks factor V, factor VII, and fibrinogen. Lysis of fibrinogen results in the liberation of degradation products.

These products are known as *fibrin degradation products (FDP)*; they interfere with platelet aggregation and have anticoagulant activity.

Through these various coagulation inhibitors, a well-controlled balance between clotting and lysis is established in humans. Diagrammatically, a see-saw plank depicts coagulation control (see Fig. 23-3). On one side of the plank are the clotting factors (CF) and on the other side are the fibrinolytic factors (FF). Note that the plank may oscillate in a normal range. It is important to remember that the range of fluctuation may increase to a point at which laboratory tests are abnormal, but clinical evidence of pathologic bleeding or clotting is not seen. Ob-

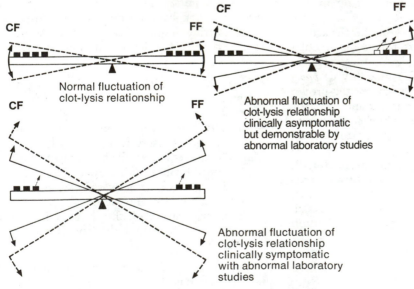

CF   FF

Normal fluctuation of
clot-lysis relationship

CF   FF

Abnormal fluctuation of
clot-lysis relationship
clinically asymptomatic
but demonstrable by
abnormal laboratory studies

CF   FF

Abnormal fluctuation of
clot-lysis relationship
clinically symptomatic
with abnormal laboratory
studies

FIGURE 23-3.
Normal and abnormal fluctuations in clot-lysis relationships.

viously, when this warning fluctuation range is exceeded, the person will demonstrate overt clinical evidence of thrombosis or hemorrhage.

The balance may be upset by

- Decreasing clotting factors, as in classic hemophilia, in which clotting factor VIII is low and the person has a bleeding tendency
- Increasing fibrinolytic factors, causing excessive bleeding
- Decreasing fibrinolytic factors, causing pathologic thrombosis
- Increasing clotting factors, causing hypercoagulopathy (still debated)

DISSEMINATED INTRAVASCULAR COAGULATION SYNDROME (DIC)

Pathophysiology

DIC is a syndrome of transient coagulation, causing transformation of fibrinogen to fibrin clot, often associated with acute hemorrhage. Paradoxically, DIC is a bleeding disorder resulting from an increased tendency to clot. The syndrome is secondary to a host of diseases and a diversity of etiologic factors. These etiologic factors and diseases include crush syndrome, hemorrhagic shock, snake bite, abruptio placentae, septic abortion, malignant hypertension, incompatible blood transfusion, pulmonary hypertension, idiopathic sepsis, carcinoma, leukemia, and cardiopulmonary bypass, to name a few.

Regardless of the etiologic agent, the syndrome of DIC has many common factors. The precipitating factors in DIC frequently cause the release of procoagulant substances into the bloodstream, including free hemoglobin, bacterial toxins, thrombosis-promoting placental tissue, amniotic fluid, and cancer-tissue fragments. These procoagulant substances provide the stimulus activating the coagulation mechanism. The activation of the coagulation mechanism results in diffuse intravascular fibrin formation and deposition of fibrin in the microcirculation.

Almost uniformly, persons have arterial hypotension often associated with shock, resulting in arterial vasoconstriction and capillary dilatation. Blood is then shunted to the venous side, by-passing dilated capillaries due to the opening of arteriovenous shunts (see Fig. 23-4). The dilated capillaries now contain stagnant blood, which accumulates metabolic by-products (pyruvic and lactic acids), rendering the blood

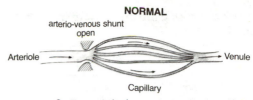

NORMAL

Capillary perfusion is normal, blood flow is rapid.

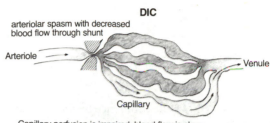

DIC

Capillary perfusion is impaired, blood flow is slow, intracapillary thrombosis occurs with blood stagnation and acidosis. Cells nourished by capillaries die of ischemia due to blood clotting.

FIGURE 23-4.
Arteriole-capillary-venule relationship in normal circulation as opposed to the DIC patient. The diagram shows the effect of A-V shunting in DIC.

acidotic. We thus have three concomitant procoagulating effects in capillary blood: (1) acidosis, a potent coagulation activator; (2) blood stagnation, which promotes increased concentration of activated coagulation factors; and (3) presence of coagulation-promoting substance in the blood.

The result of DIC to this point is the accumulation of clot in the body's capillaries, the length of which exceeds 100,000 miles in the average adult. Thus, the amount of blood clot sequestration in capillaries in acute DIC is enormous.

Because of the rapidity of the process, clotting factors are effectively used up in the capillary clotting process at a rate exceeding factor replenishment. Circulating blood becomes depleted of clotting factors. With such depletion, the person can no longer maintain normal hemostasis; therefore, bleeding follows. Hemorrhage starts from needle and incisional sites and from the respiratory, genitourinary, and gastrointestinal tracts. Blood cells now become suspended in serum rather than in plasma—serum being the liquid portion of blood minus the clotting factors used up in clotting. Not all clotting factors are used up in clotting, although the platelet blood cell is totally removed in clotting.

Table 23–1
Distribution of Clotting Factors in Serum and Plasma

Clotting Factors	Plasma	Serum
XII	†	†
XI	†	†
IX	†	†
VIII	†	0
X	†	†
V	†	0
Prothrombin	†	0
Fibrinogen	†	0
XIII	†	†
(Platelets)	(†)	(0)

† present; 0 absent; ( ) cellular component of blood.

Table 23-1 shows the difference between serum- and plasma–clotting factor distribution.

The DIC person bleeds not only as the result of consumption of clotting factors but to some degree because of increased fibrinolysis and diminished antithrombins, particularly antithrombin III. As mentioned earlier, the activation of the coagulation mechanism results in the generation of thrombin, which accelerates the coagulation activity, forming more fibrin and additional thrombin. *In vivo,* the thrombin con-

centration is regulated by antithrombins, particularly antithrombin III. Antithrombin III causes progressive irreversible destruction of thrombin in plasma, but in DIC the excessive thrombin formation exceeds antithrombin's ability to control thrombin, and coagulation proceeds uncontrolled.

The rapidly produced intravascular thrombin expedites the conversion of fibrinogen to fibrin clot and the conversion of plasminogen to plasmin. Activation of the fibrinolytic system not only brings about lysis of clots already formed but also causes production of fibrin degradation products, which further add to the bleeding diathesis because of their anticoagulant activity.

When, in the course of DIC, fibrinogen is entirely used up, circulating thrombin persists in the intravascular space, waiting for its substrate fibrinogen to arrive, converting it to clot. This arrival occurs either by additional body production of fibrinogen by the liver or by transfusion of blood, plasma, or fibrinogen, all of which serve to perpetuate the syndrome and worsen clinical hemorrhage. A summary diagram of the vicious cycle of DIC is given in Figure 23-5.

Laboratory Results. Now that the pathogenesis of DIC is understood, let us discuss how the laboratory can aid clinicians in diagnosing

Table 23–2
Laboratory Findings in Classic DIC

Test	Direction of Abnormal Values	Rationale
Prothrombin time	Prolonged	Factor V and prothrombin are measured
Partial thromboplastin time (PTT)	Prolonged	Factors V and VIII are measured and to a lesser degree — fibrinogen
Platelet count	Low	Thrombocytopenia present
Fibrinogen level	Low	Patient with DIC has reduced fibrinogen
Euglobulin lysis time (ELT)	Shortened	ELT measures fibrinolytic activity
Antithrombin III level	Low	Antithrombin III is absent in patient with DIC
Thrombin time	Prolonged	Fibrinogen is indirectly measured by thrombin time
Fibrin degradation products	Elevated	These products are increased in DIC

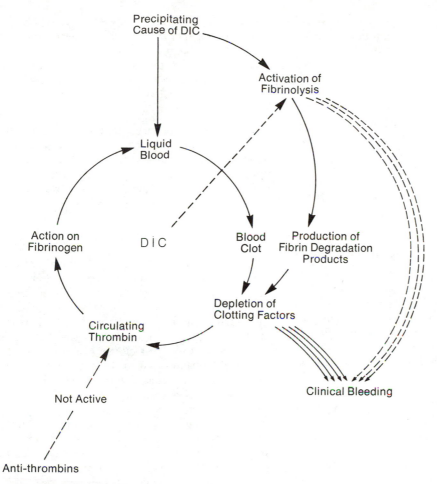

FIGURE 23-5.
Self-perpetuating cycle of clotting and hemorrhage in DIC.

DIC. Below is a list of the clotting factor and cell abnormalities found in DIC:

- Clotting factor-depleted plasma; hence, the following clotting factors are reduced:
  Fibrinogen
  Factor VIII
  Factor V
  Prothrombin
- Platelets markedly reduced (thrombocytopenia)
- Absence of antithrombins
- Abnormally high blood-thrombin levels
- Abnormally increased fibrinolytic activity
- Abnormally increased fibrin degradation products

In classic DIC, the tests given in Table 23-2 are abnormal.

Management of DIC

The management of DIC consists of treating the underlying disease, inhibiting the effects of thrombin with heparin, replacing the depleted clotting factors, and correcting the processes that may impede the clotting function.[5] The backbone of therapy consists of removing the cause of DIC. If one's basement is flooded by a broken pipe, the flooding will not be averted by mopping alone. He must turn off the water supply to the broken pipe.

Attention should also be directed at correcting hypovolemia, hypotension, hypoxia, and acidosis, all of which have procoagulant effects, depleting further the clotting factors. Correction of these imbalances should be part and parcel of the treatment of DIC bleeders. Additionally, correction of hemostatic deficiencies that compromise the clotting mechanism is necessary. Folic acid deficiency causes thrombocytopenia, and the formation of prothrombin is hindered by a vitamin K deficiency.

HEPARIN

If the underlying cause of DIC cannot be removed (as in intravascular dissemination of cancer), therapy of the syndrome may control but not cure it. Control of DIC is brought about by stopping the vicious cycle of thrombosis-hemorrhage as shown in Figure 23-5. Heparin is generally considered to be the agent of choice.

Heparin helps prevent further thrombus formation, but it does not alter clots that have already formed; it slows coagulation and permits restoration of clotting factors. It does this in three ways:

- It is antithrombin in activity and will neutralize free circulating thrombin. Heparin combines with antithrombin III and in the presence of thrombin, forms a reversible combination in which the thrombin is inactivated.
- It prevents propagation of thrombi that have formed in capillaries — in which capacity, heparin is functioning as an anticoagulant.
- It has an inhibitory effect on the activation of blood clotting *in vivo*, principally due to its effect on factor X. *Heparin,* as a powerful inhibitor, *prevents* the *activation* of *factor X* and thus blocks the progression of the sequential activation of the coagulation mechanism at factor X level.

As previously mentioned, the intrinsic and extrinsic coagulation pathways merge into a final common pathway at the activated factor X level; therefore, coagulation through either the intrinsic or extrinsic pathway can be inhibited by heparin.

Heparin also inhibits platelet aggregation that is mediated by thrombin by its neutralizing effects on thrombin. The administration of heparin therefore inhibits (1) thrombin formation, (2) thrombin-fibrinogen interactions, and (3) platelet aggregation.

In DIC, heparin should be given *intravenously* for four reasons:

- Dose regulation is far easier by intravenous rather than subcutaneous administration because the absorption rate from tissue is affected by the amount given, depth of injection, body temperature, and cardiovascular status.
- Local hematoma formation when given subcutaneously may severely alter absorption of the drug.
- The dose in severe, acute cases may be too large for proper blood levels to be attained by any route except intravenous.
- The time lag for therapeutic effect of subcutaneous heparin is too great compared to the immediate effect of the drug when administered intravenously.

The *dosage* of heparin required to treat DIC must be tempered by the clinical status of the patient and tailored to the individual as determined by sequential coagulation studies. Coagulation studies are necessary to regulate the heparin dose and to evaluate the patient's response to the therapy.

In acute DIC, heparin is administered intravenously by continuous drip in doses of either 500 to 1000 units of heparin per hour or 100 units per kg body weight every 4 hours.[6,7] The total heparin dose should be titrated at the minimal dose that will establish adequate anticoagulation by determining the disappearance rate of heparin in the patient. The goal of heparin therapy is usually attainment of a clotting time prolonged two to three times that of the normal controls.

Patients with renal failure, inadequate liver perfusion, or both will require far less heparin to control DIC because heparin is normally eliminated from the body by renal excretion (in both an altered and unaltered state) and by heparinase activity in the liver. Thus, persons with these pathologies will have an abnormally prolonged heparin half-life because of their decreased ability to metabolize heparin to an inactive form or to excrete it.

Heparin should be continued until the primary precipitating cause of DIC has been removed and clinical and laboratory evidence suggest that the patient is on the way to recovery. In early, acute DIC, a single large dose of heparin will arrest the DIC process if the primary factors have been eliminated.

TRANSFUSION THERAPY

After heparin therapy has been initiated, appropriate blood products may be administered to replace depleted clotting factors.

Blood products should not be administered until after heparin therapy is initiated, so that the infused coagulation factors will not add fuel to the fire of circulating thrombin in the intravascular space. If blood is needed, fresh whole blood should be used because it will provide platelets and all the coagulation factors that are deficient in stored blood. If red cells are not needed, fresh frozen plasma or platelet transfusions will provide the coagulation factors and platelets for hemostasis.

ANTIFIBRINOLYTIC DRUGS

Antifibrinolytic drugs, ε-aminocaproic acid (eACA [Amicar]) should, with rare exception, *not* be given in DIC. The rationale for giving eACA is to take advantage of the potent antifibrinolytic effect of eACA, hence reducing the fibrinolytic component of bleeding in acute DIC. Let us not forget that eACA is a double-edged sword. It inhibits not only pathologic but also normal fibrinolysis, hence inhibiting a protective mechanism in the clot-lysis balance. DIC is, after all, a hypercoagulable state, and eACA may render a patient even more hypercoagulable by destroying the lytic side of the balance. Certainly, if one desires to control the pathologic element of fibrinolysis, eACA must not be given unless the patient is adequately heparinized, and then only with great caution.

FOR SUBACUTE AND CHRONIC BLEEDING

Thus far we have discussed the acute bleeding episodes of DIC. However, this syndrome occurs in both a subacute and a chronic phase.

In the *subacute stage,* bleeding may not be clinically obvious; however, at this stage the patient is in great danger of becoming an overt bleeder (acute DIC). Treatment of the subacute is important only to prevent the acute stage from occurring.

The *chronic form* of DIC is usually unassociated with hemorrhage or abnormal clotting tests. The only clue may be a sudden drop in hematocrit in the absence of any demonstrable blood loss. It is assumed that hemoglobin is sequestered as clot in capillaries. Due to the slow replacement of red cell mass in circulating blood, the only manifestation of chronic DIC is a *drop* in *circulating blood hemoglobin.* Blood volume is kept normal with rapid plasma replacement. The typical chronic DIC patient is the one with a sudden episode of coronary shock, with hemoglobin loss as a single occurrence.

MIMICKING SYNDROMES

"All that glitters is not gold." Likewise, all that bleeds is not DIC. All too often every bleeding crisis is diagnosed as DIC. There are numerous bleeding situations that mimic DIC, and they should not be forgotten. A few of these are acute fibrinolytic activation, clotting factor depletion secondary to massive hemorrhage, and acquired clotting factor inhibitors. Unfortunately, routine laboratory data do not differentiate these syndromes with ease. Because treatment of the different bleeding disorders varies, correct diagnosis is essential if the person's life is to be prolonged. Incorrect diagnosis, and hence improper treatment, will hasten death.

Implications for Nursing Care

Any critically ill person is at risk for developing DIC, but an increased awareness of this potential problem has resulted in earlier recognition and intervention. The critical care nurse with an understanding of the normal physiological mechanisms involved in maintaining hemostatic hemostasis may be the first to identify the early signs of coagulation dysfunction. Recognition of the signs of dysfunction depends upon knowing what to look for, based upon a knowledge of physiological norms, and using a systematic approach to assessment. Remember: all that bleeds is not DIC. The nurse must be suspicious of the subtle signs of bleeding that may be heralding the onset of this medical catastrophe. Clues to the onset of DIC, such as the appearance of petechiae, ecchymosis, or prolonged bleeding from injection or venipuncture sites, may be so subtle that they are overlooked until the patient manifests overt signs of bleeding.

The patient with DIC presents a challenge to any competent, creative, compassionate critical care nurse. He exhibits a varied constellation of problems and has the potential for developing more, all of which will test the nurse's ingenuity when planning nursing care and interventions to meet his needs.

The critical care nurse will be confronted with a patient bleeding from the nose, gums, and injection sites, and thus a patient who must be handled with care lest other bleeding be stimulated; a patient covered with purpura, petechiae, and ecchymosis; a patient immobilized by a variety of drainage tubes, IV lines, and hemodynamic monitoring equipment and often attached to a mechanical ventilator; a patient frightened by the loss of blood, stressed from the numerous venipunctures and arterial punctures required for lab tests; a family frightened by their loved one's appearance, and his bleeding, and with no understanding of this catastrophic event.

All three — patient, family, and staff — will need emotional support.

The remaining pages will emphasize some of the complications, nursing assessments, and interventions peculiar to the person with a bleeding diathesis from DIC. The reader is referred to the appropriate chapters in this book for lengthier discussions and review.

ASSESSING FOR POSSIBLE COMPLICATIONS

The DIC patient is at risk for developing the following problems: increased bleeding or thrombosis, pulmonary complications, fluid-electrolyte and renal problems, intravascular and extracellular fluid volume depletion or overload, and cardiac dysrhythmias and infection. The DIC patient already has a bleeding diathesis that may be compounded by the administration of heparin to treat the syndrome. Thus, an integral part of the nursing care plan is to continually monitor the patient for signs of increased bleeding, noting the sites and amount of bleeding. Since bleeding may occur in any system, a systems approach is necessitated.

1. Assess for bloody drainage

    Not only does persistent oozing from injection sites, venipuncture, or arterial puncture sites require close monitoring, but also surgical sites, mucous membranes, drain sites, and chest tube sites need to be carefully checked for bleeding and the amounts carefully noted. Monitoring the drainage from the genitourinary and gastrointestinal tracts, as well as tracheal aspirates, includes checking the urine, stool, emesis, nasogastric drainage, and sputum for the presence of blood.

2. Observe for signs of thrombosis

    The formation of thrombus may also be evidenced, and if it does occur, the symptoms exhibited are also associated with the system involved. Often arterial and venous thrombi occur at the sites of intravascular cannulization; thus, the distal and proximal pulses should be ascertained frequently, noting the quality of the pulse and capillary filling.

    Frequent assessment of the patient's neurologic status — level of consciousness, orientation, pupillary reaction, and movement and strength of extremities — will indicate manifestations of intracranial bleeding or thrombosis. The use of any painful stimulus should be tempered with caution, since it could initiate a new bleeding site.

    The kidneys are most often affected by thrombosis; decreased urinary output is the warning sign. Remember, there are other etiologic factors of decreased urinary output such as dehydration, hypovolemia, or hypotension that must also be addressed in the assessment.

3. Check for petechiae, ecchymosis, or cyanosis

    Many of the signs of bleeding are manifested in the integumentary system, and the patient should be inspected for petechiae, purpura, ecchymosis, and peripheral and central cyanosis.

    Petechiae are pinpoint-size, flat lesions caused by hemorrhage into the skin, and purpura are larger skin hemorrhages. These signs may be obscured in the ethnic person of color; however, the nurse who is an alert observer and knows where to look, won't miss them.

    Petechiae appear as reddish purple pin points on the buccal mucosa and also in the conjunctiva. They may be observed on the volar surface of the forearms in moderately dark-skinned individuals. *Ecchymosis* can also be observed on the buccal mucosa, and neither it nor petechiae will blanch when momentary pressure is applied.

    Evidence of *cyanosis* may be observed in the sclera, conjunctiva, buccal mucosa, tongue, lips, nailbeds, palms, and soles. In order to recognize early changes, the nurse must be familiar with the patient's color before the onset of cyanosis and should adapt her assessment to the dark-skinned person lest these signs of bleeding be missed.

4. Provide meticulous care to avoid infection

    Infection predisposes the patient to bleeding. All IV, hemodynamic monitoring, and incisional sites, as well as open bleeding areas, require meticulous care to prevent infection.

5. Assess for fluid volume

    DIC patients usually lose large quantities of blood and receive frequent transfusions and other fluids to maintain the intravascular and extracellular fluid volume at a level that provides optimum blood pressure, cardiac output, and urinary flow. It is important to be alert for signs of fluid overload because these patients already have fragile capillaries.

6. Assess for respiratory and cardiovascular problems

    Assessment of the respiratory and cardiovascular systems must be made at frequent intervals. It is important to detect as soon as possible the presence of basilar rales, cyanosis or pallor, hypoxia or hyperventilation, tachycardias, dysrhythmias, gallop rhythm, and increases in central venous pressure and pulmonary artery wedge pressure.

7. Provide gentle care to avoid trauma

    Another nursing goal is to protect the patient from trauma or stresses that may predispose him to further bleeding. All nursing procedures and interventions should be carried out with extra *gentleness*. Particular, gentle care is necessary for the patient's skin, as an inadvertent scratch or removal of a scab on an old bleeding site may initiate another episode of bleeding. Skin care should be such as not to disturb scabs. Fingernails and toenails should be trimmed to prevent scratches. Electric razors should be used to shave male patients. Mouth care should be performed with cotton swabs and diluted mouthwash to avoid injury to the mucous membrane.

Medication should be given intravenously, but if a medication must be given by injection, the smallest gauge needle possible for the solution being injected should be used. The same is true of venipuncture and arterial puncture procedures. Following injections or punctures, pressure must be applied to the site for a minimum of 15 minutes and frequent inspections made for evidence of continued bleeding.

8. Attend to IV therapy lines and heparin infusion

If the patient has an arterial line, it may be tempting to draw blood samples for coagulation tests from this heparinized line, but it must be remembered that any heparin picked up from the line can distort the values. If hospital protocol permits the aspiration of blood from central venous lines, lab work may be drawn from these lines without picking up heparin. When invading a catheter for blood, strict aseptic technique must be observed.

Because the administration of heparin is of prime importance in the care of the DIC patient, the continuous infusion rate must be carefully monitored. The use of a self-regulating IV infusion apparatus, such as an IVAC, assists in controlling the rate of fluid infused. Machines are prone to dysfunction and are dependent upon the operator to ensure the proper rate of infusion.

9. Provide psychosocial support

In assessing and planning nursing care for the patient with DIC, the critical care nurse's knowledge, skill, resourcefulness, creativity, and decisiveness will be challenged. Any illness requiring hospitalization stresses an individual, and when an illness requires placement in an intensive care unit, the patient is exposed to additional stress. The nurse's assessment must include the patient's psychosocial status and nursing interventions directed at preventing or alleviating stresses resulting from unmet psychosocial needs that may stimulate the fibrinolytic system.

Just as the patient with DIC requires extra gentleness, so also does the patient's family. Nursing interventions should be directed at allaying their anxieties by explaining simply what is happening to their loved one and providing emotional support by encouraging the family to verbalize their fears without being judged.

REFERENCES

1. Minna JD et al: Disseminated Intravascular Coagulation in Man, p 6. Springfield, Charles C Thomas, 1974
2. MacIver JE: The physiology of blood coagulation. In Israels MCG, Delamore IW (eds): Haematological Aspects of Systemic Disease, p 105. London, W.B. Saunders, 1976
3. Ibid., p 103
4. McKay DG: Disseminated Intravascular Coagulation: An Intermediary Mechanism of Disease, p 15. New York, Harper & Row, 1965
5. Coleman R et al: Disseminated intravascular coagulation: A problem in critical care medicine. Heart Lung 3, No. 5:793, 1974
6. Coleman R et al: Disseminated intravascular coagulation (DIC): An approach. Am J Med 52:685, 1972
7. Silver D, Daniel TM: Diagnosis and management of nonmechanical bleeding. In Berk JL et al (eds): Handbook of Critical Care, p 360. Boston, Little, Brown & Co, 1976

BIBLIOGRAPHY

Berk JL et al (eds): Handbook of Critical Care. Boston, Little, Brown & Co, 1976
Beyers M, Dudas S: The Clinical Practice of Medical-Surgical Nursing. Boston, Little, Brown & Co, 1970
Coleman RW et al: Disseminated intravascular coagulation (DIC): An approach. Am J Med 52:679–689, 1972
Coleman RW et al: Disseminated intravascular coagulation: A problem in critical care medicine. Heart Lung 3, No. 5:789–796, 1974
Deykin D: The clinical challenge of disseminated intravascular coagulation. N Engl J Med 283, No. 12:636–644, 1970
Ganong WF: Review of Medical Physiology. Los Altos, Lange Medical Publications, 1973
Groer ME, Shekleton ME: Basic Pathophysiology: A Conceptual Approach. St. Louis, C.V. Mosby, 1979
Israels MCG et al: Haematological Aspects of Systemic Disease. London, W.B. Saunders, 1976
Lerner RG: The defibrination syndrome. Med Clin North Am 60, No. 3:871–880, 1976
Mant MJ, King EG: Severe acute disseminated intravascular coagulation. Am J Med, pp 557–563, October 1979
McKay DG: Disseminated Intravascular Coagulation: An Intermediary Mechanism of Disease. New York, Harper & Row, 1965
Mielke HC, Rodvien R (eds): Mechanisms of Hemostasis and Thrombosis. Miami, Symposia Specialists Publications, 1978
Minna JD et al: Disseminated Intravascular Coagulation in Man. Springfield, Charles C Thomas, 1974
Shafer KS et al: Medical-Surgical Nursing, 6th ed. St. Louis, C.V. Mosby, 1975

Patricia A. Diehl

Burns
24

People who receive burns present one of the most demanding of all health-care crises. One who is presumably well can, within minutes, become the victim of extensive burns. A grim reality! Fraught not only with dramatic physiological changes, burns also generate a stark psychological component. The physical and emotional devastation suffered by a severely burned patient is unparalleled by any other ailment known to man.

The picture is not as bleak as it once was, however. Within the past 25 years, great strides have been made in burn care. The prognosis has changed from *expecting death* to *expecting life*. Thus, helping the burned person cope with his precarious state of equilibrium is a challenge to all care givers. Nurses, in particular, need to understand the interrelated changes in all body systems and to be able to provide the therapeutic interventions and the supportive and maintenance care necessary in all stages of recovery.

NORMAL STRUCTURE AND FUNCTIONS OF THE SKIN

Sometimes it is hard to remember that the skin is the body's largest organ and is indispensable to life. A thorough understanding of the normal skin and its functions will help the reader to understand the effects created when the skin is destroyed by burns.

Structure

The skin consists of three layers: the epidermis, the dermis, and the subcutaneous fat (see Fig. 24-1). The epidermis is the thin outer layer of

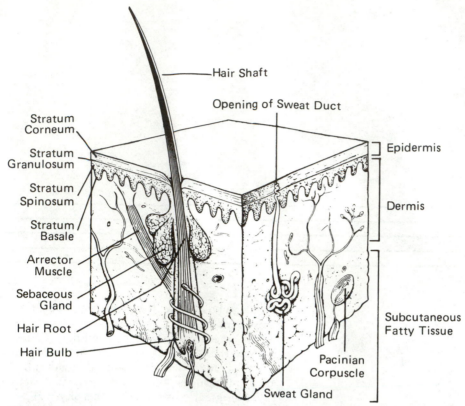

Hair Shaft

Opening of Sweat Duct

Stratum Corneum

Stratum Granulosum

Stratum Spinosum

Stratum Basale

Arrector Muscle

Sebaceous Gland

Hair Root

Hair Bulb

Epidermis

Dermis

Subcutaneous Fatty Tissue

Pacinian Corpuscle

Sweat Gland

FIGURE 24-1.
A three-dimensional view of the skin.

epithelial cells that are continuously being replaced. Important elements of this layer are keratin, an insoluble protein that waterproofs the skin, and melanin, which pigments the skin in varying shades of brown. The total color of the skin is created by a combination of the yellow keratin, brown melanin, and a pinkness from the underlying vasculature.

The dermis is a thicker layer richly endowed with blood and lymph vessels. It contains sebaceous glands, which lubricate the skin by their oily secretions, and hair follicles. The hair follicles play two important roles — cosmetic appearance and perception of tactile stimulation. Also contained in this layer are the sensory receptor cells for touch, temperature, pain, and pressure.

The deepest layer is the subcutaneous fat, which insulates the body, protects the underlying muscles, and gives the body form and shape.

Function

The skin is the body's first line of defense from invasion by microorganisms and environmental

radiation. The pH of the skin ranges from 4.0 to 6.8, retarding the growth of microorganisms on its surface. As a barrier, it has a second function: to contain body fluids, thereby preventing dehydration and electrolyte imbalances.

It is, however, an excretory organ as well. Sweat glands continually secrete insensible perspiration, which contains water, sodium chloride, and some metabolic products, notably ammonia. This function is closely related to maintenance of the core body temperature. The metabolic processes of the body produce heat, which must be maintained in a carefully controlled range to avoid thermal cellular damage. The hypothalamus controls body heat by sending stimuli to the cutaneous blood vessels, causing them to dilate or constrict. When they dilate, more blood flows through vessels near the skin's surface, losing heat by conduction, convection, and radiation into the external environment. Large amounts of additional heat may be lost if sweating occurs simultaneously. It is estimated that 576 calories are required to evaporate 1 liter of perspiration. Heat is conserved when the hypothalamus causes the blood vessels in the skin to constrict. Vasoconstriction allows less blood to flow near the skin's surface, and consequently less heat is lost.

Neurologically, sensory receptor cells located in the dermis react to a multitude of environmental stimuli and relay their reactions to the brain; the body reacts accordingly. For example, exposure to the sun's rays on a warm spring day creates a pleasant, glowing feeling, but touching a hot stove causes pain.

Finally, by virtue of its shape, color, and texture, the skin gives the body its cosmetic appearance, which plays a major role in self-identity.

BURN DEPTH

Partial-Thickness Burns. A partial-thickness burn involves the epidermis and the upper part of the dermis (see Fig. 24-2). A sunburn is a familiar example. The skin looks pinkish red. It blanches in response to pressure because the underlying vasculature is intact. It feels painful at first and later itches because sensory receptors

for pain are sufficiently functional to relay these messages. Although peeling will occur within 3 to 6 days, this burn will heal spontaneously without scarring because an adequate number of epithelial cells exist to generate a new epithelial cover. A deeper partial-thickness burn will also be pinkish red and painful. In addition, it will form blisters and subcutaneous edema.

Depending upon the depth and other factors, these burns may heal spontaneously or may convert to full-thickness wounds. To heal spontaneously, sufficient epithelial cells must remain, and the wound must be clean. If the wound becomes infected, traumatized, or the blood supply compromised, these burns will convert to full-thickness wounds.

Full-Thickness Burns. Deep dermal wounds extend well into the dermis; full-thickness burns extend down into subcutaneous and deeper tissues (see Fig. 24-3). Very deep dermal and full-thickness burns may appear white, red, brown, or black. Reddened areas do not blanch in response to pressure because the underlying blood supply has been interrupted. Brownish

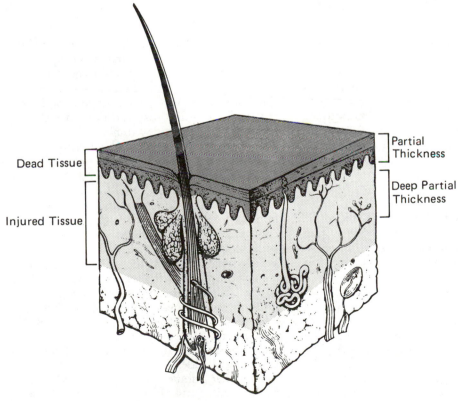

FIGURE 24-2.
Partial-thickness burn.

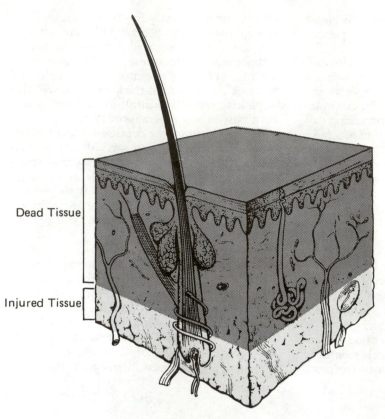

Dead Tissue

Injured Tissue

FIGURE 24-3.
Full-thickness burn.

streaks are evidence of thrombosed blood vessels.

These burns are completely anesthetic because the sensory receptors have been totally destroyed. In addition, they may appear sunken because of the loss of underlying fat and muscle. Regeneration of the skin is impossible, and grafting is necessary to restore normal skin function.

SYSTEMIC REACTIONS TO BURNS
Severe burns affect virtually every body system at some time in the course of recovery. The most immediate changes occur in the respiratory and circulatory systems.

Respiratory System
Inhalation injuries are seen in approximately 30% of all patients with major burns. Respiratory involvement should always be suspected if the burns are about the head and neck or if the person had been trapped in an enclosed space. Inhalation of hot air, soot particles, and gases given off by the burning materials irritates the respiratory tissues and leads to edema and tissue destruction. This in turn leads to inadequate circulation through the lungs and hypoxemia.

Respiratory symptoms may occur at varying times following the original injury. Some patients who develop respiratory complications will show symptoms within the first 24 hours after the burn is sustained. These symptoms include dyspnea, inspiratory wheezing, copious amounts of mucous secretions, and laryngeal or bronchial spasms and edema (see Table 24-1).

Other patients develop pulmonary complications in 1 to 7 days. They suffer from alveolar collapse and increased lung water. The alveolar collapse leads to a decrease in the functional residual capacity of the lung and a decrease in tissue compliance. Transpulmonary shunting around the nonfunctional portion of the lungs leads to ventilation-perfusion inequalities (see Chapter 13). Simultaneously, fluids accumulate in the extravascular spaces at the bases of the lungs and further contribute to ventilation-perfusion inequalities.

A smaller number of the patients who suffer respiratory complications do so after 1 week. These problems tend to be pneumonitis or, more rarely, pulmonary embolism.

Table 24–1
Respiratory Complications of Burns

24 Hours	*1–7 Days*	*Later Than One Week*
Dyspnea	Alveolar collapse	Pneumonitis
Inspiratory wheezing	Increased lung water	Pulmonary embolism
Copious mucous secretions		
Laryngeal or bronchial spasms and edema		

Circulatory System

The circulatory system undergoes both physical and chemical changes.

Fluid Loss. The most remarkable change is the tremendous *"fluid shift"* created by a rapid outpouring of fluids from the vascular system into the interstitial spaces. This rapidly leads to hypovolemic shock. The fluid shift begins soon after the injury and may continue up to 48 hours. The burn injury destroys blood vessels and other cells, causing a release of a histaminelike substance. This increases the permeability of the capillary walls, allowing the fluid portion of the blood to escape into the interstitial spaces. Severe edema is created both at the burn site and in more remote areas of the body. It is important to remember that *this fluid loss is from the circulating blood volume* rather than from the body *per se*. It largely remains in the body as increased interstitial fluid (edema).

Loss of Plasma Protein. Soon after the burn, plasma protein will also start to leak through injured capillary membranes. This leakage is not as rapid as that of water and electrolytes because the protein molecule is larger. The patient frequently has an altered albumin/globulin (A/G) ratio, indicating that of the proteins, more albumin than globulin has escaped from the vasculature. This is true because the albumin molecule is the smaller of the two. Loss of protein from the circulating volume also contributes to the development of hypovolemic shock if untreated. It should be remembered that normally the osmotic pressure exerted by the plasma protein opposes the hydrostatic filtering forces existing in the capillaries and that filtration of water is opposed by the retaining action of the protein. However, when the protein concentration is decreased, these opposing forces are weakened, and more water is filtered out of the vascular system.

Reduced Circulatory Volume. The loss of fluid from the intravascular space results in a thickened, sluggish flow of the remaining circulatory blood volume. The effects reach to all body systems.

DECREASED CIRCULATING BLOOD VOLUME⟶ ↓ *cardiac output*.
LOW CARDIAC OUTPUT⟶ ↓ *tissue perfusion*.
POOR TISSUE PERFUSION⟶*metabolic acidosis and stasis of blood*.

This slowing of circulation allows bacteria and cellular material to settle to the lower portion of the blood vessels, especially in the capillaries, resulting in sludging. The inactivity of bed rest further contributes to this state.

The *antigen-antibody reaction* to burned tissue adds further to the circulatory congestion by the clumping or agglutination of cells. Simultaneously, *coagulation problems* occur as a result of the release of thromboplastin by the injury itself and the release of fibrinogen from injured platelets. If *thrombi* occur, they may cause ischemia of the affected part and lead to necrosis. Since this is a widespread occurrence, any organ in the body—heart, lung, liver, kidney, brain—may be involved, and organ failure can occur. The increased coagulation process may also develop into disseminated intravascular coagulation (DIC) (see Chapter 23).

The initial compensatory mechanism that occurs in relation to fluid loss is *vasoconstriction*. Simultaneously, the protein concentration in the blood vessels draws fluid from interstitial spaces in unburned areas of the body into the vascular system in an attempt to offset some of the lost volume. The blood pressure may appear normal at first, but if fluid replacement is inadequate and plasma protein loss ensues, hypovolemic shock soon occurs.

Blood Cell Count. In relation to blood cells (CBC), the leukocyte count is initially high because of the hemoconcentration. If *leukocytosis* persists after one week, it is usually indicative of infection by a gram-positive organism, often *Staphylococcus aureus*. The *erythrocyte* count in severe burns is decreased, and the patient is anemic. Some of the red cells are hemolyzed by the effects of the heat as they pass through the burned area at the time of the injury. Other red cells are simply trapped in engorged capillaries. Hence, they are unavailable to the general body. Anemia is also due to bleeding at the burn site initially as the wound is sustained and later as debridement is performed.

Electrolyte Alterations. Electrolyte concentrations are altered not only from the leaking process but also from direct injury to burned cells. Chemical changes are due to shifts in the composition of various fluids as they move from one body compartment to another. Electrolyte studies at first show an increase in serum potassium because of intracellular potassium release. After about 48 hours the capillary walls have healed sufficiently to stop the fluid shift from the vascular tree. Fluid is then drawn back into the blood vessels, edema subsides, the plasma volume expands, and diuresis begins. At this time large amounts of potassium are lost, and replacement may be necessary. In severe burns, the alterations in potassium levels must be carefully monitored to avoid cardiac failure. The plasma level of both sodium and chloride is normal or slightly elevated at first but increases rapidly as excessive interstitial fluid is reabsorbed. The blood urea nitrogen (BUN) may be elevated if excessive protein catabolism occurred. Blood glucose levels may be temporarily increased as a result of the action of epinephrine, which is released in reaction to the stress of the burn injury. The epinephrine acts on amino acids to produce glucose (gluconeogenesis) required to meet the body's demands during stress.

Cardiac Function. Changes in cardiac function are not as clearly understood as circulatory changes. Most of the changes that are known relate to therapy rather than to the original burn insult. It is known that the cardiac output may be decreased even without a significant decrease in circulating blood volume. Cardiac assessments become particularly important later in fluid replacement; care must be taken to avoid circulatory overload, which can lead to ventricular failure and pulmonary edema.

Renal System

At first, a temporary *oliguria* is seen. The two major contributors to the decreased urinary output are

- Decreased glomerular filtration rate (GFR). With hypovolemia, the renal vasoconstriction results in a decrease of GFR.
- Increase of antidiuretic hormone (ADH). The shock of the burn injury causes an increase in ADH from the posterior pituitary gland.

Continued oliguria may be caused by tubular necrosis. Hemolysis of red blood cells at the time of the injury causes hemoglobin pigment to be released into the bloodstream. If fluid replacement is not sufficient to flush the hemoglobin through the kidney, tubular necrosis occurs (see Chapter 17).

Gastrointestinal System

Gastric dilatation and paralytic ileus may be present early. If they occur in the first 24 hours, they are believed to be due to a decrease in intestinal mobility created by vasoconstriction in the splanchnic area or to the stress of the injury itself. If they occur after a few days, invasive burn-wound sepsis is probably the cause of this phenomenon. Bright red blood may be present in the gastric secretions due either to the presence of a gastritis or to the congestion of fragile capillaries that rupture easily. Multiple gastric or duodenal ulcers, known as Curling's ulcers, may develop at any time in the postburn course. Their exact etiology has not been established.

CARE OF THE PERSON WITH BURNS

Treatment of the person with burns is divided into several sequential steps:

1. Initial assessment
2. Intensive critical care
3. Wound management
4. Rehabilitation

Initial Assessment

It is of utmost importance to obtain an accurate *history* of the burn incident and to determine the *severity* of the burns.

The degree of burn injury is determined by temperature of the heat source and duration of the exposure. Prolonged contact with a relatively low-temperature heat source can cause more tissue damage than flash burns of a shorter duration.

Five factors determine the severity of the burn wound.

- The size of the burned area
- The depth of the burn
- The location of the burn
- The age of the person
- Concomitant illness and injury

Burn Area Size. Several possible rules are available for estimating the extent of a burn in percentages of the total body surface. The *Rule of Nines* divides the body parts into multiples of 9% (see Fig. 24-4). The head is considered to account for 9% of total body area, each arm for 9%, each leg 18%, and the anterior and posterior trunk 18% each. The perineum accounts for 1%, making a total of 100%. It is important to remember that burns may be either circumferential or involve only one surface of a body part: a circumferential burn of an arm is 9%, whereas if only the anterior surface were burned, the value would be 4½%.

While the Rule of Nines is the most commonly used method, Berkow's method is more accurate, particularly for infants and children, because it allows for proportionate growth (see Fig. 24-5). Small scattered burns can be estimated by comparing the size of the examiner's hand to the victim's hand. Allowing for differences, the palmar surface of the hand equals approximately 1% of an adult's total body surface.

Burn Depth. Burn classifications are based on the anatomic structures (as discussed previously) or classified as first, second, third, and fourth degree burns (see Table 24-2).

Burn Location. The location of the burn is important to healing and general rehabilitation. Burns of the face, head, neck, hands, feet, and genitalia create particular problems. Although they may be limited in surface area, these burns usually require hospitalization of the person and special care because they are in important areas where rapid, uninfected healing with minimal scarring is desired. Burns of the head that involve the external ear and burns of the hands that involve the distal phalanges are particularly difficult to heal because these structures are primarily composed of cartilage, which lacks a good blood supply.

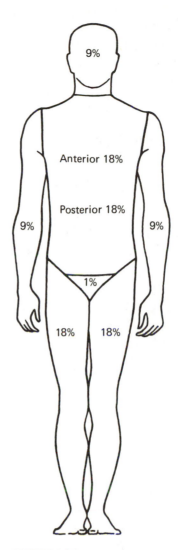

FIGURE 24-4.
The "Rule of Nines" method for determining percentage of body area with burn injury.

If burns in any of these special areas do not heal well, serious psychosocial and economic problems related to appearance, self-concept, manual dexterity, and locomotion occur.

Person's Age. Although burns occur in all age groups, the incidence is higher at both ends of the age continuum. Persons under 2 years and over 60 years of age have a higher mortality than other age groups with burns of similar severity. A child under 2 years is more susceptible to infection because of his immature immune response. The older person may have degenerative processes that complicate his recovery and that

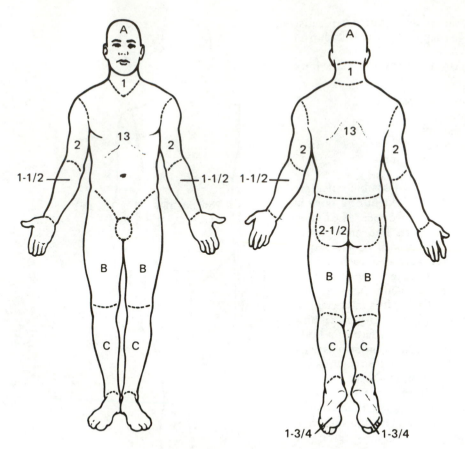

Relative Percentage of Areas Affected by Growth

	Age in years					
	0	1	5	10	15	Adult
A—1/2 of head	9-1/2	8-1/2	6-1/2	5-1/2	4-1/2	3-1/2
B—1/2 of one thigh	2-3/4	3-1/4	4	4-1/4	4-1/2	4-3/4
C—1/2 of one leg	2-1/2	2-1/2	2-3/4	3	3-1/4	3-1/2

FIGURE 24-5.
Berkow's method for determining percentage of body area with burn injury.

may be aggravated by the stress of the burn. As a general rule, children with burns of 10% or more and all adults whose injuries account for 12% to 15% or more of total body surface will require hospitalization.

Concomitant Illness and Injury. A complete medical history should be obtained as soon as possible to determine if the person has any known illnesses. Some diseases, such as diabetes and kidney failure, may become acute during the burn process. If inhalation injuries were sus-

tained in the presence of cardiopulmonary pathology (congestive heart failure, emphysema), the respiratory status is tremendously complicated. Or the person may have sustained other traumatic injuries in the burn accident, particularly if an explosion occurred.

The overwhelming magnitude of the burns may overshadow the possibility of other internal injuries and fractures. A complete physical examination should be done as soon as it is feasible to determine the full extent of the person's injuries.

Table 24–2
Burn Classifications

Classification	Tissues Involved	Characteristics
1st degree Partial-thickness	Epidermis and upper part of dermis	Pinkish red skin color Blanches from pressure Painful → itching
2nd degree Deeper partial-thickness	Epidermis and dermis	Pinkish red skin color Painful Blisters Subcutaneous edema
3rd degree Full-thickness	Epidermis, dermis, and subcutaneous tissue	Skin color—white, red, brown, or black No blanching from pressure No pain Brownish streaks Sunken appearance
4th degree All tissues	All above tissue plus muscle and bone	Extremely deep wounds Charred or free dead tissue Edema Immobility of area

Intensive Critical Care

Care and therapy in this period closely parallel the tissue and systemic changes resulting from the burn insult. Hopefully, immediately following the crisis, someone *stopped the burning* by removing the hot clothing and cooled and cleansed the skin with large amounts of cool water. Even though the burn may be the most obvious presenting bodily insult, treatment of respiratory distress, hemorrhage, or shock takes priority.

RESPIRATORY ASSESSMENT/ MANAGEMENT

The person himself provides the best defense against alveolar collapse by hyperventilating and moving about. If he is unable to move, deep breathing and passive postural changes may be sufficient. If the person has inhaled flames, smoke, or toxic chemical fumes, some degree of respiratory distress can be expected.

Frequent observation for dyspnea, inspiratory wheezing, increased hoarseness, use of accessory muscles of respiration and restricted movements of the thorax, and character and quantity of sputum are essential. Equally important is monitoring arterial blood gases. The patient who is experiencing laryngeal/bronchial spasms or edema has decreased air movement and exchange. Pulmonary drug therapy, such as bronchodilators and steroids, may be indicated and initiated. Continued or rapid deterioration requires more aggressive action—endotracheal intubation or tracheostomy. A mechanical ventilator may or may not be necessary, depending upon the location and severity of the obstruction (see Chapter 13).

If severe lung edema is present, dehydration is forced by administration of salt-poor albumin and Lasix. This improves pulmonary function but may lead to such other problems as hyponatremia, renal insufficiency, and central nervous system (CNS) deterioration.

CIRCULATORY ASSESSMENT/ MANAGEMENT

Immediately, the patient requires rapid administration of large amounts of intravenous fluids to control burn shock from fluid shift. Regardless of etiology, the shock syndrome remains the same. A marked reduction of blood flow through tissues leads to cellular hypoxia, which leads to tissue death.

The hypotension, reduced blood flow, and hypoxia stimulate compensatory mechanisms in the body; for example, stimulation of the aortic and carotid pressor receptors increases pulse rate and selective vasoconstriction. These pressure receptors will maintain normal blood pressure until approximately 20% of the blood volume has been lost. The adrenal glands release epinephrine, which augments the above responses, and the patient becomes restless and anxious. Respirations increase in rate and depth in order to promote venous return and cardiac filling. Changes in circulatory hydrostatic and osmotic pressures, due to decreased volume, pull fluids from the interstitial spaces into the blood vessels. It is easily seen why, in a severe burn, rapid fluid replacement is necessary to prevent the shock process from continuing.

Fluid Replacement Therapy. Fluids are administered through one or more large bore intravenous catheters or cannulas, which allow rapid administration. Since veins are usually at a premium, it is desirable to establish a good intravenous route early and maintain it for some time.

Several formulas are available for calculation of fluid replacement for the burned patient. In general, rigorous replacement of lost crystalloid and colloid solutions must be made. Free water, given as 5% dextrose/water with or without added electrolytes, is regulated to cover insensible fluid loss. Ringer's lactate is used as the crystalloid solution because it is a balanced salt solution that closely approximates the composition of extracellular fluid. In addition, it has large molecules, which serve to expand the circulating plasma volume.

Tables 24–3 and 24–4 show two of the many methods available for calculation of fluid needs. It is important to remember that formulas are simply *guides*. The exact amount of fluid administered should be based on the clinical response of the patient.

The following example may help illustrate the very large amounts of fluid required. The Baxter formula for a patient weighing 75 kg, who received burns over 50% of his body, would be stated:

$$4 \text{ ml} \times 75 \text{ kg} \times 50\% = 15,000 \text{ ml}$$

Of this, 7500 ml is to be administered the first 8-hour period and 3750 ml is to be administered the second and third 8-hour periods. Hence, it is extremely difficult to avoid fluid overload and pulmonary edema when it is necessary to infuse fluids so rapidly. Consequently, severely burned patients may be given digoxin to create maximal function of the left ventricle and to minimize the chances of transient increases in left atrial pressure. Isoproterenol infusions may be used for symptoms of decreased cardiac output.

Adequacy of fluid replacement is judged clinically for adults by a urinary output of 30 to 70 ml per hour, pulse rate below 120, blood pressure in normal to high ranges, central venous pressure (CVP) readings less than 12 cm

Table 24–3
Fluid Replacement in an Adult Burn Patient
Brooke Formula

FIRST 24 HOURS
1. Colloids solution — 0.5 ml/kg/% of burn
2. Crystalloids solution — 1.5 ml/kg/% of burn
3. Electrolyte-free solution — According to age and size of patient

SECOND 24 HOURS
One-half of the amount of colloid and crystalloid solutions. Same amount of the electrolyte-free solution.

Table 24–4
Fluid Replacement in an Adult Burn Patient
Baxter Method

First 24 hr — Crystalloids solution 4 ml/kg/% of burn
Infusion rate — ½ total volume — 1st 8-hr period
¼ total volume — 2nd 8-hr period
¼ total volume — 3rd 8-hr period
24–36 hr — Administer plasma
36–48 hr — Administer free water with electrolytes as needed
OR
Water by mouth
48 hr–10 days — Regulate fluids by need

H_2O or a pulmonary capillary wedge pressure (PCWP) reading below 18 torr, clear sensorium and clear lung sounds, and the absence of intestinal symptoms such as nausea and paralytic ileus (see Table 24-5).

ADDITIONAL MEASURES

Other important aspects of care are

- Control of pain
- Administration of tetanus antitoxin or toxoid
- Insertion of a nasogastric tube
- Insertion of a Foley catheter
- Initial wound care

Pain control is usually by intravenous administration of analgesics and narcotics in small but frequent doses. The intravenous route is preferred because absorption rates of other routes are unpredictable. The aim is to control pain without decreasing respirations. The nurse who differentiates the restlessness of hypoxia from the symptoms of pain will respond accordingly.

Tetanus antitoxin is a mandatory treatment in emergency rooms unless the patient has had a booster within the last year. If the patient has had at least two DPT (diphtheria, pertussis, tetanus) injections, a booster of 0.5 ml of DPT or tetanus toxoid is given. If the patient has had no previous tetanus immunizations, immune human globulin (Hyper-tet) is given.

A *nasogastric tube* is inserted if the patient is nauseated or vomiting. Initially, it prevents aspiration of vomitus and allows for observation and testing of gastric contents. Later it serves as an avenue for tube feedings.

The *Foley catheter* facilitates accurate measurement of output and prevents incontinence, which might contaminate the wounds or create additional skin problems.

Initial wound care constitutes cleansing and debridement of the burn. Charred clothing that adheres to the wound must be soaked off. For extensively burned persons, wounds are washed with large amounts of warm saline because a great deal of body heat is lost through the wound. Body temperature is monitored hourly. The dead skin is simply cut away. When working with the wound, the nurse should note the adequacy of circulation to all body parts. Stiff, inelastic layers of dead tissue, *eschars,* are created by the drying of burned skin. When edema occurs rapidly under the eschar, circulation may be impaired. A surgical incision (escharotomy) may be necessary to relieve the constriction and reestablish adequate circulation.

Table 24-5
Clinical Manifestations of Adequate Fluid Replacement

Blood pressure	Normal to high normal ranges
Pulse rate	<120
CVP	< 12 cm H_2O
PCWP	< 18 torr
Urinary output	30–70 ml/hr
Lungs	Clear
Sensorium	Clear
GI tract	Absence of nausea and paralytic ileus

Burn Wound Management

Once the patient is out of all life-threatening situations, a regular regime of wound care is instituted. Wound care has two purposes: prevention of infection and assistance to the body's own healing process.

INFECTION

One of the greatest and most devastating dangers to the patient with burns is infection. The body, now open and vulnerable, can be invaded by all types of microorganisms. These organisms thrive and multiply in a "dirty" wound. With impaired body resistance to infection, a localized wound infection may spread throughout the body. Septicemia and pneumonia are the two leading causes of death.

If wound infections do occur, they are primarily treated with topical antibiotics. Since the vasculature is impaired and the drugs cannot reach the organisms in the wound, some authorities believe systemic antibiotics are ineffective. If antibiotics are given, their primary purpose is to clear the blood and eradicate any satellite lesions.

Septic shock, seen mostly in patients with extensive full-thickness burns, is caused by invading bacteria from the wound entering the bloodstream. Clinically, the patient should show a fever, but the range of temperature elevation is extremely variable. The usual febrile reaction is altered when great heat losses from fluid loss are occurring. Other symptoms are a rapid yet regular pulse (140 to 170; sinus tachycardia), decreased blood pressure, oliguria, paralytic ileus, petechiae, frank bleeding from wounds, and disorientation (see Table 24-6).

WOUND CARE

Several methods of wound care are possible, and hydrotherapy may be coupled with any of the

Table 24-6
Symptoms of Septic Shock

Temperature (varies)
Pulse (140 to 170 — sinus tachycardia)
Blood pressure decreased
Paralytic ileus
Petechiae
Frank bleeding from wounds
Disorientation

other methods of treatment. The patient is placed in a whirlpool bath for 20 to 30 minutes, for the purpose of loosening exudates, cleansing wounds, removing dressings, or applying topical medications. Bath solutions are plain warm water, normal saline, balanced electrolyte solutions, or nonirritating cleansing agents. Since the baths are usually quite painful, patients receive an analgesic 20 to 30 minutes prior to tubbing.

Open Wounds.   These are wounds left exposed to the air on the premise that bacterial growth is minimized in the absence of moisture. Although this treatment allows for easy inspection, it requires very careful nursing care — usually reverse isolation. The room temperature is maintained at approximately 82°F (31°C) to prevent loss of body heat and shivering, which would increase the patient's basal metabolic rate. If the burn is circumferential, special nonadherent coverings on turning frames may be necessary. The wound is kept free of exudate by frequent cleansings, performed either at the bedside or in the whirlpool. On partial-thickness wounds, crusts are lifted off and cut away if it can be done without causing bleeding. Full-thickness burns have a leathery eschar that will loosen slowly as collagen fibers gradually disintegrate. They may also be surgically removed.

The open method may be used to treat grafted areas because it allows direct observation of the graft site. Protection of the graft by special positioning or restraints may be necessary. Donor sites heal well by open exposure.

Semi-open Wound.   Topical antimicrobial creams may be used alone or in combination with a thin layer of gauze to create a partial cover for the open wound. Burns of the face are often treated this way. Wounds are still cleansed and debrided at prescribed intervals, and a thin layer of the medication is reapplied. The most commonly used antimicrobial creams are silver sul-

fadiazine 1% and Sulfamylon Acetate 10%. The choice of medication is largely a personal preference of the physician, for both are highly effective.

Silver sulfadiazine (Silvadene) acts on the cell membrane to inhibit bacterial growth. It is painless, creates a soft, pliable eschar, provokes few allergic responses, and has no effect on the patient's electrolyte balance.

Sulfamylon Acetate is especially effective in deep burns because it penetrates through avascular areas to help control infections. Unlike Silvadene, it causes a stinging pain due to its acidity and may cause a rash in sensitive patients. Careful nursing assessments of both the patient and his laboratory data are necessary, because Sulfamylon is a renal anhydrase inhibitor. It can lead to impairment of the renal buffering mechanism, resulting in bicarbonate diuresis and retention of chlorides and ammonia. Clinically, the symptoms are tachypnea of 35 to 45 or arterial blood gases with pH 7.45 to 7.50 and PCO_2 below 30. Neither reaction may be sufficient to warrant discontinuation of the medication because supplemental therapy may be initiated.

Another antimicrobial cream is *gentamicin sulfate* 0.1% (Garamycin). This agent is extremely effective against many microorganisms and yet not widely used. Because organisms become resistant to it, it is usually reserved for life-threatening situations.

Silver nitrate 0.5% is still used extensively for its antimicrobial actions. While it may be used as a cream, it is primarily applied as a soak (see the section below on wet dressings).

Occlusive Dressings.   Dry occlusive dressings are used much less frequently because many authorities feel they add to difficulties in infection control. When used, a layer of fine mesh gauze is applied directly to the wound to avoid adherence to the new epithelium. *Remember: two burn surfaces should never touch because the epithelialization will create "webbing" of the skin.* Next, several layers of dry fluffy gauze are applied for drainage absorption. These are held in place by an outer wrapping of Kling gauze or elastic bandages loosely applied to prevent constriction. Occlusive dressings are very warm and thus are uncomfortable to the patient. They may be used especially to protect graft sites.

Wet Dressings.   Useful during all stages of wound care, a wet dressing consists of (1) a thin layer of wet gauze applied directly to the wound or graft site, (2) a covering of many layers of gauze saturated with normal saline or silver nitrate 0.5% solution, (3) a dry covering, which holds the gauze in place. Because wet dressings are messy, there is a temptation to use plastic protection. The nurse needs to keep in mind that plastic increases heat retention, fostering bacterial growth in the wound and creating a hyperthermic effect in the patient. Wet dressings need to be "wet down" at least every 2 hours, but need not be completely changed more often than every 12 hours. If silver nitrate is used, it must be started within 72 hours because it cannot penetrate through an eschar. Being very hypotonic, it causes a leeching of the sodium ion into the dressing and precipitation of silver chloride onto the wound. This creates an alkalotic state characterized by hyponatremia and hypochloremia, which may require replacement therapy. Other associated problems are maceration of the skin from constant moisture and black staining of linens, clothes, and furniture by the silver nitrate's exposure to light.

Biologic Dressings. Various types of grafts may be applied at different times. It is desirable to apply a graft as early as possible to provide a cover that prevents fluid loss and creates a barrier against invading organisms. Temporary coverings, called *heterografts* or *xenografts,* are from animal sources or man-made films (*e.g.,* porcine grafts and Teflon grafts). Permanent grafts are applied when all epithelial elements are lost or in reconstructive surgery for cosmetic or functional reasons. If the skin to be grafted is taken from the patient's own body, it is known as an *autograft.* Occasionally a burn victim has an identical twin whose skin is histocompatible for an *isograft.*

Usually skin for grafting is scarce and so must be extended. Using both split-thickness and full-thickness layers of skin, the grafts can be done in many ways. Examples are (1) transplanting only small pieces of skin and allowing epithelial tissue to fill in between or (2) mechanically creating lacelike slits in the skin to be grafted, which can be stretched to cover a larger area. Graft sites must be protected against trauma and slippage and frequently observed for detection of infection. Infections will cause the graft to slough off.

Rehabilitation

Patients who have sustained extensive burns will obviously require many months for recovery and rehabilitation. Physical and psychological rehabilitation measures are begun in the critical care unit and carried through the entire recovery period.

PHYSICAL REHABILITATION

Two very important physical measures are nutrition and prevention of scarring and contractures.

Nutrition. An old adage, "The burn patient who can eat will survive," may well be true. In addition to fluid replacement, the severely burned patient may need as much as 50 to 80 calories per kg of body weight to meet his metabolic requirements. This includes 2 to 3 g of protein/kg and supplementary vitamins, especially B, C, and iron if anemia is present. As an example of the huge caloric intake needed, a patient weighing 75 kg would require 3750 to 6000 calories per day. Even though the patient is usually started cautiously, as intake increases a difficult cycle may be created. While he needs a large intake, he isn't hungry, feels full, and furthermore, may have diarrhea. Prevention of excessive weight loss in adults and allowances for growth in children must also be considered, and nutritional formulas may be added to their diets.

To augment the caloric value of oral intake, intralipid therapy may be used. There is some controversy over *hyperalimentation* in burn care. The tendency is to reserve it for patients who have extensive injuries and who cannot tolerate other means of feeding. Major arguments against it are the possibility of infection and the number of other procedures it necessitates.

Avoiding Scarring and Contractures. Once regarded as inevitable, hypertrophic scarring and joint contractures are now largely preventable. Preventive measures start when the person is admitted to the hospital and continue for at least 12 months or until the scar is fully mature.

These preventive measures are not new to the nurse: positioning the body and range of motion exercises. Positioning the body with extremities extended is extremely important. Patients prefer tightly flexed positions for comfort, but if permitted they will lead to severe contractions. Range of motion exercises should be carried out with each dressing change or more often if indicated. Special splints are used to maintain arms, legs, and hands in extended yet functional positions. Later, when the wounds have healed sufficiently, the person is custom-fitted for special pressure garments. The garment, by continuous uniform pressure over the entire area of the burn, prevents hypertrophic scarring and must be worn 24 hours a day for approximately one year. The smooth elastic garment forms a shield that permits the person to wear normal clothing and resume ordinary activities much sooner.

PSYCHOLOGICAL REHABILITATION

Psychological care of the burned patient is extremely difficult; he may, in the course of his therapy, run the full gamut of behavioral responses. Early in the care, a combination of physical pain and emotional disturbances may lead to abnormal behavior. The injury itself has created many primary problems to which the patient must adapt. It has created a threat to his survival, possible disfigurement, a great deal of physical discomfort, repeated operations, and a long and tedious convalescence. Secondary to the burn incident, emotional reactions result from separation from family and loved ones, fear of rejection, emotional pain and guilt related to the accident, and inner conflict over dependency now and in the future. Guilt may be particularly severe if the patient feels that his carelessness was the cause of injuries to himself or others, especially if others died as a result of the accident.

If burns involve the face, eyes, or hands, additional emotional support will be needed, for damage to these structures will have a long-term effect on the patient's life and livelihood.

At first, a severely burned patient may be euphoric and firmly believe that he will be well enough to leave the hospital in a few days. The fact that he has little pain in deep burns adds to this effect. As time goes on, however, the patient's behavior will change. He may become withdrawn, regress to childish habits of speech and body position, or become wild and abusive; he may want to die and beg his care-givers to let him do so. With sustained care and support, his normal personality with a more futuristic orientation will slowly begin to emerge.

A consistent and truthful team approach that includes the patient and his family is necessary. Supportive measures that will allow the patient time to assimilate what has happened to him and to grow in his ability to cope are

- Staff should be stabilized as much as possible to increase their familiarity with the care and to create a sense of identification between patient and nurse.
- Family members can be very helpful if incorporated into the overall plan of care and instructed in selected procedures.

- Diversional therapy (*i.e.,* reading, watching television, listening to music) should be encouraged as soon as possible.
- Occupational therapy should be started as soon as the patient is able.

Obviously, a concerted effort is necessary to coordinate all of the services required by an extensively injured patient.

In addition to the emotional support for the patient, it is advisable to provide support for the nursing staff. Faced with long and arduous care of these patients, where progress is slow and setbacks are common, staff quickly develop "burnout" unless some of their emotional reactions and problems can be aired and solved (see Chapter 6).

Summary

The skin serves multiple physiological functions that render it indispensable to life. When a large amount of total skin surface is destroyed by burns, severe systemic reactions occur in nearly every body system. After initial burn care, these may take priority over the actual burn area. It is essential that the nurse understand the interrelatedness of these reactions and be alert to the signs of impending crisis. Once the immediate crises precipitated by the burn injury are under control, the patient faces a long and tedious recuperation. A firm, compassionate team approach will help the patient accept the physical and emotional pain and stress that must be endured.

The care of a patient with burns truly requires that we look beyond the scars and disfiguration to that part of the person that is more than the sum total of his parts.

BIBLIOGRAPHY

Artz CP (ed): Burns: A Team Approach. Philadelphia, W.B. Saunders, 1979

Bartlett H, Allyn P: Pulmonary management of the burned patient. Heart Lung, September/October 1973, pp 710–718

Busby HC: Nursing management of the acute burn patient and nursing management of optimal burn recovery. J Contin Educ Nurs 10, No. 4:16–30, 1979

Hunt JL: Burn wound management. Heart Lung, September/October 1973, pp 690–695

Jacoby FG: Nursing Care of the Patient with Burns. St. Louis, C.V. Mosby, 1976

McCrady V (ed): Burn Management. Crit Care Quart 1, No. 3: 1978

Selkurt EE (ed): Basic Physiology for the Health Sciences. Boston, Little, Brown & Company, 1975

Helen C. Busby and
William Seiffert

Hepatic Failure 25

Liver function is essential to life. The production and storage of certain essential elements and the detoxification of many harmful substances occur within this organ. Fortunately, the liver has an exceptional functional ability and regenerative capacity. Liver disease may be acute or chronic, and dysfunction may be reversible or irreversible, depending upon the amount of tissue involved and the nature of the insult.

ANATOMY

The liver is the largest glandular organ in the human body. This two-lobed (right and left lobes) organ lies just below the diaphragm with its greatest portion located to the right side of the body. Its superior (rounded) surface fits into the curve of the diaphragm and is in contact with the anterior wall of the abdominal cavity. The inferior surface is molded over the stomach, the duodenum, the pancreas, the hepatic flexure of the colon, the right kidney, and the right adrenal gland.

In keeping with its function as a gland, the liver removes certain elements from the blood and converts them into forms the body can use. The functional unit of the liver is called a *lobule*. In the tissues surrounding each lobule are found the terminal branches of the portal vein, the hepatic artery, and the bile ducts (see Fig. 25-1).

The *portal vein* is formed behind the head of the pancreas by the union of the superior mesenteric and the splenic veins. At its entrance to the liver, the portal vein divides into two trunks, which supply both lobes of the liver. The

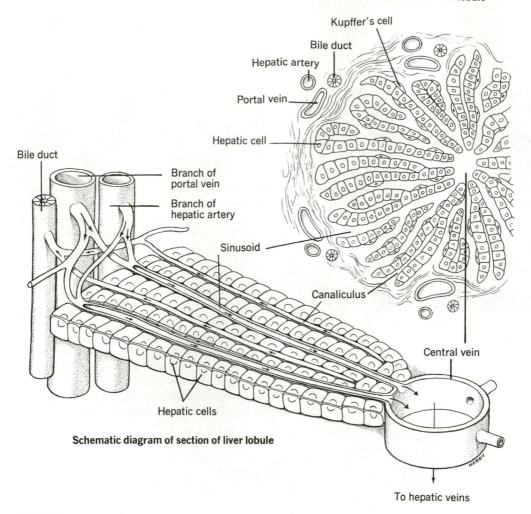

Cross section of liver lobule

Kupffer's cell

Bile duct

Hepatic artery

Portal vein

Hepatic cell

Bile duct

Branch of
portal vein

Branch of
hepatic artery

Sinusoid

Canaliculus

Central vein

Hepatic cells

Schematic diagram of section of liver lobule

To hepatic veins

FIGURE 25-1.
Liver lobule and sinusoids. (Chaffee EE, Greisheimer EM: Basic Physiology and Anatomy, 3rd ed, p 397. Philadelphia, J.B. Lippincott, 1974)

branches of the portal vein then disperse throughout the tissue of the liver and become the interlobular veins as they encircle each lobule. The blood sinusoids then pass toward the center of each lobule where they unite and form the central veins, which in turn form the sublobular veins, which then become the hepatic veins. The two hepatic veins drain into the inferior vena cava.

The *hepatic artery* supplies the liver with nutrients. This artery, along with the left gastric and splenic arteries, is the terminal branch of the celiac artery. The branches of the hepatic artery within the lobule of the liver form capillaries that communicate with the sinusoids from the interlobular veins.

The *bile ducts,* which carry the bile secreted by the liver cells to the duodenum to aid in the digestion of fats, originate within the liver cells as bile canaliculi. They anastomose to each other and then pass to the periphery of the lobule where they form the primary bile ducts. These bile ducts from both lobes of the liver then unite to form the hepatic duct. The hepatic duct becomes the common bile duct after its connection with the cystic duct (see Fig. 25-2).

The *cystic duct* and the *gallbladder* are just an enlargement in the biliary system in which excess bile secretion may be stored. The gallbladder concentrates bile and then empties its contents, by way of the common bile duct, into the duodenum during digestion.

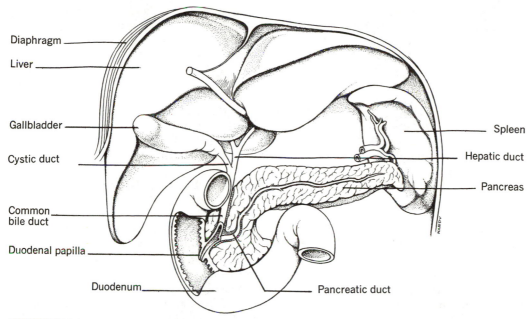

FIGURE 25-2.
Liver and biliary system. (Chaffee EE, Greisheimer EM: Basic Physiology and Anatomy, 3rd ed, p 398. Philadelphia, J.B. Lippincott, 1974)

The common bile duct and the main duct from the pancreas usually unite just before the duct enters the lumen of the duodenum. There is often a dilation of the tube after this junction (the ampulla of Vater). The opening of the common bile duct in the duodenum is about 8 to 10 cm from the pylorus.

PHYSIOLOGY

The physiological processes that occur in the liver are multiplex. This is probably due to the extremely high permeability of the cell membranes in the hepatic sinusoids and to the large volume of blood that is exposed to these sinusoids. In this area the large protein molecule diffuses almost as easily as the smaller fluid molecule; hence, a rapid exchange of substances between blood and liver cells occurs.

A vast array of biochemical reactions that are vital for continuation of the metabolic process occur in the liver. We will not undertake the explanation of these chemical reactions but rather will concentrate on four major functions of the liver that we have labeled (1) storage and distribution, (2) conversion, (3) secretion, and (4) detoxification.

Storage and Distribution

The liver very efficiently stores essential elements needed by the body and releases them according to bodily needs. Besides the glucose and protein, the liver stores trace metals such as iron and copper and the vitamins B_{12}, A, D, and many of the B–complex group.

Whenever we think of vitamins that are concerned with the liver, we must include vitamin K. Although vitamin K is not stored in the liver, it is closely related to liver function. This fat-soluble vitamin is absorbed from the intestinal tract, and adequate absorption is dependent upon the liver's ability to secrete bile into the intestinal tract. More importantly, vitamin K is a vital coenzyme in the liver's ability to produce the plasma proteins, prothrombin and factors IX and X. These two proteins are necessary for blood coagulation (see Chapter 23).

The liver plays a major role in replenishing the blood's supply of glucose when the blood concentration falls below normal. Liver cells are highly permeable to glucose (digested carbohydrate) and will absorb 75% of all excess glucose entering the blood. This is accomplished by the enzyme glucokinase, which accelerates the rate of glucose uptake by the liver cell. Glucokinase production is regulated by levels of insulin in the bloodstream. The absorbed glucose is stored in the liver as glycogen.

The liver is the largest storehouse for amino acids in the body. The amino acids derived from protein digestion travel to the liver by way of the portal vein. Intracellular enzymes in the parenchymal cells of the liver convert the excess amino acids into cellular proteins. These proteins are then stored in the liver and released as needed to maintain equilibrium between the body's cellular and plasma proteins. The rate at which the liver converts its cellular proteins into plasma proteins is dependent upon metabolic needs. In the normal body approximately 30 g of stored protein are used every day. However, if large amounts of plasma proteins are being lost, as in severe burns, the liver can increase its production of plasma proteins to as much as 4 g per hour or 100 g per day.

Conversion

The liver plays an active role in the conversion of carbohydrates, proteins, and fatty acids into energy. Energy is required for all chemical reactions to occur. The compound adenosine triphosphate (ATP) is the basic source of energy at the cellular level. The energy released from the metabolism of carbohydrates, proteins, and fatty acids is eventually oxidized into ATP. All three nutrients are progressively degraded to acetylcoenzyme A (acetyl-CoA), which is further degraded to ATP, CO_2, and H_2O.

Glucose. Glucose is the end product of digested carbohydrates and is the main source of energy for the body. The liver closely monitors the level of glucose in the bloodstream and releases stored glucose as necessary to maintain a normal blood level. When the concentration of blood glucose falls below normal, the concentration of blood insulin also falls. The low blood level of insulin has an inhibitory effect on glycogenesis, allowing glucose to remain in the bloodstream.

If this action alone is not sufficient to raise the blood glucose level to normal, the glycogen stored in the liver is converted back into glucose by the enzyme glucose 6-phosphatase and released into the bloodstream. Glucose 6-phosphatase is activated by blood levels of epinephrine and glucagon. The liver can also increase blood glucose concentration by the process of gluconeogenesis, which is conversion of certain amino acids into glucose.

Protein. The end product of protein digestion circulates in the blood as amino acids. These amino acids are resynthesized by the liver to form the three major plasma proteins: albumin, fibrinogen, and the globulins. *Albumin* is necessary to maintain the colloid osmotic pressure

throughout the body, thereby preventing excess loss of fluid from blood capillaries. *Fibrinogen* is necessary in the coagulation process, and the *globulins* are necessary for the formation of antibodies. Of these three major plasma proteins, the liver produces all the body's albumin and fibrinogen and 50% of the body's globulins. In addition, the liver, with the help of vitamin K, synthesizes all the body's prothrombin and blood factors V, VII, IX, and X which are essential for fibrinogen to be activated.

Fatty Acid. When cellular and plasma proteins are in equilibrium, and the protein storage cells are saturated, certain amino acids are degraded by the body and stored as fat. These amino acids are ketogenic, and when the amine radical is split from the carbon skeleton, ammonia is released (deamination). The liver converts this ammonia into urea and releases it into the bloodstream. It is then secreted into the urine by the kidneys. The fatty acids that remain after deamination are synthesized into triglycerides.

Triglycerides, phospholipids, and cholesterol are the principal lipids, or fats, of the body. A large portion of the triglycerides, most of the phospholipids, and essentially all of the cholesterol are formed in the liver. *Triglycerides* are composed of one, two, or three fatty acid molecules bound to one glycerol molecule. Triglycerides become the body's source of energy when glucose is not available. After the initial breakdown of the triglyceride molecule to fatty acids and glycerol, the liver degrades the fatty acid molecule to acetyl CoA. The final conversion to ATP, CO_2, and H_2O follows the same pathway as acetyl CoA derived from the metabolism of glucose.

Phospholipids are complex triglyceride compounds. They are a component of the myelin sheath and are used in the formation of thromboplastin, in chemical reactions requiring the phosphate radical, and in the formation of elements necessary for the structure of cells.

Cholesterol is a sterol formed from the degradation products of a fatty acid and is the main component of bile. It is an important element in maintaining the permeability of cell membranes throughout the body and in forming certain steroid hormones such as aldosterone and cortisol.

Secretion

The only substance actually secreted by the liver is bile. The bile solution contains bile salts, cholesterol, bilirubin, fatty acids, and plasma electrolytes. The secretion occurs in the canaliculi of the lobule and produces about 1000 ml of bile per day. Hepatic bile is diverted into the gallbladder, where water and electrolytes are reabsorbed. The final solution of bile in the gallbladder is five to ten times more concentrated then that originally secreted by the liver. The bile is stored in the gallbladder and is emptied into the intestine whenever the gallbladder muscle is stimulated to contract by the hormone cholecystokinin. Cholecystokinin is released from the intestinal mucosa following the ingestion of fat into the intestine.

Bile salts are formed from bile acids that occur in the liver during the degradation of fatty acids. The bile salts create a detergent effect on the fat globules in the intestine, which causes them to break up into small globules that are more easily attacked by the fat-splitting enzymes. More importantly, bile salts increase the solubility of the digested fats, thereby allowing their passage through the intestinal wall. If bile salts are absent, the fat globules are excreted in the stool, and a metabolic deficit of lipids will occur. The bile salts themselves are mostly reabsorbed along with the fat and recirculated through the liver and into the bile. A small amount of bile salt is lost in the feces, but the liver will replace this.

Cholesterol in the bile is probably due to the fact that it is a by-product of bile salt secretion; its presence in bile performs no known function. Normally insoluble in water, cholesterol is held in solution in the bile by the hydrotropic action of the fatty acids and the bile salts. Under abnormal conditions it may precipitate and form gallstones. The amount of cholesterol present in bile is dependent upon the amount of cholesterol in the diet. The more cholesterol ingested, the higher the concentration of it in bile. The cholesterol in solution is readily reabsorbed from the intestinal tract.

Bilirubin is the end product of metabolism of the heme portion of the hemoglobin molecule. When worn out or defective erythrocytes are phagocytized, the resultant bilirubin attaches itself to a plasma protein, mainly albumin. This bilirubin circulates in the plasma until it comes in contact with a liver cell that absorbs it; separates it from its protein; conjugates (joins) it with glucuronic acid, which makes it highly soluble; and secretes it into a bile canaliculus. When the bile is in transit through the intestines, the bilirubin glucuronide is converted into urobilinogen by intestinal bacteria. Most of this urobilinogen makes its exit from the body in the feces. Some urobilinogen is reabsorbed into the bloodstream, and some of this is excreted by the kidneys into the urine. The remaining urobilinogen is reconverted by liver cells back into bilirubin and secreted in the bile.

Detoxification

The detoxification process that occurs in the liver protects the body from many harmful substances that enter the bloodstream. Each sinusoid of the liver is lined with a layer of reticulum cells called *Kupffer's cells*. These phagocytic cells are very efficient in digesting bacteria, viruses, and other foreign matter that are brought to them by the blood flow. They are also capable of forming antibodies against the invader, if necessary. These cells are particularly important because they destroy bacteria that are constantly entering the portal blood flow directly from the gastrointestinal tract. Over 99% of the bacteria entering the body in this manner are destroyed before they can do any harm. The Kupffer's cells also destroy other particulate matter in the bloodstream (*i.e.*, worn-out red blood cells).

The liver also absorbs most drugs that enter the bloodstream. Since the liver is the center for chemical reactions in the body, it is not surprising that drugs entering the liver will be modified and excreted in a different form. This reaction is not clearly understood, but it is believed to occur in one of two ways: (1) the drug may activate a hepatic enzyme that changes the chemical makeup of the drug or (2) the drug may be made more water-soluble by microsomal enzymes in the Kupffer's cells. The time required for the drug to be cleared from the bloodstream depends upon the rate of blood flow through the liver and the absorption efficiency of the liver cells.

PATHOPHYSIOLOGY

As previously discussed, the liver is made up of four major components: the parenchyma, Kupffer's cells, bile ducts, and blood vessels. All are suspended in a fibrous stroma. Disease processes can affect these components, and if severe enough, can lead to liver failure. Knowledge of the pathophysiology creating the clinical situations is helpful in caring for persons with liver disease.

Hepatitis

Diffuse inflammation of the liver (hepatitis) can be caused by infections from viruses and by

Table 25–1
Liver Function Tests

Tests	Normal Values	Comments
1. *Protein Studies*	*g /100 ml*	
Total (Serum)	6.5–8.0	
Albumin	4.0–5.5	Albumin is a major part of total blood proteins. It is important in the maintenance of osmotic pressure between blood and tissue.
Globulins	2.0–3.0	Globulins are needed for the production of antibodies as well as helping maintain osmotic pressure.
Fibrinogen	0.2–0.4	Fibrinogen is necessary in the coagulation process.
Electrophoresis	*Percent of 100% Total Protein*	
Albumin	53%	Electrophoresis separates the various protein fractions by an electric current. In parenchymal liver cell disease, the amounts of serum proteins will be depressed or the ratio of the proteins to each other will be altered.
Alpha globulins	14%	
Beta globulins	12%	
Gamma globulins	20%	
Prothrombin Time	12–15 sec	Prothrombin is synthesized to thrombin (in the absence of vitamin K) by the liver. This test is a good index of prognosis, as a prolonged pro-time is indicative of severe functional loss.
2. *Enzyme Studies*		
SGOT	10–40 units	Transaminases are a catalyst in the breakdown of amino acids. SGPT is the specific enzyme released by damaged liver cells. LDH is present in large amounts in liver tissue.
SGPT	5–35 units	
LDH	165–300 units	
Alkaline phosphatase	2–5 Bodansky units	This enzyme hydrolyzes phosphate esters and is useful in differential diagnosis if jaundice is present. It is excreted through the biliary tract. If it is elevated, nucleotidase and leucine amino peptidase will determine if elevation is due to biliary obstruction.
Gamma glutamyle transferase	0–30 IU	Endothelia enzyme is found in the liver and closely follows elevations in alkaline phosphatase.
3. *Bilirubin*		
Total	0.9–2.2 mg/100 ml 0.8 mg/dl	This test measures the ability of the liver to conjugate and excrete bilirubin. If the conjugated bilirubin is low and the unconjugated high, it indicates a preliver block. If the conjugated bilirubin is high and the unconjugated normal or low, it indicates a postliver block.
Conjugated (direct)	0.5–1.4 mg/100 ml 0.6 mg/dl	
Unconjugated (indirect)	0.4–0.8 mg/100 ml 0.2 mg/dl	
4. *BSP* (bromsulphalein dye clearance	95%–100% excretion in 1 hr	This test measures the ability of the liver to conjugate BSP and clear it from the organ. A normal clearance is dependent upon good hepatic blood flow, functioning liver cells, and lack of obstruction in the biliary tract. This is the most sensitive of the liver function tests. It is the first test to become abnormal and the last to return to normal. False readings may be due to CHF, bleeding, previous contract dye injection, extravasation of dye at time of injection, and the patient not being in a fasting state (postprandial increased hepatic blood flow produces increased excretion).

toxic reactions from drugs and chemicals. When this occurs, the parenchymal cells are injured, and various intracellular enzymes called *transaminases* are released into the blood. The most common of these transaminases are the serum glutamic-oxaloacetic transaminase (SGOT) and serum glutamic-pyruvic transaminase (SGPT). Obviously, if enough liver cells are injured, the important metabolic and detoxifying processes of the liver are lost.

The viral infections of the liver parenchyma have been classified according to their specific infecting agent. There are three types of acute viral hepatitis—type A, type B, and non A, non B.

Type A Hepatitis. Type A, often referred to as *infectious hepatitis,* is transmitted by the fecal—oral route. It has a high prevalence in low socioeconomic regions. It can be epidemic in nature, and shellfish are often implicated in its transmission. The clinical course of type A hepatitis usually runs 1 to 3 months. Recovery is usually complete and does not lead to chronic hepatitis or cirrhosis. However, in rare instances type A hepatitis may lead to fulminating liver failure.

The diagnosis of type A hepatitis is made by the finding of high transaminase levels (see Table 25-1) and the presence of rising hepatitis A antibody (anti HAV) in the serum. It is important to note that by the time the patient presents with symptoms of hepatitis, he is no longer shedding the virus in his stool and is generally not infective.

Type B Hepatitis. Type B hepatitis is usually spread by a parenteral route. Some of the more common mechanisms of transmission are blood transfusions, needle-stick accidents in medical personnel, and the use of contaminated needles by drug addicts. However, there are a significant number of patients who contract type B hepatitis from nonparenteral routes. The antigen has been identified in body secretions such as semen, mucus, and saliva, and exposure to a person with type B hepatitis can result in infection. There is a high incidence of type B hepatitis in male homosexuals. It appears that a break in the skin or the mucous membrane is necessary for the transmission to occur.

There are three antigens identified with type B hepatitis. These antigens are (1) surface antigen, (2) core antigen, and (3) E antigen.

Hepatitis B surface antigen (HBSAG) is the first antigen to rise in the patient's blood and is usually present at the time the transaminase levels are rising. As the patient improves, the transaminase levels and the level of HBSAG decrease. Chronic active hepatitis is seen in 10% of the patients who have type B hepatitis. They continue to have levels of HBSAG and can be infective to others. The degree of liver impairment in chronic active hepatitis is variable from mild to serious and can progress to cirrhosis. This type of hepatitis is the leading cause of fulminant liver failure and is implicated in approximately 60% of all cases. Usually, as the patient's clinical con-

dition improves, the surface antigen titer falls, and the antibody to the surface antigen rises. Because of a persisting antigen–antibody reaction taking place, these patients may develop an immune complex disease such as glomerulo-nephritis.

E antigen may be very helpful in determining who is the most infective. Patients with high E antigen tend to be much more infective than those with high antibody to E antigen. Patients with E antigens usually have very active liver disease, which may be either acute or chronic. Those with high antibody to E antigen may have a tendency to be carriers for a long time.

Core antigen and core antibody titers, at the present time, have not been found to be significantly useful in clinical practice. They may be of some benefit in epidemiologic studies.

Non A-non B Hepatitis. The third type of hepatitis is designated *non A-non B hepatitis.* When type A and type B hepatitis have been ruled out by the various blood tests and the patient has an acute episode of hepatitis, especially following blood transfusions, non A-non B hepatitis is the most likely diagnosis. There are no specific tests for this, and it often becomes a diagnosis of exclusion. Its transmission and clinical course are similar to type B hepatitis. However, patients with non A-non B hepatitis tend to develop chronic hepatitis with a greater frequency than patients with type B hepatitis. A significant percentage of patients with non A-non B hepatitis develop fulminant hepatitis, but the percentage is somewhat less than patients with type B hepatitis.

Drug-Induced Hepatitis. The picture of viral hepatitis can be mimicked both clinically and pathologically by a drug-induced hepatitis. This actually results from a toxic reaction to the liver cells from either the drug itself or one of its metabolites.

The major drugs involved in toxic reactions include the halogenated anesthetic agents such as halothane, the antihypertensive medication methyldopa, the antituberculous medication isoniazid, and the phenytoins such as Dilantin. Most of these medications cause their toxicity through intermediate metabolites of the drug and rarely by their direct effect on the hepatocytes. There may also be a hypersensitivity reaction to the drug or to one of its metabolites. Acetaminophen and aspirin are other medications that can cause some degree of hepatic toxicity. The acetaminophen toxicity can be overwhelming and fatal due to the toxic effect of its metabolites on the liver cells (see Chapter 29).

"Fatty Liver"

Toxic effects on the liver, or multiple nutritional deficiencies in the diet, may cause an increase in fat accumulation within the parenchymal cells. The net result is an enlarged liver referred to as *fatty metamorphosis,* or a *fatty liver.* The cause of the fatty changes in the parenchymal cells is unclear, but it may be a response to alterations in enzymatic function responsible for normal fat metabolism.

Alcoholism.   One of the more classic examples of fatty infiltration of the liver, and subsequent hepatitis, is seen with alcohol ingestion. Initially, the first response of the liver to alcohol ingestion is one of fatty metamorphosis. If the alcohol ingestion is discontinued, the fatty metamorphosis decreases and the liver normalizes. This happens in nutritionally deficient, as well as in nutritionally normal, patients. However, if the alcohol ingestion continues, further toxic effects occur, leading to necrosis of liver cells. Interestingly enough, this necrosis occurs around the central vein rather than the portal triads as seen in viral hepatitis and other toxic reactions.

The patient with alcoholic hepatitis also shows elevated transaminase levels. His prothrombin time may also begin to elevate, and he may have a very low albumin due to significant loss of liver function. (Refer to Table 25-1.) The loss of function may progress to cirrhosis as long as the toxic effect of alcohol is present, and this may eventually lead to liver failure.

The exact nature of the toxic effect of alcohol is unknown, but it appears to be related to the quantity of alcohol ingestion over a significant period of time. Other factors, such as nutrition, do not seem to play a part. It has recently been reported that the alcohol may induce immunologic response with a secondary inflammatory reaction. Continued exposure to the alcohol simply prolongs and propagates this immune response with its attendant inflammatory reaction.

Other Liver Disorders and Symptoms

Jaundice.   Jaundice is often the presenting clinical sign of liver disease. It can occur from the liver cells' inability to excrete bile (intrahepatic cholestasis) or from obstruction of the bile ducts (obstructive jaundice). Drugs and sepsis are often implicated in intrahepatic cholestasis, while stones and tumors may cause obstructive jaundice.

Tumors.   The liver parenchyma can be disrupted extensively by either primary tumors, such as hepatomas, or by metastatic tumors. This extensive replacement of liver tissue can lead to hepatic failure. Remaining hepatocytes are unable to carry on normal metabolic processes, and hypoprothrombinemia and hypoproteinemia often result. These patients may also present with severe obstructive jaundice due to tumor infiltration and subsequent compression of the bile ducts.

Arterial Insufficiency.   Blood flow to the liver generally protects the hepatocytes from anoxic injury. Portal venous blood has a high oxygen concentration, and coupled with the arterial supply, provides good protection against anoxic injury. However, in the event of traumatic or surgically induced arterial insufficiency, previously injured hepatocytes are extremely susceptible to anoxic insults.

With progressive inflammatory injury to the parenchyma, the normal architecture of the liver becomes deranged by fibrous bands of scar tissue. In between these bands of fibrous tissue are regenerating liver cells. The result of this architectural derangement is impaired blood flow to the sinusoids of the liver. The portal blood is unable to flow through the liver; thus, portal vein pressures rise. With sufficient back pressure on the portal system, collateral circulation develops and allows blood flow to go from the intestines directly to the vena cava. The increased blood flow to the veins of the esophagus leads to esophageal varices; of the spleen, splenomegaly; of the hemorrhoidal veins, hemorrhoids.

Ascites.   Another consequence of portal and sinusoidal hypertension is ascites. This entity represents a large collection of hepatic lymph within the abdominal cavity. In patients with portal hypertension, the production of hepatic lymph is increased and frequently is produced at a greater rate than can be reabsorbed by the thoracic duct. Two other factors are involved in the formation of ascites: (1) Elevated venous pressures in the portal system increase the transudation of fluid into the abdomen. This is often potentiated by hypoproteinemia, which causes a decreased osmotic pressure in the blood. (2) Elevated aldosterone levels increase sodium retention, and this tends to aggravate ascites and edema.

Hepatic Failure. When extensive damage to the liver parenchyma occurs, regardless of its etiology, the patient may develop hepatic failure. These patients may present with high fevers and severe abdominal pain. Their liver cells often necrose to such an extent that the liver shrinks in size. Hepatic encephalopathy may develop, and drowsiness, irritability, confusion, and finally, stupor and coma may be seen. Laboratory studies often reveal elevated prothrombin times and elevated blood ammonia levels. Such patients may also be significantly hypoglycemic, due to loss of the liver's crucial role in glucose metabolism.

The hypoglycemia may well add to the neurologic signs of delirium and confusion — seizures may even occur. Decreased clotting factor production may lead to a disseminated intravascular coagulopathy (DIC) (see Chapter 23).

An interesting phenomenon called *hepatorenal syndrome* may also develop in fulminant liver failure. In this entity, the kidneys no longer function, and the patient becomes uremic. There is an oliguric renal failure. However, the kidney morphology is normal, and if these kidneys are transplanted into a person with a normal liver, they begin to function immediately and normally.

Hepatic Encephalopathy. Patients with severe liver disease may progress to hepatic encephalopathy. Clinically, they start with a quiet delirium or stupor and then may progress to profound coma. Sometimes they become very agitated and difficult to manage. Often they have a characteristic hyperventilation syndrome with a respiratory alkalosis.

The etiology of the hepatic encephalopathy and the hyperventilation syndrome is probably related to toxic agents absorbed from the intestinal tract. Elevated serum ammonia and some amino acids have been implicated as these agents. The amino acids may act as false neurotransmitters and contribute to the encephalopathic state.

Those with portal systemic shunts may develop hepatic encephalopathy quite rapidly, and they often hemorrhage from esophageal varices or other sites in their gastrointestinal tract. The hemorrhage produces a significant nitrogenous load to the intestinal tract in the form of blood, in which bacterial deamination produces the ammonia. Normally, this ammonia is detoxified to urea by the liver. When the liver is unable to perform this detoxification, or when a good portion of the portal blood is shunted around the liver, the circulating level of ammonia rises. If ammonia and the other toxic agents can be reduced through effective therapy, the encephalopathy will gradually clear.

MANAGEMENT

The liver cells have a remarkable capacity for regeneration following injury. There is very little that can be done therapeutically to enhance this natural healing process. In general, patients with liver disease require careful supportive care during their illness and recovery, and care of the patient with severe liver disease often becomes the realm of the critical care unit. These patients require careful attention and nursing care that is based on sound judgment, for they often arrive in some state of unconsciousness. The skin and sclera will be jaundiced. Coagulation times will be prolonged, and bleeding is apt to occur from many sources. Mild sores, if not present, may develop due to the debilitated state of the patient.

Treatment of these patients consists of

- Maintaining those bodily functions not impaired by the disease (*i.e.*, respirations)
- Intervening when assistance is required to maintain specific function (*i.e.*, fluid balance)
- Taking over the function of those systems in which failure may be complete (*i.e.*, replacement of clotting factors)

1. Fluid and Dietary Requirements

Because of the patient's inability to maintain fluid and electrolyte balance, and the everpresent possibility of impaired renal function, an accurate intake and output record must be kept. Weighing the patient daily will assess fluid retention. Dietary restrictions of sodium and protein are necessary. Because of the tendency for fluid retention with sodium and aggravation of the encephalopathy with protein metabolism, carbohydrates, by way of the intravenous or oral routes, will help prevent hypoglycemia reactions.

2. Replacement Therapy

Patients with hepatic failure require a large stable intravenous line because of the need for large quantities of blood, plasma, albumin, and fluids necessary to maintain bodily functions until the diseased liver cells are regenerated. Maintenance of electrolyte balance is also achieved by the intravenous route. These patients tend toward potassium depletion due to

- Diarrhea induced by the enemas, laxatives, and antibiotics administered to evacuate or sterilize the bowel
- Diuretics to reduce water retention and edema
- Elevated aldosterone levels

3. Prevention of Infection

Because of the generalized deteriorating health state, the patient is very susceptible to infection. All the invasive equipment and procedures used — intravenous lines, bladder catheters, gastrointestinal tubes — must be treated as a source of infection. An alert and conscientious nurse can prevent many of the complications possible from these procedures by application of quality nursing skills.

4. Prevention of Respiratory, Circulatory, and Possible Skin Problems

Disturbances of the respiratory system (*i.e.,* pneumonia), of the circulatory system (*i.e.,* thrombophlebitis), and of the skin (*i.e.,* decubitus ulcers) need to be avoided. Constant nasogastric suctioning as well as frequent and careful oral-pharyngeal suctioning may be required to prevent aspiration pneumonia. Skin care must be meticulous! Subcutaneous edema, immobility, and poor nutrition are all present and are all prime factors in the development of decubitus ulcers.

5. Assessment for Evidence of Bleeding

Bleeding is a common complication due to clotting factor deficiencies. Routine testing for the presence of blood in the stool, urine, and nasogastric drainage leads to early detection. Vitamin K can be administered to help correct the hypoprothrombinemia, while prothrombin times are used to follow this abnormality.

6. Caution in Drug Administration

The use of medication poses a particular danger owing to the diseased liver's inability to detoxify many drugs. The nurse must be particularly attentive to the amount of medications administered and the level of responsiveness both before and after administration. This is true especially for sedatives, analgesics, and narcotics. As mentioned, these patients are often agitated and very combative, and since they do not metabolize sedative medications very well, the best care many times is physical restraint rather than sedation. In these circumstances, the nursing staff and the family need a great deal of support because dealing with such patients can be very difficult.

7. Assessment of Neurologic Signs

Presence and progression of the neurologic signs of hepatic encephalopathy should be noted. Two of these are "liver flap" (asterixis) and loss of spatial orientation and inability to write (apraxia). Asterixis is assessed by having the patient place his hands in full extension. Due to the lack of ability to concentrate (encephalopathy), a flapping motion occurs at the wrist or at the metacarpal-phalangeal joints. Apraxia is evaluated by asking the patient to draw a star or write his name.

8. Bowel Cleansing to Promote Ammonia Excretion

Treatment of patients with severe hepatic encephalopathy centers on a lowering of the toxic substance —*ammonia*—from the blood. This is done by thorough cleansing of the bowel to rid it of all its protein and then maintaining that state with constant nasogastric suctioning. The use of nonabsorbable antibiotics in the form of neomycin aids in lowering the bacterial count in the colon, which thereby reduces the amount of ammonia produced by protein deamination. This can be potentiated by the use of strong cathartics in the form of magnesium citrate. Another very effective method is the use of high colonic enemas. Lactulose (Cephulac) is a nonabsorbable carbohydrate that can be used to lower the ammonia levels. It works by altering the intestinal pH, making it more acidic, and thereby increasing the ammonia excretion in the stool. It also has a laxative effect.

Recovery from hepatic failure is neither rapid nor easy. There are frequent setbacks and an apparent lack of improvement. Survival for this patient is greatly dependent upon optimum medical and nursing management.

BIBLIOGRAPHY

Beeson PB, McDermott W, Wyngaarden JB: Cecil — Textbook of Medicine. Philadelphia, W.B. Saunders, 1979

Boyer JL et al: Patient care goes to a liver symposium. Patient Care 13, No. 18–19, 1979, 14, No. 4, 1980

Brunner LS, Suddarth DS: Textbook of Medical-Surgical Nursing, 4th ed. Philadelphia, J.B. Lippincott, 1980

Davidson C: Liver Pathophysiology: Its Relevance to Human Disease. Boston, Little, Brown & Co, 1970

Guyton AC: Basic Human Physiology. Philadelphia, W.B. Saunders, 1977

Holvey DN (ed): Merck Manual of Diagnosis and Therapy, 12th ed. Rahway, Merck & Co, 1972

Meltzer LE et al: Concepts and Practices of Intensive Care for Nurse Specialists, 2nd ed. Bowie, Charles Press, 1976

Plum F, Posner JB: The Diagnosis of Stupor and Coma. F.A. Davis, 1972

Schaffner F (ed): The Liver and Its Disease. New York, Intercontinental Medical Book Corporation, 1974

Helen C. Busby and
William Seiffert

Acute Gastrointestinal Bleeding

26

PATHOPHYSIOLOGY

Bleeding in the gastrointestinal tract is caused primarily by gastric ulcers or gastritis. However, duodenal ulcers, esophageal varices, carcinoma, ulcerative colitis, polyps, diverticuli, and hemorrhoids can erupt in a bleeding episode. Since bleeding that occurs from the lower gastrointestinal tract is usually not severe enough to warrant the person's admission to a critical care unit or else is treated surgically, the following pages concentrate on upper gastrointestinal tract bleeding.

The appearance of the person presenting with upper gastrointestinal tract bleeding varies considerably, depending upon the amount and rapidity of blood loss. Gastrointestinal bleeding that is the result of an erosion through an artery will be profuse and will not stop with medical management. Bleeding that is caused by gastritis or oozing from granulation tissue at the base of an ulcer will be smaller in quantity, transient in nature, and will usually respond to medical management.

Hematemesis. The patient who is vomiting blood is usually bleeding from a source above the ligament of Treitz (at the duodenojejunal junction). Reverse peristalsis is seldom sufficient to cause hematemesis if the bleeding point is below this area. The vomitus may be bright red or coffee-ground in appearance, depending upon the amount of gastric contents at the time of the bleeding and the length of time the blood has been in contact with gastric secretions. Gastric acid converts bright red hemoglobin to brown hematin, accounting for the coffee-ground appearance of the drainage. Bright red blood results from profuse bleeding and little contact with gastric juices.

Melena.   Tarry stools will consistently occur in all persons who accumulate 500 ml of blood in their stomach. A tarry stool may be passed if as little as 60 ml of blood has entered the intestinal tract. Massive hemorrhage from the upper gastrointestinal tract, along with the increased intestinal motility that occurs, may result in stools containing bright red blood. It will take several days after the bleeding has stopped for melena stools to clear.

MANAGEMENT

The *immediate medical care* of the person admitted with gastrointestinal bleeding includes four steps:

1. *Assessment* of the severity of the blood loss
2. *Replacement* of a sufficient amount of blood to counteract shock
3. *Diagnosing* the cause of bleeding
4. *Planning* a definitive type of treatment

A decision for surgical intervention is based upon many factors in the medical history and the physical examination. A person who has repetitive bleeding episodes, a history of a gastric ulcer, or sclerotic blood vessels will likely require surgery as soon as possible.

Assessment of Blood Loss and Shock

To assess the severity of blood loss and to prevent or correct deterioration into hypovolemic shock, it is necessary for the nurse to assess the person frequently. In the first stage of bleeding — less than 500 ml of blood loss — the person may show signs only of weakness, anxiety, and perspiration. Following a significant bleed, the body temperature will elevate to 101° to 102°F (38.4°–39°C) in response to the bleeding, and bowel sounds will be hyperactive due to the sensitivity of the bowel to blood.

If the intravascular volume decreases due to continued blood loss, a sympathetic nervous system response will cause a release of the catecholamines, epinephrine and norepinephrine. These will initially cause an increase in heart rate in an attempt to maintain an adequate blood pressure. Following a blood loss of 1 to 2 pints, the signs and symptoms will begin to present a picture of shock.

As the shock syndrome progresses, the release of catecholamines triggers the blood vessels in the skin, lungs, intestines, liver, and kidneys to constrict, thereby increasing the volume of blood flow to the brain and heart. Because of the decreased flow of blood in the skin, the person's skin will be cool to the touch. With decreased blood flow to the lungs, hyperventilation will occur to maintain adequate gas exchange. As blood flow to the liver decreases, metabolic waste products accumulate in the blood. This, plus the absorption of decomposed blood from the intestinal tract and a decrease of blood flow through the kidneys, causes an increase in the blood urea level. In fact, the blood urea nitrogen (BUN) may be used to follow the course of a gastrointestinal bleed. A BUN above 40 — in the setting of a gastrointestinal bleed and a normal creatinine level — is indicative of a major bleed. The BUN will return to normal approximately 12 hours after the bleeding has stopped.

An excellent parameter in assessing shock is urinary output, which *must* be measured hourly. As the intravascular volume decreases, urine output decreases due to the reabsorption of water by the kidneys in response to the release of antidiuretic hormone (ADH) by the posterior lobe of the pituitary gland (see Chapter 16 on the effects of hypovolemic shock on the kidneys).

A drop in the person's blood pressure is an advanced sign of the shock syndrome and indicates that the body's own protective mechanisms have been overwhelmed.

Every nurse must always be alert for changes in this patient's condition. The patient must be monitored closely, assessed with knowledge and skill, his events anticipated, and significant changes reported immediately. The nurse must also allay the fears and apprehension of the patient. The sight of the blood alone is very upsetting to him, as he probably sees it in larger quantities than it really is, and he may well feel that he is going to bleed to death. If the nurse displays competency, efficiency, and the ability to answer his questions satisfactorily, she will provide a calming effect while the necessary procedures are carried out.

Blood Transfusion and Gastric Intubation

The patient admitted with gastrointestinal bleeding needs an immediate intravenous infusion route by means of a large caliber intracatheter or cannula. Blood is typed and cross-matched, and transfusion treatment is based on the presence of shock as well as on the blood count and blood volume levels. A central venous pressure (CVP) line may be placed to facilitate monitoring intravascular volume (see Chapter 10 on hemodynamic pressure monitoring).

A levine tube may be inserted into the person's stomach to assist with the diagnosis, to assess the rate of bleeding, to remove irritating gastric secretions, to prevent gastric dilatation, and to lavage with an iced solution to decrease bleeding tendencies by reducing blood flow.

Iced Saline Irrigation. If the person is presenting with hematemesis, the stomach is irrigated with iced saline until the returned solution is clear. It is important to keep accurate records of the amount of fluid used for irrigation so that this fluid can be subtracted from the total amount of aspiration to ascertain the true amount of bleeding.

Another method that may be used to control gastric bleeding is a continuous irrigation of the stomach with iced saline containing *levarterenol* (Levophed). The usual dilution is two ampuls of levarterenol per 1000 ml of normal saline. The principal action of this agent is vasoconstriction. Following absorption in the stomach, levarterenol is immediately sent to the liver by way of the portal system, where metabolism of the drug takes place; therefore, a systemic reaction is prevented.

Instillation of Topical Thrombin. If continuous irrigation with iced saline does not decrease the amount of bleeding, the instillation of topical thrombin into the stomach may be ordered. Thrombin clots blood at the site of bleeding by acting directly with fibrinogen. Because of this action, topical thrombin is used only on the surface of bleeding tissue and is never injected into blood vessels where extensive intravascular clotting would result.

The speed with which thrombin clots blood is dependent upon its concentration; for example, 5000 units of topical thrombin in 5 ml of saline is capable of clotting 5 ml of blood in 1 second. Remember, to clot the site of bleeding in the stomach, the topical thrombin must come in contact with the capillary that is bleeding. This may not be possible; therefore, topical thrombin will not be beneficial in every case of upper gastrointestinal tract bleeding.

The procedure for instillation of topical thrombin is more time consuming than difficult.

1. Aspirate stomach contents and measure.
2. Instill per nasogastric tube 2 oz (60 ml) of a buffer solution and clamp the tube. Dilute acid is detrimental to thrombin activity; therefore, stomach acids must be neutralized prior to administration of thrombin. Milk may be used until the pharmacy can prepare a buffer solution. This phosphate buffer solution is stable only for 48 hr, so solutions cannot be stored for future use.
3. After 5 min, instill 2 more oz of the buffer solution, containing 10,000 units of topical thrombin. Clamp tube.
4. After 30 min, aspirate stomach. If no fresh bleeding is evident, instill 2 oz of the buffer and clamp the tube.
5. Repeat instillation of 2 oz of the buffer solution every 1 to 2 hr for 24 to 48 hr.
6. If bleeding is not controlled after the 30 min, or if bleeding begins again, repeat steps 1 through 4. Repeat this procedure until bleeding is stopped.
7. Remember to total the aspiration and mark as output. Since the buffer solution is absorbed, mark this amount as intake.

Administration of Pitressin

Intravenous vasopressin (Pitressin) may be instituted, especially if the bleeding is due to esophageal varices or gastritis. This drug lowers portal hypertension and therefore decreases the flow of blood at the site of bleeding. It is sometimes infused by means of selective arterial catheter placement. Pitressin needs to be used with caution because it can cause a hypertensive state. It may also affect the urinary output by its ADH properties.

Vitamin K may be administered if it is indicated by a prolonged prothrombin time.

Sengstaken-Blakemore Tube

Esophageal varices should be suspected in the patient who has been addicted to alcohol and who presents with upper gastrointestinal bleeding. To control the hemorrhge from the varices, pressure is exerted on the cardia of the stomach and against the bleeding varices by a double-balloon tamponade (the Sengstaken-Blakemore tube) (see Fig. 26-1).

Once the tube is positioned in the stomach, the stomach balloon is inflated with no more than 50 ml of air. The tube is then slowly withdrawn until the gastric balloon fits snugly against the cardia of the stomach. Once it is determined by radiograph examination that the gastric balloon is in the right placement at the cardia and not in the esophagus, the gastric balloon can be further inflated—up to the desired amount without surpassing the balloon's capac-

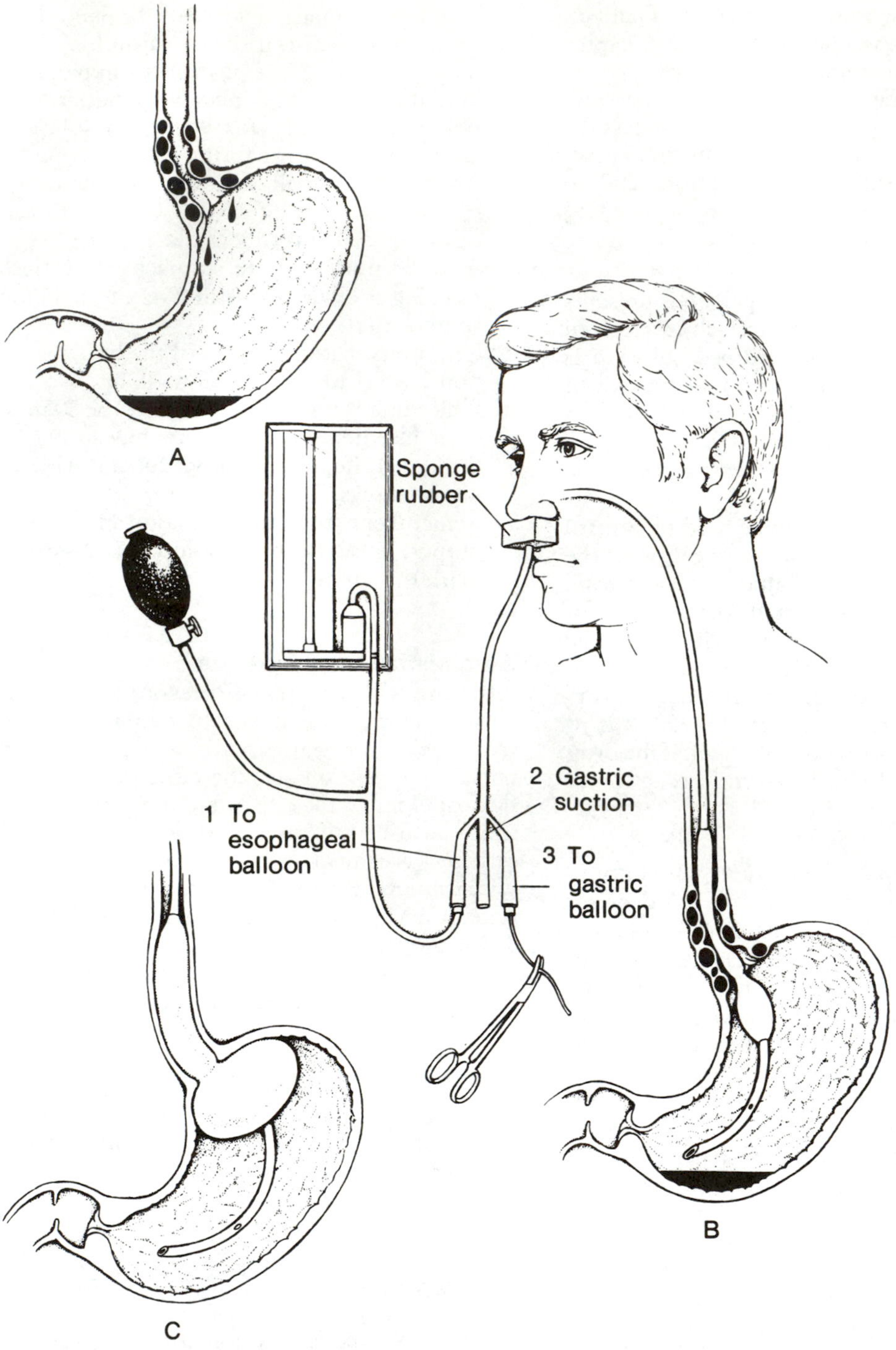

FIGURE 26-1.
Diagram showing esophageal varices and their treatment by a compressing balloon tube (Sengstaken-Blakemore). (A) Dilated veins of the lower esophagus. (B) The tube is in place in the stomach and the lower esophagus but is not inflated. (C) Inflation of the tube and the compression of the veins which can be obtained by inflation of the balloon. (Brunner LS, Suddarth DS: Textbook of Medical-Surgical Nursing, 3rd ed, p 609. Philadelphia, J.B. Lippincott, 1975)

ity. Traction is then placed on the tube where it enters the patient and is achieved by means of a piece of sponge rubber, as shown in Figure 26-1. This procedure may be sufficient to control the bleeding if the varices are in the cardia of the stomach. In fact, a Linton tube may be tried before the Sengstaken-Blakemore tube is inserted (see Fig. 26-2).

If bleeding continues, the esophageal balloon is inflated to a pressure of 25 to 40 torr and maintained at this pressure for 24 hours. Pressure for longer than 24 hours could cause edema, esophagitis, ulcerations, or perforation of the esophagus.

If bleeding still persists, traction is applied to the end of the balloon. This may consist of suspending a weight from the end of the tube or putting a football helmet on the patient and securing the tube, under traction, to the face bar.

The potential dangers of this treatment require constant observation and intelligent care. It is essential that the three tube openings be identified, correctly labeled, and checked for patency prior to insertion. The pressures in the balloons must be maintained, and the balloons must be kept in their proper position. If the gastric balloon ruptures, the entire tube may rise into the nasopharynx and completely obstruct the airway. A pair of scissors should be readily available at the bedside. The tube should be cut immediately to rapidly deflate the balloons and the entire tube removed whenever a question of respiratory insufficiency or aspiration occurs. It is wise to prophylactically restrain the patient's arms if he is agitated and restless to prevent him from dislodging the tube.

Nursing care of a patient with a Sengstaken-Blakemore tube in place involves skillful application of knowledge.

- The person is kept at complete rest because exertion, such as coughing or straining, tends to increase intra-abdominal pressure that predisposes to further bleeding.
- The head of the bed is kept elevated to reduce the flow of blood into the portal system and to prevent reflux into the esophagus.
- Since the person is unable to swallow, saliva must be suctioned frequently from the upper esophagus.
- The nasopharynx also needs frequent suctioning owing to the increased secretions resulting from irritation by the tube. A nasogastric tube may be inserted into the esophagus to the top of the esophageal balloon to control these se-

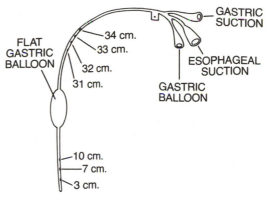

FIGURE 26-2.
Linton tube. (Courtesy of Davol, Inc.)

cretions and to prevent their aspiration into the lungs.
- The nasogastric tube should be irrigated every 2 hours to assure its patency and to keep the stomach empty.
- The nostrils are checked frequently, cleansed, and lubricated to prevent tube-caused pressure areas.

Persons with liver damage tolerate the breakdown products of blood in the intestinal tract very poorly. Therefore, it is imperative that blood *not be* allowed to remain in the person's stomach because it will migrate into the intestinal tract. Bacterial action on the blood in the intestinal tract produces ammonia, which is absorbed into the bloodstream. The ability of the liver to convert ammonia to urea is impaired, and ammonia intoxication ensues (see Chapter 25).

After the crisis is reversed, surgery for a portal systemic shunt may be indicated. If not, medical management continues.

Reducing Gastric Acid
Since gastric acid is extremely irritating to bleeding sites in the upper gastrointestinal tract, it is necessary to decrease the acidity of the gastric secretions. With the introduction of the drug cimetidine (Tagamet), it is possible to actually decrease the production of gastric acid. At a gastric pH of 2.0, the mechanism for stimulating gastric secretions is totally blocked. Cimetidine raises the gastric pH by inhibiting the action of histamine. A single dose will decrease acid secretion for up to 5 hours. To neutralize the remaining gastric acid, antacids are given in sufficient

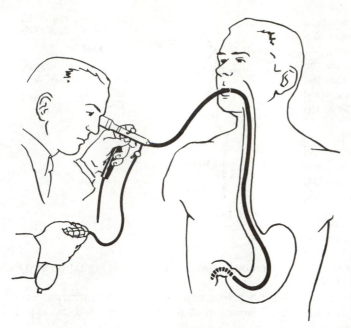

FIGURE 26-3.
Patient undergoing gastroscopy. Note the extreme flexibility of the tube with the patient in the sitting position. (Adapted from McNeer G, Pack GT: Neoplasms of the Stomach. Philadelphia, J.B. Lippincott, 1967)

quantity and often enough to be effective (*i.e.*, Maalox, 60 ml every 2 hr).

Diagnostic Studies

Diagnostic studies are performed as soon as possible for the purpose of establishing a definite diagnosis.

A *prothrombin time* is performed to rule out (1) the presence of long-term anticoagulant therapy (which may not immediately be made known in the excitement of admitting a patient during an episode of gastrointestinal bleeding) and (2) liver disease. A prolonged prothrombin time may be indicative of liver disease.

As soon as the person's clinical condition stabilizes, an upper gastrointestinal series or gastroscopy may be performed (see Fig. 26-3). Both are of immense value to the physician in deciding definitive treatment.

Summary

Treatment of the upper gastrointestinal bleeding episode is continued until there is no further evidence of active bleeding. The nurse will probably experience many frustrations while caring for such patients; however, constant observation and expert nursing care are essential to stabilizing them.

BIBLIOGRAPHY

Brunner LS, Suddarth DS: Textbook of Medical-Surgical Nursing, 4th ed. Philadelphia, J.B. Lippincott, 1980
Given BA, Simmons SJ: Gastroenterology in Clinical Nursing, 2nd ed. St. Louis, C.V. Mosby, 1975
Guyton AC: Basic Human Physiology. Philadelphia, W.B. Saunders, 1977
Holvey DN (ed): Merck Manual of Diagnosis and Therapy, 13th ed. Rahway, Merck & Co, 1977
Meltzer LE et al: Concepts and Practices of Intensive Care for Nurse Specialists, 2nd ed. Bowie, Charles Press 1976
Watson JE: Medical-Surgical Nursing and Related Physiology, 2nd ed. Philadelphia, W.B. Saunders, 1979

Helen C. Busby and
William Seiffert

Hyperalimentation: Total Parenteral Nutrition
27

One of the breakthroughs in the medical management of persons who have lost their ability to eat or absorb nutrients is hyperalimentation or total parenteral nutrition (TPN). Through this process, sufficient calories and nitrogen to sustain life can be supplied to the body. With the present feasibility of this treatment, the person's nutritional status is considered early in his illness and is treated more aggressively than ever before. The patient with a long–term postoperative course, the patient with multiple trauma, the patient receiving chemotherapy, and the patient being treated with acute hemodialysis are but a few candidates for this sophisticated therapy (see Table 27-1). The increased energy required by

Table 27–1
Indications for Total Parenteral Nutrition

Malnutrition	Diverticulitis
Malabsorption	Alimentary tract fistula
Chronic diarrhea	Alimentary tract anomalies
Chronic vomiting	Reversible liver failure
Failure to thrive	Acute and chronic renal failure
Gastrointestinal obstruction	Burns
Ulcer disease	Hypermetabolic states
Granulomatous enterocolitis	Complicated trauma or surgery
Ulcerative colitis	Short bowel syndrome
Pancreatitis	Protein-losing gastro-enteropathy
Severe anorexia nervosa	Nonterminal coma
Indolent wounds and decubitus ulcers	Malignant disease (adjunctive therapy)

Dudrick SJ: Total intravenous feeding: When nutrition seems impossible. Drug Therapy, Hospital Edition 1, No. 2:92, 1976 the body to handle the stresses imposed on it by these conditions will lead to the starvation state without nutritional support.

Protein-sparing nutrition alone may be used for short-term therapy in persons with no nutritional deficiencies and little change in their metabolic rate (*i.e.,* elective surgery). The administration of isotonic amino acid solutions by way of a peripheral vein will preserve body protein by supplying amino acids for normal protein synthesis. It will not assist in tissue repair. If the person progresses to protein/calorie malnutrition, as in hypermetabolic states or faulty nutrition, TPN should be instituted.

SOLUTION ADMIXTURE
The solution of TPN therapy begins as an admixture containing 20% to 30% glucose and 3.5% to 5.0% amino acids. The ratio of the calories (glucose) to the nitrogen (amino acid) should be 200:1. This ratio will preserve the nitrogen balance of the body; the hypertonic glucose will be used for calories, allowing the amino acids to be used for protein synthesis. If this ratio is not preserved, excess amino acids will be lost in the urine when adequate glucose is present, or amino acids will be used for calories if adequate glucose is not present. To achieve optimal therapy, 200 calories to 1 g of nitrogen is necessary.

Daily additions to the base solution should include potassium, sodium, and chloride. The daily requirements of these elements are greatly increased because of the increased volume of water intake and output. With the increased intake of glucose and amino acids, hypokalemia will soon result if additional potassium is not administered in sufficient quantities to maintain normal serum potassium levels. Potassium is also necessary for the transport of glucose across the cell membrane. Magnesium, calcium, phosphorus, and other trace elements are added as deficiencies occur. Since cations are poorly absorbed in the intestinal tract, the intravenous requirements of these elements are less than one would suspect. A multiple vitamin preparation is usually mixed in 1 liter of base solution per day. A unit of albumin may also be included daily to supplement protein intake.

Decisions concerning the amount of additives necessary to maintain the patient's electrolyte balance are determined from serial blood tests. Positive nitrogen balance is monitored by serial blood urea nitrogen (BUN) and creatinine levels. A hyperalimentation panel as shown in Table 27-2 is done daily until the electrolytes are stabilized. Once stabilization is achieved, the serum levels may be checked every other day.

Glucose intolerance may occur at the onset of treatment if the pancreas does not respond to the increased glucose load. Fractional urines must be performed every 4 hours on every patient receiving hyperalimentation therapy. Parenteral insulin, either by continuous intravenous infusion or by intermittent subcutaneous injections, should be administered when necessary to maintain the quantitative urine glucose at the 2% level.

FLOW RATE AND VOLUME
The rate of infusion of the hypertonic solution must be constant over a 24-hour period to achieve maximum assimilation of the nutrients and to prevent hyperglycemia or hypoglycemia.

Table 27-2
Tests That May Be on a Hyperalimentation Panel

Chemistry	Normal Ranges	Results
pH	7.35-7.45	
Sodium	135-149 mEq/liter	
Potassium	3.5-5.3 mEq/liter	
Chlorides	100-109 mEq/liter	
Calcium	4.5-5.7 mEq/liter	
Phosphorus	1.45-2.76 mEq/liter	
Magnesium	1.5-2.4 mEq/liter	
Glucose	70-115 mg/dl	
BUN	8-22 mg/dl	
Creatine	0.8-1.6 mg/dl	
Bicarbonate	22-26 mEq/liter	
Total protein	5.5-8.0 g/dl	

The flow rate cannot be increased to compensate for interruptions or slowing of the infusion because glycosuria with osmotic diuresis (diuresis from body compartments and cells leading to dehydration) can occur. Headache, nausea, and lassitude are early symptoms of too rapid an infusion. Too slow an infusion results in the administration of fewer nutrients, and hypoglycemia with a rebound of insulin may occur.

The aim of treatment is a continuous infusion that meets the caloric requirements of the patient by allowing maximum use of the carbohydrate and protein substrates with minimal renal excretion. The flow rate must be checked faithfully every 30 to 60 minutes. If a slowing does happen to occur (as from an obstruction in the infusion line from a kink in the tubing), an increase of flow not to exceed 10% of the original rate may be instituted to bring the caloric intake back to the desired level. An infusion pump will help ensure continuous accurate infusion. However, because such pumps are mechanical devices subject to malfunctions, the nurse must keep a close watch on the flow rate.

Volume is given according to established water metabolism levels (2500 ml/24 hr in adults and 100 ml/kg/24 hr in infants) and carbohydrate metabolism (0.5 g/kg/hr). One thousand to 2000 ml in 24 hours is the initial intake with a gradual increase according to the patient's tolerance, as established by careful clinical and chemical monitoring. Three liters is generally the maximum daily volume. However, patients undergoing massive catabolism, such as that occurring in severe or extensive burns or severe traumatic injuries, often require 4 to 5 liters per day.

In these severe nutritional deficiencies, where excess calories are required, the intravenous infusion of lipids in adjunct with the hyperalimentation solution may be employed. The 10% fat emulsion delivers a fat particle comparable to a chylomicron (normally digested fat particle) and provides 1:1 calorie per milliliter of solution. These calories do not require insulin for use by the body; therefore, the danger of hyperinsulinemia or rebound hypoglycemia is eliminated.

Intralipids are isotonic and can be infused in a peripheral line. The person must be monitored by observing his serum for turbidity 4 to 6 hours post infusion to make sure the fat is being cleared from the blood.

If there is a problem with the integrity of the kidneys or heart, fluid volume must be carefully calculated to prevent cardiopulmonary overload. A special hypertonic solution, nephramine, may be used in this setting. This solution provides the eight essential amino acids in 250 ml, and when diluted with the 500 ml of the hypertonic glucose solution, provides the necessary calories and proteins for 24 hours without an excess of water.

If the patient is receiving adequate nutrition, his weight gain should be ¼ to ½ pound (100 to 300 g) per day. If he is gaining much more, it is probably water retention and not tissue gain, and the volume infused needs be adjusted downward.

INFUSION SITES

Knowing the nature of the hyperalimentation solution, one can easily understand why the usual normal intravenous routes are not used. This hypertonic solution would rapidly cause thrombosis at the tip of the intravenous catheter. Since this high caloric nitrogen solution must be rapidly diluted and dispersed within the blood vessels, the superior vena cava is an excellent site. Figure 27-1 indicates the different routes that can be used. Passing the intravenous catheter into the superior vena cava by way of the subclavian vein is the route of choice because it allows the patient the greatest freedom of movement without disturbing the injection site, and the incidence of infection at this level of the body is lower. Jugular veins may be used but are not as comfortable for the patient. Basilic vein routes are too prone to irritation and infection for long-term therapy. The femoral vein as a route to the inferior vena cava is rarely selected because it is highly susceptible to contamination from body pathogens, such as abdominal wound drainage, urine, and stool.

INFECTION POTENTIAL

Two key factors are involved in the success of hyperalimentation therapy: (1) the long-term presence of the indwelling catheter directly in the superior vena cava and (2) the hypertonic solution. Both are prime sites for the source of infection.

Insertion Site. The puncture site is a potential portal of entry of organisms, and the solution is an excellent culture medium for many species of bacteria and fungi. Meticulous asepsis in the care of the line and in the preparation of the solution cannot be overstressed.

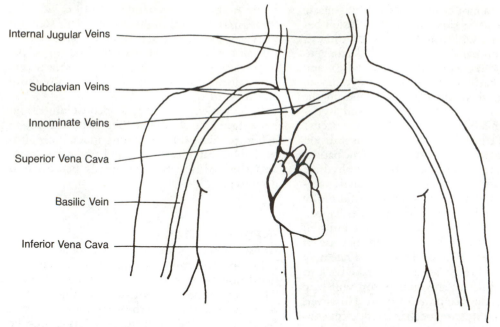

FIGURE 27-1.
Venous anatomy for hyperalimentation routes.

Asepsis starts with the insertion of the indwelling catheter. This is performed under strict sterile technique, and a sterile dressing is applied to the site. This dressing should be changed every 24 to 72 hours. At the time of the dressing change, the site should be examined for signs of leakage, edema, or inflammation, and the catheter should be checked for any kinking of the tube. The skin should be cleansed with a solvent such as acetone to remove surface skin fat that harbors pathogenic organisms and adhesive tape which, if allowed to accumulate, will cause irritation and skin breakdown. A large area surrounding the catheter is cleansed with an antibacterial solution (*e.g.,* an iodine preparation) and a broad-spectrum antibiotic ointment is applied to the puncture site. An occlusive dressing or an "op site" dressing is applied over the area. Open or draining wounds around the area or a tracheostomy require extra precautions to ensure sterility of the site. A transparent plastic waterproof surgical drape over the entire dressing will help prevent contamination from fluid or exudates if the op site dressing is not used. With sound infection control procedures, the sterility of the insertion site can be maintained for the length of the treatment, even if the treatment lasts for months.

Solution Sterility. Maintaining sterility of the solution is mandatory. As stated above, it is an excellent culture medium for pathogens. The solution should be prepared in the pharmacy by a pharmacist. Preferably, additives are added under a laminar air-flow hood to assure a particle-free environment. If the nurse must add electrolytes and other elements to the base solution, she must be aware of any contamination that may occur from syringes, needles, medication vials, and so forth. A new solution hung every 8 hours (with disposal of any solution left in the container after 8 hours) may be employed. Solutions are inspected for clouding or particular matter when the flow rate is checked every 30 to 60 minutes.

All of the intravenous tubing should be changed once a day at the time a new solution is hung. If dressings are changed daily, the new tubing, the new solution, and the dressing change should be correlated to take place at the same time. If dressings are changed every 48 to 72 hours, the indwelling catheter and tubing connection sites should be situated so the change of tubing does not interfere with the integrity of the dressing. The tubing change is made with the patient in a low Fowler's position or flat in bed to prevent an air embolism from occurring with a deep inspiration.

Drug Administration Precautions. No intravenous push or piggyback medications should be given in the same line as the hyperalimentation solution. No steroids, pressor drugs, antibiotics, or other parenteral drugs are ever added to the base solution because they may interact with the fibrin hydrolysate or with one another, forming a precipitate that would not be visible to the naked eye. In addition, the mixing of drugs (other than the electrolytes) in the solution could necessitate adjusting the flow rate according to their requirements rather than those of the nutritional hypertonic solution. If any intravenous medication or blood transfusions are necessary, an alternate route should be started for their administration. Only the hyperalimentation solution with its electrolyte additives added under aseptic conditions should be administered through the central line. The subclavian catheter should not be used to draw blood samples, either. Any break in the system is an entrance for infection; maintaining the sterility of the system is of the utmost importance.

NURSING CARE

Nursing care is based on the patient's individual requirements. The degree of illness may vary from that of the severely burned, critically ill person to that of the postoperative gastrectomy person who is up and about, progressing satisfactorily. Daily weights are recorded; the patient should be weighed with the same scale at the same time each day. Accurate intake and output records give a picture of the patient's fluid balance. Vital signs are taken and recorded depending upon the problems of the patient. Any elevation of body temperature is reported immediately. The intravenous tubing and solution are changed and cultures taken from the discarded tubing and solution. If the fever persists, the treatment may be discontinued and the central catheter removed. A culture is taken immediately from the tip of the catheter. An elevated temperature may be due to an allergic reaction to the nutrients, an infection around the catheter, contamination of the fluid or infusion tubing with resulting septicemia, or the person's own disease process.

Close observation for signs of solution infiltration is a *must*. Any pain or swelling in the area of the catheter insertion must be reported. Activity and ambulation are encouraged whenever possible to decrease the risks of phlebitis, cardiopulmonary problems, and muscle wasting. Lack of exercise and muscle inactivity also lead to a catabolic state with protein breakdown and excretion.

Many persons receiving hyperalimentation therapy are afraid, worried, and anxious. Their reactions to their illness vary greatly, and they need help and support with their psychological needs as well as with their physical and physiological needs.

An expert team is essential for this therapy — the physician, the pharmacist, the nurse — and the nurse is the one who must have the expertise in the administration of TPN.

BIBLIOGRAPHY

Ivey MF: Status of parenteral nutrition. Nurs Clin North Am, June 1979, pp 285–304

Lumb PD et al: Aggressive approach to intravenous feeding of the critical ill patient. Heart Lung, January–February, 1979, pp 71–80

Millam DA: Intravenous therapy. Crit Care Update, December 1979, pp 5–10

Priestnal KW et al: Parenteral nutrition by a subclavian line. Nurs Times, January 1980, pp 78–81

Wilson J et al: Meeting patients' nutritional needs with hyperalimentation. Nursing, September 1979, pp 62–69

Frank Davidoff

Diabetic Emergencies 28

DIABETES: A DISEASE OF DISORDERED NUTRITION

Critically ill diabetic patients present a bewildering array of signs and symptoms: stupor, hyperventilation, vomiting, falling urine output, and unstable blood pressure may all be present and clamoring for attention. The number and complexity of laboratory measurements flashing past may be intimidating. Yet there is a basic coherence to all this metabolic "violence." The route to understanding the disorder lies through an understanding of the physiology of nutrition, for diabetes is a disease of disordered nutrition.

Feeding and Fasting

Nutrition faces two major challenges related to each other but fundamentally different: storage and rerelease. The first arises because ingested nutrients are absorbed from the gastrointestinal (GI) tract over a relatively brief period of time. Under the usual circumstances of daily living, for example, glucose absorption occupies roughly a 3-hour period following each meal, or about one-third of the 24 hours. Most tissues, however, use nutrients fairly constantly, particularly for energy, over the 24 hours. The body must therefore jealously guard the excess nutrient being absorbed, storing it away for use in between feeding times, in order to maintain a relatively constant internal environment. Preventing wastage of ingested nutrient must have been extremely important for survival during evolution, for it led to extraordinarily efficient storage mechanisms. Nutrient storage in the feeding phase of nutrition is appropriately referred to as an *anabolic* state.

After storing incoming nutrient, the body faces an entirely different nutritional task: feeding the tissues from stored reserves. This task is a delicate one: nutrients must be released from storage depots at exactly the right rate. If release is too slow, other tissues may "starve in the midst of plenty." If release exceeds consumption by even a small amount, nutrients are lost, primarily in urine, leading to accelerated depletion of body reserves. If release becomes totally uncontrolled, both consumption and excretion mechanisms become swamped; nutrients accumulate in extracellular fluid, distorting and disfiguring the physiochemical environment that bathes every cell, leading to physiological malfunction, symptoms, and ultimately death.

A key concept in understanding the physiology of the fasting state is the dynamic balance that regulates the release of nutrients. Thus, in general, nutrient release from tissue storage sites does not depend upon a positive signal, such as a hormonal trigger, to call it into action. Rather, the storage tissues left to themselves (*i.e.,* isolated tissues deprived of both nutrient [substrate] input and hormonal signals) spontaneously break down and release their stored nutrients, almost as though it were their fundamental condition to sacrifice their own constituents for "more important" functions elsewhere. Control of this process is achieved by a second, negative hormonal signal, which restrains the rate of nutrient release, setting it precisely to meet the required rate of nutrient demand. It should now be clear why the dynamic balance between spontaneous tissue nutrient release and hormonally controlled damping down of this release in the fasting phase of nutrition is sometimes referred to as an *anticatabolic* state.

It is apparent from our discussion of nutritional physiology so far that at any one moment in the course of a normal 24-hour day the human body can almost never be said to be in nutrient balance. Rather, balance shifts from hour to hour, from moderately positive to moderately negative, and it is only over the course of the entire day that the sum of these positives and negatives begins to approach balance (zero). Indeed, in free-living, healthy adults, energy balance probably approximates zero only in the course of 1 to 2 weeks.[1]

The "Big Head Problem" and the Central Role of Glucose

Apart from a clear understanding of the feeding-fasting duality and its control, one other major concept is necessary to make sense of diabetes and diabetic catastrophes, namely the unique metabolic role of the brain. In humans, the brain is not only disproportionately large, it is also virtually completely dependent upon glucose for its energy supplies, in contradistinction to most other large organs that can easily switch to long-chain free fatty acids and indeed appear to do so in preference to glucose when both substrates are presented together.

This selectivity of the brain for its energy source, sometimes referred to as the *"big head problem,"* is compounded by the fact that, at least in adults, the brain stores almost no glucose (as glycogen).[2] As a result, normal brain function depends from minute to minute upon a supply of glucose from the bloodstream, as evidenced by the almost immediate appearance of cerebral dysfunction when blood sugar falls below normal levels and equally dramatic restoration to normal when blood sugar is raised again. The brain also seems to need its glucose-derived energy at the same rate day and night, waking and sleeping, working and resting, at a rate of about 5 g (1 tsp) per hour, which represents about half of the average daily adult glucose intake.

A number of other tissues are also either relatively dependent (*e.g.,* white blood cells, kidney medulla) or totally dependent (*e.g.,* red blood cells) upon glucose-derived energy, although glucose deprivation does not have such immediate, obvious, or potentially harmful consequences for them as it does for the brain. The problem of feeding the brain thus looms as a task of central importance in human nutritional physiology. In the course of evolution, preserving brain function appears also to have emerged as a development of highest priority, judging from the number and importance of the physiological mechanisms directed primarily at providing energy to the brain, sometimes at the expense of other organs.

In point of fact, the brain, as we shall see, can use one other major energy source, namely *ketone bodies.* These are not a normal dietary constituent, but rather are generated within the body from its own fat stores as a kind of emergency fuel especially adapted to the fasting state.

An understanding of the changing tissue fuel requirements and fuel sources over time (from the fully nourished condition during a meal, through the three phases of increasingly stringent adaptation, to prolonged fasting) provides a high power view of the physiological mechanisms involved in the maintenance of normal nutrition and fleshes out the metabolic scenario needed to understand diabetes.

The Four Phases of Nutrition

THE FED STATE

From the first mouthful of a meal through the absorption of the last of the ingested nutrients from the GI tract, the fed state is characterized by a condition of metabolic plenty. Since most meals for free-living subjects contain a mixture of the three macronutrients, with carbohydrates usually predominating, three different physiological mechanisms are required to store these nutrients, which enter the body in several-fold excess of minute-to-minute need. A limited fraction of carbohydrate not burned immediately is stored as glycogen, both in liver and in muscle; the remainder is promptly converted to fatty acids and glycerol and ultimately packed away as triglyceride in the fat droplets of adipose tissue. Feeding the brain its requisite ration of glucose is obviously no problem under these circumstances.

Dietary fat enters the circulation as chylomicrons, a complex microdroplet fat emulsion, which is cleared primarily for storage directly into adipose tissue. Amino acids are taken up into most tissues in proportion to their need, while amino acids in excess of immediate need are probably stored at least temporarily in a depot of skeletal muscle proteins.[3]

If the meal contains even small quantities of carbohydrate, the metabolic storage response to feeding results in a shutting down of nutrient release from storage depots, and a more or less complete switchover, therefore, to a carbohydrate economy (*i.e.,* primary dependence upon glucose for the energy needs of nearly all tissues). As measured by studies of glucose influx rates, this tide of nutrient influx appears to be largely ended about 3 hours after the meal is started.[4]

THE POSTABSORPTIVE STATE

The term *postabsorptive* is well chosen not only because it describes the timing of this nutritional phase but also because it clearly marks this condition as a normal or physiological daily event, a condition of "noninput" of nutrients, to be distinguished from the rigorous and stressful condition of more prolonged fasting. Once glucose is no longer entering the circulation from the GI tract, the brain must be fed from glucose stored in a tissue that can release it into the circulation for use elsewhere in the body. Liver glycogen is the only such store, and since the glycogen content of the whole liver amounts to only about 75 g, at a utilization rate that decreases slowly from its initial 5 g/hour, this source lasts only about 18 hours. Defined in terms of reliance on liver glycogen, the 15-hour period, from 3 to 18 hours after the last meal, constitutes postabsorptive metabolism.

During these 15 hours, long-chain free fatty acids are released at an increasing rate from adipose tissue, and when presented to most tissues (other than brain, red cells, renal medulla, etc.) are metabolized for energy in preference to glucose. Over the period of the postabsorptive state the body progressively makes the switch from a predominantly carbohydrate to a primarily fat economy. While this change is in part brought about by the decrease in available glucose supplies, it also has the secondary effect of "sparing" glucose from use by most tissues other than the brain.

SHORT FASTING

Gluconeogenesis. As fasting progresses beyond the point of liver glycogen depletion, the brain now must rely on an alternative glucose supply, one in which new glucose is created from precursor substances. The details of this process of *gluconeogenesis* (*neo* = new; *genesis* = creation) and its regulation are extraordinarily complex, but the essentials can be outlined fairly briefly. Glucose, a 6-carbon molecule, can be created anew only from 3-carbon fragments. In mammalian metabolism, this structural constraint has important nutritional and physiological consequences because such 3-carbon compounds can be supplied only from sources other than fatty acids. The 2-carbon units that form the basic structure of fatty acids cannot be combined or rearranged to make new glucose.

Therefore, despite the abundant fat stores in fasting humans, gluconeogenesis must depend upon three nonfat sources for these 3-carbon building blocks: (1) lactate, from partial breakdown of glucose in several peripheral tissues; (2) glycerol, from the degradation of triglyceride stored in adipose tissue; and (3) certain amino acids derived ultimately from tissue proteins. All of these are brought centrally to the liver, the only organ capable of converting these smaller precursors back into glucose and rereleasing it into the bloodstream.

Gluconeogenesis from the first two of the 3-carbon precursors, lactate and glycerol, represents a strict recycling of carbons without a net loss to the body because these 3-carbon molecules are derived in the first place from peripheral glucose metabolism. In contrast, that portion of gluconeogenesis that uses amino acids puts a net drain on body protein stores, since the nitrogen is not reused for the most part, but converted to urea in the liver and excreted in the urine. The overall result of the amino acid-to-glucose conversion is the sacrifice of structural and functional tissue proteins for the primary purpose of providing the brain with its obligatory glucose substrate.

Ketogenesis. The reassembly of 3-carbon fragments to glucose within the liver requires energy, which the liver, like the other tissues, at this point finds most easily available by oxidizing fatty acids from the abundant supply present in the circulation. During fasting, however, the liver uniquely and progressively alters its fatty acid metabolizing mechanism. It no longer oxidizes fatty acids all the way to CO_2 and water, but rather to their constituent 2-carbon fragment, acetate. These acetate molecules recombine, still in the liver, into 4-carbon fatty "by-products," the ketone bodies, acetoacetate and hydroxybutyrate. The ketones then leave the liver and enter the circulation, representing a kind of water-soluble fat, which is used very efficiently for energy by most peripheral tissues. The rate of ketone body consumption by most tissues, particularly the brain, increases in proportion to their level in the circulation.

Ketogenesis and gluconeogenesis are thus seen to be critically important physiological adaptations to the metabolic stress of fasting, and under the usual conditions of fasting the two processes are tightly coupled. The net result of these adaptations is the increasing flow of lactate, glycerol, amino acids, and long-chain fatty acids into the liver, and the net release from the liver of glucose, ketone bodies, and urea.

As fasting progresses beyond 18 hours, the time at which liver glycogen is depleted, the rates of both gluconeogenesis and ketogenesis increase rapidly, reaching a maximum at about 48 to 72 hours following the meal. The circulating level of ketone bodies at this point has risen 10- to 20-fold, from its "fed state" level of about 0.1 mEq/liter to a level of about 1 to 2 mEq/liter, high enough to exceed the renal threshold and produce the characteristic *ketonuria* of fasting. Beyond this time, ketogenesis continues at a steady, rapid rate in the liver, but the consumption of ketone bodies by muscle and adipose tissues diminishes slowly and progressively. As a result, the circulating ketone level continues to rise, reaching a 6 to 7 mEq/liter if fasting is prolonged to 3 weeks, a rise of some 50- to 75-fold above its initial fed level.

PROLONGED FASTING

After about 3 weeks of total fasting, the level of circulating ketone bodies plateaus and remains relatively constant thereafter. Metabolism then enters the phase of prolonged fasting, a more-or-less steady state of adaptation to the most serious metabolic challenge of all, starvation. This adaptation is characterized by its exceedingly tight regulation, geared to maximal preservation of body stores, while at the same time not permitting the composition of nutrients circulating in blood to become too greatly displaced from normal.

The most important result of the many-fold increase in circulating ketones is to make available to the brain an energy alternative to glucose. After 3 to 4 weeks of complete fasting, ketones provide about 60% of the brain's energy supply. The demand for glucose production in the liver is thus lessened by at least this amount, which in turn reduces the drain on body protein stores. As a result, urinary nitrogen excretion drops progressively from 10 g/day in the postabsorptive state to about 3 g/day after prolonged fasting. This spares about 42 g of tissue protein or 150 g of lean tissue weight per day, an adaptation that is obviously critical to prolonged survival. In addition to this specific drop in gluconeogenic requirement, the body adapts to fasting in a more general way by lowering its overall resting metabolic energy requirement about 20%, further sparing endogenous energy and protein reserves.

The circulating level of free fatty acids, which rises to a maximum during the period of short fasting, remains quite constant thereafter, supplying a greater and greater proportion of energy needs in muscle and most visceral tissues other than the brain. Blood glucose levels, in contrast, fall during the first 3 to 4 days of fasting and then remain constant thereafter. The blood sugar levels may go remarkably low during fasting, generally somewhat lower in women than in men, sometimes as low as 25 to 30 mg/dl, without any accompanying symptoms of cerebral disturbance. This is presumably because ketone bodies have partially replaced glucose as the energy supply to the brain.[5,6]

Hormonal Control of Nutritional Physiology

Insulin. Understanding the control of nutritional balance is very much simplified by the realization that both feeding and fasting metabolism are primarily regulated by a single hormone, *insulin*. After a meal, insulin levels rise rapidly into the anabolic range of $50\mu U$ to $100\mu U/ml$, then decline as the surge of entering nutrients is stored (see Fig. 28-1, *A*). At its tissue target sites, these large amounts of insulin directly stimulate a variety of important biochemical storage steps including the rate of glucose entry into insulin-sensitive cells across the plasma membrane and the rate of glycogen, fatty acid, and protein synthesis.

As the postabsorptive state draws on, insulin levels fall into their anticatabolic range of $5\mu U$ to $10\mu U/ml$, about tenfold below the anabolic

range, passing through a "null-point" poised between these two different insulin actions (see Fig. 28-1, *A*). In the anticatabolic range, insulin no longer stimulates storage mechanisms, but rather provides the negative signal that suppresses the otherwise self-sustaining breakdown of glycogen, triglycerides, and protein in a variety of tissues and gluconeogenesis in liver. Of course, insulin in its higher, anabolic range maximally suppresses these catabolic events at the same time it turns on storage mechanisms.

Other hormones besides insulin also play some role in the "fine tuning" or modulation and smoothing of metabolic control. In particular, *glucagon* provides a counterregulatory "pull" to insulin's "push," since glucagon directly stimulates glycogenolysis, lipolysis, and gluconeogenesis in the liver. On a minute-to-minute basis, then, the rates of the major opposing nutrient storage and release processes are regulated by the balance between insulin versus glucagon levels. Moreover, glucocorticoids from the adrenal cortex, catecholamines from the adrenal medulla and peripheral adrenergic neurons, and growth hormone (somatotropin) from the anterior pituitary provide "permissive" control of metabolism both by direct effects on tissues and

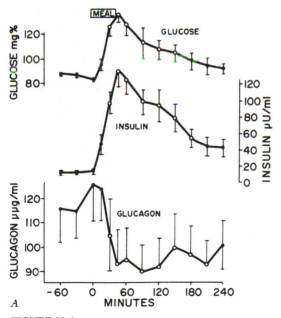

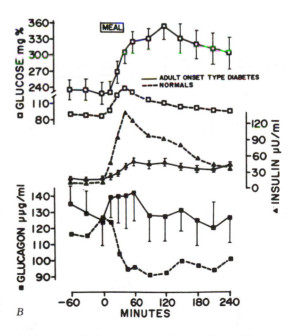

FIGURE 28-1.
Insulin and glucagon responses to eating a large carbohydrate meal. *(A)* Normal subjects. Note the large, early, rapidly rising increase in insulin level, the simultaneous drop in glucagon level, and the moderate, well-damped excursion of blood glucose level. *(B)* Comparison of normal vs. moderate diabetic subjects. Insulin level rises late, sluggishly, and relatively little; glucagon level increases paradoxically, and blood glucose remains at abnormally high levels for a long time in diabetic subjects. (From Müller W et al: Abnormal alpha cell function in diabetes. N Engl J Med 283:109–115, 1970, with permission)

indirect effects on insulin/glucagon release. As a group, these other hormones, like glucagon, all work to stimulate tissue breakdown and nutrient release, in essence, a part of the "stress response."

Despite the importance of these catabolic, or counterregulatory, hormones in normal physiology, the absence of one or another of them seems to be well tolerated, apparently because the presence of the others can compensate for the loss. In contrast, insulin emerges as the only "storage hormone" and hence is uniquely important as the prime regulator of metabolism. Insufficiency of insulin produces a series of disruptions in metabolism collectively referred to as "diabetes mellitus."

THE TWO FORMS OF DIABETES: MILD AND SEVERE

The Basic Disturbance

When insulin secretion becomes slightly impaired, the insulin-secreting β-cells of the pancreatic islets have no difficulty providing the low levels of insulin required to regulate fasting metabolism. Hence, in the mildest forms of diabetes (various terms for this form of diabetes include *chemical diabetes, adult onset-type diabetes, noninsulin-dependent type diabetes*), fasting blood sugar remains *normal*. It is only when the challenge of feeding calls for anabolic levels of insulin that the insulin secretory mechanism of the β-cells is insufficient to a degree. The rate of glucose (and other macronutrient) storage therefore is diminished, and it is this lag in storage that permits glucose to rise to *higher* levels and to return to baseline levels more *slowly* than normal.

These alterations characterize an abnormal glucose tolerance test, the major diagnostic tool for detecting mild diabetes, standing in sharp contrast to the brief, tightly-damped excursions of blood sugar in nondiabetic subjects (see Fig. 28-1, *B*).[7] In the mildest diabetics, all of these nutrients are retained within the body and ultimately taken up into tissues. Overall glucose utilization rates remain normal, and many of these patients therefore can, and do, continue to gain weight.

As insulin secretion capacity declines further, the β-cells cannot even supply the small amounts required in the postabsorptive or fasting states. Fasting metabolism becomes progressively unregulated, resulting not only in complete loss of nutrient storage capacity but in uncontrolled catabolism. Thus, even in the absence of any ingested food, blood sugar rises above normal owing to inappropriately accelerated glycogenolysis and gluconeogenesis. Concomitantly, the rates of lipolysis and ketogenesis become uncontrolled, leading to spiraling levels of ketones in the circulation. As the concentrations of glucose and ketones rise above the renal threshold, these nutrients are lost into the urine, imposing a calorie drain on the body and giving rise first to the glycosuria characteristic of moderate diabetes and, ultimately, the ketonuria of severe diabetes.

In the most severe diabetes (other terms for which include *insulin-dependent diabetes, juvenile onset-type diabetes, ketosis-prone diabetes*), body weight may not be maintained, despite large calorie and protein intakes, and the flesh may be literally melted down and lost through the siphon of the urine (the word *diabetes,* from the Greek meaning "siphon," was first applied to the disease several thousand years ago).

In summary, insulin possesses both anabolic and anticatabolic functions. The anabolic functions of insulin seem to be widely appreciated, since it is intuitively obvious that a storage regulator would be needed to control nutritional physiology during the feeding phase. In contrast, the anticatabolic effects of insulin, which prevent excessive mobilization of stored glucose, fat, and protein, as well as excessive glucose and ketone production during fasting, are generally more difficult to conceptualize. It is therefore somewhat ironic that a defect in secretion of feeding phase insulin produces relatively minimal disruptions in metabolism, while loss of the unimpressive, basal, fasting insulin levels permits the intrinsic catabolic processes of the body to become so unregulated that body substance is lost, distorting the amount and composition of body fluids to the point at which serious illness or even death results. This most extreme form of diabetic abnormality, ketoacidosis, represents the major diabetic emergency.

gone hypophysectomy (thereby removing growth hormone and adrenocorticotropic hormone [ACTH]) or those rendered diabetic by complete pancreatectomy (thereby removing glucagon).

DIABETIC KETOACIDOSIS

For reasons that should now be obvious, diabetic ketoacidosis is sometimes referred to as a state of "accelerated fasting" or "superfasting." Although there are many metabolic complications of this state, the major damage to the patient occurs through pathophysiological changes in three distinct areas: (1) hyperosmolarity, (2) ketoacidosis, and (3) volume depletion (see Fig. 28-2, *A*). These three disturbances interact with one another in certain ways that will soon become apparent (see Fig. 28-2, *B, C, & D*). Initially, however, they can and should be understood separately, not only because each affects the patient in a highly specific manner, but because in any one patient the degree of severity may vary separately from very slight to very severe. Indeed, many patients exhibit a severe abnormality in one area but none at all in the others. In one sense these patients represent metabolic conditions separate and distinct from diabetic ketoacidosis, but in another sense the conditions overlap diabetic ketoacidosis very closely. They will be discussed at the end of this section to highlight each of the component parts of the diabetic ketoacidosis syndrome.

Precipitating Events

While diabetic ketoacidosis can and does occur in patients who have completely lost their capacity to secrete insulin, without other obvious triggering or precipitating factors, it is quite common for stressful events, most commonly infection, sometimes emotional turmoil, to provide the "last straw" that sets the process in motion. The hormonal responses to stress include release of glucagon, glucocorticoids, and catecholamines, all of which, as indicated, drive catabolic processes at accelerated rates. The mechanism by which stress operates to initiate diabetic ketoacidosis is not difficult to envision, therefore. Indeed, even in the virtual absence of insulin secretion it is unusual for diabetic ketoacidosis to develop if these other hormones are also lacking, as in diabetic patients who have under-

Hyperglycemia and Hyperosmolarity

In contrast to normal subjects, whose blood sugars never rise above about 150 mg/dl, or even mild diabetics, in whom the level rarely exceeds 350 to 400 mg/dl, it is not uncommon for patients in diabetic ketoacidosis to exhibit blood sugars of 1000 to 1500 mg/dl. It is clear that the mechanisms that usually protect the body from such catastrophic rises in blood sugar must have broken down completely in such patients. The central mechanism that protects against hyperosmolarity turns out to be renal glucose excretion, the very same mechanism that causes the second type of abnormality in diabetic ketoacidosis, volume depletion (see Fig. 28-3).

As long as the circulating blood volume remains relatively normal, glucose is filtered at the kidney glomerulus into the renal tubules; as long as the filtered glucose load remains relatively small, all of this glucose is reabsorbed back into the bloodstream. When the filtered load increases above a certain level, however, as when the blood sugar exceeds the normal threshold of about 180 mg/dl, glucose begins to escape into the urine because the reabsorption capacity of the tubules is exceeded. As the filtered load increases further, urinary glucose loss increases very rapidly, and nearly all extra glucose put into the circulation thereafter is lost into the urine. This renal "escape valve" serves as a very powerful protective device to prevent extreme accumulation of glucose in blood. Indeed, in diabetic subjects whose circulating blood volume is well maintained, it is extremely unusual to find blood sugar levels in excess of 500 mg/dl because of the intense glucose diuresis.[8] Conversely, *any patient whose blood sugar is higher than this level must be suspected of having either a severely reduced circulating blood volume, renal damage, or both.*

As we shall see, it is glycosuria itself that is largely responsible for volume depletion. In a diabetic patient who is badly out of control and in whom oral replacement of sodium and water has been insufficient to compensate for urinary losses, a vicious cycle is set up in which hyperglycemia leads to volume depletion, which, uncompensated, in turn reduces urinary glucose losses, which again permits the blood sugar to rise even higher.

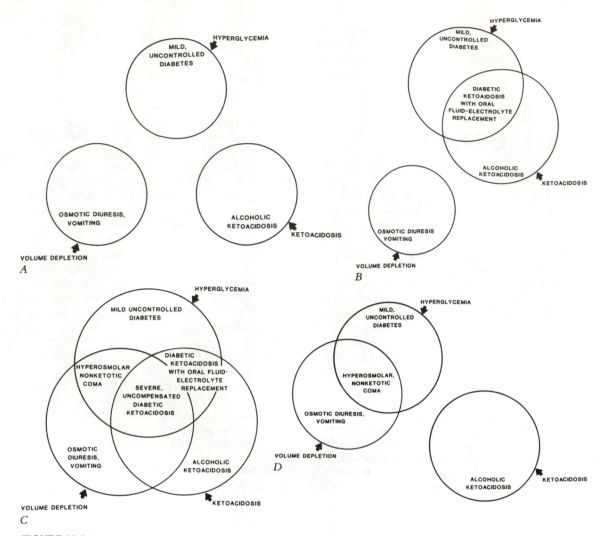

FIGURE 28-2.
The pathophysiological components of diabetic ketoacidosis and their several interactions. *(A)* The three major pathophysiological components, viewed as distinct elements. *(B)* Modified diabetic ketoacidosis: hyperglycemia and ketoacidosis are present, but volume depletion is minimal. Volume depletion may be prevented either because oral water and electrolyte intake have been sufficient to replace losses or because the syndrome developed very rapidly. Blood sugar and ketone levels can rise quickly, while it takes considerable time for osmotic diuresis to deplete the body of water and electrolytes. Therefore, patients seen early may be less volume depleted than those who have been developing the condition for many days or even weeks. *(C)* Full-blown diabetic ketoacidosis. All three pathophysiological elements make major contribution. *(D)* Hyperosmolar nonketotic coma: hyperglycemia, hyperosmolality, and volume depletion always are present, often to extreme degree, but ketosis is absent or trivial, by definition.

It appears to be the hyperosmolarity of body fluids itself, resulting from this upward spiral in blood sugar, rather than ketosis, acidosis, or volume depletion that primarily accounts for the lethargy, stupor, and, ultimately, coma that occur as diabetic ketoacidosis worsens. The evidence for this conclusion rests on the general correlation between degree of hyperosmolarity and degree of coma, in contrast to preserved mental function in states in which pure ketoacidosis exists without hyperosmolarity.[9,10]

The development of hyperglycemia, hyperosmolarity, and coma in diabetic ketoacidosis is schematically outlined in the left and center portions of Figure 28-3.

Ketosis and Acidosis
The second major consequence of severe insulin deficiency is uncontrolled ketogenesis. As ketoacids enter the extracellular fluid, the hydrogen ion is stripped from the molecule (see Equation 1

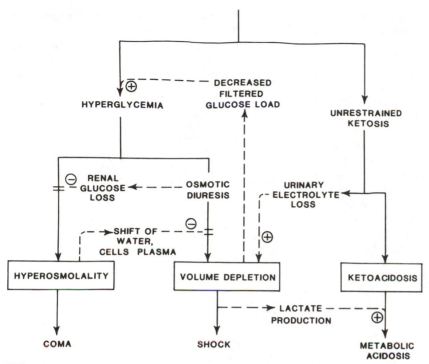

FIGURE 28-3.

The metabolic consequences of severe insulin deficiency and their interrelations leading to diabetic ketoacidosis. Dashed arrows represent secondary interactions which reduce (−) or aggravate (+) the severity of primary disturbances.

below) and neutralized by combining with bicarbonate ion buffer, thus protecting the pH of extracellular fluids and leaving behind ketoacid anion residues. The resultant carbonic acid (see Equation 2) breaks down into water and CO_2 gas, which literally "fizzes" out through the lungs.

Equation 1:
$$\text{H}^+\text{-acetoacetic acid} \atop \text{H}^+\text{-}\beta\text{-hydroxybutyric acid} \Big\}$$
$$= \text{HCO}_3^- \rightarrow \text{H}_2\text{CO}_3^+$$
$$\Big\{ \text{acetoacetate}^- \atop \beta\text{-hydroxybutyrate}^-$$

Equation 2:
$$\text{H}_2\text{CO}_3 \rightarrow \text{H}_2\text{O} + \text{CO}_2 \text{ gas } (\uparrow)$$

Therefore, as ketoacid anions accumulate, they progressively displace bicarbonate from extracellular fluid. The usual laboratory determination of electrolytes does not measure ketoacid concentrations directly. However, an excess of total measured cations (sodium plus potassium) over total measured anions (chloride plus bicarbonate) provides a clue to the presence of these so-called unmeasured anions. This excess, sometimes referred to as the *anion gap,* can serve as an indirect measure of the quantity of ketoacids present.

A total of 6 to 7 mEq/liter of ketoacids, which would reduce serum bicarbonate from its usual 25 mEq/liter down to 18 to 19 mEq/liter, seems to be well tolerated by most diabetic patients. Since, as we have seen, prolonged fasting alone can cause a physiologic, starvation ketosis of this degree, it seems logical to consider this a *mild* degree of ketoacidosis when it is produced by uncontrolled diabetes rather than by starvation.

In the range of 6 to 15 mEq/liter of ketone bodies, with corresponding bicarbonate levels of 10 to 19 mEq/liter, the buffering and acid-compensating mechanisms of the body become more seriously stressed, but in this range pH usually remains at least partially protected. Ketoacidosis of this degree is never physiologic, and when due to diabetes it can therefore be considered to be *moderate* in degree. Once the bicarbonate level goes below 10 mEq/liter owing to ketoacid accumulations greater than 15 mEq/liter, the protection against acidosis rapidly reaches its outer limit, and even slight interference with compensating mechanisms can send body pH plummeting down to very low levels. Ketoacidosis of this degree (15 mEq/liter of ketoacid accumulation) is obviously severe and life-threatening.

HYPERVENTILATION

The neutrality of body fluids is primarily protected by the bicarbonate buffering system, which determines the pH at all times by the ratio of bicarbonate anion to CO_2 gas in plasma. If bicarbonate anion is lost due to its displacement by ketoacid anions, extra CO_2 gas must be driven off at the lung by hyperventilation in order to keep the ratio at or close to its usual value of 20:1 and to maintain pH close to its physiologic value of 7.4. Hyperventilation, gradual at first, then rapidly more vigorous and more obvious as arterial pH drops below 7.2, is therefore a characteristic physical finding in diabetic ketoacidosis. This dramatic increase in ventilation, which occurs more by an increase in the *depth* than in the *frequency* of breathing, is known as *Kussmaul breathing*. The presence of clear-cut Kussmaul breathing is therefore a signal that extracellular fluid pH is at or below 7.2, a relatively severe degree of acidosis.[11]

The outer limit of compensation for a declining bicarbonate buffer reserve is imposed by the maximal rate of hyperventilation that the lungs can achieve. At the usual rates of total CO_2 production by the body, the lungs breathe fast enough to drive the total CO_2 gas level in blood down to about one-fourth of its normal value but not lower. Hyperventilation can therefore compensate, at least partially, for bicarbonate levels as low as 6 to 8 mEq/liter, one-fourth of its normal range of 24 to 32 mEq/liter. As bicarbonate drops below that level, however, CO_2 gas remains disproportionately high relative to bicarbonate, and pH then drops at an alarming rate. It is for this reason that bicarbonate levels below 10 mEq/liter are taken as an indicator of severe acidosis and call for more aggressive therapy.

TESTING FOR SERUM KETONES

Serum ketones can be measured semiquantitatively at the bedside by testing progressive dilutions of serum with *nitroprusside reagent* (powder or crushed tablets).[12] This maneuver serves several important purposes: first, it rapidly helps to confirm the *diagnosis* of diabetic ketoacidosis once it has been suggested by history, physical exam, and urine testing; second, it is possible to make a rough assessment of *degree* of ketoacidosis, at least to the extent of categorizing it as mild, moderate, or severe; and third, a major discrepancy between the amount of ketones estimated by the serum nitroprusside procedure and the total anion gap calculated from the electrolytes determined in the laboratory suggests the presence of a *second unmeasured anion,* usually lactate, contributing to the acidosis in addition to ketoacids.

KIDNEY ACTION

Finally, since ketoacids are excreted in the urine largely as their sodium, potassium, and ammonium salts, the loss of ketones through the kidneys contributes to the problems of water and electrolyte losses, the third important category of physiological damage in diabetic ketoacidosis. The development of metabolic acidosis in diabetic ketoacidosis is outlined on the right side of Figure 28-3.

Fluid and Electrolyte Losses: Volume Depletion

OSMOTIC DIURESIS

While glucose loss through the kidneys helps to protect against the ravages of extreme hyperosmolarity, the diabetic patient developing ketoacidosis pays a price for this glycosuria. Glucose remaining in the glomerular filtrate, after the renal tubules have reabsorbed all they can, forces water to remain in the tubules. This glucose-rich filtrate then sweeps on out of the body, carrying with it water, sodium, potassium, ammonium, phosphate, and other salts. The resulting rapid urine flow and obligate loss of water and electrolytes that would otherwise be reabsorbed is known as an *osmotic diuresis*. Salts of ketone bodies, as well as the urea resulting from rapid protein breakdown and accelerated gluconeogenesis, also contribute to the solute load in the renal tubule, further aggravating the diuresis.

SALT AND WATER LOSS

The average amounts of salts and water lost to the body through osmotic diuresis during the development of diabetic ketoacidosis have been measured directly. These numbers serve as important markers for understanding the degree of physiological damage done to the patient.[13] Overall water loss in a 70-kg adult patient presenting in diabetic ketoacidosis amounts to about 6 to 7 liters, or 15% of total body water. Of this, about 3 liters are derived from the extracellular compartment, judging from the accompanying average loss of 420 mEq of *sodium* and assuming the sodium concentration of normal extracellular fluid is 140 mEq/liter. This represents a loss of at least 20% of extracellular water, which is a very major insult to the integrity of the body fluids. Another 3 liters is derived from the intracellular space, as indicated by the loss of 300 mEq of *potassium,* the major intracellular cation, since the potassium concentration within cells is normally about 100 mEq/liter.

The fluid lost to the body is slightly hypotonic, meaning that it contains a slight excess of water over salts, as would be expected from an osmotic diuresis due to glucose and urea. These figures, as noted, represent averages. The *net* losses found in any particular patient will be the result of many different factors, among them the intensity and duration of the hyperglycemia and, hence, the intensity of osmotic diuresis; the amount of water and electrolyte replaced by mouth during this time; the presence of other fluid and electrolyte losses such as vomiting, diarrhea, or sweating; and the integrity of renal function (see Fig. 28-2, *B*).

COMPENSATORY MECHANISMS

Sodium and water make up the central structure of the extracellular fluid, including the vascular volume. Removal of these large quantities of sodium and water from the body is therefore perceived as a serious threat to the maintenance of the circulation, and a variety of compensatory mechanisms are called into play to prevent vascular collapse and shock. For example, an increase in pulse rate usually occurs, which helps to maintain cardiac output in the face of shrinking intravascular volume.

Much more important, however, is a protective shift in body fluid brought about by the hyperglycemia itself. Because free glucose is limited almost entirely to the extracellular water, an osmotic pressure gradient is set up across the cell membrane, between the extracellular compartment and the interior of the cells. Therefore, the higher the blood sugar, the more water is drawn out of cells and into the extracellular space. Thus, as sodium and water are lost into the urine, shrinking the extracellular fluid, they are, in effect, "replaced," at least as to their osmotic effect, by glucose entering from the liver and by water entering from all cells, which reexpand the extracellular fluid again (see Fig. 28-3, *left*).

The very hyperosmolarity that produces damaging central nervous system (CNS) effects and osmotic diuresis therefore provides at least a partial and temporary mechanism for preventing vascular collapse, an important "prop" to the structure of the extracellular fluid in ketoacidosis. It is, however, a rather shaky one because of its rapid reversal when blood glucose is lowered again.

ADVERSE EFFECTS

Despite these efforts at compensation, circulatory integrity is progressively compromised as diabetic ketoacidosis progresses, leading ultimately to a series of secondary pathologic changes, some of which, in turn, develop into self-perpetuating, vicious spirals.

Decrease in Glomerular Filtration. First, loss of vascular volume produces a fall in glomerular filtration, which is why the usual measures of renal function, including blood urea nitrogen (BUN) or creatinine levels, are characteristically elevated in ketoacidotic patients. We have already seen how decreasing renal function permits blood glucose levels to spiral to extreme values (see Fig. 28-3, *center*), but other consequences, particularly difficulty in controlling potassium excretion, also result from this change. Since the excretion of potassium by the kidney occurs by the exchange of potassium for sodium, adequate sodium must be present at the exchange site in the kidney for the rate of potassium excretion to keep pace with the need for excretion. When vascular volume is diminished and renal perfusion reduced in consequence, not enough sodium may be available for this exchange. Despite a total body depletion of potassium, the serum potassium level may therefore rise above normal, even to dangerous or lethal levels.

Decrease in Tissue Perfusion. A second major consequence of diminished vascular volume is a generalized decrease in tissue perfusion. Well before the drop in volume has reached the point at which blood pressure actually falls and full-blown shock is said to be present, blood is shunted away from many tissues, and the perfusion of nearly all tissues suffers. The resultant decrease in oxygen delivery causes those tissues to shift to some degree of anaerobic glucose metabolism, resulting in the increased production of lactic acid. The release of this second organic acid into the circulation simply lowers the bicarbonate further, aggravating the already existing metabolic acidosis (see Fig. 28-3, *right*). A combined lactic acidosis and ketoacidosis is not an uncommon finding, therefore, in patients with diabetic ketoacidosis.

Phosphate Loss. Tissue hypoxia due to decreased tissue perfusion may be aggravated indirectly in ketoacidosis as the result of urinary loss of another electrolyte, phosphate. As body phosphate stores are depleted, circulating phosphate levels fall quite low in plasma, depriving the red cells of an essential reactant used to form a variety of organic phosphate compounds. Under these circumstances, red cells become depleted of certain key phosphate derivatives, which in turn increases the tightness of oxygen binding to the hemoglobin within those cells. As these cells pass through the poorly perfused tissues, less oxygen is given up than from red cells with a normal complement of phosphate compounds, and tissue hypoxia is worsened.

Shock. Finally, if vascular volume falls low enough, compensation mechanisms fail, blood pressure drops, and true shock supervenes. A rapidly worsening cycle of acidosis, tissue damage, and deepening shock may then occur, leading ultimately to irreversible vascular collapse and death. The full-blown syndrome of diabetic ketoacidosis is characterized by major contributions from all three major pathophysiological disruptions (see Fig. 28-2, *C*), each of which is primarily responsible for one of the major clinical features: coma, shock, and metabolic acidosis (see Fig. 28-3).

THERAPY

Rational and effective therapy for diabetic ketoacidosis must be based on an understanding of the mechanisms of metabolic damage, both primary and secondary, as outlined above. Each therapeutic maneuver is directed primarily at one of the three areas of physiological disruption. However, it should be clear by now (see Figs. 28-2 and 28-3) that none of these disruptions exists completely separate from the others. Hence, therapy which reverses one abnormality may also have important *benefits and risks* in other areas because of their interlocking nature.

Volume: Salt and Water Replacement

The most immediate threat to life in a critically ill ketoacidotic patient is *volume depletion*. Once the diagnosis is even seriously considered, the first priority is always to get a large, secure intravenous line in place. A cutdown may be necessary in a severely dehydrated patient almost in shock because veins may be collapsed and hard to find. As soon as this line is estab-

lished, 0.9% (normal) saline is rapidly infused. The goal is to reverse the worst of the extracellular volume depletion as soon as possible. Infusing the first liter in one hour is not too fast a rate, since this will replace only one-third of the extracellular loss in the average patient and even less in others who are more dehydrated. Other plasma expanders, such as albumin or plasma concentrates, may be necessary if low blood pressure and other clinical signs of vascular collapse do not respond properly to saline alone.

Assessment. Once volume replacement is initiated, there is time to plan the remainder of therapy in a somewhat more considered fashion. At this point, an assessment of the severity of total volume depletion can be made. The history, intensity, and duration of symptoms; amount of oral intake; presence of other fluid losses through vomiting and so forth; and documentation of the amount of weight actually lost will all provide important clues to the seriousness of volume depletion. The physical examination provides additional information: decreased tissue turgor (sometimes even to the extent of softened consistency of the eyeballs in severely dehydrated patients), tachycardia, decreased sweating, and postural or supine hypotension all help to confirm the extent of volume loss. A numerical estimate of total body fluid loss is extremely valuable in planning phased therapy (*e.g.*, the fraction of loss to be replaced over each time interval).

Goals of Volume Replacement. Volume replacement is not only critical to preserving the integrity of the circulation, it is also instrumental in treating hyperglycemia, preventing hyperkalemia, and reducing lactic acidosis. Because any patient with a blood sugar significantly above 450 to 500 mg/dl became that way in large part because of volume depletion severe enough to prevent compensatory renal glucose loss, it makes physiological sense to rely on volume replacement for restoration of that glucose excretory mechanism. Quite recently, it has been conclusively demonstrated that the fall in blood sugar during treatment of diabetic ketoacidosis is about 80% attributable to glucose loss into the urine, rather than being primarily the result of insulin-induced changes in glucose production and comsumption.[14] This is not to say that insulin effects are trivial in treating ketoacidosis, but rather that in the earliest phases of treatment insulin therapy *complements* proper fluid and electrolyte replacement.

Finally, it is well to remember that volume losses will continue throughout the first several hours of therapy as long as glycosuria and the osmotic diuresis are not completely controlled. Volume replacement must therefore restore not only the deficits that *exist* at the time of the patient's arrival, but also those that continue to be *created* during therapy, before full metabolic control is achieved.

Insulin

Since the primary deficit leading to diabetic ketoacidosis in the first place is severe insulin deficiency, insulin obviously stands as a key component of successful therapy. Indeed, until the advent of insulin, diabetic ketoacidosis was almost never fully reversible and was usually fatal.

Several metabolic effects of insulin are of special importance to therapy of ketoacidosis. First, insulin promptly shuts off the supply of free fatty acids emerging from adipose tissue, thereby restricting the production of ketones at its source. Second, insulin directly inhibits hepatic gluconeogenesis, preventing further addition of glucose to an already overburdened extracellular fluid. Simultaneously, hepatic ketogenesis is further reduced, which assures the ultimate reversal of the ketoacidosis itself. Third, insulin restores cellular protein synthesis. Although this effect occurs more slowly, it in turn permits the restoration of normal potassium, magnesium, and phosphate stores within tissues.

Insulin induces a relatively limited increase in tissue glucose uptake during the therapy of diabetic ketoacidosis.[15] It is therefore primarily the *anticatabolic* effects of insulin, the reduction of glucose and ketone *inflow,* which are important in the early part of therapy. When glucose and ketones are no longer entering the extracellular fluid, the body is then in a position to reduce hyperglycemia and ketonemia both by urine losses and continuing tissue consumptions. The *anabolic* effects of insulin have little role early in the therapy of ketoacidosis, becoming much more important in later phases.

Cautions. The extremely high glucose values found initially in patients with diabetic ketoacidosis are psychologically distressing to contemplate. It is always tempting, therefore, to choose a course of therapy that will reduce the blood sugar as quickly as possible. However, there are two good reasons to avoid dropping the blood sugar too fast or too far, particularly if the approach to its lowering is primarily to rely on insulin without sufficient simultaneous volume replacement.

In the first instance, recall that large quantities of glucose in the extracellular space draw water out of cells; glucose and water together partially reexpand the volume lost from osmotic diuresis of sodium and water (see Fig. 28-3). Sudden and rapid lowering of the blood sugar with insulin, through a combination of increased tissue uptake plus decreased gluconeogenesis, allows water to move very rapidly back into cells, withdrawing the prop to extracellular volume and provoking potentially catastrophic vascular collapse.[16] The sequence of events highlights in yet another way *the importance of early volume replacement with sodium and water,* preceding or concurrent with insulin therapy.

The second problem arises in patients with prolonged, severe hyperglycemia, in whom large quantities of glucose (or glucose-derived compounds) accumulate slowly within the brain.[17] Compared with water, these compounds are only poorly permeating. Hence, if the blood sugar is lowered too fast and too far (below about 250 mg/dl), particularly without sufficient electrolyte replacement in extracellular fluid, water is freed up to move into the brain, drawn by the accumulated intracerebral glucose metabolites. The result may be cerebral edema, with a worsening of coma instead of the expected improvement as the blood sugar falls.

High vs. Low Dosage. In the past, insulin was used in relatively large doses, such as 200 to 400 units in the first 24 hours, usually in intravenous bolus doses, in treating diabetic ketoacidosis; this was based on the theory that "insulin resistance" was present. Although such high-dose insulin therapy was generally quite successful, it has become apparent with further experience over the years that lower doses are often equally effective, particularly when given by continuous intravenous infusion or intramuscular injection rather than by the conventional intravenous bolus or subcutaneous doses.[18] As the trend toward ever lower doses has grown, considerable controversy has developed concerning the optimal dose and route of insulin therapy.

Perhaps the most useful position at this point is to be aware of the pitfalls of both the high- and low-dose approaches and to adopt general guidelines to therapy of ketoacidosis that are necessary to avoid the worst of these. When looked upon in this fashion, the controversy appears to be somewhat of a "tempest in an IV bottle."

The following set of principles may be applied in attempting to achieve optimal therapy:

- An initial loading dose of insulin is rational to fill tissue insulin binding sites and to assure initiation of insulin action.
- The major drawback of low-dose insulin therapy is the possibility of undertreating: some patients are much less responsive to insulin than others, and at the outset there is no way to distinguish those who will be, in fact, somewhat more insulin-resistant. It therefore cannot be assumed that all patients will respond appropriately to low doses. Moreover, there is no intrinsic virtue to using the lowest possible dose: insulin is cheap and nontoxic.
- The major drawbacks of high-dose therapy are as listed above and are less a function of excessive insulin *per se* than of insufficient recognition of volume depletion and insufficiently aggressive volume replacement. Although late hypoglycemia is also somewhat more likely with high-dose insulin, hypoglycemia is easily prevented if intravenous glucose is added to the regimen at the appropriate time; it is easily detected if the patient is carefully watched, and it is easily treated.
- Whatever insulin dose and route are chosen, changes in blood sugar and clinical state should indicate a clear-cut, beneficial response before it can be assumed that the chosen therapy is effective. If blood sugar does not drop, and blood pressure and urine output do not stabilize, insulin or fluid therapy may not have been adequate. There is *no* substitute for the ancient and honorable practice of close patient monitoring.

Potassium and Phosphate Replacement

All patients in diabetic ketoacidosis are deficient in total body potassium stores to a greater or lesser degree. Yet because the renal handling of potassium excretion is the main minute-to-minute determinant of the serum potassium level, patients may have initial serum potassium levels ranging all the way from very low to very high. Potassium replacement must be withheld until an accurate measurement of this level is reported back from the laboratory. Beginning intravenous K^+ therapy in the presence of unrecognized hyperkalemia and inadequate renal mechanisms for handling potassium loads can rapidly lead to a fatal outcome. Although the electrocardiogram (ECG) can provide bedside clues to the presence of high or low K^+ levels, there is enough room for error in its interpretation to discourage a decision about K^+ therapy based on the ECG alone.

If the initial serum potassium level is low, intravenous K^+ is generally begun right away. This is particularly important because both insulin and saline can be predicted to drive the K^+ even lower, possibly to dangerously low levels at which skeletal muscle paralysis and cardiac arrest may occur. If the initial K^+ is normal or high, intravenous K^+ is generally withheld until it is clear that the level has begun to drop *and* that urine flow is established.

Failure of the K^+ to fall can occur because of (1) persistent, uncorrected acidosis (which drives K^+ out of cells and into extracellular fluid); (2) as we have discussed, intrinsically impaired renal function; or, (3) perhaps most importantly, insufficient restoration of circulating volume.

Phosphate levels generally also drop during therapy, aggravating any preexisting tendency of red cells to bind oxygen more tightly. Although in most patients this is not felt to be an effect of major importance, some phosphate replacement seems reasonable. Therefore, many patients now receive phosphate in the middle and later phases of therapy, usually combined with K^+ replacement, by adding potassium phosphate salts to the intravenous infusion.

Bicarbonate: Pro and Con

Patients with mild or moderate ketoacidosis who are properly and promptly treated with salt, water, and insulin will eventually excrete and metabolize the ketone bodies remaining in extracellular fluid. As this process continues, bicarbonate anions are increasingly reabsorbed from the renal tubules to replace the disappearing unmeasured anions, and the bicarbonate deficit is slowly repaired. This self-induced recovery is quite satisfactory in the majority of ketoacidotic patients. Sometimes the large amounts of chloride administered along with the sodium in intravenous saline may produce a confusing but transient hyperchloremia and delay for several days the full return of the bicarbonate level to normal.

For patients with the most severe degrees of acidosis, whose bicarbonate levels are initially 10 mEq/liter or lower, concern arises about a relatively sudden decompensation of buffering capacity, with resultant rapid worsening of the acidosis. In these patients it makes sense to infuse bicarbonate intravenously early in the course of therapy. The deficit in bicarbonate can be calculated quite exactly and an appropriate amount given intravenously over several hours to raise the level at least to the 10 to 12 mEq/liter range.[19]

Possible CNS Acidosis. The major risk to rapid correction of the acidosis by bicarbonate replacement arises from yet another imbalance or disequilibrium between the extracellular fluids of the body and those surrounding the brain, resulting from unequal rates of movement of certain molecules across the blood-brain barrier. In this instance, bicarbonate moves into the brain-associated fluids much more slowly than CO_2 gas (plus H_2CO_3). As a result, the expected and desired parallel rise of both HCO_3^- and CO_2 that occurs elsewhere in the body during treatment does not occur in the cerebral compartment, but CO_2 (and H_2CO_3) rises more quickly than HCO_3^-. The net result is a shift in the HCO_3^-/CO_2 ratio that drives the cerebral fluid pH down, producing a paradoxical, though again transient, worsening of cerebral acidosis. This CNS acidosis may then be manifested clinically by deepening stupor or coma in a patient whose arterial pH seems to be improving. Fortunately, a major degree of cerebral impairment due to this pH disequilibrium is unusual, and the central acidosis corrects itself with time if the patient is otherwise supported.

General Care

LOOKING FOR PRECIPITATING CAUSES

Proper metabolic management alone does not assure a favorable outcome in patients with diabetic ketoacidosis: a number of aspects of general care are at least as critical. To begin with, a careful search for precipitating causes is always necessary, not only with an eye to preventing future episodes, but because the ketoacidosis may not respond well even to aggressive metabolic therapy if an underlying problem, particularly infection, remains undetected and untreated.

Two of the most difficult and confusing areas in clinical assessment are the frequent occurrence of abdominal symptoms (nausea, vomiting, abdominal pain, tenderness, and rigidity) and the interpretation of stupor or coma.

ABDOMINAL SYMPTOMS

Gastric motility is greatly impaired as diabetic ketoacidosis develops; gastric distention with stagnant, dark, heme-positive "crankcase oil" fluid is therefore quite common. Vomiting, with the ever-present threat of aspiration, particularly in the stuporous patient, can be a significant problem. Nasogastric intubation for decompression may therefore be very useful, both in reducing discomfort and in minimizing the risk of aspiration, as long as it is done with proper care to avoid aspiration during passage of the tube.

Conscious patients are often *extremely* thirsty, but it is a mistake to give in initially to their pleas for water: adding fluid to an already distended stomach inevitably leads to worsening of abdominal distress and usually to vomiting. Reassurance that the thirst will pass as therapy progresses and providing ice chips to minimize the sensation of thirst are more humane and appropriate in the long run.

Severe abdominal pain, tenderness, and ileus frequently prove to be due to the ketoacidosis itself, but initially may be hard to distinguish from an intra-abdominal catastrophe such as perforated viscus, which may have precipitated the ketoacidosis. A similar problem arises in interpreting stupor or coma: did intracerebral bleeding or infection precipitate both the acidosis and the coma, or did the acidosis produce coma? Lumbar puncture may be the only way to obtain reassurance on this point, primarily by looking for evidence of infection: meningitis, encephalitis, or brain abscess. Blood, urine, and throat cultures are almost always appropriate in the general search for infection.

COMA CARE

The principles of coma care are really no different for the severely ill ketoacidotic patient than for any other. The primary point of emphasis during this care is the concern for vomiting and aspiration. Proper positioning on the side, continuous close observation, and the ready availability of a nasopharyngeal suctioning apparatus are the keys to avoiding aspiration. Nasogastric intubation may safely be carried out in patients who are conscious and who have a good gag reflex, but for stuporous or comatose patients a cuffed endotracheal tube should be in place before any attempts are made to pass a nasogastric tube.

MANAGING BLADDER FUNCTION

A similarly knotty problem arises in managing bladder function in ketoacidotic patients. On the one hand, early access to bladder urine is of extreme importance: first, it may be of tremendous help in making the earliest possible diagnosis; second, urinary tract infection is not uncommonly the trigger event, and must be sought; third, knowing that urine flow is established is critical to assessment of circulatory competence and to the decision for potassium therapy. Later in treatment, monitoring urine flow, sugar, and acetone levels is a very useful complement to measurements of plasma metabolites and fluid balance.

On the other hand, catheterization of the bladder always introduces the risk of urinary infection and may not be necessary for achieving the above goals. In the conscious patient who can voluntarily void, catheterization is really not necessary. Therefore, every effort should be made to obtain urine samples in such patients without catheterization, recognizing that in long-standing diabetes, a neurogenic bladder with incomplete bladder emptying is commonly present. Urine specimens in such patients may provide imperfect sampling of their metabolic condition, and interpretation of volumes or tests should be appropriately cautious.

If catheterization is absolutely necessary, an indwelling catheter connected to closed drainage is perfectly acceptable and certainly useful. Its presence should never be ignored, however, and a conscious effort should be made to remove it at the earliest possible opportunity; the longer it remains in place, the greater the risk of bladder sepsis. Repeated straight catheterizations may provide the requisite information with less risk of infection, but whatever catheterization program is chosen, scrupulous aseptic technique for insertion is of prime importance.

FLOW SHEETS

It should be apparent by now that management of diabetic ketoacidosis depends on an unusually large and complex amount of numerical information. Measurements are needed in many separate but interacting areas. These measurements must be expressed in fairly precise numbers and must be repeated over time. Important therapeutic decisions depend upon trends in these numbers and their response to treatment.

There is no way in which information of this amount and importance can properly be handled if it is kept largely in the physician's head, on the individual lab reports, or even in the progress notes in the body of the record. A separate flow sheet must be set up that displays the key data,

including vital signs, blood chemistries, urine tests, fluid balance, and medications, in neat and orderly fashion according to time. The flow sheet serves a more general secondary function as well, by focusing attention on the *need for continuous monitoring until the patient is clinically and chemically improved.*

Phases of Care

Although there are no sharp lines between them, the course of management of diabetic ketoacidosis naturally divides itself into several phases.

First Phase.   The first phase consists of the immediate effort to establish the diagnosis and, once ketoacidosis is even strongly suspected, to assure that life-preserving therapy is begun. An abbreviated history from family or friends of an unconscious patient, a search for a diabetic identification card or jewelry, a rapid assessment for clinical clues of volume depletion and Kussmaul respiration, and blood drawing for initial chemistries should not take more than a few moments. Blood sugar by glucose oxidase strip (Dextrostix) and serum ketone measurements at the bedside may really be all that are required to clinch the diagnosis. While these are being performed, the best possible intravenous line is established, and volume replacement is begun.

Second Phase.   Once this first phase is completed a second phase of more considered assessment and therapy begins: details of the history and physical exam, including the careful search for precipitating causes, should be obtained while awaiting the more complete laboratory assessment. Cultures, ECG, and appropriate roentgenograms are performed at this point. The flow sheet is set up, and decisions made about coma care, intubation, and catheterization.

Third Phase.   A third phase is then entered in which the worst of the metabolic damage is repaired. This phase lasts roughly 8 to 24 hours, depending upon how sick the patient is on admission and how responsive he proves to be to therapy. The goal during this phase is *not* to achieve complete correction of all the abnormalities. Indeed, as we have seen, excessive speed of correction can be hazardous, particularly in patients in whom ketoacidosis has been developing gradually over a long period of time, since the body's adaptations to the metabolic insults are not all immediately reversible and overly aggressive therapy may actually make some problems worse.

The key difficulties to be watched for during this phase are

- *Worsening stupor or coma.* Aside from the possibility of CNS infection or stroke, the major concerns are for osmotic or *p*H disequilibrium from excessively rapid correction of blood sugar or bicarbonate. The most important clue here is clinical worsening of mental state in the face of "chemical" improvement.
- *Hypotension.* Certainly sepsis, myocardial infarction, and other causes of shock must be looked for, but again, rapid reduction of blood sugar without sufficient sodium and water replacement may be responsible.
- *Hyperkalemia.* Early occlusion of the arterial supply to a limb, not rare in diabetics with severe peripheral vascular disease and easily overlooked in a comatose, hypotensive patient, can permit leakage of large amounts of potassium into the circulation, producing or aggravating hyperkalemia. The limbs should therefore be monitored for asymmetric pallor, coldness, rubor, and so forth. More often, hyperkalemia results from premature K^+ infusion, persistent acidosis, and insufficient volume replacement.

Fourth Phase. Finally, a fourth phase arrives in which the patient's clinical state is stable or improving and the majority of the metabolic abnormalities are reversed. The completion or recovery then takes place over a period of about 12 days and includes repletion of body stores of many nutrients, including magnesium, protein, phosphate, and so forth, as cell constituents are resynthesized.[20]

Once it is clear that GI tract function is restored, oral replacement is not only desirable but necessary to provide all of the complex nutrition required for recovery, but oral feedings should be withheld until gastric distention is gone and intestinal motility clearly present. It is during this phase that attention should be directed at *preventing* future recurrences of diabetic ketoacidosis.

Prevention

Often overlooked, prevention is really one of the most important aspects of diabetic ketoacidosis management. In fact, it can easily be argued that not only is diabetic ketoacidosis unpleasant, dangerous, and expensive, it is also unnecessary,

since, in theory, it should always be preventable. In practical terms, of course, there is probably no way in which all episodes can be prevented, particularly in previously undiagnosed diabetics in whom the disease is not even suspected. In many other patients, however, the recurrence of ketoacidosis represents an admission of failure in management.

Prevention of diabetic ketoacidosis breaks down into two aspects: outpatient and inpatient.

AMBULATORY CARE

In outpatient settings, there are no great mysteries to successful prevention: what is needed is not sporadic application of complicated measures but consistent use of a few simple rules. The most important of these are the following:

Patient Education. Ideally, patients and their families should understand enough about the mechanism and meaning of ketoacidosis to be able to avoid those things that are likely to bring it about, to recognize its approach, to slow it down or minimize its development, and to go for help fast, if it does begin to happen.

Perhaps the most common avoidable mistake arises from lack of appreciation of the importance of insulin's *anticatabolic effects.* Most ketosis-prone patients easily and intuitively accept the need for insulin injections if they are hungry and eating well but have considerable difficulty in recognizing their insulin need when they are ill, anorectic, not eating, or actually vomiting.

Every such patient needs to be instructed repeatedly that

- His body, like that of any nondiabetic person, *must have insulin, even if no food is being taken in.*
- The amount of insulin required in the postabsorptive or fasting state alone is about half of the total he would need if he were eating, although when fasting, it must be spread out as an insulin "trickle" rather than given in insulin "bursts."
- Illness generally increases insulin need, so that even if not eating, he may actually require more than 50% of his usual daily dose.
- If insulin is taken in restricted doses (two split doses of intermediate-acting insulin in 24 hours), insulin reactions are unusual.

An "illness" regimen should be laid out ahead of time, discussed, and rehearsed, including

- Religious injection of reduced-dose, intermediate-acting insulin at least once, possibly twice a day

- A call to the patient's nurse or physician early rather than late
- Urine testing for ketones
- Injections of small, supplemental doses of short-acting insulin several times daily if necessary, according to the results of the urine tests, until glucose levels come under control

Refills. The second most frequent communication problem is a misunderstanding about insulin refills and logistic problems in obtaining refills or the necessary advice about crisis management. Most pharmacies now will sell insulin to patients without a rigid requirement for a current prescription, but "Murphy's Law" (If something can go wrong, it will) seems to apply to insulin regimens. Accordingly, it is not unheard of for a patient to miss several days of insulin therapy because "I ran out and my doctor's appointment was only a few days away"; because "in the excitement of the horse show, I skipped a few doses" . . . the examples go on and on. Similarly, difficulty in reaching a medical person for advice by phone or limited access to a medical care facility may interfere with timely therapy in such a way as to permit unnecessary episodes of ketoacidosis. A relatively simple measure such as establishment of a "diabetes hot-line" can have a dramatic impact in reducing the number of episodes.[21]

Individual Patterns. Beyond these general causes, certain diabetic patients seem to develop their own individual patterns for recurrent episodes of ketoacidosis: the patient who is mentally incompetent and without an adequate caretaker network; the alcoholic patient who develops ketoacidosis during sprees; the adolescent patient in whose battle with his parents, neglect of his diabetes has become his "ultimate weapon"; the patient who has denied the existence of his diabetes so firmly that its care is viewed with utmost lack of concern. For these patients the ingenuity, persistence, and professionalism of the entire health-care team is challenged, but many patients will eventually respond.

Inpatient Settings. Prevention of diabetic ketoacidosis in inpatient settings is a different matter entirely. Here the key is close monitoring in patients known to be ketosis-prone and a high index of suspicion in patients not previously known to be diabetic. Regular urine testing in known diabetics will always permit ketoacidosis to be prevented, as long as the materials for sugar and acetone testing are known to be fresh and active, the testing is properly done, and abnormal results promptly reported. Of course, not all urinary ketosis is diabetic ketosis, since fasting regularly produces ketonuria. The main differential clue is, of course, the absence of concurrent glycosuria with fasting ketonuria, but if there is any doubt, the matter should be investigated right away with the proper confirmatory blood testing.

In hospitalized patients not known to be diabetic who develop unexplained extreme thirst, negative fluid balance, stupor, or hyperventilation, diabetic ketoacidosis is a part of the differential diagnosis, particularly in those with obvious triggering stresses such as severe infection, trauma, CNS bleeding, and so forth. A high index of suspicion and proper testing will exclude or make the diagnosis, and in the latter instance may be lifesaving.

HYPEROSMOLAR COMA
Not infrequently, patients develop the marked hyperglycemia and hyperosmolarity of diabetic ketoacidosis, but without the ketoacidosis: the syndrome of so-called hyperosmolar nonketotic coma (see Fig. 28-2, *D*). The syndrome is important because of (1) its similarities to and its differences from full-blown diabetic ketoacidosis, (2) the differential diagnosis, and (3) differences in management.

Manifestations
Characteristically, such patients are elderly and not previously known to have diabetes. They become a bit drowsy, take in less and less by mouth, are noted over several days to slip ever deeper into stupor, and are finally brought to the hospital in a state of extreme volume depletion. Blood sugar in these patients is more or less by definition over 600 mg/dl, and in addition to the total extracellular sodium and water losses, a large additional "free water" deficit exists probably because of failure of the thirst mechanism and consequent lack of oral intake. These patients therefore often have very high serum levels of both sodium and glucose, the latter sometimes in excess of 2000 mg/dl, and extraordinarily high serum osmolarities.

From our discussion of the mechanism of extreme hyperglycemia, it might be expected that poor renal function must contribute even more greatly to the development of the hyperosmolar nonketotic syndrome than to diabetic ketoacidosis itself and, indeed, renal function is generally much worse in the former. As in most things related to diabetes, the hyperosmolar syndrome is not always "pure": some patients have a degree of ketosis as well. However, it seems logical to consider the diagnosis to be the hyperosmolar syndrome only if the anion gap attributable to ketoacids is less than about 7 mEq/liter, and full-blown ketoacidosis if greater than 7 mEq/liter.

Causes

Although the reason that some patients develop hyperosmolar coma without acidosis is very intriguing, it is usually not known. In experimental animals, a combination of mild diabetes, large doses of glucocorticoids, and extreme water deprivation is required to produce a model of the disease.[22] The model may have important similarities to the human situation, since the patient's history frequently includes extremely poor water intake in the face of continuing insensible and urinary water loss, and upon recovery the patient's diabetes is usually mild and noninsulin requiring.

In some patients, it is clear that the syndrome is iatrogenic, induced by one of a variety of medications including glucocorticoids, diazoxide, and diuretics, by dialysis against hyperosmolar glucose solutions, or by prolonged intravenous hypertonic glucose infusion, as in central hyperalimentation regimens.

Management

In a general way, therapy for the hyperosmolar syndrome is very similar to those aspects of therapy for diabetic ketoacidosis that are directed at the hyperglycemia and volume depletion. The major difference is the extent or degree of the volume depletion, which is, on the whole, considerably greater in the hyperosmolar syndrome, and which calls for extremely vigorous replacement. Moreover, these patients not only seem to require less insulin to control their hyperosmolar state, they are even more vulnerable to sudden loss of circulating blood volume with rapid, insulin-induced blood-sugar reduction than are ketoacidotic patients. It has even been suggested, therefore, that the hyperosmolar nonketotic syndrome be treated with saline alone, omitting the use of insulin altogether, but small doses of insulin are generally given.

Prognosis

Patients who develop the hyperosmolar nonketotic coma syndrome do not do very well: complications are frequent and mortality rates may be 25% to 50%. The multiplicity of associated diseases in what is mostly an elderly population; inability of the cardiovascular system to handle the rapid volume shifts during the development and treatment of the syndrome; and intravascular thrombosis as well as focal seizures, presumably due to extreme hyperconcentration of blood and poor local blood flow, all seem to contribute to this rather bleak outlook.

ALCOHOLIC KETOACIDOSIS

At the opposite metabolic extreme from patients with diabetic hyperosmolar nonketotic coma are an entirely different group with severe ketoacidosis but no hyperglycemia (see Fig. 28-2,*A*). Strictly speaking, these latter ketoacidotic patients do not belong in this discussion because they do not have diabetes: their ketoacidosis is induced by heavy alcohol intake, and their glucose tolerance is quite normal. They are, nonetheless, important to the discussion for the light they shed on pathogenesis and on clinical manifestations of diabetic ketoacidosis and because alcoholic ketoacidosis may figure prominently in the differential diagnosis of certain patients. Moreover, because the therapy of the two conditions is very different, the distinctions must be clearly recognized.[23]

Manifestations

Patients who develop alcoholic ketoacidosis are almost invariably women. They are usually chronic drinkers who, just before they become ill, suddenly increase their drinking, then just as suddenly, begin vomiting and stop drinking. Vomiting usually then continues, abdominal pain develops, and 2 or 3 days later they seek care: awake, alert, only slightly dehydrated, often with Kussmaul breathing, and usually with a silent, tender, distended, and resistant abdomen. Urinalysis initially shows strongly positive ketones but no sugars, and the blood sugar is usually normal or low, although it may be *slightly elevated*. However, the anion gap is very large, serum ketones are positive at higher dilutions, and arterial *p*H is decreased, sometimes to extremely low values.

Management

In striking contrast to diabetic ketoacidosis, the most effective therapy for alcoholic ketoacidosis consists initially and primarily of simple intravenous dextrose and water, without insulin. Modest amounts of saline may be added to the regimen if vomiting has been severe and volume depletion is significant. During therapy, serum phosphate concentration may drop extremely low. The level should be monitored, and phosphate salts administered accordingly, lest a "low phosphate" syndrome develop.[24]

Causes

The development of alcohol ketoacidosis seems to depend upon a combination of several factors whose relative importance and mechanism remain speculative. Certain biologic "host" characteristics are probably required, since only a small minority of all alcoholic patients develop the syndrome, and, more importantly, if they later resume drinking, ketoacidosis often develops repeatedly in these same patients. Moreover, the hormonal milieu may contribute, since the predominance of female over male patients is striking. In addition, several environmental factors are so constant that they almost certainly play a role. Alcohol is obviously involved, although alcohol by itself is necessary but not sufficient. Vomiting may also be a cause rather than a result of the syndrome, possibly by provoking a marked stress hormone release, including catecholamines, and judging from the rapid and complete response to glucose therapy, glucose deprivation may also figure into production of the syndrome.

HYPOGLYCEMIA

While it may be apparent to medically trained people that, of the two diabetic emergencies, ketoacidosis is actually far more life-threatening, from the patient's point of view, even mild hypoglycemia is usually seen as a much greater problem.

Manifestations

To begin with, hypoglycemia in diabetics, while occurring mostly in the insulin-dependent group, is much more common than ketoacidosis. Second, the onset of hypoglycemia is much more rapid and its manifestations much more variable, often occurring in such subtle ways as to evade the victim's notice until he is unaware of what is happening and unable to seek the proper remedy. Insulin-induced hypoglycemic reactions therefore often occur in the midst of the patient's daily life, which can be, at the very least, embarrassing and at worst highly dangerous. Third, even though measurable recovery from hypoglycemia is rapid and complete within minutes after proper treatment, many patients remain emotionally (and possibly physiologically) shaken for hours or even days following insulin reactions. Finally, in extreme, severe situations, prolonged or recurrent hypoglycemia, while uncommon, does have the potential for permanent brain damage and can even be fatal.

Preventing, treating, and generally coping with each of the diabetic emergencies is difficult enough even when a clear distinction is made between them and their mechanisms are fully understood. Unfortunately, as anyone who has worked with diabetic patients can testify, the problem is further compounded by an almost universal confusion between ketoacidosis and hypoglycemia. Most patients lump the two together under the common heading of "diabetic coma." Repeated explanations based on physiology, the use of graphic material as much as possible, clear and practical instructions on how to respond in each situation, and infinite patience are the minimum requirements for handling this confusion.

Neurologic Responses to Hypoglycemia

Cerebral Responses. As blood sugar falls below normal, the CNS responds in two distinct fashions: first, with impairment of higher cerebral functions and soon thereafter with an "alarm" response in vegetative functions.

Patients most commonly describe the symptoms of mild or early insulin reactions as fuzziness in the head, trouble thinking or concentrating, shakiness, light-headedness, and giddiness. These changes occur when the cerebral cortex is deprived of its main energy supply. This part of the brain is apparently the most sensitive to the loss of glucose.

Almost as common, but usually inapparent to the patient, are changes in personality and behavior during insulin reactions. As with alcohol and other agents that affect cerebral function, these changes in personality vary with the person, the situation, the rapidity of onset, and other unknown factors. They range from silly, manic, inappropriate behavior through withdrawal, sullenness, or truculence, to grumpy, irritable, suspicious or, in the extreme, paranoid and even, rarely, violent behavior. It is no wonder that, particularly when combined with difficulties in motor function such as trouble walking and slurred speech, patients who are well into insulin reactions may closely resemble people who have been drinking alcohol. It is for this reason that diabetic identification cards and jewelry indicate that such findings in the bearer may represent hypoglycemia rather than drunkenness.

The major lesson from all of this is that *any patient taking insulin whose behavior or personality becomes inappropriate or uncharacteristic for him should be suspected of having an insulin reaction and treated accordingly.* The index of suspicion should be particularly high if such changes are episodic, occur at a time when the particular form of insulin used is expected to have its maximum activity, and are accompanied by consistently negative urine tests for sugar.

A major source of anxiety for many diabetics taking insulin is concern for unrecognized hypoglycemia during sleep, leading to possible brain damage, such that they may "never wake up." Many patients having insulin reactions are wakened by the reaction, so it is possible to be realistically reassuring about this. However, some patients seem not to waken consistently and must rely on the presence or availability of a family member or partner to detect and treat nocturnal reactions.

While the manifestations of cerebral cortical dysfunction from hypoglycemia are usually diffuse rather than focal, some patients develop focal signs or symptoms such as aphasia, vertigo, localized weakness, or even focal seizures with their insulin reactions. Such focal changes usually occur when there is prior focal damage to the specific area of the cortex, as from a previous stroke or head injury. Occasionally these focal symptoms occur without any obvious predisposing factor, which makes for an extremely confusing diagnostic puzzle.

Vegetative Responses. Close on the heels of the cortical changes follows a series of vegetative neurologic responses. The primary response is discharge from the centers that control adrenergic autonomic impulses, with the resultant release of norepinephrine throughout the body and epinephrine from the adrenals. The resultant tachycardia, pallor, sweating, and tremor are characteristic of hypoglycemia and usually serve as an important early warning sign by which many patients recognize an oncoming reaction. This adrenergic discharge is part of a larger stress response including release of large quantities of the "counterregulatory" hormones such as glucocorticoids, growth hormone, and glucagon, which attempt to drive the blood sugar back up primarily by stimulating hepatic glycogen breakdown.

Other vegetative signs and symptoms may occur during hypoglycemic reactions but are less constant. Despite myths to the contrary, hunger is not a prominent feature of insulin reactions in most patients, though it does sometimes occur; headache may be seen; and the stress response may on occasion trigger secondary sequences of symptoms, including angina or pulmonary edema in patients with fragile cardiovascular disease.

Ultimately, as hypoglycemia persists and worsens, consciousness is progressively impaired, leading to stupor, then coma. The vegetative centers controlling fundamental systems of respiration, blood pressure maintenance, and so forth are the most resistant to hypoglycemia and will continue to function even when most other cerebral functions are lost.

The more profound the hypoglycemia and the longer it lasts, the greater the chance of transient or even permanent cerebral damage after blood sugar is restored. There does not seem to be a clear duration threshold for such damage, but severe hypoglycemia lasting more than 15 to 30 minutes not uncommonly results in at least some symptoms that persist for a time after glucose is given.

Pathophysiology

The minute-to-minute dependence of the brain on glucose supplied by the circulation results, as we have noted, from the inability of the brain to burn long-chain free fatty acids, the lack of glucose stored as glycogen within the adult brain, and the unavailability of ketones under fed or postabsorptive conditions.

There is little doubt that when blood sugar falls abruptly, the brain recognizes its energy deficiency once the serum level goes much below about 45 mg/dl. The exact level at which symptoms occur varies widely from person to person, however, and it is not uncommon for levels as low as 30 to 35 mg/dl to occur, as during glucose tolerance tests, with no symptoms whatsoever.[25]

More controversial is the question of whether symptoms develop in response to a rapidly falling blood sugar even before it has gone below the usual lower limit of normal. Since certain physiological responses, such as growth hormone release, occur with declining but still normal blood sugars, it is likely that symptoms may occur on this basis, but the stimulus of a falling level is probably less strong and consistent than reduction below an absolute threshold. On the other hand, the brain seems to adapt at least partially to lowered blood sugar levels, particularly if the decline is slow and chronic. It is not unusual for patients with extremely low blood sugars, such as those with insulin-secreting tumors, to exhibit perfectly normal cerebral function in the face of blood sugars that are persistently below the normal range.

Diagnosis

In principle, the diagnosis of hypoglycemia should be relatively simple and clear-cut. Because of the extreme *nonspecificity* of its manifestations and the extraordinary *biologic variation* in response to a low blood sugar, the diagnosis, in actual practice, is often subtle and complex. A serum sugar found to be below 25 mg/dl may always to held responsible for accompanying symptoms. Even in the range from 25 to 45 mg/dl, however, symptoms may not always be attributable to the hypoglycemia (particularly in spontaneous or reactive hypoglycemia), and between 45 and 65 mg/dl the relationship becomes even more difficult.[26,27]

Making a reasonably secure diagnosis of *symptomatic hypoglycemia* therefore depends on three elements:

- Documentation by an independent observer that symptoms are occurring, at a time when the blood sugar can be determined
- Correlation of the symptoms with a blood sugar level that is either absolutely low or declining very rapidly
- Prompt reversal of the symptoms upon administration of glucose, with a correlated rise in blood sugar level

In the absence of any of these three criteria, the diagnosis, although it may be strongly suspected, is less certain. It is therefore of prime importance that a blood sugar level be drawn (or determined by glucose oxidase strip at the bedside) if at all possible *prior* to giving glucose.

While measuring blood sugar is easily done in the hospital, it is much less feasible in outpatients, in whom the diagnosis often rests on suspicion plus the response to glucose.

Urine sugars are an unreliable indicator on which to make a diagnosis of hypoglycemia because the bladder urine represents an "integral" sample of blood sugar levels over time. The sample voided just before or after an insulin reaction may well contain glucose from a prior glucose peak several hours previously, thus giving a *false positive* impression. On the other hand, uniformly negative urine tests are consistent with the diagnosis and help to increase its likelihood.

Management

The treatment of insulin reactions is always glucose: if the patient can swallow, the glucose is most conveniently gives as a glucose- or sucrose-containing drink, since in this form it probably gets through the stomach and into the absorbing intestine in the fastest possible time. Several teaspoons of sugar in a small volume of liquid produces excessive sweetness that is nicely masked by the tartness of the traditional "O.J." (orange juice) therapy. If the patient is too groggy, stuporous, or uncooperative to drink, 30 to 50 ml of 50% glucose solution is given intravenously from a syringe over several minutes. If this route or dosage is unavailable, 1 mg of glucagon given subcutaneously or intramuscularly will reverse the symptoms by inducing a rapid breakdown and release of glucose into the bloodstream from hepatic glycogen stores.

The amount of glucose needed to reverse an insulin reaction acutely is not large: in order to raise the blood sugar from 20 up to 120 mg/dl, less than 15 g (3 teaspoons of glucose) will suffice in an average sized adult. Glucose in almost any oral form will serve: starch, as in crackers or cookies, once through the stomach, is broken down to free glucose and absorbed so rapidly that blood sugar rises virtually as fast as with free glucose or sucrose.

As an extension of their fears that they might "never wake up" from nocturnal insulin reaction, patients are frequently concerned about what to do if they don't respond to the initial therapy. They must be reassured that if the first bolus of glucose consumed doesn't seem to work, the sensible thing to do is to take in more;

insulin reactions are *always* reversible with enough glucose. The response to oral glucose, of course, takes time, perhaps 5 to 15 minutes, while with intravenous glucose the response should occur within a minute or two at most.

Failure to respond fully in the appropriate time indicates either that not enough glucose has been given, that the diagnosis is in error, or that the hypoglycemia has been long and severe enough to produce persistent, though not necessarily permanent, cerebral dysfunction.

Prevention

Occasional insulin reactions can and do happen in even the most stable insulin-requiring diabetic. As long as they are mild, they can usually be tolerated without difficulty and are not cause for alarm or for changes in regimen. Frequently the permissive event is clear: a skipped meal, an unusually strenuous bout of exercise.

When reactions are relatively frequent, recurrent, or severe, however, it is a different matter entirely. Unless the reactions are prevented, the patient may be functionally disabled: always terrified that one is about to occur; unwilling or unable to drive a car; overeating to prevent them from happening; and so forth.

The search for causes and for corrective measures is a complex and individual matter for each patient, but it is usually rewarded by finding one of several underlying mechanisms at fault. Perhaps the most common and most important mechanism is an atypical response to the usual intermediate-acting insulin that serves as the mainstay of therapy in most diabetics. Such "early" or "late responders" are quite common, and frequently not recognized as such.[28] When the nature of their response pattern is properly defined, some relatively simple adjustments in insulin regimen often virtually eliminate both insulin reactions and excessive spill.

A related problem is the patient whose urine glucose appears to be getting progressively worse, particularly in the morning, despite higher and higher insulin doses. Such a paradoxical response may be a clue to undetected nocturnal insulin reactions, followed by a counter-regulatory response of such intensity that the blood sugar overshoots, leading to the increasing spill by the next day, the so-called Somogyi effect.

A second mechanism must be sought when a previously stable, reaction-free patient begins to experience hypoglycemic episodes. Certain bio-logic explanations must, of course, be excluded, including increased insulin sensitivity due to weight loss, the onset of azotemia, and so forth. More often than not, such a physiological phenomenon is not discovered, and a meticulous search for problems with insulin dosage or administration should then be undertaken.

Murphy's Law applies to insulin excesses as well as deficiencies, and *nothing* should be taken for granted: every detail of insulin therapy from insulin purchase, appearance, unitage of insulin and syringes, injection sites, injection technique, and especially any recent change in any part of the regimen should be explored in detective fashion, looking for the flaw or the inconsistency. Prescription errors, mismatched syringe and insulin unitages, use of new injection sites, and other errors as yet unheard of may very well emerge.

Finally, the administration or withdrawal of other drugs may be the precipitating event for recurrent insulin reactions.

Alcohol is by far the worse offender: not only do patients often eat less when they have a few drinks, but alcohol shuts off gluconeogenesis by interfering with intermediate biochemical steps within the liver. When combined with injected insulin, this combination not infrequently leads to hypoglycemia, which may be tricky to sort out clinically because of concurrent inebriation.

Salicylates in large doses can reduce blood sugar and again, in combination with insulin, can produce hypoglycemia when either drug alone would not do so in the doses employed.

Since *glucocorticoids* used therapeutically cause insulin resistance, insulin doses are often raised to meet the increased insulin demand. If the steroids are then tapered without appropriate downward adjustments in insulin dose, frequent reactions may supervene.

These are the major but by no means the only examples of drug-insulin interactions relevant to hypoglycemic episodes. It must not be forgotten, moreover, that oral hypoglycemic agents (sulfonylureas), which are still used in a great many patients, can also produce severe and long-lasting hypoglycemia.

Typically, patients who experience such episodes tend to be elderly and undernourished with impaired renal or hepatic function. Virtually any patient on oral agents may become hypoglycemic, especially in the presence of another potentiating agent such as phenylbutazone, salicylates, or above all, alcohol.[29]

REFERENCES

1. Garrow JS: Energy Balance and Obesity in Man, 2nd ed. New York, Elsevier/North Holland Biomedical Press, 1978
2. Cahill G: Starvation in man. N Engl J Med 282:668–675, 1970
3. Daniel PM, Pratt OE, Spargo E: The metabolic homeostatic role of muscle and its function as a store of protein. Lancet 2:446–448, 1979
4. Service FJ, Nelson RL: Characteristics of glycemic stability. Diabetes Care 3:58–62, 1980
5. Cahill: Starvation in man
6. Fajans S, Floyd JC: Fasting hypoglycemia in adults. N Engl J Med 294:766–772, 1976
7. Service: Glycemic stability
8. Daughaday WH: Diabetic acidosis. In Williams RH (ed): Diabetes, pp 516–548. New York, Paul Hoeber, 1960
9. Fulop M, Tannenbaum H, Dreyer N: Ketotic hyperosmolar coma. Lancet 2:635–639, 1973
10. Cooperman M, Davidoff F, Spark R et al: Clinical studies in alcoholic ketoacidosis. Diabetes 23:433–439, 1974
11. Daughaday: Diabetic acidosis
12. Alberti KGMM, Hockaday TDR: Rapid blood ketone body estimation in the diagnosis of diabetic ketoacidosis. Br Med J 211:565–568, 1972
13. Daughaday: Diabetic acidosis
14. Clements RS Jr, Vourganti B: Fatal diabetic ketoacidosis: Major causes and approaches to their prevention. Diabetes Care 1:314–325, 1978
15. Ibid
16. Brown RH, Rossini AA, Calloway CV et al: Caveat on fluid replacement in hyperglycemic, hyperosmolar nonketotic coma. Diabetes Care 1:305–307, 1978
17. Clements RS, Blumenthal SA, Morrison AD et al: Increased cerebrospinal-fluid pressure during treatment of diabetic ketosis. Lancet 2:671–675, 1971
18. Fisher JN, Shahshahani MN, Kitabchi A: Diabetic ketoacidosis: Low-dose insulin therapy by various routes. N Engl J Med 297:238–240, 1977
19. Garella S, Dana CL, Chazan JA: Severity of metabolic acidosis as a determinant of bicarbonate requirements. N Engl J Med 289:121–126, 1973
20. Daughaday: Diabetic acidosis
21. Miller LV, Goldstein J: More efficient care of diabetic patients in a county hospital setting. N Engl J Med 286:1388–1391, 1972
22. Bavli S, Gordon EE: Experimental diabetic hyperosmolar syndrome in rats. Diabetes 20:92–95, 1971
23. Cooperman: Alcoholic ketoacidosis
24. Lentz RD, Brown DM: Treatment of severe hypophosphatemia. Ann Intern Med 89:941–944, 1978
25. Hofeldt FD: Reactive hypoglycemia. Metabolism 24:1193–1208, 1975
26. Fajans: Fasting hypoglycemia
27. Hofeldt: Reactive hypoglycemia
28. Marler E, Bressler R, Styron C: The use of insulin in unstable diabetes mellitus. South Med J 57:1447–1451, 1964
29. Seltzer HS: Severe drug-induced hypoglycemia: A review. Compr Ther 5:21–29, 1957

**Mary Ellen McManus and
Deborah Moisan**

Drug and Poison Overdose 29

The daily emergence of new chemicals and drugs and the consequences of their use, misuse, and abuse present special challenges for nurses practicing in critical care environments. In the past, acute poisonings have largely gone unrecognized in nursing. This is no longer the case. Present societal exposure to numerous compounds makes it imperative that health professionals have some basic knowledge of toxicologic emergencies and the subsequent care necessary to maintain life.

The incidence of poisoning within the United States is estimated at 2 to 5 million per year, with this number steadily increasing. Approximately 5000 of these cases result in death. Although all age groups are affected, pediatric contacts account for 85% of human accidental poisonings. The remaining 15% includes adolescents and adults involved in intentional (suicide/abuse), accidental, or industrial exposure. While pediatric contacts involve the majority of poison center calls, it is the adult attempting suicide who will most often be seen and cared for in a critical care environment. The intent of this chapter is to present basic guidelines for assessment and treatment management of the acutely poisoned patient, followed by selected commonly observed poisonings, their clinical course, and advance management.

THE DILEMMA OF MANAGEMENT

When the person presents with poisoning or drug overdose, it can be a management dilemma, a dilemma that begins with the history taking.

Frequently, neither the person nor his family is able to accurately relate the circumstances surrounding the exposure. Sometimes the person, family member, or friend feels guilty about the incident and gives incomplete information. Or, as a result of the drug's effects, the person may arrive comatose or delirious, thus leaving the history surrounding the exposure an enigma.

Three areas of information are needed: general history, basic exposure information, and possible first aid that might have been given.

History. Included in the history are name, age, weight, address, phone number, and health history. An initial recording of weight is indicated because the toxicity of many agents can be predicted on a milligram per kilogram basis. The address and phone number are important if both the patient and family are unable to provide a verbal history. A relative may have access to the residence and can explore possible sources of poisoning. The health history is most useful because illnesses and medication regimes can influence the severity of the poisoning.

Poison Overdose/Exposure. The product's name, ingredients, amount, route, and time of exposure are vital to poison treatment. While the majority of acutely poisoned patients in the critical care unit involve intentional ingestion, other routes of exposure include inhalation; ocular, dermal, and parenteral exposure; and envenomation through bites and stings. Knowing the approximate time of the exposure will determine *when* and *what* treatment is indicated. When used concomitantly, alcohol can be a potentiating agent to the initial poison. Thus, multiple substance exposure must be anticipated.

Initial First Aid. It is always wise to question what was done as first aid by family, paramedics, or emergency room personnel. Surprisingly, initial measures are overlooked in the haste to admit the person to critical care.

If verbal history and clinical status conflict or when history is lacking, laboratory analysis of blood, urine, and emesis may prove helpful in making the diagnosis. Again, the time post-exposure is important to note, for some drugs do not peak in the system for several hours, and a toxic level could be missed if analysis is performed too soon.

Many times the patient plus the poisoning create a large range of potential problems and

arrive in the unit with varying degrees of clinical emergencies. Equally as important as the history and sometimes more crucial is the initial assessment of the core systems. Emergency support measures to maintain life must take priority.

BASIC SUPPORTIVE CARE
Initial evaluation of the patient's immediate danger and good supportive care form the basic management of any poisoned patient. Basic supportive care consists of six steps:

1. Establishment and management of the airway. *There is no contraindication to breathing.* It is essential to intubate the patient if the gag reflex is lost, if seizures are present, or if the patient has lost consciousness. Frequent suctioning may be necessary (see Chapter 13).
2. Control bleeding. Prevent and treat shock with whole blood or fluids if necessary. Fluids should be given only to hydrate the person, and caution taken for the amount given in order to prevent pulmonary edema.
3. Determine if there are any associated injuries or other disease processes.
4. Establish and manage an acid-base and electrolyte status.
5. Naloxone (Narcan) is never harmful to administer. In suspected narcotic overdoses it may be necessary to give 10 to 20 times the usual recommended dose to reverse the narcotic effects. Naloxone can be repeated frequently, since the half-life is relatively short—approximately 60 minutes.
6. Cardiac monitoring is essential in a comatose patient. Many overdoses predispose the patient to cardiac irregularities and dysrhythmias (see Chapter 9).
7. Glucose administration may be warranted.

Most poisoned patients require the above supportive care in combination with a poison protocol.

MANAGEMENT OF THE ACUTELY POISONED PATIENT
Only after the patient has been sufficiently stabilized and supportive care established can further measures to prevent absorption or to enhance excretion be carried out.

Prevention of Absorption
Although there are several treatments that prevent or minimize absorption, the poison, the

amount, the route, and the time of exposure will all contribute to the decision as to which methods are best.

Ocular Exposure. For an ocular exposure, a lukewarm water or saline irrigation must be done as soon as possible. The eye should be flooded from a large glass 2 or 3 inches from the eye. Continue the washing for 15 minutes. Do not hold the eye open but rather have the patient blink the eye open and closed. A lukewarm shower may also be used. Be sure to use low pressure.

Dilution. If there is the slightest suspicion of an insecticide or pesticide exposure, the first consideration should be a thorough decontamination of the skin. After all the person's clothes have been removed and placed in a plastic bag to prevent further contamination to others in the area, three separate showers should be given:

1. Soap washing
2. Rubbing alcohol washing
3. Soap washing

By performing such washings, 90% of an organophosphate or carbamate insecticide can be removed even 6 hours after the exposure. A gasoline or chlorine bleach exposure can result in serious burns, and a 20-minute skin decontamination with soap and water should be performed.

For all ingested poisonings, dilutions can be done safely at home or enroute to the hospital. The recommended diluents are milk and water. These can be beneficially used unless the patient is experiencing a seizure, has lost the gag reflex, or is unconscious. The amount recommended is 15 ml/kg body weight to a maximum amount of 200 to 300 ml. Fruit juices, vinegar, or oils are contraindicated, especially if the substance ingested is an acid or alkaline. When fruit juice or vinegar is given, it can cause an exothermic heat reaction. This reaction can lead to further burning and damage of the esophagus.

Emetics. A constant dilemma facing the emergency personnel is when to vomit or not to vomit. Vomiting is contraindicated in a patient who has lost the gag reflex, has seizures, has lost consciousness, or has oropharyngeal burns. The use of emetics in a hydrocarbon exposure will be discussed later in this chapter.

Syrup of Ipecac. Syrup of ipecac (not ipecac elixir) is the preferred method of gastric empty-ing. The recommended dose of ipecac for children is 15 ml orally, which can be repeated one time if necessary. The recommended dose for adults is 30 ml. It should be followed with 15 ml/kg of clear fluids to a maximum of 200 to 300 ml. The child should be kept ambulatory. If no emesis results in 15 to 30 minutes, one repeat dose may be given. Fluids should be given after each consecutive emesis until the emesis is clear, as the person may need to vomit three or four times. Once the emesis is clear the person should be kept NPO (not allowed to eat or drink) for 1½ hours. This will produce a cessation of emesis.

Apomorphine, Salt, Mustard Powder. Other emetics are not recommended. Apomorphine depresses the central nervous system and creates respiratory depression. Other emetics such as salt water have produced fatalities, and the therapeutic/toxic ratio for such substances as mustard powder and copper sulfate may be too narrow to judge.

Lavage. Gastric lavage has been considered the standard method of emptying the stomach for many years. As stated earlier, emesis is now preferred to gastric lavage because of the frequent poor recovery of the poison or drug. This may be due to the inadequate size of the bore in the lavage tube. If a No. 16 or No. 18 French nasogastric tube is used in an adult, no intact pieces will be recovered. A No. 36 French tube is recommended.

Gastric lavages are indicated when the patient is comatose, having seizures, has no gag reflex, or when a decrease in consciousness is expected. The airway should be cleared, a cuffed endotracheal tube inserted for airway protection, and the patient placed in a left lateral head-down position. Again, to obtain maximum efficacy, a large bore lavage tube must be used.

Repeated washings should be conducted until the returns are clear—10 to 15 washings. For each washing, 100 to 200 ml of fluids are used for an adult and 10 to 15 ml/kg to a maximum of 200 ml for a child. Lukewarm water or normal saline is recommended, and it is important to recover any lavage fluid that is instilled. At the completion of the lavage, the tube should be kept in the stomach for activated charcoal or a cathartic instillation, if needed. When there is no further need for the tube, it should be pinched off and removed. Remember: keep suction close at hand for the possibility of aspiration!

Absorbant. Activated charcoal is an inert ingredient with tremendous absorbant properties.

There is no contraindication to giving it, but it is not recommended in case of a strong alkaline or acid. At the very least, it will act as a gastrointestinal marker. Because it absorbs syrup of ipecac, the two should not be given together. Activated charcoal should be given only after the emesis is clear and the patient has been NPO for one hour.

In theory, the recommended dose is 5 to 10 times the amount of the toxin ingested. In practice, the adult dose is 30 to 100 g, approximately 10 to 30 tablespoons. It can be premixed with water to form a thick soup or catsuplike consistency, and when the bottle is tightly sealed, it can be stored indefinitely. The following chart lists the drugs well-absorbed by charcoal.

CHARCOAL-ABSORBED DRUGS
Alcohol
Amphetamines
Aspirin
Barbiturates
Camphor
Chloroquine ipecac
Chlorpromazine
Digitalis
Ethchlorvynol
Glutethimide
Malathion
Mercuric chloride
Morphine
Opium
Oxalates
Parathion
Phenothiazine
Propoxyphene
Quinine
Salicylates
Strychnine

Cathartics. To prevent further absorption and to speed elimination, a saline cathartic should be used. It is preferred to oil base cathartics because a saline cathartic does not leave the patient at risk to aspiration pneumonitis. Saline cathartics such as magnesium sulfate, magnesium citrate, and sodium sulfate provide safe and effective intestinal evacuation. Administered orally or by nasogastric tube, the dosage is as follows:

- Magnesium sulfate: adults—30 g with a maximum of 100 g in 24 hr
- Magnesium citrate: 4 ml/kg to 300-ml dose
- Sodium sulfate: adults—30-g dose with a maximum of 100 g in 24 hr child—250 mg/kg

The dose should be repeated every 4 hours to the maximum dose or until a charcoal stool is present. Be sure to confirm presence of bowel sounds.

Enhancement of Excretion
The pharmacologic characteristics of a drug greatly influence the severity and the length of clinical course of the acutely poisoned patient. These properties—absorption rate, body distribution, and elimination rate—are taken into consideration when choosing methods that will enhance a drug's excretion from the body.

Forced Diuresis. Forced diuresis is beneficial for severe poisonings in which the drug is primarily excreted in the urine in its active form. If this method is used, careful monitoring must be done to ensure that cerebral edema does not occur. Some drugs are best excreted when urine is made alkaline; others, when the urine is made acidic. Frequent pH testing and electrolyte monitoring are indicated if these methods are employed.

Hemodialysis and Peritoneal Dialysis. Hemodialysis and peritoneal dialysis are used as supportive care when more conservative methods (gastric emptying, charcoal, cathartics, antagonists) have failed (see Chapter 17). If a drug or poison is highly bound to the body's tissues or widely distributed throughout the body, attempts to dialyze the drug will be futile. Therefore, it may be necessary to consult a pharmacologist to determine a drug's characteristics. The rate of removal of a dialyzable substance is usually five to ten times greater with hemodialysis than with peritoneal dialysis. However, peritoneal dialysis is easier to perform and can be initiated more rapidly.

Universal Antidote
"The universal antidote," with which you may be familiar, *should be considered useless!* It consists of

2 parts burnt toast	= activated charcoal
1 part milk of magnesia	= cathartic
1 part strong tea	= tannic acid

Burnt toast is burnt carbohydrate and not activated charcoal. Milk of magnesia is not as effective as saline cathartics. And a sufficient amount of tannic acid would cause liver impairment.

The following chart lists the only recognized

effective antagonists for specific intoxicants. Caution must be taken with dosage and route of administration because if given incorrectly, some antagonists will cause further complications.

EFFECTIVE ANTAGONISTS FOR SPECIFIC INTOXICATIONS

Intoxications	Antagonists
Carbon monoxide	Oxygen
Cyanide	Amyl nitrite
	Sodium nitrite
	Sodium thiosulfate
Nitrites	Methylene blue
Organophosphates	Atropine
	Protopam (2-PAM)
Narcotics	Naloxone (Narcan)
Anticholinergics or tricyclic antidepressants	Physostigmine
Acetaminophen	N-acetylcysteine (Mucomyst) (investigational)
Ethylene glycol and methanol	Ethanol

COMMONLY OBSERVED POISONINGS

Benzodiazepines

Benzodiazepines are minor tranquilizers that exhibit central nervous system depressant effects. Because of the long half-life, these drugs may cause prolonged drowsiness in the overdose situation. No documented fatalities have occurred from the ingestion of these agents alone, but frequently they are involved in the multiple overdose, most notable with alcohol. Ingestions of 500 to 1500 mg have occurred with only minor toxicity. Physical dependence can occur with chronic ingestion; therefore, withdrawal may be anticipated if a person arrives with an acute oral benzodiazepine overdose.

Substances/Examples
- Valium
- Librium
- Dalmane
- Ativan
- Tranxene
- Serax

Clinical Effects
- Lethargy — stage 1 coma
- Hypotension
- Tachycardia
- Decreasing bowel sounds
- Decreasing respirations

Lab Work
- Plasma screen
- Urine

Treatment
- Ipecac/lavage/charcoal/cathartic
- Ventilatory support
- Fluids for hypotension — vasopressor
- Treat withdrawal

Amphetamines

Amphetamines are drugs that have a stimulant effect on both central and peripheral nervous systems and also have analeptic properties. The response is variable and dependency can occur with chronic abuse. Clinical effects are easily seen within an hour of ingestion, and death occurs from cardiac arrhythmias and circulatory collapse. Because of the rapid excretion of these drugs, treatment of acute intoxication is achieved in 24 to 36 hours.

The withdrawal for chronic abusers requires psychiatric intervention, as these persons are often suicidally depressed. Withdrawal should take place over 2 to 3 weeks because rapid withdrawal will lead to seizures.

Substances/Examples
- Diet pills
- Illicit drugs (MDA, STP, DMT)

Clinical Effects
- Restlessness — seizures
- Coma
- Cardiac arrhythmias
- Hypotension
- Hypertension

Lab Work
- Urine for amphetamines

Treatment
- Ipecac/lavage/charcoal/cathartic
- Forced acid diuresis for severe overdose
- IV Valium for seizures
- Oral chlorpromazine for hypertension
- Fluids for hypotension
- Suicide precautions

Methanol

Methanol is an alcohol commonly found in antifreeze, windshield washer fluid, and sterno. After rapid absorption by ingestion, inhalation, and dermal exposure, it undergoes hepatic metabolism to formaldehyde and formic acid, both of which are much more toxic than methanol itself. These two end products produce severe acidosis and blindness, with the onset of symptoms in several hours to several days.

The administrtion of intravenous alcohol (ETOH) is the treatment of choice. Alcohol competes with methanol at the enzyme site in the liver, blocking the formation of toxic metabolites and allowing methanol to be excreted unchanged. The drip must be continued for 2 to 3 days or until the blood methanol level is less that 20 mg/dl and acidosis is corrected.

Substances/Examples
- Antifreeze
- Windshield washer solvent
- Varnish
- Sterno
- Wood alcohol

Clinical Effects
- Marked acidosis
- Blindness
- Gastrointestinal symptoms
- Coma
- Respiratory failure

Lab Work
- Blood methanol
- Arterial blood gases
- While on drip: glucose
                    blood alcohol

Treatment
- Ipecac/lavage/charcoal/cathartic
- Correct acidosis with sodium bicarb 0.5 to 1.0 mEq/kg
- Correct potassium depletion
- Ethanol drip if symptoms or if blood methanol greater than 20 mg/dl
- Hemodialysis for marked acidosis or blood methanol 50 mg/dl
- Do *not* stop drip if dialyzed

Ethylene Glycol

Ethylene glycol is an alcohol found primarily in antifreeze and solvents and is rapidly absorbed upon ingestion. Hepatic metabolism produces organic acids, which cause severe acidosis, and oxalic acid (crystals), which leads to renal tubular necrosis.

As with methanol, the administration of intravenous alcohol will compete with ethylene glycol at the enzyme site and prevent the formation of toxic metabolites. The alcohol drip should continue 1 to 3 days until acidosis disappears and crystaluria resolves.

Substances/Examples
- Antifreeze solvents

Clinical Effects
- Acidosis
- Persistent vomiting
- Lethargy-coma
- Seizures
- Renal tubular necrosis
- Myocardial failure

Lab Work
- Blood ethylene glycol
- Arterial blood gases
- Urine for crystals
- While on drip: glucose
                    blood alcohol

Treatment
- Ipecac/lavage/charcoal/cathartic
- ETOH drip
- Hemodialysis for uncorrected acidosis

Propoxyphene

Propoxyphene is a weak synthetic narcotic found in a variety of preparations and acts directly on the central nervous system. Its rapid action allows for observable symptoms within 30 minutes of ingestion, and effects may be exhibited for 8 to 12 hours. Because narcotics decrease gastrointestinal motility, pill fragments may be recovered several hours later. A diagnostic clue to propoxyphene overdose is that the person will present with seizures and pinpoint pupils.

The propensity toward seizures makes lavage preferable to ipecac. Large amounts of naloxone (2 to 20 ampules as a bolus) have been required to reverse the effects of propoxyphene overdose.

Substances/Examples
- Darvon
- Darvon compound
- Darvocet N-100

Clinical Effects
- Seizures
- Pinpoint pupils
- Coma
- Respiratory arrest
- Hypotension
- Cardiac arrhythmias

Lab Work
- Arterial blood gases

Treatment
- Lavage with protected airway/charcoal/cathartic
- Narcan 0.4 to 0.8 mg IV (may bolus with 5 to 10 amps if no initial response)
- Valium for seizures unresponsive to Narcan
- Maintain fluids

Organophosphates

Organophosphates are insecticides that are widely used in agriculture and for home/garden pest control. Well absorbed through ingestion and percutaneously, these agents exhibit their main effects by preventing the breakdown of the neurotransmitter acetylcholine. This enzyme accumulates at nerve synapses and creates a cholinergic crisis—all symptoms being the result of acetylcholine stimulation.

The efficient dermal absorption requires a rigorous skin decontamination. Leather products cannot be decontaminated; therefore, leather shoes, watchbands, belts, and so forth must be discarded.

Atropine blocks the effects of excessive acetylcholine if it persists in high enough concentrations, and the administration of 2000 mg has been required to reverse the symptoms of a severe poisoning. Atropine is not effective for reversing muscular manifestations (respiratory paralysis) and, if this occurs, the additional administration of *protopam* (2-PAM) may be required. Because many organophosphates are in combination with hydrocarbon propellants, the toxicity of both agents demands attention.

Substances/Examples
- Parathion
- Tepp
- Dursban
- Diazinon
- Malathion
- Insect sprays
- Pest strips

Clinical Effects
- Muscarinic (secretions)
    increased salivation
    increased lacrimation
    increased urination
    diarrhea
    vomiting
- Nicotinic (muscles)
    muscle weakness
    respiratory paralysis
- Central nervous system
    psychotic behavior
    coma

Lab Work
- Red blood cell (RBC) cholinesterase

Treatment
- Ingestion: ipecac/lavage/charcoal/cathartic
- Dermal: decontamination washings
        personnel must protect themselves
            from contamination
- Atropine: 1 to 2 mg IV—repeating 2 to 3 minutes until secretions dry
- Treat hydrocarbon pneumonitis
- 2-PAM if: atropine ineffective
            RBC cholinesterase 50% of normal

Hydrocarbons

Hydrocarbons are substances with various numbers of carbon atoms and are found in numerous products. Their toxicity is largely dependent upon their viscosity and votility, with main clinical effects on the pulmonary bed. Hydrocarbons of low viscosity are easily aspirated, spread quickly over lung surfaces, and cause a chemical pneumonitis within 8 to 12 hours. Thicker hydrocarbons do not spread easily and therefore have a lower degree of toxicity. Some hydrocarbons have systemic toxicity associated with them and can cause central nervous system depression and renal and hepatic damage.

When a hydrocarbon causes systemic symptoms or when it is in combination with other ingredients that have systemic toxicity, it is best to remove it from the stomach. *Ipecac* is highly preferred, and contrary to earlier beliefs, aspiration occurs upon ingestion and *not* in the process of inducing emesis. Lavage, on the other hand, increases the chance of aspiration because hydrocarbons cling to the tube and on withdrawal more easily enter the trachea. When treating aspiration, the use of steroids is contraindicated. They inhibit the natural immunosuppressive response of the cell.

Substances/Examples
- Gasoline
- Kerosine } vomit if 1 ml/kg
- Turpentine
- Toluene
- Xylene } always vomit
- Benzene
- Heavy greases
- Motor oil } no need to vomit
- Furniture polish

Clinical Effects
- Aspiration pneumonitis
- Central nervous system depression
- Albuminuria
- Hematuria
- Hepatic damage
- Cardiac arrhythmias

Lab Work
- Arterial blood gases
- Chest roentgenogram with a repeat in 12 to 24 hr
- Renal studies
- Hepatic studies

Treatment
- Induce emesis, if appropriate
- Cathartics
- Supportive care
- *Avoid* steroids, epinephrine, analeptics

Iron

Iron is found in a number of preparations including multivitamins with iron and prenatal vitamins. Iron has a direct effect on the gastrointestinal mucosa. In less than 2 hours there can be severe hemorrhagic necrosis with large losses of blood and fluid. The plasma iron concentration and total iron-binding capacity may vary and are regulated by hemoglobin synthesis. In children, iron preparations have been fatal. Careful calculations must be made of the amount of elemental iron ingested.

Substances/Examples
- Multivitamins with iron
- Ferrous gluconate
- Entron
- Fergon
- Ferralet plus
- Ferrous sulfate
- Mol-Iron
- Feosol
- Fer-In-Sol
- Ferrous fumarate

Clinical Effects
- 1st phase—30 min to 2 hr
     lethargy
     restlessness
     hematemesis
     abdominal pain
     bloody diarrhea
- 2nd phase—immediately following period of apparent recovery
- 3rd phase—2 to 12 hr after the first phase
     onset of shock
     refractory acidosis
     cyanosis
     fever
- 4th phase—2 to 4 days
     possible hepatic necrosis

Lab Work
- STAT—serum iron
           total iron binding capacity
- Flat plate of abdomen
- Type and crossmatch for blood
- Electrolytes

Treatment
- Support life
     correct shock with fluids or blood
     electrolytes as indicated
- Ipecac: if not contraindicated
- Lavage—sodium bicarbonate or Fleet Phosphate Enema Solution
- Deferoxamine for severe symptoms or if serum iron is greater than 350 mg/dl

Acetaminophen

Acetaminophen is an antipyretic and minor analgesic commonly found in households for those who cannot or would prefer not to take aspirin. Because it is so common, people often confuse aspirin and acetaminophen. One needs to be cautious as to which medication was taken when there is an accidental or intentional overdose. Acetaminophen overdose is considered to be an acute ingestion of 7.5 g or more.

There are no unique signs or symptoms in the first 24 hours following the exposure that would make the diagnosis definite. Persons present with general symptoms commonly seen with medical problems as well as with overdose.

Treatment with N-acetylcysteine must be initiated within 16 hours. If not, acute hepatocellular necrosis will result and 1 out of 10 cases of massive overdose will cause death. It should be noted here that those patients who die from severe Darvocet-N ingestion most likely expire from propoxyphene effects rather than from the effects of acetaminophen.

Substances/Examples
- Tylenol
- Datril
- Liquiprin
- Nyquil

Clinical Effects
- Nausea
- Malaise
- Vomiting
- Right upper quadrant pain
- Hepatic necrosis—48 to 72 hr

Lab Work
- Serum glutamic-oxaloacetic transaminase (SGOT), serum glutamic-pyruvic transaminase (SGPT)
- Blood urea nitrogen (BUN) q 24 hr
- Total bilirubin
- Prothrombin time (P.T.)
- Acetaminophen level 4 hr post ingestion and repeat in 4 to 8 hr*

Treatment
- Acetaminophen only—lavage
- Mixed—charcoal and cathartic lavage after 1 hr

*4-hr toxic level equals 150 μg/ml

- Mucomyst (N-acetylcysteine) oral 20% — loading dose 140 mg/kg; maintenance dose 70 mg/kg q 4 hr x 17

Salicylates

Salicylates are used as antipyretic, analgesic, anti-inflammatory, and antirheumatoid medications. Absorption is erratic, and a lag up to 28 hours can occur. Salicylates obey a zero order of kinetics; that is, doubling the dose may more than double the plasma level. Half-life may be increasingly prolonged. A plasma level before 6 hours after ingestion is useless. In children, chronic ingestions cause hypoglycemia, but hyperglycemia is more common with overdose in adults. Salicylates interrupt prothrombin production and inhibit platelet function and other clotting factors.

Substances/Examples
- Aspirin
- Bufferin
- Anacin
- Bayer aspirin
- Aspergum
- Decaprin
- Ecotrin

Clinical Effects
- Mild—asymptomatic
    tinnitus
    deafness
- Moderate to Severe—
    hyperventilation
    severe vomiting
    hyperthermia
    coma
    hypoglycemia
    hyperglycemia
    acidosis
- Very Severe—
    pulmonary edema
    convulsions
    severe acidosis
    acute renal failure

Lab Work
- Aspirin level 6 hr after exposure and repeat 12 hr
- Electrolytes
- Clotting factors
- Arterial blood gases
- Urine *p*H

Treatment
- Ipecac/lavage/charcoal/cathartic
- Maintain respirations
- Alkalinization of urine
- Hemodialysis, if indicated

- Hyperpyrexia should *not* be treated with alcohol sponging or salicylates

Barbiturates

Barbiturates are of two basic types: short-acting and long-acting. They are used as anticonvulsants, sedatives, and hypnotics. The effects seem to be primarily due to the interference with impulse transmission to the cerebral cortex—central nervous system depression. They have no analgesic properties. They are metabolized in the liver. Short-acting barbiturates have little excretion in the kidney whereas long-acting barbiturates are primarily cleared in the kidney in overdosage. The drug is generally highly protein bound. Addiction is frequently a possibility.

Short-Acting Barbiturates

Substances/Examples
- Pentobarbital
- Nebralin
- Nembutal
- Night-caps
- Pental
- Secobarbital
- Seconal

Clinical Effects
- CNS depression—respiratory/cardiac arrests
- Coma
- Hypotension
- Hypoxia
- Hypothermia
- Bullae
- Withdrawal symptoms
    tremors
    nausea
    anorexia
    vomiting
    muscular weakness
    convulsions

Lab Work
- Plasma levels—repeated
- Electrolytes

Treatment
- Establish airway
- Prevent absorption:
    ipecac/lavage/charcoal/cathartic
- Charcoal perfusion, forced diuresis, and hemodialysis *not* effective
- Valium for seizures

Long-Acting Barbiturates

Substances/Examples
- Phenobarbital
- Methabarbital
- Mysoline (15% converted to phenobarbital)

Clinical Effects
- Same as short-acting barbiturates
- Varying degrees of coma and CNS depression — respiratory/cardiac arrest
- Aspiration pneumonia

Lab Work
- Plasma levels — repeated
- Electrolytes
- Urine pH

Treatment
- Establish respirations
- Prevent absorption:
    ipecac/lavage/charcoal/cathartic
- Forced alkaline diuresis (hemodialysis if unresponsive)
- Hypotension/shock — fluids first, then vasopressors
- Bullae — burn treatment
- Seizures — Valium

Tricyclic Antidepressants
Tricyclic antidepressants are used in the treatment of endogenous depression. The tricyclic antidepressants are rapidly distributed once they are absorbed from the gastrointestinal tract. They are highly lipid and protein-bound, which is very important to remember when treating this type of overdose. Tricyclic antidepressants have both central and peripheral effects resulting from the blockage of the re-uptake of norepinephrine, an atropinelike anticholinergic effect and a direct myocardial depressant effect. The major cause of mortality is the cardiotoxicity. Ventricular, supraventricular, and atrioventricular delay dysrhythmias may result.

Substances/Examples
- Triavil
- Etrafon
- Impramine
- Amitriptyline
- Doxepin
- Desipramine
- Nortriptyline
- Nordoxepin

Clinical Effects
- Decrease gastrointestinal motility
- Respiratory depression
- Cardiac arrhythmias
- Hypertension
- Hypotension
- Abnormal deep tendon reflexes
- Seizures
- Coma
- Hallucinations

Lab Work
- Plasma levels
- Electrolytes
- Arterial blood gases

Treatment
- Airway management
- Ipecac/lavage
- Charcoal q 4 hr for 24 hr
    (Hemodialysis and charcoal hemoperfusion are *not* effective)
- Cardiac monitoring — especially for prolonged QRS
- Physostigmine for life-threatening symptoms
- Hypotension — fluids first, then vasopressors
- Seizures — Valium

Carbon Monoxide
Carbon monoxide is an odorless and tasteless gas. It is found in the exhaust of automobiles, in the emissions of backyard barbecue devices, after the inhalation of methylene chloride, and when gas burns incompletely. Carbon monoxide is not found in natural gas but can be contained in the gas produced from coal. It has a strong affinity to and combines quickly with hemoglobin to produce carboxyhemoglobin. In persons with a compromised cardiovascular system, 15% saturation of carboxyhemoglobin or greater can produce a heart attack.

Substances/Examples
- Incomplete combustion
- Automobile exhaust

Clinical Effects
- Earliest signs:
    headache
    tightness across forehead
    throbbing in temples
- Weakness — collapse
- Dizziness — syncope
- Nausea
- Vomiting
- Increased pulse rate
- Increased respiratory rate

Lab Work
- Plasma levels
- Liver function tests
- Arterial blood gases

Treatment
- Remove from environment
- Establish respirations
- Oxygen at high flow
- *No* analeptic drugs
- Convulsions — Valium
- *Monitor all* vital signs

BIBLIOGRAPHY

Berkowitz BA: Relationship of pharmacokinetics to pharmacological activity: Morphine, methadone, naloxone. Clin Pharmacokinet, January 1976, pp 219–230

Brown J et al: Experiment kerosene pneumonia: Evaluations of some therapeutic regimes. J Pediatr, March 1974, pp 396–401

Csajka PA, Duffy JP: Poisoning Emergencies, p 5. St. Louis, C.V. Mosby, 1980

Extension of Assistance of Emergency Medical Services System: Report by Committee on Interstate and Foreign Commerce. U.S. Goverment Printing Office, Washington, D.C., May 15, 1979

Jacobs J et al: Acute iron intoxication. N Engl J Med, 273, No. 21:1124–1127, 1965

Matthew H, Lawson A: Treatment of Common Acute Poisonings, 3rd ed. Edinburgh, Churchill Livingstone, 1974

Peterson RG, Rumack BH: Treating acute acetaminophen poisoning with acetylcysteine. JAMA 237:2406–2407, 1977

Picchioni AL et al: Activated charcoal versus 'universal antidote' as an antidote for poison. Toxicol Appl Pharmacol 8:447–454, 1966

Robertson WO: Iron poisoning: A problem of childhood. Top Emerg Med 1, No. 3:57–62, 1979

Rumack BH (ed): Poisindex. Englewood, Micromedex, 1979

Rumack BH, Burrington JB: Caustic ingestions: A rational look at diluents. Clin Toxicol, November 1977, pp 27–34

Rumack BH, Sullivan JB: Management of the Acutely Poisoned Patient. The Rocky Mountain Poison Center, September 20, 1979

Spiker DG et al: Tricyclic antidepressant overdose: Clinical presentation and plasma levels. Clin Pharmacol Ther 18, No. 5:539–546, 1975

Sullivan JB et al: Management of tricyclic antidepressant toxicity. Top Emerg Med 1, No. 3:65–71, 1979

Barbara Lockwood

Flight Nursing: Care of the Critically Ill Patient at Altitude 30

Persons experiencing a medical emergency have, in the past, had to await treatment until they arrived at a hospital or clinic. Now, what once was dreamed of in fantasy is a reality at St. Anthony Hospital Systems, Denver, Colorado.

Prior to October 1972, the only "flight nurses" most people had heard of were Air Force officers. However, during the past several years, a number of people in Colorado and across the nation have come in contact with a hospital flight nurse from St. Anthony's "Flight For Life" program. This program came about because a small group of people were dedicated to the idea of delivering quality emergency care to the victim at the scene, no matter where the situation occurred.* Typically, nurses had very little to do with the planning of the program, even though the registered nurse was to play the vital role. As the primary care deliverer, the nurse developed into the focal point of the endeavor—the ultimate factor which determined its success or failure.

The most significant aspect of the "Flight For Life" program is that it is not primarily a transportation system. It is a system that responds to victims wherever they are and continues to care for them until they are placed in the care of a

---

*The "Flight For Life" program would not have been possible without the continuous encouragement and support of the medical staff, the Administration, and the Board of Directors of St. Anthony Hospital Systems, and the Sisters of Saint Francis. Their innovative ideas and input were vital to the development of the nurse's role as it is today. Their willingness to support such a program and the participating nurses is truly unique.

physician in a medical facility. This system delivers sophisticated medical equipment and a highly trained, well-educated nursing team. Symptomatic reversal of the crisis begins as soon as the team arrives at the scene. Once the victim is stabilized, he is transported by helicopter or fixed-wing aircraft under the close supervision and care of the nursing team.

The need for rapid transportation and easy access to the scene, as well as the rugged terrain of the Rocky Mountains, made the helicopter the perfect vehicle for this service. As the service expanded, regulation fixed-wing aircraft were added to accommodate longer flights. The concept underlying the flight nurse program has been realized. Today the program transports 272 patients per month and continues to grow. Now an international program, the longer fixed-winged flights have taken the nurses into 32 states, to both coasts of the country, and to Costa Rica, Canada, and Mexico.

The purpose of this chapter is to explore the role of the flight nurse and to outline the qualifications that nurses assuming this role must possess. Background training and education, special knowledge and skill, personality characteristics, and the personal commitment necessary to fill the role will be discussed. This exploration would be incomplete without a discussion of the mechanisms incorporated into the program for maintaining reliability and ensuring accountability of the nurse.

The flight nurse is a critical care nurse practitioner, skilled in intervening in emergency situations of all kinds. The ultimate aim, of course, is to get the patient to a hospital alive. She is well versed in all aspects of critical care and crisis intervention. Therefore, a generalist approach to nursing is an absolute necessity. The flight nurse is able to care for the cardiopulmonary arrest victim as well as for the patient with crushing trauma or the child with epiglottitis. The care she delivers is directed at the immediate crisis. *Longer term care* will be undertaken by others upon arrival at the hospital.

Preparation of the Flight Nurse

In order to meet the above expectations, a broad experience base is helpful. This gives the nurse basic knowledge that she can build upon so that she can develop, over several months, into an excellent flight nurse. Nurses of various professional backgrounds have become flight nurses. They have all worked several years in emergency rooms, intensive care units, or coronary care units. One requirement is experience with critically ill patients with both medical and surgical problems. Expertise in trauma makes it easier to assimilate all the new material the nurse is required to learn. Another desired experiential element is having worked with patients of all ages — newborn to aged.

Assimilating past clinical experiences and education into the skills and theoretic knowledge required for flight nursing is accomplished by several processes. The desired end result is to develop a critical care nurse practitioner, capable of assessing all emergencies, choosing the appropriate method of intervention, and reversing the crisis in unpredictable, unstable surroundings. In order to develop this expertise, the flight nurse undergoes an intensive, rigorous orientation period.

Much of this orientation involves an "unlearning" process. She must learn to work outside of the more comfortable hospital surroundings, where equipment is stable and where there are many experienced people on whom to rely. The typical working environment of the flight nurse is ever changing. It may be a vibrating helicopter, a small fixed-wing airplane in turbulent weather, a bathroom floor, a garage, an interstate highway, the interior of an overturned vehicle, or a small rural hospital with very limited facilities. Her supplies and equipment must be portable and are packed away into a multitude of small cases. The people the flight nurse must rely on will probably have less expertise than she does. These people also change with the location of the crisis. Most likely those who are at the scene will be emergency medical technicians, firemen, paramedics, law enforcement agents, onlookers, and the family of the victim.

During the early phase an enormous amount of learning is still going on, both on and off the job. For example, each flight nurse must complete a nine-month critical care practitioner course offered at the hospital. The course is directed at preparing the nurse who will work in areas where sophisticated facilities are nonexistent and where physicians are not immediately available. It stresses a systems approach to illness and injury and a review of physiology, common and not-so-common emergencies and the appropriate interventions that a nurse may initiate in these situations. After the orientation process is completed, the nurse begins to fly on her own.

None of her education and training lies fallow. The flight nurse must have her entire knowledge base at her disposal at all times. There is no way to second guess what types of patients will be seen in an eight-hour shift. One rule everyone learns early is "always expect the worst." The chances of being unprepared are minimized by this philosophy.

While the knowledge base of the flight nurse has been described in general, a review of her specific areas of expertise gives a more complete picture of what makes her as effective as she is.

A solid understanding of anatomy and physiology, as well as of anatomical abnormalities and pathophysiology, of all body systems is essential. In order to determine where a victim is bleeding internally one must know what organs lie under the injured exterior. For example, several crushed lower left ribs should alert the nurse to a possible splenic injury. Anticipation of this potential problem may save the victim's life. It is also extremely difficult to assess a distressed newborn if one has had no experience in caring for a normal infant.

Role of the Flight Nurse

MAINTAINING A PATENT AIRWAY

The flight nurse must have a firm command of the care of the patient with respiratory embarrassment, whatever the cause. She must be able to recognize and clear an obstructed airway. The obstruction may be caused by emesis or blood, a foreign body, or trauma, and it may be of the upper or the lower airways.

Once the nurse has cleared the airway, she must be sure that it remains open. This may simply involve positioning the victim on his or her side and applying frequent suctioning, or it may require intubating the patient and assisting ventilation with a hand ventilator (Ambu bag).

Intubation. The intubation procedure is taught by anesthesiologists in the calm controlled environment of the hospital. It is up to the flight nurse to become proficient enough to intubate in any circumstance. Most people do not collapse in "convenient" places. They are usually on the floor, requiring the nurse to intubate on her knees or stomach, or outside in the bright sunlight, where it is difficult to visualize with a laryngoscope's small bulb. (The latter problem can be solved by having a large person block the sunlight during the procedure.)

Regardless of where or under what circumstances intubation is done, the same principles apply. All the necessary equipment must be available. The procedure must be done quickly to reduce the risk of hypoxia. The intubator must be accurate and must recognize immediately if the endotracheal tube is correctly positioned. Trauma must be kept to a minimum. These principles require the nurse intubating in untoward circumstances to possess the greatest expertise possible.

The most important aspect of intubation, however, is not performing the skill well, but knowing when and when not to intubate. It is difficult to maintain a tight seal on a face mask when bagging a patient and moving him or her from the scene to the helicopter, flying in high winds, and moving him or her from the helicopter to the hospital. When the patient requires constant ventilation and transport is difficult, intubation may be indicated prior to transport. The unconscious patient with emesis or bleeding into the oral cavity obviously needs intubation to maintain a patent airway. Swelling of the neck from burns or hematomas may warrant intubation as a prophylaxis against an occluded airway, particularly if the trip to the hospital is long.

Regardless of the problems inherent to transporting the critical patient, some patients are better off if intubation is not attempted in the field. The child with epiglottitis may experience complete upper respiratory occlusion once the laryngoscope blade is placed in the mouth. Unless the nurse is prepared to do a tracheostomy, and she is not, the better plan is to support respiratory status as well as she can with a partially open airway and avoid intubation. To prevent the risk of injury to the spinal cord, patients who may have cervical spine fractures are not always intubated. A tracheostomy done at the hospital will be safer for such patients.

Each patient is different, and whether or not the nurse intubates is dependent upon her judgment of the patient's condition, the time transport will take, and other factors such as weather conditions and mode of transportation. Flight nurses try to avoid intubating the patient in flight. Hitting an air pocket during the procedure may rid the patient of his front teeth, or worse. The nurse's skill, judgment, and anticipation of problems that may occur in flight can save the patient from unnecessary complications or further injury.

AUSCULTATION SKILLS

In order to interpret placement of the endotracheal tube without the benefit of a radiograph, the nurse has expertise in using auscultation to evaluate breath sounds. This skill is also useful for determining the extent of pulmonary congestion from chronic lung disease, pulmo-

edema, or fluid overload, and for recogniz-
g pneumothorax and ruptured diaphragm.

One obstacle frequently prevents the use of
auscultation: noise. The helicopter and fixed-
wing aircraft are very noisy. Even the atmosphere outside the aircraft may be so perme-
ated with the sounds of traffic, extrication
equipment, and the aircraft itself that the ears are
rendered useless. The flight nurse learns to adapt
other senses to make up for this loss. The senses
of sight and touch become primary assessment
tools. If the sides of the chest are not rising
equally, there is probably a pneumothorax, or
the endotracheal tube is in the right mainstem
bronchus. A deviated trachea can alert the nurse
immediately to a pneumothorax or hemo-
pneumothorax.

The nurse develops the ability to *feel* rales and
rhonchi. The color of the patient's skin is observed closely for the slightest change that may
indicate improvement or deterioration of respiratory status. Should the nurse discover a pneumothorax, she can "needle" the affected side of
the chest with an angiocath to evacuate the
trapped air.

OXYGEN THERAPY

Reversing acute problems of the respiratory system requires an in-depth understanding of
oxygen transport problems. The nurse must
know when to apply oxygen and how much is
appropriate. Since Denver, Colorado sits one
mile above sea level, the amount of oxygen is less
than that of sea level communities, and the resi-
dents' blood gas levels are different. Many people served by the "Flight For Life" program live
in mountain communities at higher elevations.
Colorado also has a large tourist trade, bringing
people from all over the country.

The flight nurse must be familiar with oxygen
transport variances caused by altitude changes.
The history taken from the patient or family
should include place of residence. Many oxygen
transport problems occur in people from sea
level communities when they come to Colorado. Some chronic illnesses, like emphysema,
are aggravated. The most common problem occurs on the ski slopes. The cold, in combination
with relative hypoxia in individuals accustomed
to a more heavily oxygen-laded atmosphere,
frequently produces high altitude pulmonary
edema. Hypoxia also causes high altitude psychosis. Each flight nurse cares for several of these
victims each ski season. Problems peculiar to
transporting the critically ill at high altitudes in
unpressurized aircraft will be dealt with later in
this chapter.

CARDIAC EMERGENCIES

As would be expected, the flight nurse is also
proficient in intervening in cardiac emergencies.
Many patients with acute myocardial infarctions
are treated every year. This requires that the
nurse interpret electrocardiograms and treat life-
threatening arrhythmias. The appropriate drugs
(lidocaine, atropine, isoproterenol [Isuprel], sodium bicarbonate, adrenalin, and morphine sulfate) are carried for these emergencies. A
portable monitor-defibrillator is always on
board the aircraft for the observation and treatment of these patients.

While the electrocardiogram is an important
aspect of monitoring the acute infarct patient,
the flight nurse cannot always rely on her equipment. Altitude plays tricks with portable medical equipment. Very few such machines work
reliably above 10,000 feet. The rotor blade action of the helicopter and radio communications
can also cause inaccurate readings.

Because of these variables, the flight nurse
learns to watch the patient. She rarely takes her
eyes off the patient, or her fingers off the femoral
pulse. Talking to the patient constantly, she explains the flight, outlines what will happen at the
hospital, and monitors patient perceptions of
what is happening minute by minute.

Many people have expressed concern that
transporting the victim of acute myocardial infarction by air is dangerous and anxiety-producing for the patient. Surprisingly, most of the
awake patients do very well in flight. The close
monitoring and one-to-one relationship with
the nurse seem to comfort the patient and ease
anxiety.

Cardiopulmonary Resuscitation. The flight
nurse must also participate in many cardiopulmonary resuscitations (CPR). These may
occur in small rural hospitals, in the aircraft, on
the golf course, and in every other conceivable
location. The cause may be ventricular fibrillation due to acute myocardial infarction, cerebral
vascular accident, poisoning, drowning, elec-
trocution, or trauma. The victim may be an
infant, a child, a teenager, or an adult of any age.

Most of the arrests are not witnessed by the
flight nurse, for they have occurred before she
arrives on the scene. When the flight nurse arrives, she follows the protocol outlined by the
hospital for CPR. She becomes the team leader

and assigns duties to paraprofessional personnel or persons on the scene; one fireman to do closed chest massage, one to bag the victim after she has intubated, and so on. She carries out the protocol where appropriate, starts intravenous fluids, and gives the appropriate drugs. When all that is feasible is done at the scene, she prepares for transport.

CPR is continued enroute to the hospital while the nurse receives and carries out instructions from the emergency room physician. Upon arrival at the hospital, she and the patient are met by the "Cor Zero" team who continue resusciation efforts if indicated.

At the scene, the leadership abilities of the flight nurse can determine the outcome for the victim. If she can direct the people at the scene effectively, the chances of saving the victim increase. This requires all her knowledge and expertise, a calm approach, and continual observation of the procedure. She must correct ineffective closed chest massage, teach at the spur of the moment, and coordinate every person's activity for the benefit of the patient. In a highly charged emotional atmosphere, this takes a great deal of patience and is not easily done. Experience helps the nurse turn an excited crowd of parapro fessionals and laypeople into a very effective life-support team.

TRAUMATIC ACCIDENTS

Accidents are one of the foremost causes of death for all ages. The intervention of the flight nurse can significantly decrease morbidity and mor tality caused by accidents. All aspects of traumatic injury are in the nurse's repertoire.

Of primary importance to the well-being of the victim is an initial, thorough assessment from head to toe. All injuries are noted and treated when appropriate. In order to properly evaluate the patient's condition, the nurse must elicit as complete a history as possible. She must know how long ago the accident occurred, if there were witnesses, if the victim was moved, how much blood there was, whether or not seat belts were worn, and specific body areas which were bluntly injured.

Many times, the victim is still trapped in the vehicle upon arrival of the nurse. This necessitates initiation of appropriate therapy prior to extrication. After climbing into the vehicle, she makes her assessment and establishes the airway, stops any visible bleeding, and begins replacing fluid for hypovolemic shock, if indicated.

It has been mentioned above that the flight nurse's ears often become useless in the field. For this reason, blood pressures are difficult to obtain. One can still palpate to assess blood pressure, but this is extremely time-consuming if the victim is bleeding to death. Most flight nurses rely more upon the rate and quality of peripheral and central pulses. Young adults can maintain their blood pressures until exsanguination occurs. A rapid thready pulse will indicate impending death much earlier than a change in blood pressure.

Only absolutely necessary procedures are done at the scene. Many victims of trauma will die if surgery is delayed. In such cases, the airway is opened, IVs are started, and large fractures are immobilized. This type of emergency requires the nurse to call on all her experience and best judgment. If a hospital can be reached within 10 minutes, fluid resuscitation can wait until nurse and patient are airborne. Longer flights require the nurse to do more for the victim at the scene, but she must work quickly and deftly while the patient is still bleeding. Air transportation of these victims expedites the trip; often the helicopter is used for this type of injured patient. Upon arrival at the hospital, the surgeon and surgical team take over.

Flight nurses also see a large number of victims with head or spinal cord injuries. Besides immobilization and transportation, a thorough assessment is extremely important. The condition of the patient—level of consciousness, degree of sensation, motor abilities, vital signs, and pupillary reaction—must continually be monitored. Any changes must be noted. When the patient arrives at the hospital, the physician will be better able to assess his or her neurologic status if an accurate record has been kept.

In order to care for the victim of neurotrauma more effectively, each flight nurse has received additional instruction at the regional center for neurotrauma in Denver. Nurses have learned to insert Gardner-Wells tongs to immobilize cervical fractures, apply traction, pad and use a portable Stryker frame. Instructions for this sophisticated therapy are received from a physician in Denver by telephone or radio.

OTHER EMERGENCIES

Many medical emergencies in and around Denver require more than the expertise of the flight nurse. The most common of these are *poison ingestions* and *poisonous bites*. When these occur close to the hospital, the nurse treats the symptoms as indicated. Those emergencies occurring outside the Denver area require consultation with the Rocky Mountain Poison Control Center. A physician or a nurse from this team accompanies the flight nurse to the rural hospital requesting assistance.

The flight nurse administers life support while the poison control personnel initiate therapy directed at reversing the effects of the particular poison. Simultaneous use of the expertise of both teams has proved extremely effective in decreasing morbidity and mortality in poison cases.

Two other types of emergencies call into play the participation of other experts available in the city. Care of the *critical neonate* requires constant input from neonatologists and personnel in neonatal intensive care nurseries in Denver. The flight nurse is taught to assess the neonate and to correct the common problems of these tiny patients: ventilation, circulation, temperature control, and maintenance of adequate glucose levels. During transport, she receives specific instructions from a neonatologist in Denver as she relays her assessment of the infant's condition and describes the infant's symptoms. The neonatal nurseries provide the clinical experience for the flight nurses; their personnel are the instructors.

Recently, the program has also begun to participate in the transportation of *high-risk mothers* to Denver hospitals specializing in their care. Medical personnel from these hospitals accompany the flight nurse on these flights. The team is always prepared not only to treat the mother, but to deliver a distressed infant. Adding this service has required further education of flight nurses so they can appropriately evaluate the high-risk mother, anticipate problems she may have, and intervene in any potential or realized emergency during transport. Many hospital critical care nurses are required to have a good deal of the above described knowledge base and expertise.

EFFECTS OF ALTITUDE

One area of expertise unique to the flight nurse is the ability to understand and apply the principles of aerospace medicine to the care of her patients.

On the Nurse. The nurse must be acutely aware of the effects altitude has on her performance. Most of the regulation aircraft used are pressurized; however, the helicopter, which is used in the majority of flights, is not. In order to gain access into many of the mountain communities serviced, altitudes of 15,000 feet are reached. Anytime the helicopter flies above 10,000 feet, oxygen masks must be worn by the pilot and the nurse. Without oxygen, hypoxia would adversely affect the nurse's judgment, impede her ability to care for the patient, and even cause unconsciousness.

The nurse frequently works outside the helicopter at high elevations, such as on mountain rescues, or in Leadville, Colorado, which has an elevation of 10,000 feet. It is not practical to wear an oxygen mask under these circumstances, and, because she is not acclimatized to these elevations, she must conserve her strength and continually be aware of how the altitude is affecting her performance.

Other factors, such as whether or not she has eaten and the amount of sleep she has had, affect the nurse's performance at high altitudes. Flight nurses frequently work in excess of their 8-hour shifts and miss meals because of flights. If the nurse is tired and has a low blood sugar level, the effects of altitude-induced hypoxia will hinder performance more rapidly. All of these factors influence whether or not the nurse makes the right decision at the appropriate time.

On the Patient. Altitude affects the patient as well as the nurse. All patients are given oxygen if flying above 8,000 feet. The patient with an oxygen transport problem such as pulmonary edema, chronic lung disease, or flail chest has higher oxygen requirements. Hypovolemic patients also have higher oxygen requirements because they have fewer red blood cells and less hemoglobin to carry oxygen to the tissues. Patients who have received medications that depress the respiratory system, such as morphine and diazepam (Valium), require greater amounts of oxygen.

The flight nurse closely observes each patient for any signs of hypoxia during these high-altitude flights and adjusts the level of inspired oxygen accordingly. Many patients become anxious when the nurse tries to apply oxygen because they fear their condition has suddenly worsened. A brief explanation of the effects of altitude and the nurse's simultaneous use of oxygen usually allay the patient's fears.

Other Considerations of High Altitudes

Besides decreased oxygen supply, high altitudes are accompanied by an overall decrease in atmospheric pressure. This causes a number of problems for patients with specific injuries. Complications increase as altitude increases and decrease as altitude decreases. For example, increased intracranial pressure from a closed head injury rises higher as altitude increases. The patient may become stuporous and later obtunded. As altitude decreases, the level of consciousness improves. This phenomenon makes it very difficult to evaluate a closed head injury. Altitude may not be the only factor influencing the level of consciousness. The patient may truly be deteriorating independently of the effect of altitude.

Decreased atmospheric pressure also has adverse effects on open injuries. An enucleated eye may lose more vitreous humor as altitude increases. These patients should never be transported in unpressurized aircraft unless another injury will cause death before safer transportation can be arranged. Bleeding will also increase as altitude does. This may require more rapid fluid replacement at high altitudes. The nurse must take extra precautions not to overload the patient. Fluid replacement itself becomes a problem at altitudes in excess of 10,000 feet. Intravenous fluids do not run correctly. For this reason plastic IV bags are used. Blood pumps must be applied to the bags and the pressure adjusted to obtain the correct rate of flow. Edema also increases with decreased atmospheric pressure. Casts may have to be bivalved before transportation to prevent cutting off circulation to the limb.

Closed drainage systems cannot be used at high altitudes because the fluid or air will not move from the body to the receptacle. Adequate drainage is obtained by venting all drainage systems to the air—Foley bags, nasogastric tubes, and so on. Decompression of the stomach may have to be assisted manually by the nurse. Normal chest tube drainage systems are replaced with a one-way valve apparatus to release air trapped in the pleural cavity. This is extremely important because pneumothoraxes extend as altitude increases.

The complications caused by decreased atmospheric pressure and decreased oxygen supply play a continual role in the flight nurse's decision-making processes. Both she and the patient are affected. Continual observation of the patient for any adverse signs and symptoms, plus awareness of her own response to the environment, is essential. Anticipating potential problems prepares the nurse to take corrective action when necessary. All knowledge of various illnesses and injuries is collated with an indepth understanding of aerospace medicine.

SURVIVAL TRAINING

Along with the foregoing, the nurse has a healthy respect for the potential hazards that the aircraft she works on and around holds for her and her patients. She works within stated safety regulations enforced by the pilots and the Federal Aviation Association (FAA). Because she works outdoors much of the time, she must understand the influence of environment on the human body. Excessive temperatures, either hot or cold, will affect her performance as well as her patient's condition. She must be prepared to survive in the wilderness if something should go wrong with the aircraft. Survival training is part of flight nurse orientation, and a special survival kit is taken on every flight into the mountains.

It takes most nurses several months to learn the required material and skills and assimilate them into a framework within which they can perform. All the material must be readily available to the nurse in order for her to assess the patient, arrive at a conclusion, appropriately intervene in the emergency, continue to monitor the patient, and respond to any changes. The ultimate goal is to deliver the patient to the hospital in better condition than he was at the time of the crisis.

ASSESSMENT LIMITATIONS

To realize this goal, the flight nurse must be able to concentrate on several areas at once. Knowledge and skill combined with the data obtained from various sources provide the basis for the split-second decisions the nurse needs to make. The importance of excellent oservation skills cannot be overemphasized. Any overlooked symptom, no matter how minor it appears, may change the outcome for the patient. Observation of the patient has always been one of nursing's primary responsibilities. Accurate observation, however, is much more difficult for the flight nurse because of the working environment.

The flight nurse makes her assessment without the luxuries many nurses take for granted. There are no radiographs to confirm a fracture or check for endotracheal tube placement, no blood gas studies to confirm respiratory acidosis, no blood work to confirm electrolyte imbalance, hematocrit and hemoglobin levels, or serum glucose. It has been noted how useless the ears become when confronted with the high noise level at the scene and on board the aircraft. Performance of common procedures such as listening for breath sounds and measuring blood pressures is impossible. Monitoring equipment is also less reliable in the field than in the hospital. It is subject to interference, not only from the patient's movements, but also from the aircraft's vibration and radio communications. As stated earlier, equipment does not function properly above certain altitudes.

Few nurses consider working in well-lighted facilities a luxury. The flight nurse, however, will see at least half of her patients after dark. A flashlight may be the only source of light available. Once aboard the helicopter, the nurse cannot use bright lights because the pilot would be blinded and unable to navigate. After several months, the flight nurse is able to note even skin color changes in the dark almost as well as she does in light.

Observing the patient is hindered not only by the absence of light but also by the inability to examine the injured portions of the body. During the winter months, many patients' injuries are hidden under layers of bulky clothing. It is unwise to undress the patient in freezing temperatures. The nurse learns to feel for fractures and other injuries through the clothing. If she is in doubt, it is safer to immobilize a suspected fracture than to assume the limb is uninjured.

The flight nurse works around these obstacles to accurate observation of the patient. She assumes nothing and suspects the worst. To appropriately evaluate the patient requires the nurse's constant vigilance and the ability to substitute other senses when one is rendered inefficient. Most patients can save the nurse frustrating minutes by relating what is wrong. The patient's subjective appraisal of his body is extremely accurate. Nurses frequently forget this, but many times the patient can save his or her own life if someone is willing to listen. Flight nurses have learned that patients who say they are going to die will do so with extreme rapidity if the crisis is not reversed.

IMPLEMENTING PROTOCOLS OF CARE

Whether or not the crisis is reversed is the ultimate responsibility of the flight nurse. The survival of the patient is dependent upon how well the nurse interprets her observations and on what measures she takes to stabilize the victim prior to transportation. No one wants to lose a patient in the air because something was left undone at the scene. Long-term survival also depends on what is done during transport. A misplaced endotracheal tube will doom the patient to certain anoxic brain death. A fracture which is not immobilized may cause the loss of a limb.

Physicians at St. Anthony Hospital Systems have established protocols for the treatment of every imaginable emergency. These are not standing orders. Standing orders limit the nurse's judgment. Protocols allow the nurse room to incorporate knowledge, observation and assessment of the patient, and nursing judgment into treatment. Flight nurses do not make differential diagnoses. Rather, they evaluate the symptoms presented and treat them accordingly. If the patient is bleeding, they try to stop the bleeding and replace fluid loss, and so on.

No two emergencies or patients are alike. In order to make the best decision and to reverse the crisis effectively, the nurse must call on prior knowledge, past experience, all observable data, including patient history, and all the common sense available to her, and then "tailor-make" a given protocol to meet the needs of the patient.

An example of this decision-making process is the treatment of the patient with a flail chest. The protocol states that the method of stabilizing a flail chest is intubation with assisted mechanical ventilation. If the patient were comatose and had severe paradoxical respiration, the flight nurse would intubate and ventilate with a hand ventilator (bag resuscitator) until the patient could be placed on a mechanical ventilator at the hospital. However, this patient is wide awake, frightened, and having moderate paradoxical respiration. The hospital is 3 minutes away by air. The nurse cannot intubate because the patient would resist frantically. The nurse has two choices: (1) wait until the patient becomes comatose or (2) administer large amounts of oxygen by nasal cannula and mask, splint the patient, if possible, and get to the hospital as fast as possible. The second choice is clearly the best for the patient. Once at the hospital, the physician can administer a paralytic respiratory drug, intubate, and place the patient on a mechanical ventilator. Should the patient lose consciousness in flight, the trip is very short, so he can be ventilated with a bag and mask until landing at the hospital, where he can be intubated and supported properly.

DECISION-MAKING AND LEADERSHIP SKILLS

Decisions made by the flight nurse are always countered by an element of risk. Each action taken may cause yet another complication. In the example above, the nurse is counting on the patient's remaining awake and cooperative during the flight. The nurse must have alternative actions prepared if her expectations are incorrect. She must also balance one alternative against another, sometimes choosing the one least likely to harm the patient. There are no easy formulas to follow. The nurse does whatever is necessary to intercede in the crisis within the scope of her abilities.

Accountability is a word each flight nurse understands intimately. The patient's welfare is the nurse's responsibility. Each decision made must be justified and evaluated. The final analysis lies with the patient.

The most difficult decision for the flight nurse to make is to decide to do nothing. Action may harm a patient more than watching and waiting. To accompany a patient screaming in pain is terrifying. It would be easier on the nurse to medicate the patient for pain. However, that very pain will help the physician to recognize and correct the problem. In mass casualty accidents or disasters, it is extremely difficult for the nurse to leave the dying victims in order to save others.

Decision-making is vital to the flight nurse's role. If the nurse cannot mobilize others at the scene of the crisis to help carry out the decisions made, the effort is futile. The helicopter draws hundreds of onlookers everywhere it lands. The people who called for the flight nurse are anxious to help but generally are less skilled and less knowledgeable. Leadership by a calm, experienced, critical care practitioner will turn chaos into an environment conducive to the survival of the patient. Mastery of this kind of situation takes a very long time. It is the most difficult thing a flight nurse has to do and the hardest thing to learn.

prepares whatever is necessary for the patient. If the nurse communicates incorrectly, the hospital may not be prepared.

For example, the patient has a thoracic-aortic aneurysm diagnosed by a physician in a small rural hospital. The nurse phones the receiving hospital and states the patient has an aortic aneurysm. Upon the patient's arrival, a general surgeon is ready to revise an abdominal-aortic aneurysm, but a chest surgeon must be called in, delaying the operation another 30 minutes. The only thing that will save this patient is surgery, which was delayed by the nurse's faulty communication.

Much has been written about the impact a crisis has on family members and loved ones. The flight nurse must deal with this daily, for many crises occur with loved ones present. When the helicopter and flight nurse arrive, families must stand by helplessly watching the painful, sometimes almost barbaric, process of saving their loved one's life. There is no place like a hospital waiting room for the family. There are no curtains to draw around the victim. Many people cannot bear to watch and leave voluntarily. Others stand fixed, unable to move from the spot. Some are victims with their own injuries asking what happened to their son or wife. Whatever the situation, the flight nurse tries to help the family cope with the crisis. Families who lose loved ones after heroic efforts have been made by the flight team are sometimes angry. Flight nurses frequently feel guilty when the family of a deceased victim receives a bill for services rendered. Many times, however, the family thanks the team. Their loved one died, but they know that had there been any chance of survival he would have lived. They do not have to wonder, "Could something more have been done?"

COMMUNICATION SKILLS

A strong leader has to have excellent communication skills. The nurse must translate medical terminology into words the laypeople helping can understand. In order to direct patient care, the nurse must give orders that are clear and to the point. A good communicator also listens to witnesses to learn the history of the situation and the minute-by-minute changes they observed. Communication with the receiving hospital is vital to continuity of care. The nurse radios the condition of the patient to the hospital and receives orders from physicians, while the hospital

AUDIT SUPPORT SYSTEM

Flight nursing is an expanded role for the registered nurse. She has skills and makes decisions that may never be required of other nurses. All nursing roles must build in a system of checks and balances to ensure optimum care and safety for the patient; this expanded role requires an even more elaborate system. For the nurse who works under little direct supervision, the process must provide for quality control, ensure that expertise of the nurse is maintained, evaluate success or failure, and provide a continuous learning situation for all.

An elaborate audit system provides those checks and balances necessary for the flight nurse role. This consists of peer review, supervisor review, and review by the medical director and any other physician he consults. Each flight record is audited daily by the nursing supervisor and medical director. The flight nurse may be called on at any time to justify what she did for any given patient. Statistics are also kept on each patient transport, breaking down what was done for the patient, diagnosis made by the receiving physician, and outcome for the patient. It would be impossible to evaluate the actions taken by the nurses without a thorough follow-up of the patients.

Perhaps the most important part of the audit system is the bimonthly flight nurse meeting. During these meetings, the nurses review flights together. They discuss the patient's history, the crisis that required the team, the assessment the nurse made, the problem-solving process used to decide on treatment, and patient outcome. These dialogues allow the nurses to explore and rehearse alternatives with their peers. The nurses learn from one another how they might approach a problem the next time they encounter it. More experienced nurses give helpful hints to those new to the program. The atmosphere is safe for openness, allowing the nurses to question and explore without ridicule. It takes a strong nursing leader to ensure that this atmosphere is maintained and that each nurse is given the opportunity to learn and develop professionally.

The medical director also attends these meetings. Serving as a resource person, he answers questions, adds medical input to case reviews, and provides the medical support necessary for the success of the flight nurse. The flight nurse meeting is also used to provide in-service education. The statistics, the patients, the medical director, and the nurses themselves determine what subjects are to be reviewed and what new areas of knowledge need to be taught.

IMPLICATIONS

The "Flight For Life" program is successful. It has provided a system that begins to reverse the crisis before the patient arrives at a hospital, and it continues to expand its service area. Expanding the role of the nurse to the role of the flight nurse has been instrumental in developing the program into what it is today. Without the expertise of the nurse, her commitment to her beliefs, her involvement with the community, and her willingness to work long hours in extreme environmental conditions, the program could not have been as successful.

The existence of "Flight For Life" has stimulated the community's ambulance companies, fire departments, and even the state patrol to become aware that moving a patient to a hospital rapidly without treatment is not always compatible with life. People are now concentrating on stabilizing the patient prior to transportation. Many private ambulances, fire departments, and rescue squads call the helicopter when they realize that the patient is too critical for them to handle. With increasing community awareness, the "Flight For Life" program is used for the right patient at the right time. Emergency care at the scene has improved immensely in the Denver metropolitan area since the program has been in existence. Those patients who do not require the flight nurse's skills are getting better, more comprehensive care by paraprofessionals prior to hospital arrival than ever before.

Flight nursing is a new role on the horizon. Only a few women and men have had the opportunity to experience it. Flight nurses have proved that a nurse can perform in areas only physicians worked in before. They have not become, as many feared, little doctors. Instead they have brought into the role all their past education and experience as nurses and have become well-educated, highly skilled crisis/critical care practitioners. Each nurse is acutely aware of her limitations and her responsibilities. Within the framework of the role, the nurses are contributing to the well-being of the community. They are helping save lives by being the second link in the life support chain

1. Basic life support given by those first on the scene
2. Advanced life support given by the flight nurse
3. Definitive therapy administered by the physician
4. Maintenance of life support provided by intensive care nurses and other hospital personnel

Many people have asked, "Why use a registered nurse? An emergency medical technician or a paramedic could do the same thing." With this the author strongly disagrees. While skills can be taught to anyone, the commitment to use them judiciously and to maintain accountability to the patient cannot. The entire nursing educational process is directed at developing people who will be committed to the patient's welfare before anything else. It has been a relatively successful socialization process. The basic nursing material presented gives each nurse enough theoretic and experiential background to build on to develop into any nursing role. No paraprofessional is as ready to take on the extra knowledge, new skill, and formidable responsibility as is the professional nurse. The role, if held by anyone else, would cease to be a nursing role. Nurses *do* make the *difference*.

**Unit
Five**

Professional Practice in the Critical Care Unit

Patricia D. Barry

Adverse Effects of Critical Care Units on the Nurse
31

Nurses in critical care units (CCUs) often feel a special sense of pride in themselves. The level of work they perform and the knowledge required to do their jobs well are known to be the most complex of any staff nursing positions in the hospital. Accompanying this justified self-pride and positive professional self-image is another self-expectation that many critical care nurses experience: to be calm and cool under pressure. This calmness has been commented on by several authors.[1-5]

It is interesting that it is frequently the nurses themselves who impose this expectation on themselves. Physicians, whom, it should be noted, have the opportunity to go into and out of the CCU, rather than remaining for assigned tours of duty, frequently remark on the nurses' apparent ability to tolerate the very high level of stress that exists there. Many doctors believe that the environment is difficult to tolerate for any period of time.[6] This implies that physicians would find it difficult to remain for several-hour periods and still maintain an outward calm. Patients and families react well and are calmed themselves by a cool, professional nurse demeanor. Importantly, they are also comforted by nurses who are able to become emotionally involved with them and occasionally "let go" of the professional demeanor and demonstrate their caring.

If physicians, patients, and families are all willing to accept the need for the nurse to be human and occasionally slip out of the cool, professional role, why, then, do so many CCU nurses impose this rigid expectation on themselves?

STRESSORS IN THE CCU

Unquestionably, the most important reason that CCU nurses set such high expectations for themselves is to help them maintain emotional equilibrium. This is the greatest coping defense that most nurses use in dealing with the constant pressures of the CCU. Before explaining and discussing the need for coping abilities in nurses, it is important to accurately present the variety of stresses on the intensive care nurse.

Most nurses would immediately identify the unpredictability of the CCU environment as a leading stressor. Other stressors are the "incessant repetitive routine . . .; every step must be charted . . .; floating in nurses from elsewhere . . .; frequent situations of acute crisis . . .; physical dangers (inadequate protection from x-rays, needles, isolation patients and those who are delirious; lifting heavy, unresponsive patients). . .; distraught relatives . . .; (constant sounds of) moaning, crying, screaming, buzzing and beeping monitors, gurgling suction pumps, and whooshing respirators . . ."[7] Another very important stress on the nurse, and one that should not be underestimated, is also described by Hay and Oken. Everywhere there are human bodies, many of them wasted, mutilated, or discolored. There are exposed genitalia, and excretions of feces, blood, chest mucus, vomitus, and urine. Some patients' dressings are soaked with purulent discharge, serous or bloody drainage.

STOP READING

Think back to your *honest* reaction as you read each of the stressors in the preceding section. Be honest with yourself.

TAKE A BIG BREATH AND LET IT OUT SLOWLY

Now, pretend that you are on a beautiful, green hillside that slopes gently downward to a sandy beach. There are large, crashing waves that you can see and hear. The sun is shining. You are lying under a graceful old maple tree that protects you from the sun. A breeze is gently blowing your hair. Beautiful! Right? Now, slowly reread the list of stressors and let yourself *feel* a response. You may feel nothing as you read some of them. For others you may feel disgust, anxiety, or boredom. Are you able to detect a difference between your first set of responses and your second set? If not, it is possible that the coping strategies that you have unconsciously developed have resulted in an emotional detachment that is causing you to miss many of the good and positive aspects of

life in and *out* of the CCU. It is very difficult to deaden one's response to negative emotional experiences without concurrently deadening it to pleasure and joy. What a high cost! What causes it to happen?

A common personality trait in many nurses is selflessness. This trait is nurtured and praised by nursing educators and administrators. When people are selfless they deny their own physical or emotional needs in the service of others. A nurse who legitimately refuses to work a double shift, float to another unit, or take on extra assignments because of chronic understaffing is usually not as popular with supervisors as one who denies his or her own needs and acquiesces immediately.

Because in the past, selflessness has been a desired trait in nurses and because the selfless individual has received far more approval from peers and supervisors than the outspoken person who tries to assert his rights, many nurses have been socialized into denying their own needs, their own feelings — their own humanness!

Remember that nowhere on earth are people born knowing how to deny their own needs and feelings. Instead they have *learned* to deny them. The most important motivation in this process is the need for approval.

Think for a moment: if it is true that physicians, patients, and families are all able to recognize the nurse's humanness and accept that, on occasion, the professional, calm, cool exterior shell can safely slide away, revealing the real person who is underneath, why then do we hold on so tightly to the cover and instead try to stifle our own humanness?

If we are looking for approval, to whom are we looking? Nursing peers and supervisors are the obvious answer: the easy answer! The tough answer is to admit that we do it to ourselves. Sometimes nurses are their own severest critics. If they fail in their own, sometimes impossible self-expectations, the result is guilt.

Many nurses were taught that it is not good to feel grief, fear, disgust, or love when working intimately with other human beings. Despite their own humanness they were taught that it was not "professional" to feel such emotions about patients. When a person feels something he was taught not to feel, the result is guilt. Since guilt is an unpleasant feeling, the mind (the ego, specifically) helps to defend the individual so that the guilt will not occur. Repression is a defense or coping mechanism that buries the original feelings of grief, fear, and so forth so that they are no longer felt. Another device the ego uses is denial. In denial, the original feelings are not even felt initially. It is important to know, however, that in both cases the memories of the experiences that *normally* cause such feelings remain stored in our unconscious memories. The repression and denial do not get rid of those memories.

The *constant* burying of these feelings is *not* normal. Remember that the nursing educators and supervisors who have taught that it is "professional" to bury them have been socialized by other nurses. Theirs is a harmful approach. It will not change until they themselves are socialized into a more humane approach and become kinder to themselves as well as to other nurses.

BURNOUT

The result of constant denial of self is probably one of the most important, yet underrecognized, dynamics of burnout. Critical care nurses, because of the highly stressful nature of their work, are "at risk" for burnout. Burnout is the result of working in a stressful environment. The worker eventually feels resigned, ineffective, and hopeless about working in such an environment. The result of burnout is that the employee either leaves the job or remains in the position functioning ineffectively. Burnout is an energyless state.

There are other important causes of burnout. Alvin Toffler, in *Future Shock,* suggests that we live in a highly technologic environment where there is rapid change occurring at a faster and faster rate.[8] The result is that the knowledge needed by critical care nurses and the complexity of patients they care for are constantly increasing, imposing even greater stress in an already stressful milieu.

If ratios of nurse to patient were improved proportionate to the increasing complexity of care, then the nurses would be able to adapt to the stress of the CCU more readily. If this does not occur, the result is chronic understaffing. The effects of chronic understaffing are many. Frustration occurs when nurses are consistently under pressure and repeatedly feel that they are not giving the full kind of care their patients need. This type of frustration ultimately leads to burnout.

Burnout is causing ever increasing numbers of nurses to leave nursing. As a result, the problem of burnout is receiving more attention in both the professional and lay sectors. Administrators are concerned because they find it difficult to adequately staff their hospitals. Members of the public sector, in reading of this problem, are concerned about who will take care of them when they go to the hospital.

As nurses, it is important for us to understand the causes of burnout. Certainly the root problems, mentioned above, have always been there. Until the last decade or so, if nurses were victims of burnout because of overwork or because of repression of self, they frequently remained in their positions, in a diminished state. Today, however, nurses are responding to a new current in society.

The feminist movement, with its strong emphasis on selfhood, has made women increasingly aware of their right to fully experience their lives. The essential goal of this movement is to improve the quality of life for all women. It attempts to make them aware of the traditional role they have filled in society and to present alternatives that they may then choose or reject. Nursing is a predominately female profession. Its members, whether men or women, strongly represent the most traditional female qualities of caring, nurturing, and selflessness.

The women's movement has created more of an awareness in women that they are "givers." In her book, Jean Baker Miller quoted a woman who said, "I can't give anymore, but I don't feel allowed to stop."[9] Insightful women have begun to realize that the permission to stop has to come *first* from the giver—not from the takers. After all, why would anyone who is receiving good things tell the giver to stop?

This giving-taking relationship has been the traditional relationship between nurse and hospital. Intelligent nurses who value themselves as people are beginning to call a halt to this hospital-takes-all approach. A new dynamic is being observed in nurses that is probably directly related to their raised consciousness as women. In the past they became burned-out, resigned, and ineffective care-givers as a result of difficult working conditions. Today, it is far more common for nurses to feel angry and frustrated by these conditions. They leave their positions rather than allowing their selfhood and their own needs to diminish.

In most cases their anger and frustration are justifiable, and they have few options other than leaving. Frequently, however, when they move to other positions, the cycle repeats itself. It is possible that after several of these moves the nurse may still become burned-out. After all, the resiliency of any human being eventually has a breaking point.

Hopeless? No. No! There are many alternatives. The important point is that the alternatives must be considered before the breaking point is in view. Baker says, "Clearly, women need to allow themselves to take, openly, as well as give."[10] The amount of energy necessary to create this change of thinking in nurses can be likened to pulling teeth—from a whale! Or stopping a 50-ton locomotive as it is hurtling down a hill! Nurses have always been givers. It is why they entered nursing. It is okay to give. It is beautiful to give. But it is also okay and beautiful to be a full human being and to value one's own worth. Judeo-Christian teaching has frequently been the basis of giving to others. It is important to note, however, that the most basic rule is "love thy neighbor as thyself." This rule assumes that we first love ourselves, and that we should love others as much—not more than we love ourselves! This may come as a surprise to many nurses who have traditionally valued the needs of others much more than their own.

ASSERTIVENESS: A HELP OR A HINDRANCE?

One of the catchwords of the feminist movement has become "assertiveness." This movement has encouraged women to become more assertive. For many women who favor the traditional feminine characteristics, the word *assertiveness* has some negative implications. It is possible that this is due to a lack of distinction between the behavioral characteristics of assertiveness and those of aggressiveness. The differences between being aggressive, being assertive, and being passive, or nonassertive, are presented in Table 31-1.

The difference between the passive person and the assertive person is that the passive person is "done unto" by another who has no awareness of the passive person's needs or desires. Passive people seem more like nonpersons. Actually, they usually put their faith in others to know what they need, usually with unexpressed expectations (also called a *hidden agenda*). When the others fail them in any way there are usually two outcomes: (1) they further submerge their "selves" and needs. The implied meaning is "I have no worth," and (2) they feel resentment. "Why did they do this to me?" Actually, the agency or other person had no idea of the unexpressed needs.

Assertive persons, on the other hand, are always aware of their own needs and the treatment that they are entitled to as human beings. They express these needs when appropriate. When their rights are openly violated, they speak up and express their feelings. Assertive persons are not offensive and do not infringe on the rights of other people or institutions. They place value on their own thoughts and beliefs. They place value on themselves.

Aggressive persons are offensive people. They impose their beliefs on others, expecting them to

Table 31-1
Assertiveness vs. Passivity and Aggressiveness

	Characteristics	Feelings in Self	Reactions of Others
ASSERTIVE	Open Honest Does not impinge on others' beliefs	At peace inside Good self-esteem Respects others' rights	Respect
PASSIVE	Weak Yielding Self-denying Hidden bargaining Deceptive about real feelings	Uncertain Tries to please others Resentful	Pity Uncertainty Unconcern Annoyance
AGGRESSIVE	Quarrelsome Bold Degrades others Bulldozes over others' opinions, beliefs, and feelings	Anger Contempt for others Extreme self-pride Anxious when aggressiveness is out of control	Indignance Displeasure Hurt Disgust

agree, and become angry when the others do not acquiesce. They actually deny others the right to their own thoughts or opinions.

THINKING VS. FEELING: WHICH IS IN CONTROL?

As an aid to changing from passive to assertive, it is important that we learn to distinguish our thoughts from our feelings. For example, if a person feels guilty, he has a gut reaction inside. Guilt is a *feeling*. A person can't think guilt; he feels it. Accordingly, if he thinks that Henry Kissinger was a good Secretary of State, he cannot *feel* that Kissinger was a good Secretary of State. He may think that it is time to paint his house; he cannot *feel* that it is time to paint his house.

In the beginning of the chapter we briefly discussed guilt. Guilt is a strong feeling. It is not pleasant to feel guilty. Most people go to any lengths to avoid feeling guilty. As a result, guilt is a very strong motivation. For most nurses, it is a troublesome and frequent companion in the working place. There are so many things nurses *think* they have to do. When they are unable to accomplish all of them, even though the limitations are beyond their control, they *feel* guilty. In order to avoid feeling guilty they frequently push themselves harder and harder.

Nurses' work, similar to women's work, is "never done." It is impossible to make a finite list of things to be done within an 8-hour shift. For example, once the absolutely required tasks are accomplished and charted, you could still give Mrs. Jones, the woman with the postcardiotomy infection in isolation, some more time; she seemed depressed today. Or, you could update some nursing care plans; they've been neglected because the unit was so busy.

Even when nurses push themselves to do more and more, the end result is still guilt—and sometimes resentment. Remember this very important point. No one can make you feel guilty. No one! Institutions and other people can make demands on you, but only you can allow yourself to feel guilty. You *let* yourself feel guilty. Your intellect—the thinking, knowing side of you—is the greatest ally you have in overcoming unnecessary guilt. It must be consciously willed into action.

I will give you an exaggerated, nonnursing example of this. If a mother buys her youngster four electronic games for his birthday and the child demands to know why he did not receive five, the mother can either *think* to herself, "How ungrateful, I did far more than was necessary," or she may *feel* guilty. The child did not make her feel guilty. She allowed his statement to cause her guilt feelings. By not consciously guarding ourselves against guilt-inducing statements or expectations of others, we become victims of guilt.

In working with nurses I have repeatedly found that feelings of guilt are the greatest cause of nurses' inability to break away from passivity. It is necessary to understand how to suppress unnecessary guilt before we can learn to be assertive, full, actualized persons.

WILL THE REAL YOU PLEASE STAND UP?

Another concept that is important in the process of being comfortable with assertiveness is one that is explained by Bowen as the *pseudo* self and the *solid* self.[11] The pseudo self is the side of us we allow others to know. Some people are all pseudo self. They are to their family members, friends, patients, and physicians exactly what those individuals need them to be. Their own needs, desires, and so forth are submerged to meet the expectations of others.

The solid self is the real you. Many nurses have a difficult time identifying the real self. It has almost entirely been given away to meet the demands of others. The real self must be dug up and reinflated. It's still there. It can return and be bigger and better than it ever was. It requires hard work and concentration and a strong imposition of intellect to break the chains of passivity. It requires control over feelings that can quickly undermine the best intentions. The greatest challenge to your success will be the same family, friends, patients, and physicians who have previously been very successful at "pulling your strings." Being assertive means speaking up for what you need, what you think, what you believe in. It means knowing your real self.

STRESS FACTORS IDENTIFIED BY CCU NURSES

A previous section presented the factors that physicians identified as being the most stressful for nurses in critical care. Now it is time to learn the factors that nurses themselves have identified as the most stressful and then to examine the ways in which they may be alleviated or eliminated completely. It is important for nurses to remember that these adverse effects will not be lessened by nursing or hospital administrators or by physicians. Changes that improve the physical and emotional states of CCU nurses must be initiated by the nurses themselves. By understanding the underlying causes of burnout and the value of assertiveness in combating burnout, and by instituting personal change and accepting their own authenticity, nurses have the tools necessary to improve their working environment.

Huckabay and Jagla surveyed CCU nurses from six hospitals.[12] The nurses identified the factors that they found most stressful in the CCU environment. The authors ranked them in order of their stressfulness, as indicated in the following chart.

RANK ORDER OF SIXTEEN COMPONENTS OF STRESSFUL FACTORS IN THE CCU

1. Workload and amount of physical work
2. Death of a patient
3. Communicating problems between staff and nursing office
4. Communication problems between staff and physicians
5. Meeting the needs of the family
6. Numerous pieces of equipment and their failure
7. Noise level in the CCU
8. Physical setup of the CCU
9. Number of rapid decisions that must be made in the CCU
10. Amount of knowledge needed to work in the CCU
11. Physical injury to the nurse
12. Communication problems between staff members
13. Meeting the psychological needs of the patient
14. Communication problems between the staff and other departments in the hospital
15. Cardiac arrest
16. Patient teaching

At first glance the possibility of lessening any of these factors may seem to be beyond the control of the nurse. It takes firm resolve and energy to *think* that changes can occur, rather than *feeling* hopeless about being able to change anything in the environment.

Let us review the list. In the first five items, those identified as *most* stressful, there is really only one that is beyond the control of the nurse — the death of a patient (although some nurses impose such high expectations on themselves that they view the death of a patient as something they *should* have been able to prevent). The remaining four items are ones that the nursing staff in a CCU, if unified, can do something about. The key word is *unified*. If the nursing group is splintered by hopelessness, competitiveness, or disparate views, then their potential strength in negotiating the changes that would lessen these stress factors will never be realized.

The next five items (6–10) are all built into the CCU environment. They cannot realistically be changed. The stress that nurses feel as a result of them can be lessened, however, and suggestions will follow later. The last six items (11–16) contain only one item — cardiac arrest — that is beyond the control of the group.

Six items on the list can be directly attributed to understaffing — a chronic problem in many CCUs. If nurses consistently tolerate an understaffed environment without protest, it is understandable that hospital and nursing administrations will not improve the nurse:patient ratio. Many staff nurses complain loudly among themselves yet passively leave the job of persuading hospital administrators of the need for better staffing to head nurses, supervisors, and nursing administrators. Who better to stand up for their needs and proclaim the results of understaffing than the nurses who are victimized? It is rarely the patients who are victimized. Most nurses selflessly accept the chronically heavy workload in the CCU in order to save their patients' lives.

If the thought of making such demands on an institution leaves you feeling weak and asking, "How dare I even think such things," review the first five basic rights for women in the health professions written by Melodie Chanevert.[13]

1. You have the right to be treated with respect.
2. You have the right to a reasonable workload.
3. You have the right to an equitable wage.
4. You have the right to determine your own priorities.
5. You have the right to ask for what you want.

GROUP MEETINGS

If chronic understaffing is eliminated, then six of the sixteen stress factors that affect CCU nurses would be decreased. The remaining factors can be addressed and usually lessened in a group setting.

A solution unanimously presented by authors

who have addressed the problem of stress in the CCU nurse is to have the CCU nursing staff meet regularly with an objective outsider who is trained in individual and group dynamics.[14-19] The ideal leader — physician or nurse clinician — is one schooled in liaison psychiatry. Liaison psychiatry is based on the study of the effects of stress on the individual and on the social systems to which he belongs: the family, working environment, hospital, and so on. Other successful leaders reported in the literature have been psychiatrists and nurse clinicians from the field of general psychiatry, social workers, and hospital chaplains trained in group process.

These are professionals employed by the hospital who usually are willing to give an extra hour of their time to this type of group. The request for such a group should come from the nursing staff. Meetings should be held once a week, at a regularly scheduled time, when the largest number of staff members can attend. A quiet meeting place adjacent to or in the CCU should be used.

The discussion group is used to address any CCU-related issue. The time is nonstructured, with the nurses raising the issues to be discussed. In the beginning weeks of the group these issues frequently are centered around the emotional management of problem patients or families. Once the staff members feel trusting of themselves and their leader, they frequently discuss some of their own psychological reactions to specific incidents, such as the hopelessness of weaning a specific patient from a respirator, grief about the death of a long-term CCU patient, anger about house staff who are not there when needed, frustration with an insensitive nursing administration, or helplessness in dealing with the wife of a dying 30-year-old patient.

Critical care nurses invest large amounts of energy and time in the care of one or two patients a day. It is inevitable that they will lose these patients, either by discharge from the unit or by death. When patients die, their nurses are left with many emotions: grief, sadness, depression, guilt, and anger. Without a safe place to talk about these repetitive losses, nurses may unconsciously repress or deny their feelings in order to survive emotionally. Two other coping mechanisms they use are avoidance and withdrawal.[20]

Avoidance and withdrawal, though two different coping mechanisms, have the same result. They occur when nurses consciously or unconsciously become numb to their own feelings and the emotional needs of patients and families.

Another name for this phenomenon is *professional distancing*.

As a result, nurses care for the physical needs of patients but hold back from an emotional commitment. This helps them to avoid the intolerable grief that occurs when the people they care for are repeatedly lost to them.

In a liaison group meeting, these feelings of grief and loss can be talked about in a supportive setting. The nurses' needs for rigid defenses against these feelings are eventually eliminated. When it is safe for them to once again feel their own honest feelings, they usually become more aware of the emotional needs of patients and their families. Their care becomes humanistic rather than technical.

Another issue that can cause conflict in the staff and also be alleviated is intrastaff conflict. CCU staff nurses are bright, ambitious, and highly motivated. When working in close contact with others like themselves in a stress-filled environment, it is possible for competition, staff schisms, or conflicts to result. Ideally they should be resolved quickly.[21] Without an available forum this is not easily accomplished.

Another problem in the CCU is nurse-doctor relationships. Eisendrath and Dunkel suggest that this may be a masked male-female issue. "This is particularly so when, despite a broader base of experience with critically ill patients, the nurse has to defer to a junior house officer with less relevant background."[22]

In addition, a problem that causes much resentment in nurses is that some doctors consistently avoid family members who need to ask questions or need reassurance.[23] When these concerns are discussed in a liaison group and the anger is vented, nurses may learn better ways of discussing these issues directly with the doctors rather than allowing resentment to grow.

STRESS: IS THERE ANY WAY TO MAKE IT BETTER?

The final section of this chapter will include suggestions for reducing stress during off-duty hours and recommendations that can also alleviate stress during working hours in the CCU. It is important to understand that the body's normal physiological reaction to stress was designed to help cavemen fight or flee from danger. In today's CCU the nurse's response to stress causes a strong increase in tension and an increase in physical activity to help with the increased workload. There is an excess of energy available, however. When a nurse finishes work and feels tense, it is frequently a result of this unexpended energy.

Because of the sedentary trend in our society, many people live with chronic tenseness. The proliferation of tranquilizer and alcohol usage attests to the uncomfortable levels of tenseness in people. The best way to reduce physical and mental tension is by physical exercise. One mile of jogging or brisk walking every day will return the body's equilibrium to normal. Many people are also pleasantly surprised to discover that their emotional state is improved also when they begin a regular exercise program. Their depression, anxiety, or fatigue are lessened and gradually disappear.

The relationship between alleviation of physical tension and emotional disequilibrium has not been adequately researched. It is known, however, that adrenalin and the other catecholamines, which are the biochemical stimulators of the stress response, are also an integral part of the limbic system — the anatomic part of the brain that is the center of emotions. When adrenalin and the other neurotransmitters return to normal levels as a result of physical exercise, it is possible that the response of the limbic system is to regain emotional equilibrium as well.

If there is mental stress about specific patients, sadness about losing a special patient, or discouragement about the working environment, the best solution is to become involved in an activity that causes you to mentally "focus in" on something else. This could be an academic course or something like an arts and craft course; anything that requires intense concentration can be beneficial. The mental stress-reducing should always be accompanied by physical stress-reduction activities, such as the walking or jogging mentioned above.

The stress that occurs as a result of working in a CCU can also, ideally, be alleviated by changes within the CCU. These changes will not be instituted by nursing or hospital administrators unless there is the impetus of strong recommendations by the CCU nursing staff. A list of such recommendations follows.

RECOMMENDED CHANGES FOR REDUCING STRESS

1. Institute 4-day work weeks with 10-hour shifts.[24]
2. Employ a full-time physician as permanent CCU director.[25]
   a. A competent physician would always be available, especially during emergencies.
   b. He would supervise and teach house staff as they rotate into the unit.
3. Schedule automatic rotations out of the CCU every 3 months for 2 weeks. These should be to an adjacent clinical area, preferably the step-down unit to which CCU patients are routinely discharged.[26]
4. Allow nurses time to visit their "special" patients who are discharged from the CCU to other hospital units.
5. Schedule a senior staff nurse on the day shift with a light patient assignment. She can assist and teach the less experienced nursing staff.[27]
6. Pay CCU nurses an extra wage increment — especially when chronic understaffing occurs.[28]
7. Upgrade the nurse:patient ratio in direct proportion to increased technology.[29]
8. Allow 6 weeks for a comprehensive orientation and training period for new CCU nurses.[30]
9. Require orderlies or other non-CCU personnel to prepare the body of a deceased patient for the morgue.[31]

In construction of new CCUs hospitals should
1. Allow larger space between patient beds.[32]
2. Ideally, build small rooms for one or two patients or install permanent partitions between patient units.[33]
3. Build nurses' lounge out of view of patients, in the center of the CCU.
4. Install windows in the unit. Install clocks within sight of patient.
   a. These are important orienting cues for patients *and* nurses.
   b. If patients are less disoriented, the stress on the nurse will be less.
5. Seek advice from CCU nurses in the architectural design.
6. Install extra amounts of sound-deadening material.

REFERENCES

1. Alberts ME: Doctor-nurse communication. RN 39, No. 5:ICU-6, 1976
2. Gardner D, Parzen Z, Stewart N: The nurse's dilemma: Mediating stress in critical care units. Heart Lung 9, No. 1:103–106, 1980
3. Hay D, Oken D: The psychological stresses of intensive care nursing. Psychosom Med 34, No. 2:109–118, 1972
4. Nadelson T: The psychiatrist in the surgical intensive care unit. RN 39, No. 7:ICU-6, 7, 1976
5. Simon N, Whitely S: Psychiatric consultation with

MICU nurses: The consultation conference as a working group. Heart Lung 6, No. 3:497–504, 1977
6. Ibid
7. Hay and Oken: Psychological stresses
8. Toffler A: Future Shock, pp 19–47. New York, Bantam Books, 1970
9. Miller JB: Toward a New Psychology of Women, pp 50–51. Boston, Beacon Press, 1976
10. Ibid, p 51
11. Bowen M: Theory in the practice of psychotherapy. In Guerin P (ed): Family Therapy: Theory and Practice, pp 42–90. New York, Gardner Press, 1976
12. Huckabay L, Jagla B: Nurses' stress factors in the intensive care unit. J Nurs Admin 2:21–26, 1979
13. Chanevert M: Special Techniques in Assertiveness Training for Women in the Health Professions, p 20. St. Louis, C.V. Mosby, 1978
14. Baldwin A: Mental health consultation in the intensive care unit: Toward greater balance and precision of attribution. J Psychiatr Nurs 2:17–21, 1978
15. Cassem N, Hackett T: The setting of intensive care. In Hackett T, Cassem N (eds): Massachusetts General Hospital Handbook of General Psychiatry, pp 319–341. St. Louis, C.V. Mosby, 1978
16. Eisendrath S, Dunkel J: Psychological issues in intensive care unit staff. Heart Lung 8, No. 4:751–758, 1979
17. Gowan N: The perceptual world of the intensive care unit: An overview of some environmental considerations in the helping relationship. Heart Lung 8, No. 2:340–344, 1979
18. Melia K: The intensive care unit: A stress situation? Nurs Times 73, No. 5:17–20, 1977
19. West N: Stresses associated with ICUs affect patient, families, staff. Hospitals 49, No. 24:62–63, 1975
20. Eisendrath and Dunkel: Psychological issues, p 755
21. Hay and Oken: Psychological stresses
22. Eisendrath and Dunkel: Psychological issues, p 755
23. Gardiner et al: Nurse's dilemma
24. Nelson J: Intensive stress. Nurs Mirror 146, No. 3:20, 1978
25. Hay and Oken: Psychological stresses
26. Melia: Intensive care unit
27. Nelson: Intensive stress
28. Ibid
29. Huckabay and Jagla: Nurse's stress factors
30. Gardner et al: Nurse's dilemma
31. Melia: Intensive care unit
32. Nelson: Intensive stress
33. Gowan: Perceptual world

BIBLIOGRAPHY

Albierti R, Emmons M: Your Perfect Right, p 11. San Louis Obispo, Impact, 1970

Ashworth P: In the intensive care unit. Nurs Mirror 146, No. 6:34–36, 1978

Barry-Wicks M, Wicks R: The coronary care unit: Practical psychological aspects of specialized nursing. J Nurs Ed 18, No. 2:20–24, 1979

Hoover M: Intensive care for relatives. Hospitals 53, No. 14:219–222, 1979

Hutchings H, Colburn L: An assertiveness training program for nurses. Nurs Outlook 27, No. 6:394–397, 1979

Jouard S: The Transparent Self, rev. ed. New York, Van Nostrand, 1971

Mann J et al: The social worker on the critical care team. Supervisor Nurse 8, No. 9:62–64, 1977

Skinner K: Support group for ICU nurses. Nurs Outlook 28, No. 5:296–299, 1980

Smith M: When I Say No I Feel Guilty. New York, Dial Press, 1975

Vreeland R, Ellis G: Stresses on the nurse in an intensive care unit. JAMA 208, No. 2:332–334, 1969

Wiley L (ed): Depression and the A.C.U. nurse: Mutual support can ease the stress. Nursing 78:8, No. 3:60–65, 1978

Maureen Cushing

Critical Care Nursing: Applied Legal Principles 32

There are not many cases of nursing negligence in a critical care setting. Whether this is due to a low incidence of negligent acts, the competency of critical care personnel, or other factors is not certain. Nevertheless, whether a negligent act occurs in the operating room, emergency room, or the critical care unit (CCU), the legal principles are the same.*

STANDARD OF CARE

Perhaps the most difficult issue to resolve in a negligence case is the standard of care that is applicable to the situation. The expert witness is the most influential factor in determining the standard. For example, the generalist nurse would be a competent witness in the instance of determining the selection of a proper injection site; however, a nurse competent in interpreting ECG readings would be required when the negligent act centered around that particular nursing activity. The standard of care is also determined by position statements of recognized professional groups, philosophies of nusing care, job descriptions, hospital bylaws and directives, and current nursing literature.

REASONABLE CARE CONCEPT

Potential liability exists for both the hospital and the health care provider. The hospital, as a cor-

---

*None of the material in this chapter should be considered as legal advice. Consult your hospital attorney or a health law attorney in the event a legal issue arises.

poration, may be liable for an equipment failure or for failing to provide competent medical and nursing staff in a CCU, while the physician or nurse may be liable for injuries that were directly and proximately caused by poor decision-making skills or for theory and skill incompetency. The law does not, however, find liability for every mistake, but rather, applies the *reasonable care* concept. That is, the care given must be reasonable under the facts of the case and be compatible with the care that a *reasonably prudent critical care nurse would have rendered under the same or similar circumstances.* Additionally, the plaintiff must prove his case. Thus, the burden is upon the plaintiff to show that the defendant-nurse's act or failure to act was the cause of the injury. In a criminal case, the burden of proof is "beyond a reasonable doubt," while in a civil case such as malpractice, the jury is instructed to decide whether or not the defendant is guilty based "upon a preponderance of the evidence."

One of the most important factors that sets the critical care nurse apart from a generalist medical and surgical nurse is the critical care nurse's knowledge of scientific theories and nursing skills that are unique to a critical care setting and necessary to meet the needs of critically ill patients. More than in any other setting, the nurse functioning in a CCU must be competent to make immediate nursing judgments and act upon those judgments.

Decision-making is the essence of the nursing process. The unexpected is to be expected, and it is the joint responsibility of the hospital and the individual nurse to be prepared for crisis intervention. A nurse who does not possess the theory and skills required of a critical care nurse should not be rendering critical care. In the event that a generalist nurse is floated to a CCU, the nurse should inform her nursing supervisor that she lacks the necessary critical care skills. The nurse should make it clear that she can carry out only nursing care activities in which she is competent. The practice of staffing, even for short periods, a CCU by floating staff nurses who do not possess the necessary competencies should be discouraged. Because events in a CCU are unpredictable, the generalist nurse should be sent to assist the CCU staff only in unusual circumstances and should not be delegated any care that the delegating nurse should reasonably know the generalist nurse is not competent to perform. It is reasonable to expect that any hospital that has a CCU will take precautionary measures to assure that it is adequately staffed. Increasingly, nurses view the adequacy of staff as a professional practice issue and are bringing this issue to the attention of hospital administration.

PROTOCOLS
When the critical care nurse is required to carry out medical acts and is not under the direct and immediate supervision of a delegating physician, the activities must be based upon established protocols. These protocols should be created by medical and nursing departments and require frequent review to determine whether they reflect current medical and nursing standards of care. It is likely that, in the event of a malpractice suit, the critical care protocols and procedures will be introduced into evidence to help establish the applicable standard of care. While it is important that protocols provide direction, unnecessary detail may be difficult to overcome when a nurse does not comply.

THE QUESTIONABLE MEDICAL ORDER
In addition to protocols, a policy statement should exist (by hospital bylaw or executive directive) that indicates the manner of resolving the issue of "questionable" medical order. This is important for all medical orders, but particularly for those for critically ill patients because of the unusual doses of medication that are frequently ordered. The nurse who questions a particular order should express her specific reasons for concern to the physician who has written the order. This initial approach frequently results in an explanation of the order and a medical justification for the order in the patient's medical record. Many hospitals have a policy that states that the chief of the service may be consulted about "questionable" medical orders. It is important for the critical care nurse to understand that if there is a judicial review of any medical activity, including a treatment order, the court will look to the medical professional to ascertain whether the order was in compliance with prevailing medical practice. An order that is patently wrong may subject both the physician and nurse to liability in the event that a patient suffers harm as a direct result of its implementation.

PRINCIPLES OF LIABILITY
The basic legal principles that relate to malpractice are not difficult to understand, and an

awareness of the elements of a negligence suit can reinforce some of the fundamental tenets of competent nursing practice.

A mere undesirable event or outcome does not constitute negligence. Not every fall from a hospital bed is a result of some negligent act on the part of a health-care provider. The facts or incidents surrounding the event must be examined in light of the nurse's professional obligation to the patient. Negligence is a breach of a duty to exercise care that the defendant (nurse) owed to the plaintiff (patient) under given circumstances and that resulted in harm to the plaintiff. It includes acts of omission as well as acts of commission. Therefore, either a failure to take blood gases as ordered or drawing the blood gases in a negligent manner may constitute negligence.

The elements of a negligence suit are frequently referred to as the "4 Ds":

- Duty
- Dereliction of duty
- Direct causation
- Damages

For example, a nurse owes the patient a duty to administer the medication Dilantin by slow intravenous push. That duty is breached when it is injected too rapidly, when the patient suffers harm, and when the harm is attributed to the intravenous push.

There are degrees of negligence, such as ordinary negligence and gross negligence. Ordinary negligence is associated with carelessness, whereas gross negligence connotes willful negligence. In a suit in which it is alleged that the defendant failed to render ordinary care, the question becomes, "was *reasonable* care rendered under the circumstances?" When a nurse fails to put up the bed rails of an unconscious patient and the patient is injured in a fall from the bed, the jury must determine whether this omission was reasonable or not. Conversely, by statutory provision, when a nurse stops at the scene of an automobile accident to render medical assistance, the degree of negligence is measured in terms of "gross negligence."[1]

A recent case serves to illustrate a number of legal and professional principles.[2] The suit alleged that hospital employees (a resident and nurses) caring for an infant were negligent in monitoring his condition because they failed to assess a life-threatening postoperative complication.

The 4-month-old boy was admitted for correction of a congenital trachea condition and underwent a tracheotomy. The surgery was uneventful and he was last examined by the surgeon in the CCU at 11 PM. The physician left orders and went home. At that time the infant's condition was satisfactory and he had no manifestations of postoperative complications. At 3:55 AM he stopped breathing and suffered devastating and irreversible brain damage when the resuscitation team was unable to quickly restore respirations or a heartbeat. The cause of the arrest was a massive pneumothorax from the gradual accumulation of trapped air beneath the skin (subcutaneous emphysema), which had entered the body at the site of the tracheotomy and had subsequently worked down until it broke through the surface of the lung. Expert testimony determined that the infant had exhibited signs and symptoms of the complication for almost 2 hours before the crisis occurred. The jury found the hospital liable for the negligence of the nurses and the resident.

This case emphasizes a well-recognized legal duty frequently addressed in malpractice cases. That is, the duty to monitor care. The infant's status was that of a fresh postop patient, and an ordinary standard of care would require diligence in observing his postoperative progress, including the prevention and treatment of complications. It is noteworthy that the American Nurses' Association Code of Ethics identifies an obligation that the nurse "maintains competence in nursing."[3] The statement embodies the concept that a nurse, whether generalist or specialist, not undertake any nursing responsibility that she is not prepared to manage. Additionally, there is a requirement that the nurse avail herself of continuing education to update and expand theoretic and skill components of nursing practice. It is unlikely that liability would have been found if the hospital employees had monitored the infant for this potential complication and intervened to protect the safety and well-being of the child. The court in essence held that although the complication itself was perhaps unavoidable, the failure to recognize and deal with it constituted negligence.

A patient had surgery for acute gallbladder disease. He fell from his bed during his first postoperative night. Twenty-four hours after the fall, he went into shock, and the drug Levophed was ordered. He had infusions running into both arms, but they were discontinued when they infiltrated. An IV was begun in the patient's leg, infiltrated, and caused a permanent partial disability. Evidence at the trial determined that the infusion containing the Levophed had been infusing into the tissues for a period of 2 hours. The court found the evidence sufficient to warrant a finding of negligence for failing to detect the situation within a reasonable time.[4] Infiltration of intravenous fluids is fairly common, and tissue necrosis is an acknowledged and not uncommon complication with the administration of Levophed. Generally, the courts have held that so long as the drug is indicated by the patient's condition and the patient has constant attention during the infusion, the occurrence of tissue necrosis is an unavoidable side-effect and damages will not be awarded.[5]

VICARIOUS LIABILITY

The doctrine of *respondeat superior* or "let the master answer" is an important concept for nurses functioning in a critical care setting. It is based upon an agency relationship, that is, a relationship in which one person acts for another. The relationship between a nurse and the institution is generally that of employee and employer. So long as the nurse acts within the scope of her employment, the employer is held to answer for her negligent acts. This is based upon the principle that in an employee-employer relationship, the employer has a right to control the nurse's actions. The doctrine has its roots in the concept of vicarious liability.

When the employee functions outside the authority identified by policy and directive, the employer will not be liable for the nurse's negligent acts and will not be a party to the suit. A physician not employed by the hospital is an independent contractor and is individually liable for his own negligent acts. There are many occasions when the physician "borrows" the employee-servant, thus assuming responsibility for the nurse's negligent acts. Although some states by case law recognize that the nurse-employee may be servant of both the hospital and the physician, most courts find the nurse was serving one or the other. This is a frequent legal issue for nurses functioning in an operating room setting, but the doctrine has been applied to a number of situations in an acute care setting.

A 1975 case that found the physician liable for failing to inform the patient of critical information also discussed the nurse's employment relationship issue. The suit was against three physicians and the hospital as the employer of the operating room nurse. The patient was admitted to the hospital in August 1968 for surgery to correct a disorder of his internal sex organs.

His work-up revealed a large mass that was later determined to be a sarcoma in the pelvic region. A laparotomy determined that the mass was not removable. Although many postoperative roentgenograms revealed the presence of two hemostats and this fact was known, none of the attending physicians advised the patient or his wife. The patient learned of the foreign bodies 7 months after the surgery when an x-ray technician alerted the wife to their presence. The patient's condition at that time was too precarious for any surgery, and he died in July 1968 as a result of the sarcoma, with the hemostats still in his body. A suit was brought by the wife alleging negligence during the operation and failure to disclose the presence of the clamps. The wife's expert witness testified that the presence of the clamps caused or contributed to the patient's pain status and that their early removal would have eased his suffering. The defendant's expert testified that the patient's pain was due entirely to the sarcoma and that the clamps did not contribute to his discomfort. The defendant-physicians said their decision to conceal the error from the patient and family arose not from a desire to protect themselves, but was based upon a well-recognized medical practice of keeping from the patient those facts of his condition that in the physician's opinion may upset him. No excuse was offered for not disclosing the finding to the wife.[6] The three physicians were held liable for both the original negligent surgery and for failing to disclose the presence of the foreign bodies. The nurse was not the borrowed servant of the physicians and was not liable for either the instrument loss or concealment.

The case illustrates the potential liability for concealment of information from the patient or a family member. Concealment from the patient may be justified under the "therapeutic privilege" concept; however, a failure to inform the spouse or other immediate family member may not be justifiable. Therapeutic privilege supports the position that if the patient would suffer harm because of disclosure of aspects of his condition, including diagnosis, in some circumstances the physician may decide not to disclose the information.

A suit against the hospital and a manufacturer of IV equipment illustrates the duty of a nurse to be knowledgeable regarding the operation of complex machinery and use of products commonly seen in the unit.[7] There is a duty not to use any equipment that has patent defects. Generally, where the defect is latent or hidden and not subject to reasonable discovery, no liability on the part of the hospital employees using it will be found. Hospital protocol should identify the person who is primarily responsible for checking electrical sources and equipment. Generally, it is the hospital engineer. While it is doubtful that a nurse would be held liable for a defect in equipment that she had no way of detecting, if the equipment suddenly ceased to do what it was intended to do, made unusual noises, or had a history of malfunction that was not repaired, it is likely that some degree of liability would accrue to the hospital. All literature that accompanies the equipment should be available as reference, and a representative of the company should indicate the means for resolving sudden equipment failures and emergency replacement.

As in all cases of negligence, the duty of the individual defendants must be ascertained. A case dealing with the liability of the nurse, the manufacturer, and the distributor of an IV infusion set ultimately absolved the distributor, and although it found negligence on the part of the nurse, no liability was attached to the negligent act. During the insertion of an intracath into a patient's arm by a nurse, a portion of the catheter broke off and was carried through the venous system, where it lodged in the right atrium of the heart. The patient incurred serious injury, and open-heart surgery was necessary. The court found that the administering nurse did not follow the sequence of steps as shown and explained in the accompanying instructions. The nurse did not extract the needle, as recommended by the manufacturer, before allowing the solution to infuse into the vein. She waited until she observed that the solution was running into the vein and then applied pressure to withdraw the needle, at which time the catheter separated from the unit. The jury found the nurse negligent but exonerated her employer by finding that her negligence was not a direct cause of the injury. The manufacturer was liable for the full amount of the damages awarded.

A hospital may be liable for negligence on two legal theories: respondeat superior and corporate liability. The well-known *Darling* case is an example of a situation in which the hospital was liable for corporate negligence, as well as vicarious negligence on the part of its nurses.[8] Darling was injured in a high school football game. A plaster cast put on his leg in the emergency room was not monitored, resulting in amputation of the leg after he developed gangrene. The hospital, as a corporation, was liable for failing to require a general practitioner to consult with available orthopedists. The hospital was also liable for the nurse's negligence in failing to monitor the status of the youth's limb. A more recent case dealt with liability relating to equipment.[9] A woman who had a complex pancreatic condition was being transferred from one hospital room to another. The room was a short distance from her old room, and during the transfer she experienced severe respiratory distress. It was known that she had previously experienced respiratory difficulty. When the nurses reached the new room and attempted to attach the oxygen supply to the wall outlets, they discovered that they did not fit. She expired before emergency oxygen could be obtained. The court held that the cause of death was attributed to the negligence of the hospital as a corporation for failing to standardize the outlets and the oxygen plugs. There was no liability upon the part of the nurses. If the facts were that the woman was experiencing respiratory problems before the transfer was begun or the rooms were separated by a great distance, there may have been a duty to have the woman transferred with portable oxygen or to delay the transfer until her status improved.

There is extensive case law on negligence in administering blood transfusions. A woman had a successful operation for kidney disease and was scheduled for discharge in 48 hours.[10] A hospital intern and a nurse gave the woman a blood transfusion that was intended for another patient on the same floor. When the patient complained that her doctor had not told her of the treatment, the intern and the nurse informed her that her daughter donated it. In spite of her objections and statement that she did not have a daughter, it was administered. The plaintiff had severe chills, high temperatures, headaches, and subsequently became mentally ill. She spent a long time in a state psychiatric institution. The hospital was liable for the negligence of the intern and the nurse.

The importance of always checking labels cannot be emphasized enough. A woman had an uneventful delivery, but her uterus failed to contract, and severe bleeding necessitated performing a hysterectomy.[11] A nurse's aide who was a friend of the patient and an employee of the hospital went to the blood bank to donate blood. When the technician saw her, he handed her 2 units of whole blood. The nurse's aide understood him to say that it was to go to the operating room, whereas the technician testified that he instructed her to take it to another unit for another patient. The aide gave the blood to the operating room circulating nurse, and both checked the numbers on the blood container against the original lab slips. They both failed to note that the postpartum patient's name was not the same as the one stamped on the slip. The technician, alerted by a call for the blood for the other patient, rushed to the operating room, but the plaintiff had already received 600 ml of the incompatible blood. The surgeon informed the patient 3 days later and did follow-up kidney function tests. All the tests were negative, but the patient subsequently developed hemorrhagic cystitis. The court concluded that the surgeon, although in charge of activities in the operating room, was not responsible for the negligence of the nurse and the nurse's aide, where it was shown that they were not under his immediate control when they improperly and negligently checked the units of blood. The hospital was liable for the negligent acts.

LIFE-SUPPORT MEASURES
There are two basic issues surrounding the question of life-support measures that have implication for the critical care nurse. One is the legal status of no code (cor zero) orders and the other is the circumstances under which advanced life-support measures may be withdrawn.

No Code (Cor Zero) Order
The "no code" order is a medically acceptable practice in some instances. The code technique is used to prevent a sudden and unexpected death as a result of either cardiac standstill or ventricular fibrillation. It is a highly invasive procedure and may constitute a "positive violation of an individual's right to die with dignity."[12] It is not indicated in cases in which the illness is terminal and irreversible and "where death is not unexpected."[13] A hospital should establish procedures that serve as guidelines to the physician and the hospital staff. The decision not to code is based upon a hopeless prognosis and is one for the physician to make. It may be made after consulting with another physician, but it should always be with the consent of the family if the patient is unable to be involved in the decision-making process. The inability of the patient to be consulted may be due to either a physiological or emotional impediment.

The two major concerns with a no code order are the decision-making process and communication of the order to the nursing staff and others expected to respond to the call for a code. Clearly the most important aspect of the order is the medical judgment regarding the diagnosis and prognosis. While a patient's prognosis may not always be ascertained with mathematic certainty, in those situations in which reasonable medical judgment determines that the patient's condition is hopeless and he is in a terminal stage of illness, a no code order is an acceptable treatment option. However, it must be pointed out that a physician's medical judgment must comply with existing medical standards of practice. For example, one applicable medical standard is that the patient's medical status be assessed frequently and all medical orders are to be based upon a reasonable assessment. The immediate family members should be kept appraised of the patient's status, and it would not be prudent of the physician to enter a no code order unless the immediate family members agreed with the decision.

Because of the nature of a critical patient and the foreseeability of unexpected change for the better, the order not to resuscitate should be evaluated on a daily basis. The order not to resuscitate should always be written and signed by the physician who is primarily responsible for the patient's medical treatment plan. The Standards for Cardiopulmonary Resuscitation (CPR) and Emergency Cardiac Care (ECC), recommended at the national conference on CPR and ECC in 1973, set out the position that the decision not to resuscitate should be clearly expressed in the patient's record and the order written on the physician's order sheet. The standards were updated in 1980, and the previous recommendation was affirmed.[14]

Most of the case law in the area of no code involves a failure to diagnose that a patient has arrested. This is most likely to occur in the operating room where the patient has not been monitored closely, and the first indication of an arrest is when the surgeon notes the dark appearance of unoxygenated blood. There are a number of reported cases alleging that the procedure was incorrectly carried out. An interesting Massachusetts appeals court case held that court approval of a no code order was not necessary where an incompetent patient was "irreversibly and terminally ill." The court held that coding the patient, even if successful, would not reverse her disease process or vegetative state.[15]

Withdrawal of Life Support Measures
The issues surrounding the initiation or withdrawal of life support measures are more complex than the no code issue. In 1976, the *Quinlan* case focused national attention on the

"right to die" controversy.[16] Since then, there have been a number of judicial opinions on medical treatment of both competent and incompetent patients. The problem of treating a terminally ill incompetent patient is especially troublesome because frequently there has been no prior evidence of what his wishes would be. In 1977, the Massachusetts supreme court determined that a severely retarded 67-year-old man, who had been institutionalized for all but 14 years of his life, did not have to have chemotherapy instituted for treatment of leukemia.[17] Unlike the *Quinlan* case, the court said that there should be a judicial review of similar treatment decisions. However, the Massachusetts court did not offer "guidelines" to indicate which treatment decisions would not require judicial review. In *Quinlan,* the court held that an "ethics committee" could make the decision to withdraw Karen's advanced life-support measures. In 1979, a California court allowed the removal of a respirator from a victim of an automobile accident that had left him comatose and in a vegetative state.[18] He had some brain activity and could conceivably breathe if the respirator were removed at some future date. The court allowed removal of the machine, as well as antibiotic treatment, stating that it would be a denial of a fundamental right if the court did not recognize the right of an incompetent to refuse treatment. The request was made by the man's mother. In 1978, a Florida court allowed physicians to remove the respirator of an elderly man suffering from amyotrophic lateral sclerosis.[19] The patient, who was competent to refuse treatment, requested the removal, but the physicians were reluctant to do so because of fear of civil and criminal liability. The court rejected the argument that removal would be allowing the patient to commit suicide.

A recent New York court ruled that an 83-year-old patient who was incompetent and unable to request that advanced life-support measures be discontinued should have the same constitutional protection that a competent patient enjoys.[20] Brother Fox underwent surgery for hernia repair and never regained consciousness after arresting during the procedure. A petition was brought by a religious colleague, seeking removal of the respirator. He stated that Brother Fox had indicated in the wake of the Quinlan controversy that he would not want any extraordinary life-prolonging measures performed for him if he were in a condition similar to Karen Quinlan. The opinion set out a lengthy procedure to be followed in the decision-making process. While the New York ruling requires

judicial review, as did the *Saikewicz* court,[17] the procedure is complex and unnecessarily burdensome.

In 1968, the Harvard criteria established standards for determining brain death (see Chapter 18). However, in many instances the existence of primitive reflexes precludes a finding that the patient is brain dead, according to the Harvard criteria. The criteria had been established to resolve some of the complexities of cadaver donation of kidney organs and were not adequate to meet the technologic advances that soon followed. Although a physician had medically concluded that the respirator-dependent patient was in a nonreversible vegetative state, he was unable to remove the patient from the respirator because of the presence of some reflexes. Some states adopted the Harvard criteria, by statute, while other states enacted legislation defining brain death in broader, less restrictive terms. Based upon the legal principle that one cannot kill one already deceased, hospitals and physicians were advised that in instances in which a patient met the brain death criteria, the patient should be pronounced legally dead and then removed from the support systems.

Where clinical findings preclude a brain death diagnosis, family members and hospitals frequently seek judicial review. The case of Benjamin C. is an example in which a 2-year-old child's constitutional right to privacy and freedom from nonconsensual invasion of his body integrity outweighed the state of California's interest in preserving his life.[21] The California brain death statute required "total and irreversible cessation of brain function." The child sustained extensive injury to his brain stem after being struck by an automobile. Electroencephalograms (EEGs) obtained at 3 and 6 days respectively demonstrated gross abnormalities, and he was maintained on complete ventilation. The physicians concurred that his injury was severe and irreversible but would not remove him from the respirator, as requested by the family, because he did not meet the criteria set out by the statutory definition of brain death. Additionally, the family sought to have all supportive treatment discontinued. Citing the holding in *Quinlan* and *Saikewicz,* the court held that the interests of the state were outweighed by the child's right to privacy. The court allowed the disconnection of the respirator (not ruling on other treatment orders), stating that it was an optional and extraordinary medical procedure and that turning it off would allow nature to take its course. The child died 20 minutes after being disconnected from the respirator.

The issue of the right of an incompetent patient to have life-prolonging treatment, namely renal dialysis, discontinued was considered in the *Spring* case.[22] Earle Spring was 78 years old and was receiving hemodialysis treatments three times weekly for end-stage kidney disease. He also suffered from chronic organic brain syndrome and was completely confused and disoriented. Both conditions were permanent and irreversible, and although he was alive and conscious, he was irreversibly incompetent to participate in any treatment decision. His son petitioned the court for permission to allow discontinuation of the dialysis treatments. The problem that the court had to overcome was the fact that no evidence existed that he had ever expressed a desire for continuation or withdrawal of treatment. The court again took the position that, in the area of withholding life-prolonging treatment from an incompetent patient, the decision-maker should not be an ad hoc ethics committee. After judicial review of all the facts, the judge ordered that the dialysis treatments could be stopped.

Because of advanced technology and better accident rescue measures, complex treatment decisions are an aspect of critical care nursing that a few short years ago would not have been a factor. The courts have played a beneficial role in establishing procedures by which the patients' interests and rights will be maintained.

SUMMARY

The legal responsibility of the registered nurse in the CCU does not differ from the legal responsibility of the registered nurse in any work setting. Five principles to which the registered nurse adheres for the protection of both patient and practitioner are

- A registered nurse performs only those functions for which she has been prepared by education and experience.

- A registered nurse performs these functions competently.
- A registered nurse delegates responsibility only to personnel whose competence has been evaluated and found acceptable.
- A registered nurse takes appropriate measures as indicated by her observation of the patient.
- A registered nurse is familiar with policies of the employing agency.

REFERENCES

1. Massachusetts General Laws, chapter 112, section 12B
2. Variety Children's Hospital, Inc. v. Perkins et al, 382 So. 2d 331 (1980 FL)
3. American Nurses' Association: Code for Nurses with Interpretive Statements, statement #5, 1976
4. North Shore Hospital v. Luzi, 194 So. 2d 63 (1967 FL)
5. Holder AR: Medical Malpractice Law, 2d ed, p 158. New York, John Wiley & Sons, 1978
6. Easter v. Hancock, 346 A. 2d 323 (1975 PA)
7. Vergott v. Deseret Pharmaceutical Co., 463 F. 2d 12 (1972 TX)
8. Darling v. Charleston Community Memorial Hospital, 200 NE 2d 149, 211 N.E. 2d 253 (1965 IL)
9. Bellaire General Hospital v. Campbell, 510 SW 2d 94 (1974 TX)
10. Necolayff v. Genesse Hospital 73 N.E. 2d 117 (1947 NY)
11. Parker v. St. Paul Fire and Marine Insurance Co., 335 So. 2d 725 (1976 LA)
12. Matter of Dinnerstein, 380 N.E. 2d 134 (1978 MA), ftn. #10
13. Ibid.
14. Standards for cardiopulmonary resuscitation and emergency cardiac care. JAMA 244, No. 5:507, 1980
15. Dinnerstein
16. In re Quinlan, 70 NJ 10, 355 A. 2d 647 (1976 NJ)
17. Superintendent of Belchertown v. Saikewicz, 370 N.E. 2d 417 (1977 MA)
18. In the Matter of Vincent Martin Young, #A 100863, Superior Court of Orange County, California, September 11, 1979
19. Satz v. Perlmutter, 362 So. 2d 160 (1978 FL), affirmed Jan. 18, 1980
20. Eichner v. Dillon, 426 NYS 2d 517 (NY App. Div. 1980)
21. In the Matter of Benjamin C, No. J914419, Superior Court of California, Feb. 16, 1979
22. In the Matter of Earle Spring, 405 N.E. 2d 115 (1980 MA)

Naomi Domer Medearis

Planning for the Training and Development of the Critical Care Nursing Staff

33

Would you believe . . .

> . . . A new nurse starts the first day of orientation in critical care with the instruction, "For the moment, read this (critical care protocol). I'll get back to you as soon as things are less hectic"?

It happens!

> . . . On a Cor Zero, the nurses are immobilized by high levels of anxiety because they lack sufficient "hands on experience" to feel confident of their life-supporting skills?

It happens!

> . . . A critical care unit (CCU) staff becomes overwhelmed by the constant flow of crises, and there is no plan to handle the stress, anxiety, and exhaustion generated by these day-in, day-out situations?

It happens!

> . . . A clinical specialist accepts the educator role in the CCU and has little or no preparation for developing problem-centered and people-centered programs for the staff?

It happens!

Perhaps you can identify with these situations or have similar incidents of your own. Situations like these demand new ways of training and developing staff.

WHAT IS AHEAD IN THE 1980s?

Alvin Toffler gave a preview of the future in his book *The Third Wave*. He identifies some of the changes we face as individuals and as members of organizations in the decades prior to the year 2000—changes that hold crucial implications for health care systems and CCUs! He emphasizes that one faces the task of integrating the stresses and strains created in the work setting with the multiplicity of pressures experienced in his personal life. Add to these daily living circumstances the complexity and uncertainty of issues and conflicts on the local, national, and international scenes, and the task becomes more complex. New individual and organizational approaches are necessary for survival and growth.

The integration of personal- and work-life goals for achieving a sense of wholeness is a key goal for all our lives, according to Lippitt.[1] When our personal-, social-, and work-life goals are out of balance, our effectiveness and sense of wholeness are affected. This poses a dilemma for organizations. The effective integration of organization, service unit, and individual goals and values challenges health care administration as never before. The quality of one's work life depends on how well organizations respond to these demands. In a health care system in which delivery of service depends almost exclusively upon individuals, new ways of dealing with human resources are essential.

Today's health care professionals are people who (1) hold different perceptions of the work ethic; (2) look to the organization to provide support for personal and professional growth needs; and (3) look to administration for structured opportunities to share not only their competencies but also their beliefs, concerns, and ideas. Such expectations call for innovative, appropriate, and economically feasible strategies for developing hospital personnel.

One health care area in which the impact of work and life stresses culminates is the CCU. There the staff sees some of the ravages of individual responses to life situations. Survival in this highly accelerated, ever-changing environment challenges every critical care staff member. Increasingly, hospitals are focusing on redefining the role of the educational arm of their professional staff. Organizational development and staff development are emerging as the new frontier in education programs. The health care field is beginning to respond in cost-effective ways. Training *does* occur whether it is planned or unplanned! Both cost money!

In a *Wall Street Journal* interview, Peter Drucker stated,

Let's make no mistake about it. Training is a cost! Every industry must measure its ability to cover the costs of its basic resources, its people, its physical plant

and capital. . . . Believing you can hire people who fully understand their jobs, your company, and how to competently do your business without expending any training and development effort is like looking for a free lunch. Training is a necessary expense.

Developing people is "where it is at."[2]

DECENTRALIZED EDUCATION FOR CLINICAL UNITS

The impact of many forces within and outside the hospital points to decentralization training as an educational strategy to manage change. Included in these forces are (1) increased emphasis of hospitals on critical care, (2) the establishment of standards for special care units by the Joint Commission on Accreditation of Hospitals, (3) the professional certification program of the American Association of Critical Care Nursing, and (4) the legal prerequisite for contact hours in continuing education. Thus, education has become an important issue and program in the management of CCUs.

Critical care nurses look for hospital systems that offer educational/staff development programs, that are committed to maintaining high levels of competency, that provide opportunities for personal and professional growth, and that work to prevent burnout of professionals. A viable staff development program becomes an important criterion in the recruitment, retention, and promotion of the professional nurse in special care units.

The proliferation of technical specialties, new drugs, sophisticated equipment, and medical procedures creates high levels of anxiety and frustration among the people who need to function as *inter*dependent team members. In most professional disciplines, professionals are trained to function *in*dependently. As a result, professionals, performing services for the patient, do not know how to deal with one another and to collaborate in working with the patient. Tailoring educational programs to set goals, clarify roles, and share perceptions and expectations *can* be accomplished through decentralization of education and staff development. The beginning point is orientation that is designed around the training and experience the nurse brings to the job, the level of competency demonstrated, and the particular needs the nurse has to become a member of the critical care social system.

Thirteen hospitals participated in a research study focusing on the purpose, organization, and plan for orientation and continuing education.[3] The results supported decentralization in clinical services such as critical care. Decentralization does not exclude critical care nurses from participating in *relevant* in-service and orientation programs offered by the education department of nursing service. Most important, decentralization needs solid support from administration as opposed to token compliance, relevant in-service as opposed to one-shot traditional sessions, and accountability for results as opposed to numbers and mere program visibility on paper. In return, administration will expect bottom-line results—quality assurance, stable staff, quality work-life, achievement of goals, and demonstration of critical care cost-effective education. Learn to document results!

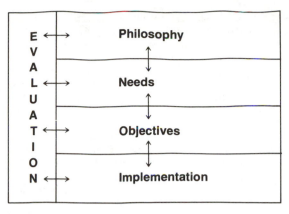

FIGURE 33-1.
Program planning model.

PROGRAM PLANNING FOR CRITICAL CARE EDUCATION

To survive organizational politics and interfaces, a well-planned decentralized educational program is essential. An effective approach to program development is diagrammed in Figure 33-1. Five components comprise the model: philosophy, needs, objectives, implementation, and evaluation.

Philosophy

To start with, a statement of philosophy should set forth the beliefs and values of staff education and development for critical care personnel, as well as the concepts and beliefs about the quality of care and the competencies of staff. It should also include statements identifying its organizational functions and its importance in achieving the organizational goals.

Examples of philosophical statements:

We believe that a quality staff education program is essential if the hospital's goals for quality assurance in patient care and cost-effective operations are to be realized.

We believe the hospital has a responsibility to support staff education by providing adequate manpower, budget, space, materials, and opportunities for personal and professional growth.

We believe each employee has a right to be oriented to the unit; to be able to use current professional skills on-the-job; to participate in continuing education programs; and to receive recognition in merit/performance appraisal programs for demonstrating increased competency based on achievement of professional goals.

We believe the quality of work-life and the genuine concern for humanizing the work setting will humanize patient care and guarantee quality care.

Needs

Educational needs occur at all levels—patient and family, individual staff members, multidisciplinary critical care committee members, and administration. Consideration of needs from all levels makes need assessment a complex and difficult task.

Determining the needs and then categorizing them will facilitate identification of essential program areas. Programs from the identified areas will become the service one delivers as nurse educator.

One method for identifying needs is (1) describe the current condition (the situation as it is now); (2) describe the desired condition (the way you would like for it to be); and (3) define the knowledge, attitudes, and skills necessary to bring about the desired condition. The following example illustrates all of these steps.

The *current condition* might be described as follows:

A "buddy" or preceptor has been assigned to orient and train new nurses. The buddy was selected because of job competence and the assumption of providing a good role model. The methods used are primarily demonstration, imitation, and providing some information on procedures and protocols. The new nurse is assigned one patient and the buddy has her regular patient load. The teaching is done on-the-job.

Several problems become evident with this method of orienting new staff nurses:

. . . Some buddies resent add-on responsibilities because they are still expected to carry a full assignment. There is no recognition or monetary reward for this additional work.

. . . Some see training as an encroachment on the quality of care they hold themselves accountable for with their own patients. This condition creates frustration or dissatisfaction with self and the job. Some feelings are communicated directly, or indirectly, to the new nurse, who then reacts to the value conflict her buddy is experiencing.

. . . Sometimes these reactions are norm setters for the new nurse — she learns to stay out of the way, keep a low profile, live with fear and anxiety about her ability to perform, use trial and error as the way to learn.

. . . The high turnover, less commitment to learning, resistance to change, low self-concept, and lack of job satisfaction make the cost of unplanned training or training by assumption ("a nurse knows . . .") very costly and increase the probability of early burnout.

The *desired condition* might be described as follows:

A buddy or preceptor will have an opportunity to discuss with the nurse educator what is involved in becoming a buddy. The buddy will willingly decide to accept the responsibility and will contract for training and assistance with the nurse educator. Assistance will include negotiating for a realistic patient load during the intensive part of the training of new staff people. The buddy will receive systematic training and feedback using the principles and concepts of adult education. The co-learner model will become the model for not only staff education but also patient and family education.

Creation of the desired condition by preparing the buddy to accept and successfully carry out the teaching-learning assignment might include the following knowledge, attitudes, and skills.

Knowledge the buddy needs:

- An understanding of the differences between adult education and traditional education principles and practice
- Characteristics of the adult learner
- An understanding of the co-learner role and how it works
- Dynamics of learner involvement
- Insight as to how the holistic approach to the learner facilitates learning and increases self-concept

Attitudes the buddy needs:

- Positive reenforcement, not constructive criticism
- Expectations that the new nurse will succeed
- Sharing of responsibility
- Positive attitudes for positive results

Skills the buddy needs:

- Contracting skills (*i.e.,* negotiating)
- Active listening
- Problem-solving
- Interpersonal skills

- Writing ability for the teaching-learning plan:
  learning needs (skills inventory)
  learning objectives
  methods to be used
  skills evaluation
  organization and planning of time
  selection of clinical experiences

This example highlights the need for a program to train buddies or preceptors who are resource people in staff education. Before plans for such a program are launched, however, the need for it must be screened against the statements of philosophy that have been approved and accepted by administration. Then priorities are determined by seeing where the proposed program fits with what is already being done. Not everything that needs to be done can be done at once. Educational programs are built around *survival needs first*.

Another approach is to look at *deficiency needs*. These are needs that may be met by improving working conditions, elevating salary, and changing policies. Then, the *inherent growth needs* should be identified. These are needs that may be met by acknowledging achievement and providing advancement. This approach will create an environment that supports a "quality-of-life" philosophy and that helps staff achieve a balance between personal and professional goals. (For specific techniques for needs assessment, see step 1 in the training cycle.)

The next component, objectives, is based on meeting the identified needs and making the statement of philosophy a dynamic power.

Objectives

Objectives are statements that describe the goal or outcomes of the educational program. These objectives are broad statements that can serve as guidelines for the structure of several different programs. Objectives provide constraints so that resources can be channeled effectively and efficiently and provide the framework for fixing responsibility and accountability for the educational activities of the unit.

Examples of program objectives:

Given adequate support and resources, develop educational programs that enable staff of the CCU to perform their roles effectively, efficiently, and with personal satisfaction.

Given information and learning activities, each critical care nurse will develop a self-directed learning contract with the nurse educator to achieve relevant continuing education that will (1) meet relicensure requirements and (2) achieve professional goals.

Each program objective must be screened through the statements of philosophy and needs, not only *prior* to implementation, but on a regular basis *after* implementation. This process permits evaluation to take place at each stage of program development. It also provides necessary checks and balances so that the unit can respond to changes and evaluations of the programs.

Implementation

The structure for implementation is a master plan with clearly stated policies and procedures and with specifically identified program areas.

There may be no precedent, with suggested policies, procedures, and programs, for initiating this plan. Even so, one is needed for the nurse educator who is responsible for staff education. Otherwise, he will find it impossible to be accountable for anything that is ill defined, ambiguous in nature, or unstructured. Perhaps you, the reader, are the nurse educator. If so, you can ensure your own need to be successful and satisfied with your work by using your competence and exercising your leadership, and by being motivated by your own beliefs, you can build your expertise and interpersonal relationships. You can be assertive through the way in which you get your peers, supervisors, and medical colleagues involved in creating the master plan. Most important, you will want to work with a mentor. As you acquire sensitivity to consensus decision-making and to timing (not moving too fast for those involved), you will need to separate rejection of ideas from rejection of self and from being discouraged and disillusioned.

To begin building the master plan structure, clearly stated policies are needed. *Policies* serve as guidelines for the administration of the staff educational programs. Thus, some areas to explore are

- Educational leave—paid or unpaid
- Reimbursement for travel, lodging, mileage incurred for approved education
- Recognition through promotion, merit increases, and performance appraisals of increased competence resulting from training and development opportunities
- Prerequisites for enrolling in core programs and advanced programs
- Requirements for participation in planning and conducting in-service programs

Policies are tested and evaluated as they are used. Criteria for testing their practicality and effectiveness include evaluating them against the philosophy, needs assessment, and objectives previously developed and implementing the program requests and situations that evolve. Examples of policy statements

Each employee in the CCU will be expected to complete 12 contact hours of continuing education as a regular part of her work schedule each year, based on anniversary date.

New employees will complete 40 hours of scheduled core orientation during the first 3 months of employment. Upon satisfactory completion of the probationary period, the new employee may apply for the critical care advanced course after 6 months of demonstrated increased competency.

Each professional nurse in critical care will develop a self-directed learning plan that will include (1) a statement of objectives; (2) proposed activities to be carried out; (3) possible resources to be used; (4) validation process to determine degree of achieving objectives; (5) contract with nurse educator, colleague, or self to carry out the plan, meet deadlines, and set checkpoints for progress reports.

Procedures are systematic and ensure some degree of uniformity in implementing certain aspects of the master plan. They are necessary to clarify the way things are to be done, such as applying for educational leave, preparing budget and justifying new programs, scheduling space for in-service, keeping records of completed training, and documenting increased competency for merit review.

Example of a procedure:

Purpose: An educational calendar will be set to log continuing education requests for training outside the hospital.

Procedure: Requests should be entered 3 weeks prior to the scheduled event.

Each person is responsible for entering requests on the calendar.

Educational requests will be determined on a first-come basis.

Exceptions to this procedure will be discussed with the nurse educator or critical care supervisor.

Prior to attending the event, the nurse will schedule a conference with the nurse educator to review expectations and how the program relates to personal and professional goals.

After the event, the nurse will share with the nurse educator how the learning experience will be used in the work situation. This will be done 1 week after the scheduled event.

Procedures need to be screened against policies to validate their feasibility and relevance and then screened with staff and others involved in the process. If procedures are cumbersome — they present obstacles rather than gateways to learning — they will need to be reviewed, revised, or eliminated.

Program areas included in the master plan will be the broad areas one expects to develop. Individual modules, units, and independent programs within each area are discussed in the following section. The broad areas will include some or all of the following, depending upon the philosophy, needs, objectives, policies, and procedures of staff education:

Examples of program areas:

Orientation programs
    Introduction to unit, unit goals, and personnel
    Introduction to role as interdependent practitioner
    Unit skills module based on skills inventory
On-the-job training
    Individualized training (*i.e.*, buddy system)
    Modules — specific basic skills for new graduate
                specific skills for general nursing R.N.
                 advanced skills for critical care nurse
In-service education
    On-going, regular training sessions to up-date staff in other areas as well as critical care
    Meet relicensure requirements
Staff development
    Interpersonal competence
    Leadership development
    Preparation for advancement
    Lateral development for mastery of critical care specialties
    Certification in American Association of Critical Care Nurses
Organizational development
    Increasing effectiveness of unit
    Role clarification and team-building
    Creative problem-solving and conflict resolution
    Planning for and implementing significant change

The last three program areas hold special significance for the nurse educator. Today's professionals set high standards for themselves and look for ways to balance their work with their personal and social lives. These program areas prepare people for the changes, improve the quality of life and effectiveness of the unit, and prevent burnout by anticipating growth needs and reducing frustration, fear, and anxiety in a prime time — the 8-hour shift.

The nurse educator generates the leadership; however, the responsibility of program development is shared with each person on the staff and with all others who have a stake in a quality care unit.

Evaluation

You will note that in the model (see Fig. 33-1) the evaluation component is a two-way feedback system. The process of evaluation constantly checks the interaction and relationship of the other four components. For instance, in order to justify certain programs, the proposed objectives are checked against the statements of philosophy, the statements of need, and the various policies and procedures to validate the "fit." The same is true of any change — the feedback process is built in to evaluate and validate the feasibility of change.

Example of an evaluation:

Situation: The state law has been changed and so have the number of contact hours for certification.
           The staff requests more than the approved number of hours of regularly scheduled work time devoted to continuing education.

The policy would have to be evaluated with the new data and its impact on the staff. This does not necessarily mean that the policy will be changed. It does mean the policy would be reviewed and evaluated for its effectiveness.

An increasingly common practice of many organizations is to set aside several days (weekends, usually) to go to a local retreat site and evaluate the elements of the program planning model and set new goals and objectives for the following year. It is very important to know where you are going and even more important to know if you really got there!

In summary, developing a staff program around this planning model gives one a foundation on which to build various educational programs. Administrative decisions regarding the program would be made within this structure. Creating the master plan, with each type of training and development program, brings the model together. The on-going process of evaluating each component in the model with the other components ensures a viable plan and one that is structurally sound.

Assessing Feasibility

If you are the one responsible for critical care, and education is decentralized, you may need to assess the feasibility of this new role. The following will enable you to look at your total job with particular emphasis on the teaching-learning role.

1. List the functions you are accountable for. By writing a detailed list, you will develop a concrete picture of what you do.
2. Next, rank-order these functions according to your own priorities. Perhaps this will be difficult to do, for most everything you do will be of equal importance. However, do number them. In so doing, you lay the foundation for the next important step.
3. Critically evaluate each of these functions. Should you delegate, discontinue, reschedule, reorganize the function or retain the function as it is? This evaluation may provide data for reallocating your time and some job functions so that you can assume new training functions.
4. Now, on your priority listing of responsibilities, insert training and staff development functions in a realistic position. By doing this, you crystallize intent to create new job functions and willingness to allocate time and effort to do so.
5. Evaluate the personal resources you bring to this new role of educator. Write down the teaching you are already doing. Find answers to questions, such as "What help do I give new employees and floats? How do I introduce new ideas, procedures, equipment, and supplies? After attending an educational event, how do I share the information? Do I work side by side with my staff in a crisis situation, and what does my staff learn from me? How do I use the time when census is low? What do employees learn in the periodic performance appraisals?"

Have you found that you are doing many of these? You may want to add questions that occurred to you and more completely analyze the teaching and learning that is going on in your unit at the present time. The process of disciplining yourself to write down what you do will help you to

• Determine the training currently occurring
• Recognize and build on the teaching you are already doing
• Clarify those areas that you may want to change

Now, following the pattern used in assessing your own resources, list the administrative resources available to you, especially those that will provide needed support for launching your educational program. Your answers to the following questions may help.

• What is the attitude of nursing service toward experimenting with new ideas, new functions, new programs?
• What position does nursing administration take when plans do not work out?
• What can I expect from the multidisciplinary committee on critical care?
• What kind of financial support would administration provide, such as additional coverage, compensatory time, overtime pay for educational program attendance, underwriting the costs for outside consultants and courses?
• What hospital space is provided for staff conferences and how available is it?

Next, assess the resources that the education department offers. What support will the director give a decentralized in-service program? What materials are available? What unique resources are available within the hospital and community?

As a result of the resource assessment, you will have a basis for deciding whether or not decentralization or nurse educator is for you. If it shows promise, you are ready to study the characteristics of decentralized programming — programming tailored for adult learners.

CHARACTERISTICS OF DECENTRALIZED CLINICAL EDUCATION

The most unique characteristics of clinically based education are its flexibility, spontaneity, timing, relevance, conscious exploitation of daily situations for learning, active involvement of everyone present, and supportive nonjudgmental climate. The following brief description of each may illustrate the dynamic nature of a small, interdependent staff, personally involved in meeting their own learning goals and the general goals of the unit.

Flexibility implies that even though there are thoughtfully developed plans to meet long-term goals, changes can be made when unexpected developments occur that offer excellent learning opportunities. It allows freedom to change the master plan and to alter priorities based on current situations and needs. If the staff can be comfortable with the freedom to deviate from scheduled plans and then exercise this freedom, flexibility to meet staff's needs becomes evident.

Spontaneity helps the staff learn from daily, on-the-spot situations as they occur. Out of these situations grows the opportunity to acquire insights, identify new knowledge, and recognize new skills. Staff will develop a sensitivity for the inherent learning that is to be found in the moment. This quality spawns unexpected opportunities to learn. It makes learning fun!

A *sense of timing* is essential in planning programs and designing individualized staff development. Developing a "feeling for the pulse of what is happening" in the unit allows you to feed-in either programmed or spontaneous learning experiences and to use time more effectively.

Relevance of potential learning is validated by identifying basic issues such as

• How the information will be used
• Why it should be offered
• What changes will be required
• What changes will individuals need to make
• What results can be expected
• What risks and payoffs can be anticipated

Taking time to articulate these issues will pinpoint their relevance to patient service and to the goals of the unit.

To *exploit daily situations for learning,* situation selection is based on frequency and uniqueness of the experience. Another criterion is the opportunity for all those involved to see the same occurrence and share their different perceptions and how they experienced it. From this, you can create new procedures, anticipate similar problems, and check out the understanding for future events. It also affords an opportunity to demonstrate role and task relationships.

Active involvement of the total person is vital in the teaching-learning process. Research shows that people remember

• 10% of what they read
• 20% of what they hear
• 30% of what they see
• 50% of what they see and hear
• 80% of they they say
• 90% of what say as they do a thing[4]

These facts encourage new methods and techniques in staff training and development.

A *nonjudgmental climate* in the clinical unit supports a creative educational program. For staff who want to grow personally and professionally while working, such a climate allows moderate risk-taking, acceptance of responsibility for experimentation, and accountability for results. It thus facilitates understanding and acceptance of team relationships and individual differences. *The emphasis is not on what is right or wrong, but rather, what is the most effective way to accomplish the task.* This attitude is the most significant one

to develop when a new training program, based on staff involvement, is undertaken.

While the preceding paragraphs describe the characteristics separately, in a well-conceived program they are blended, balanced, and counterbalanced. You can measure your degree of effectiveness by the degree to which you have integrated these components.

NEW ROLE—CO-LEARNER

Probably the most exciting part of this new role is the fact that there is little precedent for it. Part of the reason is the recent major shift in emphasis from "teaching" to "learning." Becoming a learning specialist in the CCU offers a unique opportunity to develop the role as you live it.

The eminent psychologist Carl Rogers points out that as a teacher he discovered he couldn't teach anyone anything. He believes the *student learns what he wants and needs to learn.* This fact imposes a significant change in the role of the traditional teacher. Rogers believes his role as teacher is to help the student learn. To do this, the teacher needs to assume a new role of co-learner and learn many things about the learner, from the learner, and with the learner.

All members of the staff will enter into a co-learner relationship in the teaching-learning process. The learner role for staff will change from listening passively to the teacher, to being actively involved in and responsible for what they want and need to learn and when they need to learn it.

Two important pieces of research have influenced the present approach to adult education. One is the impact of the adult stages of development, as popularly described in Gail Sheehey's *Passages,* and the other is the concept of life-long learning based on the work of Allen Tough.

Because employees are adults, they need to be thought of as adults who want to learn to be effective and successful in their work. Powell and Aker point this out in the following:

Adults do not need, nor do they wish, to be overly directed or controlled in their learning experiences. They are self-directed, autonomous human beings, and desire a strong sense of dignity and individual worth. Nothing will offend this sense of dignity more than to have an individual throw bits of information at them, like raw chunks of meat, and demand that they accept them.

The adult is a learner; as such, the responsibility for learning should be placed upon him. He will choose, if allowed, what he learns and how he learns it, and will also decide the rate and speed at which he learns best. He will need helpful advice and suggestions, however, as to how he should best continue his self-directed learning . . . and this is where the teacher comes in, as a helpful aide who is prepared, not to answer the student's every question, or to solve his problem, but to help him develop the skills to solve his own problems. *The teacher should not attempt to play God.* Her adult students are as mature as she, and in certain ways probably more so. With a deep interest in the student the teacher can help him find his own way, but find his own way he must.*

The teacher, as co-learner, does assume part of the responsibility for the teaching-learning process. This responsibility centers around planning and organizing learning activities for the satisfaction of the learner's needs by having "the right resources and materials, at the right time and in the right place" so that the learner can learn when ready.

If you embrace this concept of teacher, you will probably have to unlearn many preconceived ideas. However, the excitement of sharing responsibility for learning with your fellow professionals will bring its own rewards.

Characteristics of effective co-learners include

- Considerable time for planning
- Individualized instruction made practical in terms of interests, needs, wants, and aspirations of staff
- High degree of flexibility
- Acceptance of "people as they are" and "where they are"
- Use of a wide variety of methods and techniques
- Role model for learner behavior and resource behavior
- Holistic approach to each person—recognition of the intellectual, emotional, physical, social, and spiritual attributes of the learner that strongly influence the learning process

Planning is certainly needed in order to develop unit, staff, and individual goals; to determine which method or technique or material will facilitate the achievement of objectives; and to develop criteria for evaluating progress and change. Much of planning, however, is shared with staff members, as are the instructional responsibilities. A sensitive teacher constantly adjusts and changes the plan as new opportunities

are presented and as feedback is obtained from the staff.

Many techniques and methods are available. Choice is governed by the learning need and the situation.

- Presentation techniques: lecturettes, videotape, dialogue, interview, group interview, demonstration, slides, dramatization, cassette tapes, exhibits, trips, reading
- Discussion techniques: guided discussion, article or book-based discussion, problem-solving discussion, group-centered discussion
- Simulation techniques: role-playing, role rehearsal, critical-incident process, case method, games, participative cases, sociodrama
- Organizational development techniques: goal-setting, role clarification, negotiating, group process, sharing, support groups, experiential exercises
- Nonverbal exercises
- Skill-practice techniques: exercises, drills, coaching

Allow yourself to be a learner and develop a repertoire of techniques by experimenting. Keep in mind the objective, match it with a technique, and then evaluate its effectiveness. Certain techniques are more effective in bringing about behavioral and attitudinal changes than others. So, if you have a choice, choose the one that involves your staff in active participation.

DYNAMICS OF STAFF INVOLVEMENT

If you can trigger creativity, enhance curiosity, encourage new interests, and stimulate the desire for learning and self-fulfillment, while reducing fear of failure, you will effectively perform your tasks and fulfill your role as an adult educator.

Powell and Aker offer several principles to make the job easier. These principles are listed in the chart on page 534.

In summary, the decentralization of education and staff development in the CCU offers an opportunity to experiment with innovative ways of meeting the learning needs and to achieve a higher quality of nursing service for patients. The characteristics of a decentralized training program provide a framework upon which one can create the new co-learner role. The risks in undertaking this task should be moderate while the rewards should be great.

*T Powell and GF Aker: Teaching and learning in adult basic education. Unpublished paper, Department of Adult Education, Florida State University, Florida.

PRINCIPLES OF ADULT LEARNING

1. *Adults learn better when they are actively involved in the learning process.* The more they participate through discussion groups and in other group techniques, the more responsibility they are given for what happens in a learning situation, the more effectively they will progress.
2. *Adults can learn materials which apply to their daily work more quickly than they can learn irrelevant materials.* Adults will be receptive to new information only if they are sure it is useful to them immediately.
3. *Adults will accept new ideas more quickly if these ideas support previous beliefs.* Adults come to learning situations with a well-fixed set of values and beliefs, regardless of whether or not they verbalize them. They tend to reject information which attacks or destroys their beliefs.
4. *Adults' needs and backgrounds must be understood and integrated into their learning experiences as much as possible. Out of feelings of inadequacy, many adults believe they cannot learn.* This belief will be evident in their attitude toward learning situations and toward themselves. Before they are placed in a learning situation, adults should first feel encouraged enough to attempt to learn; otherwise they are likely to fail before they begin.
5. *To the extent possible, adults should be allowed to pursue their own areas of interest at their own rate, and to find answers to questions on their own.* Regardless of how they may react to an authoritarian learning atmosphere, adults are not likely to grasp knowledge that is forced upon them. A teacher should act as a resource person, available to guide or discuss a problem with the learner. The teacher should *not* have all the answers, or even pretend to have them.
6. *Adults, because of possible unhappy past experiences, should be prepared for learning so it will be a pleasant, rather than an unpleasant, experience.* Drill and repetition of material will not help them to learn. It will only make them dislike the learning experience even more than they did before.
7. *Adult learners should be rewarded immediately for success, and should never feel as if they are being punished for making a mistake.* When rewarded, they will want to continue the experience. If punished, they are apt to reject the entire situation either by leaving it physically or by refusing to become involved.
8. *Adults learn in a series of "plateaus";* that is, they do well for a while, then level off in performance, but they will move on again if they have not become discouraged. This is a natural process, and adults should understand that it is, so that they will not give up.
9. *Adults should always know why they are learning and toward what goal they are aiming.* They should understand what steps are necessary to reach a particular learning goal, and in what order they should come. If adults become confused about where they are going, or why they are going there, they will lose interest in going any place.*

*Powell T, Aker GF: Teaching and Learning in Adult Basic Education. Mimeographed. Tallahassee, Fla, Florida State University, 1971

THE PROCESS OF STAFF TRAINING AND DEVELOPMENT

The preceding section focused on the overall, general educational plan for decentralization. The following section focuses on a practical and systematic approach to the process of designing specific programs within the broad program areas of orientation, in-service, on-the-job, continuing education, and self-directed learning projects.

One needs to keep in mind the purposes of training and staff development.

Training's primary purposes are the discovery, development, and change of people's behaviors and attitudes to improve job performance.
Staff development's primary purposes include those of training and meeting some of the staff members' need for self-worth and satisfaction through work.

Careful thought to the blending and balancing of these two is crucial if one is to achieve the ultimate goals of improving quality of work life for staff and providing quality, effective care for the patient and the family.

Industrial Systems

To provide some background for your orientation, consider the contributions of progressive industrial management in integrating organizational and individual goals. Researchers attempted to discover the key to releasing motivational energy of employees toward achieving the company's objectives. The findings showed that management's concentrated effort and the employees' willingness to participate resulted in collaborating planning in job and staff development. Over a period of time the results of these cooperative efforts lowered operating costs and turnover, facilitated produce development and new marketing and management techniques, and increased profits — the bottom line!

Health Systems

In shifting from industrial to health care systems, and to hospitals in particular, the problem of tapping the full potential of people resources is of genuine concern. With cost containment, fewer people will be expected to do more work and do it more effectively and efficiently. With the pressure to deliver higher quality health care, control costs, and more fully use staff, hospitals must look for alternatives to the narrowly conceived industrial assembly-line way of delivering health services. The product in health care is not a *thing;* it is individualized total care.

With the multiple numbers of professional specialties and skilled technicians, the challenge to integrate persons who come with special education and varied work experiences is somewhat overwhelming. To this complex situation add the fact that these people come initially with a desire to use their special expertise and with the need to keep growing in their occupational life, as well as their personal life. It appears that the key to genuine motivation rests within the employee and is released when the need to keep growing is met.

The Training Cycle

The training cycle is the process model offered as a means to release motivational energy, to facilitate the planning of realistic and needed training that can be made manageable and measurable (see Fig. 33-2). Becoming familiar with the model enhances development of individual units of instruction within the broad general areas. It can be used for one's own personal and professional learning plan or as a guide for working and planning with each staff member. Moreover, it will provide a continuing framework for recycling as new needs emerge. The training cycle uses seven steps:

1. Identify and validate individual and group needs.
2. Set learning objectives for performance and growth.
3. Plan and contract to achieve learning objectives.
4. Select resources.
5. Manage learning activities.
6. Evaluate objectives, performance, and learning plans.
7. Recycle.

If you have made an assessment of personal resources, you may now be aware of how good you feel as a teacher and aware of the value of more active staff involvement in planning the training. Such an initial awareness is shown in the model in a kind of free form. It represents consciousness of a need but lacks validation necessary to determine whether or not it is a viable learning need.

STEP 1. IDENTIFY AND VALIDATE INDIVIDUAL NEEDS

To determine what the training needs are, the best source of information will be the people with whom one works and by whom patient care is provided. As might be anticipated, different needs will come from each shift and from persons who "float" or "relieve" on days off. Remember, all persons involved in critical care have relevant training needs, including physicians, clergy, and ward clerks.

Data on needs can be obtained in many ways. Here are four that may be familiar — interviewing, observation, periodic performance evaluations, and planned and unplanned changes. Several methods usually are employed and result in a *data base* of "conscious needs."

Interviewing individuals in the CCU can be accomplished either formally or informally and either on a one-to-one basis or in a group. Preparation prior to interviewing will facilitate gathering specific data and guide the discussion. The use of some open-ended questions will permit free-flowing input from participants. Examples of open-ended questions are

- What do you like best about your job?
- What do you like least?
- If you could, how would you change working in the unit?
- What problems bug you the most?
- How could training for the unit be improved?
- What plans do you have to earn contact hours for relicensure?

Actively listening to what is said and being aware of what is not said will help identify the needs. Taking notes verbatim while interviewing and then summarizing with the same words will assist in validating them with the person(s)

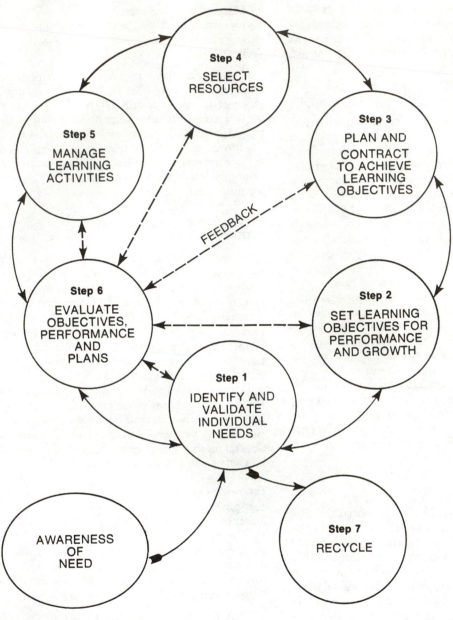

FIGURE 33-2.
Training cycle: —————, relationship of components; —————, feedback system.

involved. Or, the interviewer can ask the participants to prioritize the needs. Validation of need and priority will help in overall planning.

Observation means data based on guided observations of job performance and on interactions with patients, ancillary personnel, and one another. It also includes observing contacts with persons who provide direct services to the patients but who are not part of the critical care

staff. These perceptions will provide the criteria for determining the required level of competence for effective performance. Therefore, observations must be based on criteria set and shared prior to making the observations. The skills inventory for critical care would be a logical starting point. The quality assurance standards would be another. The observational data will reveal skill deficiencies as well as unconscious needs (needs not revealed in the interviews but evident in behavior and attitude). To validate one's perceptions, feedback to each person is necessary.

Periodic performance evaluation data may indicate needs and resources both employee and educator are aware of. In some cases, reports may cover several evaluation periods and reflect changes in the performance level. In studying this data, consider the evaluator and his perceptions and biases and the abilities and skills, as well as attitudes, that each employee demonstrates toward self, job, and others. Currently, most performance evaluations are based on goals set by the employee, the degree of achievement, and the way in which they were achieved.

A suggestion from Malcolm Knowles might help pinpoint how the educational needs, which the data produced, are defined.[5] He states that a need is "the gap between present level of competency and a higher level required for effective performance" as defined by the organization, the individual, or society. His concept is illustrated in Figure 33-3. Writing statements to describe clearly the two levels of competency will make need identification easier.

Example:

Required level of competency (standard)	The primary nurse will talk with patient's family in the waiting room a minimum of two times a shift.
Possible educational need	G A P
Present level of competency	The primary nurse has not talked with the families of patients because she is "too busy"

Gap: determine the reasons for failure to meet the standard. For example, does the nurse have difficulty managing time, is she uncomfortable with interpersonal relationships with families in crisis, or does she not accept the standard? Is it a training need?

To answer this question, a profile of each nurse's experience and some well-designed open-ended questions will help identify or validate whether or not there really is an educational need.

Planned change is more easily handled than unplanned change. People are constantly in need of obtaining pertinent information, clarification of expectations, and knowledge of the skills and competencies necessary to effectively manage the variety of changes that are occurring. Thus, the responsibility of preparing people for change whenever possible is included in the eductional package. Example

The installation of new computers at the nursing station will provide information needed for physicians' decisions. Getting staff ready for the change by providing information about the reasons for change, the new equipment, the advantages and disadvantages, and the changes in staff work, prepares people for the learning that will follow, and hopefully will lower the resistance to change.

It is important to lower the resistance before it has a strong basis. The job will be easier for those who know the staff's concerns and who have time to work with them in identifying alternatives, modifications, and suggestions that will involve them in finally accepting and implementing the change.

In the case of *unplanned change,* recognition of the fact that some people would rather not do something than fail at unfamiliar tasks is essential. Coaching them as they perform different tasks will help them meet their need to be successful. By taking the time to individualize training, one not only builds commitment to the change, but also strengthens the co-learner role with them.

Validation. To "check out and make sure the need is real" becomes the issue of validation. Validation requires that data sources are sought that will verify the reality and the extent of the need. It supports the fact that the *gap,* or educational need, exists and justifies further consideration. The best source of validation and the one most frequently overlooked is the person for whom the training is being planned—the learner(s). Sources such as supervisors, administration, research studies, and consultants also provide verification. In many instances, their input is essential; however, learners must not only be aware of the need to increase compe-

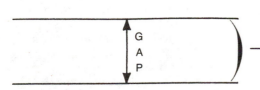

Required level of competency

Educational Need

Present level of competency

FIGURE 33-3.
Definition of an educational need.

tency, but must want to do it for their own reasons. Therefore the learner provides one of the soundest answers.

Knowles phrases it this way:

The more concretely an individual can identify his aspirations and assess his present level of competencies in relation to them — the more exactly he can define his educational needs — the more intensely will he be motivated to learn. And the more congruent the needs of the individual are with the aspirations of the organization . . . [and vice versa] the more likely will effective learning take place.[6]

Assuming the need identified and validated is an educational need, the capabilities of the unit and staff form the first criterion of whether or not the need can be met. The probability that training needs can best be met in the unit is a basic assumption. To increase the level of competency on the job, the reality situation offered by the unit provides the best learning laboratory. If the need is more long-range, staff development may be the logical approach. This may involve feasible programs outside the unit, such as a core critical care course.

The final consideration is determining the priority of needs that result from the assessment. It is wise to involve the staff in helping to establish priorities. If the first need undertaken is "bite size" and the chances of meeting it are good, one probably has a winning combination to move to the next step in the process.

STEP 2. SET INDIVIDUAL LEARNING OBJECTIVES FOR PERFORMANCE AND GROWTH

The second step is setting goals and objectives so that training and staff development efforts will have direction and achieve positive results. *Goals* will be identified as long-term targets and will be broad in scope. For instance, an educational goal might be stated:

To involve each staff member in planning and implementing the in-service program for the unit.

Another might be stated:

To provide more effective nursing care in the unit by increasing the level of competency of each person in not only meeting the physical needs, but also the psychosocial needs of critical care patients and their families.

Although these examples are explicitly stated and provide guidelines upon which to structure a training program, more specific objectives (short-range targets) are needed to ensure understanding and measurable achievement of goals.

These more specific learning objectives are stated in behavioral terms that describe outcomes or results.[7] By writing behavioral objectives, the learner has a clearer idea of what is expected, and both educator and learner can measure the results. Using active verbs (such as perform, demonstrate, master, use) sharpens statements of objectives. Writing objectives helps in determining content and learning experiences. They keep one on target.

Short-term objectives usually include these characteristics:

- They represent behaviors that are observable by others.
- They are specific, limited in scope, and include certain conditions, such as time and method.
- They are measurable.

There are three types of objectives that will need to be considered if improved performance and growth are expected outcomes.

- Cognitive objectives: information
- Affective objectives: attitudes, self-concept
- Psychomotor objectives: skills

Example of psychomotor learning objective

Given instruction on the use of monitoring equipment (information) by the head nurse, within 5 days (time) a new staff nurse will be able to prepare a patient and properly attach equipment (result/outcome).

When initiating the idea of staff writing personal objectives to increase their effectiveness and job satisfaction, a warm-up to the idea is necessary. At first it may be difficult. Determining objectives may be a new skill, and they will need training to do it successfully. Also, they may feel threatened by the idea because it represents a change and it fixes responsibility on them to achieve their objectives. To involve staff from the very beginning, it might be helpful to raise questions that stimulate their active involvement:

- What would I be doing differently if I were to set a goal?
- How might someone else know that I have changed my style in interacting with patients and their families?
- What will I need to know and do to reach my goal?
- What can I do for myself?
- What help will I need from others? Who specifically?

After each person identifies goals, co-workers can review and critique them. In the process of sharing, staff can sharpen one another's goals by asking questions. This helps determine what kind of goal is being set. Is it a "must" (a survival) goal? Is it a "want" (it would be nice) goal? Is it attainable? Is it an ideal goal that could never be attained and yet would set direction for the maker? Is it a maintenance goal? Or is it a growth goal that combines elements of the ideal and achievable reality?

With feedback, each staff member will clarify the goal, making it more specific, more realistic, more measurable, and more attainable. This process makes it possible for a person to request feedback from co-workers and to assess progress. Another outcome of this process is the building of a mutual support group, and this kind of positive reinforcement is essential in high-stress areas.

After setting the goals, it is necessary to develop a plan to achieve individual goals. Hence, objectives, or mini-goals, are defined. Each person identifies the barriers or blocks that stand in the way of attaining the goal. Along with this, each person is encouraged to identify all of his personal assets or strengths. After listing the blocks and assets, each person writes objectives to deal with each block. These objectives become short-term and comprise the bite-size steps one takes toward the desired outcome.

Example of translating a barrier into a short-term objective:

When I'm not sure what to do next, I procrastinate.
Objective: I will list all of the information I need and ask for assistance to begin moving toward my goal

This process helps each person understand how functional objectives can be in generating action that is aimed directly at the target.

The step of goal–objective formation is probably the most difficult of all, but it is essential and can never be overlooked. As staff become more comfortable with working together in planning the initial steps, goals and objectives may change. It should be remembered that this element of change is implicit when working with the concept of process.

STEP 3. PLAN AND CONTRACT TO ACHIEVE LEARNING OBJECTIVES

In order to reach objectives, staff will need assistance in developing a plan of action that will zero in on the forces that slow down learning. Kurt Lewin's force field analysis provides a model that is useful to plan effectively. There is a natural resistance to change, and the removal of this resistance is essential if the desired learning is to take place. Honestly acknowledging resistance to learning and accepting it as a normal phenomenon will remove some of it. This strategy helps the learner identify the reasons for resisting, and this awareness will make it easier to move toward building on the assets, abilities, and strengths that support new learning. Encourage learners to specifically identify resources they can use to weaken, reduce, or overcome these blocks and free energy to accomplish their objectives. Help them identify the driving forces—those things that tend to propel them into action and move them toward the learning objective. These forces provide the motivation. When a person capitalizes on these and applies personal resources to offset the resistance, that individual is ready to develop a plan. Work with each person in determining what is to be done, when it is to be done, how it is to be done, why it is to be done, what the payoffs are, what the risks are, and what degree of success is anticipated. Help each one assign specific responsibilities to himself and to other resource people that were identified. Help clarify the self-assignment of responsibilities—things the person holds himself accountable for. Encourage specific information on the person's expectations of others, including the educator.

A contract, or working agreement, is an effective device for achieving and supporting goals and objectives. The contract is not formal. It evolves as staff and individuals openly discuss expectations of one another in terms of what needs to be done to achieve learning objectives. For instance, in assigning responsibilities, dialogue clarifies what is needed, why a particular resource is best, and who does what and when. To clarify the assignment, the persons involved should discuss reasonable checkpoints and set deadlines. This practice provides specific data for mutually shared expectations. This agreement provides the mechanism to check progress, the status of assignments, and problems, as well as an opportunity to renegotiate if indicated.

If one keeps in mind a strategy that will help staff understand and accept the tension between their desire to grow and their desire to remain the same, their movement through the process of *unlearning, learning,* and *relearning* will be greatly assisted.

Adults resist unlearning things that have worked for them in the past and that were adequate for the situation. In the process of giving up familiar ways, adults will accept the necessity of learning new ways if they increase competence. However, learning is not enough; adults need to internalize the learning—make it a regular part of their behavior. Thus they need the opportunity and time to relearn, or "refreeze" the new behavior so that it becomes their typical response to a situation. Follow-up with coaching provides positive reenforcement that speeds up the refreezing process. It might be helpful to make notes on a daily schedule as a reminder to do the follow-up, for it may require only observation to measure the internalization of new behaviors.

Risks and payoffs, two basic factors, are powerful and influence the learning process. Since learning imposes change, it is important to make sure the risk is a moderate one. Moderate risks result in a fair degree of safety and a good chance for success. Knowing the degree of risk they are taking enables staff to accept responsibility for learning. (A nonjudgmental climate supports risk-taking.)

Equally important are the payoffs. Because frequently these are taken for granted, plan very carefully for genuine payoffs. An open discussion of "both sides of the coin" of the learning experience—risks and payoffs—will make it much easier for learners to buy into an experience. It will allow co-workers to give support during the learning process, and learners will have a gauge to anticipate the results of changed behavior as they strive for increased competency and self-fulfillment. Self-fulfillment is one of the most valued regards.

One further point: adults want immediate payoffs in return for learning new things. They want to be able to use the learning *now,* not at some indefinite future time. Being able to use the learning effectively and feeling competent about it is the most effective immediate payoff. Documented goal achievement through the learning objectives provides information for merit increases—another concrete payoff.

STEP 4. SELECT RESOURCES

After the action plan has been developed, and even as it is taking shape, the identification of appropriate learning resources follows. Look for situations, people, and materials that will enhance learning opportunities.

Situations offer unique resources. For example

- *Participative learning as a resource.* Unstructured learning groups provide rich resource material for learning about "people things." Task groups are useful for integrating theory inputs into operational objectives.
- *The learner as a resource for planning and implementing programs.* The creative and practical forces generated by employees who accept the role of learner release resources that can only be obtained from such involvement.
- *Daily living experiences as a resource for learning.* When employees accept role playing and role training as a way of improving their competency, daily happenings in the unit provide the content for the learning situations. These offer a rare potential for reality-checking attitudes, values, and habitual responses to situations. They afford employees the opportunity to try on different behaviors—to expand their behavioral repertoire for meeting common experiences. As resources, these are among the most stimulating and exciting.
- *Spontaneity as a resource in learning.* When spontaneity is present, learning is precious, stimulating, and fun. How does one develop spontaneity, make room for it, and capitalize on it? Spontaneity develops in a supportive, nonevaluative climate. Some norms which govern behavior in the critical care unit may inhibit the development of spontaneity.
- *Conflict as a resource for learning.* From genuine differences in values, expectations, techniques, roles, priorities, comes the grist for conflict. Working through these differences provides another viable resource for learning. Here the issue is how to develop a climate in which people can learn from conflict; to create a norm where conflict is legitimatized or sanctioned; to set ground rules so that the conflict can be resolved. Probably one of the most effective resources for learning is found in the differentness of people and their perceptions that can openly be dealt with.
- *Failure as a resource for learning.* If the staff within the unit can be desensitized, so that persons who believe they have failed can learn from the experience, failure can become a motivational force. Role training helps the learner to find new ways to approach the problem. The question, "How would you do it differently?" may help the learner develop spontaneous responses that can be capitalized on later.

Resource People. Selecting competent resource people requires careful planning. Criteria for this selection are threefold:

- The resource person's ability to adapt professional knowledge, expertise, and vocabulary to staff's background/experience

- The person's ability to adapt expertise to the objectives. Unless the resource person has been given a well-developed set of objectives prior to the session, the information will be based on his own perception of what is needed. This may subvert achieving the learning objectives.
- The resource's ability to listen to and respect the knowledge and experience staff members bring to the session. The assessment of this quality places a special responsibility on the educator. If the resource person believes in and communicates respect for the staff and their work and builds on this, he will be an acceptable resource person. Therefore, take time prior to the session to share this information.

Resource people will need well-prepared answers to questions like these:

- Why me? What do you want from me?
- How do I fit in with the overall educational program?
- What are the people like that you want me to work with?
- What will they want to know?
- What do you expect to happen when the session is over?

These or similar questions need to be answered for staff members involved in in-service and staff development programs. They, too, provide a reservoir of resources that needs to be tapped. To tap such resources, however, people will need to know honestly what is in it for them. In other words, what's the payoff for being a resource person? If they can see a payoff, they will be motivated to learn and to become involved. They will accept the change that learning creates and demands. For instance, why would a staff member take on the responsibility of becoming a preceptor or buddy in the orientation program?

Materials. With the help of the in-service educator, in-service educators in your community, manufacturer's representatives, and learning laboratories in schools of nursing, it is possible to locate excellent materials to use in group sessions or for individual work. Materials can range from programmed instruction units to reading materials for personal use or group discussion. Also, setting the expectations for staff to bring in items such as articles, cartoons, and news items enriches resources and underscores mutual responsibility.

Software (flip charts, markers, masking tape, mockups, posters, workbooks) creates a variety for pacing learning.

In summary, select the resource for achieving specific learning objectives and keep in mind the work situation, the timing, and the learners. Accommodating all of these elements becomes an art, so allow time to develop this particular ability.

STEP 5. MANAGE LEARNING ACTIVITIES

Once the potential resources have been selected, the next step in the process model is managing the activities in such a way so that both learning and unit objectives are achieved. To gear learning to the work cycle in a practical and realistic manner demands artistry in juggling the components that shape an effective and satisfying learning experience. These components include time, place, materials, equipment, situations, and human resources. One may have to settle for something less than the ideal educational setting and schedule learning in conjunction with work in progress. As these functions become more complimentary, less time and energy will be used in their integration.

Readiness of the Learner. To manage opportunities for individual learning, become thoroughly familiar with the level of performance of each staff member and his learning objectives. The skills inventory and nurse's experience data provide a baseline for determining content. Interaction observations and skill behaviors will provide data on readiness. Readiness to learn is important — physically, intellectually, and psychologically. Recognizing this, timing then becomes the vital element. Sometimes training will be scheduled for a specific time; at other times it can be done in the process of the day's activities on an unscheduled basis. The educator's responsibility is to see that training happens when the learner is prepared and ready to learn, and that appropriate techniques are used.

A long enough period of time for learning is necessary to capitalize on the learning potential of staff. Consider the fact that each time the learners experience a new behavior, they are in effect relearning it in each new situation. When it becomes evident that a new behavior has been well integrated into performance, taper off any coaching or special attention.

Situation. Tune in to the daily experiences within the CCU that offer content for learning — such readiness and spontaneity facilitates learning. Getting people together and orienting them to the situation requires presence of mind and quick action. At first this practice will be awkward. But as staff becomes comfortable with it, this cooperative effort can be directed or suggested by any person. Being sensitive to feedback (verbal and nonverbal) allows adjusting the teaching to the activity's progress. This flexibility in style of managing the situation and oneself will increase the potential for learning. It also increases the potential for unique resources.

Content.   Several cautions for managing content may save time and effort. So often the tendency is to tell learners *what you want them to know,* and rarely to take time to *find out what they already know — or even need to know.* The usual response of the learners in this situation is mixed; they feel put down, or they are bored and tune out the instructor. Thus a guideline might be to take time to find out "who knows what" and build from there. This behavior is compatible with seeing one's own self as a co-learner.

When it is necessary to provide a considerable amount of information, organize it into segments or modules that can be grasped by the learner. An overload of information with little or no breathing space between segments is discouraging. Prepare information in lecturette formats. Research on listening cites the traps that listeners fall into when listening to long lectures.[8] Twenty minutes is suggested as an effective block of time for content. Follow this with learner involvement techniques so that some internalization of content takes place and retention is enforced. Pacing facilitates absorbing information.

When extensive content in a particular sequence is indicated, look at the potential resources within the staff as presenters. If sharing responsibilities for content is expected, staff can prepare specific information in collaboration with the planner. In this way it decreases the exposure of the educator as "teaching resource," and increases the versatility of the unit's resources. This approach to managing content allows more time to manage the overall CCU and directs the resources toward both unit goals and individual growth goals.

Human Resources.   This subject is covered rather extensively in step 4. However, a point that bears repeating is this: Take time to carefully prepare all resources — be they outside or from within the hospital resources.

A great deal of the success and effectiveness of the resource depends on how the following have been managed: scheduling, objectives of the session, information announcing the session, rationale for the content and method of presenta-tion, plan to involve the learners and the preparation of the learners, and the setting for holding the session.

Attention to these details creates a climate that supports the teaching-learning activities and the people involved.

Place, Material, Time, and Equipment.   One asset of the CCU not to be overlooked is its dual function as a treatment area and as a learning area. This fact simplifies some of the management problems of providing an educational facility. The standard equipment and materials used serve the needs of both patient and staff-learner. As one begins to blend the service of nursing care to patients with on-the-spot teaching, there will also begin to develop a keen appreciation of the versatility, efficiency, and capacity of the CCU. Space for in-service sessions and team meetings poses a problem. Explore space adjacent to the unit such as classrooms, conference rooms, and board rooms. Usually, if sessions are scheduled in advance, the space can be reserved. Ask the multidisciplinary staff for the unit to assist in locating space.

The most difficult problem will be finding time for educational activities. Give up the idea that numbers mean good in-service. If the people attending can use the information, training, or discussion, the time will be spent profitably. Because the census in critical care varies, scheduling learning activities poses a real challenge! Several ideas may help stretch the imagination to discover feasible alternatives.

- What about having several "packaged" programs available so that they can be pulled out when the census is low? Working on current performance problems is another agenda.
- What about overlapping schedules at the end of one shift and the beginning of the next shift?
- What about taping sessions and planning discussion guides to go with them?
- What about occasionally conducting a special in-service during each shift?
- How about rotating staff so that everyone scheduled for the day shift has the opportunity to work with a preceptor, or attend scheduled in-service that is especially pertinent to what they want to learn?
- How about getting ideas from the staff to determine best time for all shifts and regular floats?
- How about working out a plan with another department? One example in a hospital was set

up by the operating room (OR) staff. The OR scheduled surgery one hour later than usual on Friday mornings so that prime time could be devoted to in-service, team-building, and creative problem-solving. The surgeons supported the plan. Could you hitchhike on such a schedule? Would someone care for patients in the unit while others would be free for training?

STEP 6. EVALUATE OBJECTIVES, PERFORMANCE, AND THE LEARNING PLAN

The next step is to evaluate the learning, which means measuring the degree of change in performance of persons involved in the training activities. It also means measuring the achievement of the learner's own objectives. Observing these changes in terms of overt behavior and guided observations over a period of time will result in the evaluation of the employee's ability to integrate new learning into job performance.

Another form of evaluating learning is open staff meetings. This allows staff to give feedback on the significance of the learning and how they have been able to use what they have learned. In this process, evaluation can be made of staff function effectiveness. Successes, failures, conflicts, creative solutions—all these are part of the evaluation process and contribute information essential to ongoing needs and new objectives for the next sequence of learning activities.

The action plan can be evaluated for how effectively the driving and restraining forces were identified and handled. Learner resources can be evaluated for how effectively they overcame the blocks to learning. Working agreement and deadlines can be reviewed for how effectively the contract contributed to objective achievement.

Grist for evaluation includes organization of the learning activities in terms of the working situation, readiness of learners, preparation of resource people, materials used, and timing.

Perhaps the most difficult element to measure will be the *results*. Results that are "winners" give data that support long-term effects such as lower turnover, effective patient care on a cost basis, and a high level of staff competence in less time than the former training plan.

Factors for documenting costs for training and development include some of the following. The list offers possible data for justifying budget and results of training and development.[9]

- Planning time (percentage of salary for time spent by each member of the planning team, or number of hours spent by each member multiplied by the hourly salary rate, and fees for consultants)
- Staff time (percentage of salary for time spent by each member engaged in planning and production and in gathering materials, or the number of hours spent by each person multiplied by the hourly salary rate)
- Supplies and materials
- Outside services for preparing or purchasing materials
- Construction or renovation of facilities
- Equipment
- Installation of equipment
- Testing, evaluation, redesign, reproduction of resources (including personnel time and costs of materials and services)
- In-service education for others who might participate in the in-service
- Overhead (utilities, furniture, room, or building costs)
- Miscellaneous (office supplies, telephone, travel, and other items)
- Documenting the amount of time spent directly on creating the overall education program in addition to the other functions performed with staff and patients will give one some experience in tracking supportive data.

A great deal of time and effort are already being expended in the unit on informal teaching, learning from imitation, and learning from mistakes. Gathering data for a period of time on the current level of performance and then data to support the new overall education program will help justify adequate budget.

To facilitate gathering data, use resources such as the hospital's personnel director, in-service educator, and cost accountant. There may be a researcher on the hospital staff who could help design effective evaluation tools. If not, local colleges and universities have resource people who design such evaluations. Graduate students in schools of nursing look for real research projects, and professors welcome opportunities to place students in primary research situations.

Use feedback from everyone involved in the learning activities. Data from these resources will provide viable information to use in moving into the recyling process, which is step 7.

STEP 7. RECYCLE

The last step starts the process all over again. Based on validation of new needs and unmet needs that emerge from the process and on changes that have evolved during the intervening time, recycling educational programs begins again.

All of the steps in the process model involve other people, and in the final analysis, the process model is also a participative model offering the greatest potential for working with peers and professionals.

CONCLUSION

After reading this chapter and reflecting on how people learn to cope with the significant changes in their personal and professional lives and to realize self-fulfillment and satisfaction as a result, where can they go?

WHERE CAN I GO?

If this is not a place where
    tears are understood,
Where can I go to cry?

If this is not a place where
    my spirits can take wing,
Where do I go to fly?

If this is not a place where
    my questions can be asked,
Where do I go to seek?

If this is not a place where
    my feelings can be heard,
Where do I go to speak?

If this is not a place where
    you'll accept me as I am,
Where can I go to be?

If this is not a place
    I can try, and learn, and grow,
Where can I just be me?

If this is not a place where
    tears are understood,
Where can I go to cry?

(Modified from a song by Ken Medina, "Where Can I Go?" by OD Network Newsletter, May 1978; reproduced with special permission, *Training and Development Journal,* American Society for Training and Development, Madison WI, May 1980)

REFERENCES

1. Lippitt GL: Integrating personal and professional development. Train Develop J, May 1980
2. Drucker P: "Learning from Foreign Management," Wall Street Journal, June 4, 1980, p 20
3. Innovations in In-service: Decentralized Staff Faculty. Arizona State University, Tempe, Arizona, 1975
4. Special survey/research project conducted by the Industrial Audiovisual Association
5. Knowles M: The Modern Practice of Adult Education. New York, Association Press, 1970
6. Ibid.
7. Mager R: Preparing Instruction Objectives. Palo Alto, Fearon, 1963
8. Nichols RG, Stevens L: Are You Listening? New York, McGraw-Hill, 1957
9. Kemp JE: Instructional Design, 2nd ed. Fearon, Belmont, 1977

BIBLIOGRAPHY

Argyris C, Schon DA: Theory in Practice: Increasing Effectiveness. San Francisco, Jossey-Bass, 1975

Byrne MS: The clinical specialist: Her role in staff development. In Staff Development. Wakefield, Contemporary, 1975

Buzan T: Use both sides of your brain. Saturday Rev, August 9, 1975

Clark CC: Burnout: Assessment and intervention. J Nurs Admin, September 1980

Conklin R: How to Get People to Do Things: The Key to Persuading, Leading, Motivating, Selling, Supervising, Influencing and Guiding Others. Chicago, Contemporary Books, 1979

Cooper SS (ed): Self-directed learning in nursing. In Nurses Resources. Wakefield, Concept Development, 1980

Feeney EJ: Twelve ideas toward effective training. Train Develop J, September 1980

Garry W: Integrating wellness into learning. Train Develop J, July 1980

Hennig M, Jardim A: The Managerial Woman. Garden City, Archer Press, 1977

Knowles M: The Adult Learner: A Neglected Species, 2nd ed. Houston, Gulf Publishing, 1978

Latham GP, Locke EA: Goal setting: A motivational technique that works. Organizational Dynamics, Autumn 1979

Lewis KM: In-service training and continuing education. In AACN Organizational and Management of Critical Care Facilities. St. Louis, C.V. Mosby, 1979

McGregor D: The Human Side of Enterprise. New York, McGraw-Hill, 1960

Medearis ND, Medearis DW: The uniqueness of the adult learner. AORN J, April 1975

Medearis N, Popiel E: Guidelines for organizing inservice education. In Nursing and the Process of Continuing Education, 2nd ed. St. Louis, C.V. Mosby, 1977

Mintzberg H: Planning on the left side and managing on the right. Harvard Bus Rev, July–August 1967

Sheehy G: Passages: Predictable Crises of Adult Life. New York, E.P. Dutton & Co, 1977

Tubesing DA: Wholistic Health: A Whole Person Approach to Primary Health Care. Human Sciences Press, 1979

Warr P (ed): Personal Goals and Work Design. New York, John Wiley & Sons, 1976

Woodcock M, Francis D: Unblocking Your Organization: A Practical Guide to Organizational Change. La Jolla, University Associates, 1978

Zemke R: Goal setting is the first step in any performance program. Training: The Magazine for Human Resources Development, July 1980

Index

Numbers followed by an *f* indicate a figure; *t* following a page number indicates tabular material.